Cardiovascular Disease:
From Molecular Mechanisms to
Clinical Therapies

Cardiovascular Disease: From Molecular Mechanisms to Clinical Therapies

Editor

Gaetano Santulli

MDPI • Basel • Beijing • Wuhan • Barcelona • Belgrade • Manchester • Tokyo • Cluj • Tianjin

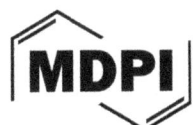

Editor
Gaetano Santulli
Albert Einstein College of
Medicine
Montefiore University Hospital
New York
United States

Editorial Office
MDPI
St. Alban-Anlage 66
4052 Basel, Switzerland

This is a reprint of articles from the Special Issue published online in the open access journal *Journal of Clinical Medicine* (ISSN 2077-0383) (available at: www.mdpi.com/journal/jcm/special_issues/cardiovascular_molecular_terapy).

For citation purposes, cite each article independently as indicated on the article page online and as indicated below:

LastName, A.A.; LastName, B.B.; LastName, C.C. Article Title. *Journal Name* **Year**, *Volume Number*, Page Range.

ISBN 978-3-0365-0993-8 (Hbk)
ISBN 978-3-0365-0992-1 (PDF)

© 2021 by the authors. Articles in this book are Open Access and distributed under the Creative Commons Attribution (CC BY) license, which allows users to download, copy and build upon published articles, as long as the author and publisher are properly credited, which ensures maximum dissemination and a wider impact of our publications.

The book as a whole is distributed by MDPI under the terms and conditions of the Creative Commons license CC BY-NC-ND.

Contents

Preface to "Cardiovascular Disease: From Molecular Mechanisms to Clinical Therapies" . . . vii

En-Young N. Wagner, Suzi Hong, Kathleen L. Wilson, Karen J. Calfas, Cheryl L. Rock, Laura S. Redwine, Roland von Känel and Paul J. Mills
Effects of Caloric Intake and Aerobic Activity in Individuals with Prehypertension and Hypertension on Levels of Inflammatory, Adhesion and Prothrombotic Biomarkers—Secondary Analysis of a Randomized Controlled Trial
Reprinted from: *Journal of Clinical Medicine* **2020**, *9*, 655, doi:10.3390/jcm9030655 1

Luca Liberale, Erik W. Holy, Alexander Akhmedov, Nicole R. Bonetti, Fabian Nietlispach, Christian M. Matter, François Mach, Fabrizio Montecucco, Jürg H. Beer, Francesco Paneni, Frank Ruschitzka, Peter Libby, Thomas F. Lüscher and Giovanni G. Camici
Interleukin-1 Mediates Arterial Thrombus Formation via NET-Associated Tissue Factor
Reprinted from: *Journal of Clinical Medicine* **2019**, *8*, 2072, doi:10.3390/jcm8122072 13

Maria-Angela Losi, Raffaele Izzo, Costantino Mancusi, Wenyu Wang, Mary J. Roman, Elisa T. Lee, Barbara V. Howard, Richard B. Devereux and Giovanni de Simone
Depressed Myocardial Energetic Efficiency Increases Risk of Incident Heart Failure: The Strong Heart Study
Reprinted from: *Journal of Clinical Medicine* **2019**, *8*, 1044, doi:10.3390/jcm8071044 29

Piero Pollesello, Tuvia Ben Gal, Dominique Bettex, Vladimir Cerny, Josep Comin-Colet, Alexandr A. Eremenko, Dimitrios Farmakis, Francesco Fedele, Cândida Fonseca, Veli-Pekka Harjola, Antoine Herpain, Matthias Heringlake, Leo Heunks, Trygve Husebye, Visnja Ivancan, Kristjan Karason, Sundeep Kaul, Jacek Kubica, Alexandre Mebazaa, Henning Mølgaard, John Parissis, Alexander Parkhomenko, Pentti Põder, Gerhard Pölzl, Bojan Vrtovec, Mehmet B. Yilmaz and Zoltan Papp
Short-Term Therapies for Treatment of Acute and Advanced Heart Failure—Why so Few Drugs Available in Clinical Use, Why Even Fewer in the Pipeline?
Reprinted from: *Journal of Clinical Medicine* **2019**, *8*, 1834, doi:10.3390/jcm8111834 39

Amalie L. Povlsen, Daniela Grimm, Markus Wehland, Manfred Infanger and Marcus Krüger
The Vasoactive Mas Receptor in Essential Hypertension
Reprinted from: *Journal of Clinical Medicine* **2020**, *9*, 267, doi:10.3390/jcm9010267 59

Iginio Colaiori, Raffaele Izzo, Emanuele Barbato, Danilo Franco, Giuseppe Di Gioia, Antonio Rapacciuolo, Jozef Bartunek, Costantino Mancusi, Maria Angela Losi, Teresa Strisciuglio, Maria Virginia Manzi, Giovanni de Simone, Bruno Trimarco and Carmine Morisco
Severity of Coronary Atherosclerosis and Risk of Diabetes Mellitus
Reprinted from: *Journal of Clinical Medicine* **2019**, *8*, 1069, doi:10.3390/jcm8071069 71

Ahmed Ismaeel, Marco E. Franco, Ramon Lavado, Evlampia Papoutsi, George P. Casale, Matthew Fuglestad, Constance J. Mietus, Gleb R. Haynatzki, Robert S. Smith, William T. Bohannon, Ian Sawicki, Iraklis I. Pipinos and Panagiotis Koutakis
Altered Metabolomic Profile in Patients with Peripheral Artery Disease
Reprinted from: *Journal of Clinical Medicine* **2019**, *8*, 1463, doi:10.3390/jcm8091463 81

Gilda Varricchi, Stefania Loffredo, Leonardo Bencivenga, Anne Lise Ferrara, Giuseppina Gambino, Nicola Ferrara, Amato de Paulis, Gianni Marone and Giuseppe Rengo
Angiopoietins, Vascular Endothelial Growth Factors and Secretory Phospholipase A_2 in Ischemic and Non-Ischemic Heart Failure
Reprinted from: *Journal of Clinical Medicine* 2020, 9, 1928, doi:10.3390/jcm9061928 99

Richard Myles Turner and Munir Pirmohamed
Statin-Related Myotoxicity: A Comprehensive Review of Pharmacokinetic, Pharmacogenomic and Muscle Components
Reprinted from: *Journal of Clinical Medicine* 2019, 9, 22, doi:10.3390/jcm9010022 115

Bettina Hieronimus, Steven C. Griffen, Nancy L. Keim, Andrew A. Bremer, Lars Berglund, Katsuyuki Nakajima, Peter J. Havel and Kimber L. Stanhope
Effects of Fructose or Glucose on Circulating ApoCIII and Triglyceride and Cholesterol Content of Lipoprotein Subfractions in Humans
Reprinted from: *Journal of Clinical Medicine* 2019, 8, 913, doi:10.3390/jcm8070913 153

Agnieszka Maciejewska-Skrendo, Maciej Buryta, Wojciech Czarny, Pawel Król, Michal Spieszny, Petr Stastny, Miroslav Petr, Krzysztof Safranow and Marek Sawczuk
The Polymorphisms of the Peroxisome-Proliferator Activated Receptors' Alfa Gene Modify the Aerobic Training Induced Changes of Cholesterol and Glucose
Reprinted from: *Journal of Clinical Medicine* 2019, 8, 1043, doi:10.3390/jcm8071043 169

Aristides Tsatsakis, Anca Oana Docea, Daniela Calina, Konstantinos Tsarouhas, Laura-Maria Zamfira, Radu Mitrut, Javad Sharifi-Rad, Leda Kovatsi, Vasileios Siokas, Efthimios Dardiotis, Nikolaos Drakoulis, George Lazopoulos, Christina Tsitsimpikou, Panayiotis Mitsias and Monica Neagu
A Mechanistic and Pathophysiological Approach for Stroke Associated with Drugs of Abuse
Reprinted from: *Journal of Clinical Medicine* 2019, 8, 1295, doi:10.3390/jcm8091295 185

Naoki Katayama, Keiichi Odagiri, Akio Hakamata, Naoki Inui, Katsuya Yamauchi and Hiroshi Watanabe
Transient Laterality of Cerebral Oxygenation Changes in Response to Head-of-Bed Manipulation in Acute Ischemic Stroke
Reprinted from: *Journal of Clinical Medicine* 2019, 8, 1739, doi:10.3390/jcm8101739 221

Giovanna Gallo, Maurizio Forte, Rosita Stanzione, Maria Cotugno, Franca Bianchi, Simona Marchitti, Andrea Berni, Massimo Volpe and Speranza Rubattu
Functional Role of Natriuretic Peptides in Risk Assessment and Prognosis of Patients with Mitral Regurgitation
Reprinted from: *Journal of Clinical Medicine* 2020, 9, 1348, doi:10.3390/jcm9051348 235

Lisa-Marie Mauracher, Nina Buchtele, Christian Schörgenhofer, Christoph Weiser, Harald Herkner, Anne Merrelaar, Alexander O. Spiel, Lena Hell, Cihan Ay, Ingrid Pabinger, Bernd Jilma and Michael Schwameis
Increased Citrullinated Histone H3 Levels in the Early Post-Resuscitative Period Are Associated with Poor Neurologic Function in Cardiac Arrest Survivors—A Prospective Observational Study
Reprinted from: *Journal of Clinical Medicine* 2019, 8, 1568, doi:10.3390/jcm8101568 247

Raluca M. Tat, Adela Golea, Rodica Rahaian, Ştefan C. Vesa and Daniela Ionescu
Resistin and Cardiac Arrest—A Prospective Study
Reprinted from: *Journal of Clinical Medicine* 2019, 9, 57, doi:10.3390/jcm9010057 259

Gaetano Santulli, Valeria Pascale, Rosa Finelli, Valeria Visco, Rocco Giannotti, Angelo Massari, Carmine Morisco, Michele Ciccarelli, Maddalena Illario, Guido Iaccarino and Enrico Coscioni
We are What We Eat: Impact of Food from Short Supply Chain on Metabolic Syndrome
Reprinted from: *Journal of Clinical Medicine* 2019, 8, 2061, doi:10.3390/jcm8122061 271

Lukas Lanser, Gerhard Pölzl, Dietmar Fuchs, Günter Weiss and Katharina Kurz
Neopterin is Associated with Disease Severity and Outcome in Patients with Non-Ischaemic Heart Failure
Reprinted from: *Journal of Clinical Medicine* 2019, 8, 2230, doi:10.3390/jcm8122230 279

Jessica Gambardella, Angela Lombardi, Marco Bruno Morelli, John Ferrara and Gaetano Santulli
Inositol 1,4,5-Trisphosphate Receptors in Human Disease: A Comprehensive Update
Reprinted from: *Journal of Clinical Medicine* 2020, 9, 1096, doi:10.3390/jcm9041096 291

Josefa Girona, Cèlia Rodríguez-Borjabad, Daiana Ibarretxe, Joan-Carles Vallvé, Raimon Ferré, Mercedes Heras, Ricardo Rodríguez-Calvo, Sandra Guaita-Esteruelas, Neus Martínez-Micaelo, Núria Plana and Lluís Masana
The Circulating GRP78/BiP Is a Marker of Metabolic Diseases and Atherosclerosis: Bringing Endoplasmic Reticulum Stress into the Clinical Scenario
Reprinted from: *Journal of Clinical Medicine* 2019, 8, 1793, doi:10.3390/jcm8111793 307

Chien-Ning Hsu, Guo-Ping Chang-Chien, Sufan Lin, Chih-Yao Hou, Pei-Chen Lu and You-Lin Tain
Association of Trimethylamine, Trimethylamine N-oxide, and Dimethylamine with Cardiovascular Risk in Children with Chronic Kidney Disease
Reprinted from: *Journal of Clinical Medicine* 2020, 9, 336, doi:10.3390/jcm9020336 319

Giovanna Gallo, Franca Bianchi, Maria Cotugno, Massimo Volpe and Speranza Rubattu
Natriuretic Peptides, Cognitive Impairment and Dementia: An Intriguing Pathogenic Link with Implications in Hypertension
Reprinted from: *Journal of Clinical Medicine* 2020, 9, 2265, doi:10.3390/jcm9072265 333

Damiano Magrì, Vittoria Mastromarino, Giovanna Gallo, Elisabetta Zachara, Federica Re, Piergiuseppe Agostoni, Dario Giordano, Speranza Rubattu, Maurizio Forte, Maria Cotugno, Maria Rosaria Torrisi, Simona Petrucci, Aldo Germani, Camilla Savio, Antonello Maruotti, Massimo Volpe, Camillo Autore, Maria Piane and Beatrice Musumeci
Risk Stratification in Hypertrophic Cardiomyopathy. Insights from Genetic Analysis and Cardiopulmonary Exercise Testing
Reprinted from: *Journal of Clinical Medicine* 2020, 9, 1636, doi:10.3390/jcm9061636 345

Filip Rolski and Przemysław Błyszczuk
Complexity of TNF- Signaling in Heart Disease
Reprinted from: *Journal of Clinical Medicine* 2020, 9, 3267, doi:10.3390/jcm9103267 361

Elena Grossini, Serena Farruggio, Daniele Pierelli, Virginia Bolzani, Lidia Rossi, Piero Pollesello and Carolina Monaco
Levosimendan Improves Oxidative Balance in Cardiogenic Shock/Low Cardiac Output Patients
Reprinted from: *Journal of Clinical Medicine* 2020, 9, 373, doi:10.3390/jcm9020373 385

Ioannis Drosos, Maria Pavlaki, Maria Del Pilar Ortega Carrillo, Adriani Kourkouli, Katja Buschmann, Fotios Konstantinou, Rajinikanth Gogiraju, Magdalena L. Bochenek, Georgios Chalikias, Christos Tortopidis, Christian F. Vahl, Dimitrios Mikroulis, Dimitrios Tziakas, Thomas Münzel, Stavros Konstantinides and Katrin Schäfer
Increased Lymphangiogenesis and Lymphangiogenic Growth Factor Expression in Perivascular Adipose Tissue of Patients with Coronary Artery Disease
Reprinted from: *Journal of Clinical Medicine* **2019**, *8*, 1000, doi:10.3390/jcm8071000 . . . . **401**

Ivana Škrlec, Jakov Milić and Robert Steiner
The Impact of the Circadian Genes *CLOCK* and *ARNTL* on Myocardial Infarction
Reprinted from: *Journal of Clinical Medicine* **2020**, *9*, 484, doi:10.3390/jcm9020484 . . . . **423**

Celestino Sardu, Jessica Gambardella, Marco Bruno Morelli, Xujun Wang, Raffaele Marfella and Gaetano Santulli
Hypertension, Thrombosis, Kidney Failure, and Diabetes: Is COVID-19 an Endothelial Disease? A Comprehensive Evaluation of Clinical and Basic Evidence
Reprinted from: *Journal of Clinical Medicine* **2020**, *9*, 1417, doi:10.3390/jcm9051417 . . . . **437**

Preface to "Cardiovascular Disease: From Molecular Mechanisms to Clinical Therapies"

According to the most updated epidemiological studies, cardiovascular disease remains a leading cause of death; in fact, despite substantial advances in the care of patients, the incidence of cardiovascular disorders continues to increase. Therefore, the search for novel mechanisms and therapeutics is desperately needed, and translational studies represent the best strategy to uncover novel therapeutic targets, reduce mortality, and improve the quality of life. This book gathers original articles and systematic reviews that have both a strong basic research background and clear translational potential. All the studies have been peer reviewed by at least two experts in the field. These contributions provide an updated systematic overview that examines, in detail, the mechanisms of the main cardiovascular and metabolic disorders, including ischemic and non-ischemic heart failure, hypertension, thromboembolism, atherosclerosis, stroke, diabetes mellitus, dyslipidemia, metabolic syndrome, valvulopathies, peripheral artery disease. In the final chapter, the functional role of the endothelium in the systemic manifestations of COVID-19 is described.

Gaetano Santulli
Editor

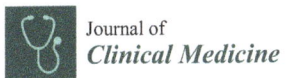

Article

Effects of Caloric Intake and Aerobic Activity in Individuals with Prehypertension and Hypertension on Levels of Inflammatory, Adhesion and Prothrombotic Biomarkers—Secondary Analysis of a Randomized Controlled Trial

En-Young N. Wagner [1,2,3,*], Suzi Hong [1,4], Kathleen L. Wilson [1,4], Karen J. Calfas [4], Cheryl L. Rock [4], Laura S. Redwine [5], Roland von Känel [2] and Paul J. Mills [1,4]

1. Department of Psychiatry, University of California, San Diego, CA 92093, USA; s1hong@ucsd.edu (S.H.); k8wilson@ucsd.edu (K.L.W.); pmills@ucsd.edu (P.J.M.)
2. Department of Consultation-Liaison Psychiatry and Psychosomatic Medicine, University Hospital Zurich, 8091 Zurich, Switzerland; roland.vonkaenel@usz.ch
3. Department of BioMedical Research, Inselspital, Bern University Hospital, 3010 Bern, Switzerland
4. Department of Family Medicine and Public Health, University of California, San Diego, CA 92093, USA; kcalfas@ucsd.edu (K.J.C.); clrock@ucsd.edu (C.L.R.)
5. College of Nursing, University of South Florida, Tampa, FL 33612, USA; lredwine@health.usf.edu
* Correspondence: en-young.wagner@dbmr.unibe.ch; Tel.: +41-(0)44-255-52-51; Fax: +41-(0)44-255-44-08

Received: 9 February 2020; Accepted: 26 February 2020; Published: 28 February 2020

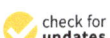

Abstract: Background: Cardiopulmonary fitness and low calorie diets have been shown to reduce inflammation but few studies have been conducted in individuals with elevated blood pressure (BP) in a randomized intervention setting. Thereby, adhesion biomarkers, e.g., soluble intercellular adhesion molecule (sICAM)-3, have not been examined so far. Methods: Sixty-eight sedentary prehypertensive and mildly hypertensive individuals (mean age ± SEM: 45 ± 1 years; mean BP: 141/84 ± 1/1 mmHg) were randomized to one of three 12-week intervention groups: cardio training and caloric reduction, cardio training alone, or wait-list control group. Plasma levels of inflammatory, adhesion and prothrombotic biomarkers were assessed. In a second step, intervention groups were combined to one sample and multivariate regression analyses were applied in order to account for exercise and diet behavior changes. Results: There were no significant differences among the intervention groups. In the combined sample, greater caloric reduction was associated with a larger increase of sICAM-3 ($p = 0.026$) and decrease of C-reactive protein ($p = 0.018$) as a result of the interventions. More cardio training was associated with increases of sICAM-3 ($p = 0.046$) as well as interleukin-6 ($p = 0.004$) and a decrease of tumor necrosis factor-α ($p = 0.017$) levels. Higher BP predicted higher plasminogen activator inhibitor (PAI)-1 ($p = 0.001$), and greater fitness predicted lower PAI-1 levels ($p = 0.006$) after the intervention. Conclusions: In prehypertensive and hypertensive patients, plasma levels of the adhesion molecule sICAM-3 and inflammatory biomarkers have different response patterns to cardio training with and without caloric reduction. Such anti-inflammatory and anti-thrombotic effects may have implications for the prevention of atherothrombotic cardiovascular disease among individuals at increased risk.

Keywords: hypertension; prehypertension; exercise; diet; adhesion molecule; sICAM; soluble intercellular adhesion molecule; inflammatory markers; intervention

1. Introduction

The pathogenesis of hypertension seems to be more complex, as it is difficult to treat despite established antihypertensive drugs and longtime cardiovascular research. Hypertension (blood pressure (BP) ≥ 140/90 mmHg) is a highly prevalent disease among United States (U.S.) citizens with a well-known impact on numerous comorbid conditions and public-health related outcomes [1–3]. On a cellular level, it is established knowledge that individuals with hypertension exhibit elevated blood levels of cellular adhesion molecules [4–6] as well as inflammatory markers [7–15]. The reason for that is mainly seen in endothelial activation [12], which explains the tight linkage between elevated BP, chronic inflammatory processes including atherosclerosis and adverse health related outcomes [7,16]. So far, studies on the effects of human hypertension on adhesion molecules have been focusing on soluble intercellular adhesion molecule-1 (sICAM-1; sCD54) [4–6] while studies measuring sICAM-3, which is potentially much more important for immune response [17], are scarce.

In treating hypertension, lifestyle modifications including adopting a regular exercise regimen are key constituents of treatment [18,19]. This recommendation might also apply to prehypertension (BP > 120/80 and <140/90 mmHg), a risk factor for the development of hypertension. The effect achieved depends on both intensity and frequency of exercise [20–22], and BP reductions of up to 15 mmHg can be achieved without using antihypertensive drugs and thus avoiding their common side effects [23]. In overweight hypertensive subjects, a combined exercise and dietary weight-loss intervention was shown to lead to even greater reductions in BP than exercise alone [22].

Meanwhile, few studies have examined the relationship between exercise and inflammation in hypertensive patients. One of the few studies showed that exercise and/or exercise plus diet interventions lead to reductions in circulating interleukin (IL)-6 and C-reactive protein (CRP) levels in obese individuals [24]. In normotensive, healthy individuals, cross-sectional epidemiological studies have shown physical activity to be negatively associated with CRP, fibrinogen, and white blood cell count [25] and inflammatory markers, including tumor necrosis factor (TNF)-α and IL-6 and prothrombotic plasminogen activator inhibitor (PAI-1) were shown to be inversely related to physical activity levels [26–28]. Furthermore, our group has shown that physical activity level and fitness are inversely related to leukocyte adhesion molecule expression [29,30].

Guided by the above described effects observed in healthy individuals, the purpose of this study was to explore the relationship of a 12-week exercise (and diet) intervention and inflammation/cell adhesion in patients with prehypertension and hypertension by measuring circulating levels of CRP, IL-6, TNF-α, PAI-1, and sICAM-1 and sICAM-3 by taking relevant cardio-metabolic confounding factors (body mass index (BMI), physical inactivity) into account. Based on these data of a randomized controlled trial (RCT), our aim was to show for the first time in vivo that exercise has not only an impact on levels of inflammatory biomarkers, but also on levels of cellular adhesion molecules. Our main hypothesis was that, compared to a 12-week wait-list control group, the 12-week exercise intervention, and especially the 12-week exercise plus diet intervention, would result in greater reduction of inflammatory biomarkers and cell adhesion molecules pre to post intervention. Second, we expected that both intervention groups would show increased fitness levels and greater BP reduction and weight reduction as compared to the wait-list control group.

2. Methods

2.1. Ethical Approval and Informed Consent

Data is taken from a clinical trial on the effects of exercise and diet on inflammation in hypertensive individuals registered in a public registry (www.clinicaltrials.gov, ClinicalTrials.gov Identifier: NCT00338572). The University of California San Diego (UCSD) Institutional Review Board approved the study protocol, to which all participants signed a written informed consent. All procedures performed in studies involving human participants were in accordance with the ethical standards of the institutional and/or national research committee and with the 1964 Helsinki Declaration and its later

2.2. Data Source, Effect of Exercise and Diet on Inflammation in Hypertensive Individuals Trial

The data of the present secondary analysis is derived from a prospective, randomized controlled intervention study examining the effect of exercise and diet on inflammation in hypertensive individuals. That study was conducted in order to compare the effect of an exercise program versus a combined exercise and diet program on reducing inflammation in hypertensive individuals. Figure 1 shows the RCT CONSORT flow diagram for participants. Of 168 eligible people, 77 individuals chose not to enter the RCT. The 91 remaining participants were randomly assigned to one of three 12-week intervention groups: aerobic cardio training and caloric reduction, aerobic cardio training alone, or wait-list control group. Participants assigned to the wait-list group were controls for at least 12 weeks until they were allocated to one of the intervention groups (exercise alone or exercise plus "Dietary Approaches to Stop Hypertension" (DASH) group). Of these 91 subjects, 9 individuals did not complete the study for personal reasons, moving away from San Diego ($n = 2$), becoming too busy or starting a new job ($n = 5$), becoming ill ($n = 2$, colon rupture, neurological concerns), and 14 individuals were not reliable/cancelled.

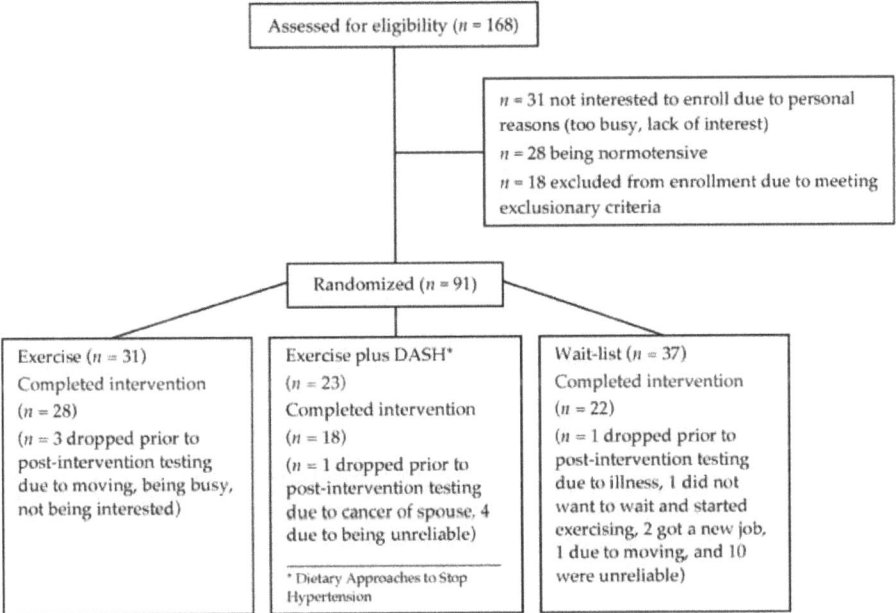

Figure 1. CONSORT flow diagram for participants.

The trial included relatively healthy, sedentary and non-medicated men and women ($n = 91$) between age 18 and 65 years with prehypertension (>120/80 but <140/90 mmHg) and stage 1 and 2 hypertension (≥140/90 but <180/110 mmHg), who were not on a current diet or had been participating in an exercise program within the past 6 months. The level of habitual physical activity was assessed using the Leisure Time Exercise Questionnaire (LTEQ) by Godin and Shepard [31] to confirm the sedentary status; individuals with LTEQ total scores above 40 were excluded. Major concomitant diseases were ruled out by blood sample, resting electrocardiogram and medical history. For each eligible participant, a trained technician or registered nurse obtained anthropometric data through standard procedures. Body weight, height and average resting BP (six measurements taken after a

15-min seated rest on two separate days using a Dinamap Compact BP® monitor (Critikon, Tempa, FL, USA)). Participants with values of high-sensitivity CRP >10 mg/L were excluded from the analyses, as values above this threshold are indicative of an acute infection.

2.3. Fitness Testing

Participants underwent a maximum oxygen intake (VO_{2peak}, mL/kg/min) treadmill exercise test to determine cardiorespiratory fitness using the standard Bruce protocol in which treadmill speed and grade were increased gradually from 1.7 mph and 10% grade every 3 min. Expired gas was analyzed by Sensormedics metabolic cart, Milano, Italy (Vmax software version 6-2A).

2.4. Aerobic Cardio Training

Since all participants were relatively sedentary at baseline, the training intervention was designed to increase exercise levels gradually to the ultimate physical activity goal: Five or more days per week of at least moderate-intensity cardiovascular physical activity (e.g., walking) for 30 to 60 min. Exercise intensity was individually adapted by the assessed heart rate (before and during exercise). Participants met with a certified personal trainer (study personnel) at the local YMCA 2 days a week for the entire 12-week intervention period. They shared with the trainer the fitness information. In-person sessions with a trainer were scheduled, as they are more likely to be completed than entirely home-based exercise and may increase the motivation for completion of the three sessions per week of exercise without a personal trainer. The sessions with the trainer included training in proper warm up, exercise and cool down and stretching. The participant was asked to do physical activity on his or her own (either in their home, neighborhood or at the YMCA) for three additional days per week. In addition to meeting a goal for the number of minutes of physical activity, participants were asked to increase incidental physical activity. To monitor their progress, participants were given a pedometer and asked to work up to an ultimate goal of an average of 10,000+ steps per day. We used the same pedometer (Omron®, Kyōto, Japan) throughout the study to warrant an adequate comparison. The inclusion of the pedometer and step goal helped to ensure that participants were not compensating for increased activity during their sessions with the personal trainer by being more sedentary throughout the rest of the day. The achievement of these goals ensured an increase in energy expenditure, which contributed to a negative energy balance. Subjects completed a log of their daily pedometer readings and presented them to the trainer each week.

2.5. Caloric Reduction

The dietary intervention was led by research dietitians at the Nutrition Services Core of the UCSD Medical Center General Clinical Research Center (GCRC) or Clinical and Translational Research Institute (CTRI). The core of the diet plan was based on the DASH clinical study [32,33]. This dietary pattern is high in fruits, vegetables, and low fat dairy foods, and low in saturated and total fat. It also is high in dietary fiber, potassium, calcium, and magnesium, and moderately high in protein. The dietary intervention aimed at reducing the individual energy intake by 500–1000 kcal/day taking into account lifestyle and dietary preferences of the participant [34]. In addition, concomitant behavioral strategies like conscious eating and stimulus control were trained. Thus, participants received intensive intervention approaches known to produce behavior change. Subjects in the experimental group met with registered dietitians and/or certified exercise trainers to establish initial dietary and physical activity goals. Regular meetings in person and by phone continued for the entire 12-week intervention. All subjects recorded their food (caloric intake in kilojoule) and provided the information to the study investigators. Diet adherence was assessed with three daily dietary recalls administered by the study dietician.

2.6. Assessment of Inflammatory Biomarkers and Cellular Adhesion Molecules

Fasting blood samples were collected within one week of, but at least two days after, the maximum exercise test at baseline. All assays were performed in the UCSD Clinical Research Biomarker Laboratory using commercially available immunoassay kits (R&D Systems products, Minneapolis, MN, or MSD Systems, Rockville, MD, USA). Intra- and inter-assay coefficients of variation (CV) were confirmed to be <5%. For subsequent statistical analyses, soluble ICAM-1 (sample size, 63), sICAM-3 (66), PAI-1 (68), CRP (62), IL-6 (65), and TNF-α (63) measures were log-transformed to normalize distributions with differing sample sizes reflecting missing biomarker data due to technical errors, etc., and we calculated the difference (Δ) from pre to post intervention levels for all biomarker measures by detracting the value before the intervention from the value after the intervention.

2.7. Secondary Analysis of Trial Data

According to the RCT protocol, $n = 18$ had been to the aerobic cardio training and caloric reduction intervention, $n = 28$ to the aerobic cardio training alone intervention and $n = 22$ to the wait-list control group. However, in reality, participants began modifying their exercise or diet behavior regardless of their intervention group assignment and modest group sizes limited statistical power. Therefore, we decided for a statistical approach with a secondary analysis of data from all 68 participants combined that may better warrant to indicate the actual behavior and inflammatory processes and consider the intervention effect described respectively.

Thus, a series of multivariate linear regression analyses were performed to examine the role of the different intervention elements (predictors). For the three predictors fitness, cardio training, and caloric intake, the differences (Δ) from pre to post intervention levels were used in the statistical analyses. We calculated these differences (Δ) by detracting the value before the intervention from the value after the intervention. Associations between the four predictors (BP, fitness, cardio training, and caloric intake) and outcomes (differences (Δ) from pre to post intervention levels of cellular adhesion molecules (sICAM-1, sICAM-3) and inflammatory biomarkers (CRP, IL-6, TNF-α)) were determined using multiple linear regression models, separately for each of the five outcome variables. Results were considered statistically significant at $p \leq 0.05$. We did not adjust p-values for multiple comparisons, as the main primary outcome was CRP; however, as we examined the potential interaction among inflammatory, adhesion and prothrombic markers, we defined one primary outcome marker in each of these three biomarker domains playing different roles in CVD: CRP for inflammation, sICAM-1 for adhesion molecules, and PAI-1 for prothrombotic factors. All other outcomes (IL-6, TNF, sICAM-3) were secondary (Il-6 and TNF) or exploratory (sICAM-3, as no study so far has been investigating sICAM 3).

For the associations between each of the predictors and inflammatory marker outcome levels, two models of increasing complexity were computed: in Model 1 we adjusted for (prehypertensive or hypertensive) BP and sociodemographic factors (age, gender) only, and in Model 2 we additionally adjusted for the other remaining predictors in one complete regression model (Table 1). Only the significant results of the five statistical models are shown for a better overview (Table 1). For our second hypothesis, mean pre and post intervention BP, fitness levels, and weight of the three groups were compared to each other. All statistical analyses were performed using IBM® SPSS® version 22.0 statistical software package (IBM Corporation, New York, NY, USA).

Table 1. First step [a] and final [b] multivariate regression analyses between inflammatory biomarkers and intervention elements (predictors) in the studied pre- and hypertensive participants.

Predictor	Δ [c] Outcome [d]	β	p [e]
SBP [e]	Δ PAI-1 ($n = 62$)	[a] 0.415 [b] 0.427	0.003 0.001

Table 1. Cont.

Predictor	Δ [c] Outcome [d]	β	p [e]
Δ Fitness (VO$_{2peak}$)	Δ PAI-1 (n = 62)	[a] −0.369 [b] −0.392	0.004 0.006
Δ Caloric intake	Δ sICAM-3 (n = 63)	[a] −0.363 [b] −0.332	0.014 0.026
	Δ CRP (n = 63)	[a] 0.317 [b] 0.342	0.025 0.018
Δ Cardio training [f]	Δ sICAM-3 (n = 63)	[a] 0.314 [b] 0.301	0.037 0.046
	Δ IL-6 (n = 66)	[a] 0.403 [b] 0.415	0.005 0.004
	Δ TNF-α (n = 68)	[a] −0.337 [b] −0.357	0.018 0.017

[a] The first step regression model included predictor, age, gender, and the difference from pre to post intervention biomarker level, and systolic blood pressure (except for systolic blood pressure as predictor). [b] The final model included the first step model and additionally the other predictors, and the difference from pre to post intervention body mass index level. [c] Δ, value difference from pre to post intervention level: We calculated the difference from pre to post intervention levels by detracting the value before the intervention from the value after the intervention. [d] PAI, plasminogen activator inhibitor; sICAM, soluble intercellular adhesion molecule; CRP, C-reactive protein; IL, interleukin; TNF-α, tumor necrosis factor-alpha. [e] SBP, systolic blood pressure. [f] Cardio training, moderate aerobic cardio training: total minutes during 12-week-intervention. [e] $p < 0.05$.

3. Results

3.1. Study Sample

The baseline demographic, metabolic and health behavior characteristics of all study participants (n = 68) included in the statistical analyses are displayed in Table 2. In the combined 68 participants, 22 subjects had reduced caloric intake and exercised regularly. These 22 participants had an average daily caloric reduction of 673 ± 594 calories (mean ± SEM) and had on average exercised 22.9 ± 2.8 h during the 12-week intervention (on average 114.5 ± 14 min per week). The intensity of aerobic cardio training of the hypertensive patients did not differ significantly from that of the prehypertensive patients (p = 0.18). Subjects who exercised regularly but had no caloric reduction (n = 38) had spent on average 21.1 ± 2.0 h on training during the 12-week intervention (on average 105.5 ± 10 min per week). Thirteen % of the participants were current smokers based on self-report.

Table 2. Demographic, metabolic and health behavior characteristics of the study participants before the intervention.

Variable	n [a]	Mean ± SEM and Range in Parentheses or Percentage Value
Prehypertension/Hypertension	68	44.1%/55.9%
Systolic blood pressure, mmHg	68	141 ± 1 (124–174)
Diastolic blood pressure, mmHg	68	84 ± 1 (69–102)
Heart rate, beats/min	68	75 ± 1 (53.0–99)
Age, years	68	45 ± 1 (25–60)
Gender, male/female	68	45%/55%
Body mass index, kg/m^2	67	30.8 ± 0.5 (22.4–38.8)
Glucose, mg/dL	64	89 ± 1 (59–120)
Total cholesterol/HDL-cholesterol ratio	63	4.8 ± 0.2 (0.5–10.8)
Smoking	68	13%
Concomitant medication	68	0%
Leisure time exercise questionnaire	65	11.7 ± 1.2 (0.0–35.0)
VO$_{2peak}$ [b] (mL/kg/min)	68	27.9 ± 0.9 (15.0–54.0)

Table 2. Cont.

Variable	n [a]	Mean ± SEM and Range in Parentheses or Percentage Value
Inflammatory measures before the intervention	n [c]	
C-reactive protein, mg/L	63	2.8 (1.1–7.1)
Interleukin-6, pg/mL	66	2.7 (1.2–4.3)
Tumor necrosis factor-α, pg/mL	68	2.7 (1.2–4.1)
Plasminogen activator inhibitor-1, ng/mL	62	41.1 (21.4–61.2)
Soluble intercellular adhesion molecule-1, ng/mL	65	306.8 (239.3–374.1)
Soluble intercellular adhesion molecule-3, ng/mL	63	2.6 (2.2–3.2)

Data are given as mean ± standard error of the mean (SEM) (range) or percentage values. Inflammatory measures are given as medians (interquartile range). [a] n, number of subjects included. [b] VO_{2peak}, peak oxygen consumption. [c] n, number of subjects who provided biomarker's measurement before and after the intervention.

3.2. Blood Pressure Classification before and after Intervention

After the intervention the mean SBP reduction for hypertensive subjects (n = 34) with 10.1 ± 2.6 mmHg was greater than the prehypertensive subjects (n = 25) with 4.4 ± 1.3 mmHg but not significantly so ($p = 0.06$). However, the average SBP of the hypertensive patients (n = 34; mean ± SEM: 148.1 ± 1.6 mmHg) decreased to the prehypertensive level of 137.9 ± 2.3 mmHg.

3.3. Cellular Adhesion Molecules and Inflammatory Biomarker Associations with Elevated Blood Pressure, Fitness and Obesity in the 68 Participants

We calculated Pearson's correlations to examine the associations of the soluble intercellular adhesion molecules and inflammatory biomarkers with BP, BMI, and fitness before the intervention. CRP was negatively correlated with fitness ($r = -0.308$; $p < 0.05$) and positively with BMI ($r = 0.327$; $p < 0.01$). IL-6 was negatively associated with fitness ($r = -0.311$; $p < 0.05$) and positively associated with SBP ($r = 0.310$; $p < 0.05$). TNF-α was negatively correlated with SBP ($r = -0.364$; $p < 0.01$). Soluble ICAM-1 was negatively associated with fitness ($r = -0.242$; $p < 0.05$) and was positively associated with CRP ($r = 0.414$; $p < 0.01$) but not with BP. Soluble ICAM-3 had no associations with BP, BMI, fitness or sICAM-1.

3.4. Behavioral Change by Intervention Elements, Change of BMI and Fitness and Its Role in Inflammation in All Participants with Elevated Blood Pressures

The higher the SBP the higher were PAI-1 levels ($\beta = 0.427$; $p = 0.001$), and the more the fitness level had improved during the intervention the lower were PAI-1 levels ($\beta = -0.392$; $p < 0.01$) after the intervention (Table 1). Aerobic cardio training was a significant independent predictor of sICAM-3, IL-6, and TNF-α levels after controlling for sociodemographic variables and SBP in a first step regression model (Table 1), meaning the greater the amount of total moderate exercise was, the higher were the levels of sICAM-3 and IL-6, and the lower were the levels of TNF-α (Table 1) after the intervention. From earlier analyses [35,36], BMI decreased in the exercise groups, and fitness increased in those groups. These results remained statistically significant, even after adjusting for changes in BMI, fitness, and caloric reduction in the final model (sICAM-3 ($\beta = 0.301$; $p < 0.05$), IL-6 ($\beta = 0.415$; $p < 0.01$), and TNF-α ($\beta = -0.357$; $p < 0.05$); Table 1). Caloric reduction (to reduce caloric intake) predicted significantly higher sICAM-3 ($\beta = -0.332$; $p < 0.05$) and lower CRP ($\beta = 0.342$; $p < 0.05$) levels in the first step and final model (Table 1).

4. Discussion

We examined the differential effects of aerobic cardio training and caloric reduction on inflammatory, adhesion and prothrombotic biomarkers in prehypertensive and hypertensive subjects. Our study adds to the existent body of literature in the context of behavioral (aerobic exercise and diet) intervention and hypertension for inflammatory biomarker outcomes. The more comprehensive approach of lifestyle changes including exercise and diet behavior change of this 12-week-intervention study might explain the differential changes of inflammatory (CRP, IL-6, TNF-α) and prothrombotic (PAI-1), and adhesion (sICAM-1 and -3) biomarkers.

The key finding is that aerobic cardio training and/or caloric reduction had differential effects on IL-6 and adhesion molecule sICAM-3 in vivo. In particular, the latter finding is novel showing a prospective association between exercise and caloric reduction respectively and sICAM-3 levels. Thereby, this is the first study to our knowledge that shows that aerobic exercise has not only an impact on inflammatory biomarkers but also on levels of cellular adhesion molecules. Until now, it was unclear how they might interact, although it is well known that aerobic exercise reduces inflammatory processes.

The increase of sICAM-3 and IL-6 in subjects with elevated BP was independently predicted by the intensity of aerobic cardio training and caloric reduction. We think that this finding may be initially counter-intuitive but is important for the following reasons: First, this finding is consistent with prior studies, which showed that exercise was associated with a significant increase in IL-6 [37,38]. In this study, however, increased IL-6 levels after intervention and its positive correlation with both exercise levels and caloric reduction may be explained by potentially anti-inflammatory effects of IL-6 [39]. IL-6 is a pleiotropic cytokine released by skeletal myocytes under contraction, mediating anti-inflammatory effects by stimulating the production of anti-inflammatory cytokines and suppression of TNF-α production [39] with all these mechanisms concurring with the results of this study. Second, this is the first study to highlight the potential role of sICAM-3 in vascular inflammatory effects of exercise and/or diet intervention among prehypertensive and hypertensive subjects. To date, studies on the effects of human hypertension on adhesion molecules have been focusing on sICAM-1 levels, which are increased in hypertensive individuals [4–6]. Soluble ICAM-1 levels reflect ICAM-1 expression on activated endothelial cells [40] and are associated with the degree of atherosclerosis [41]. Although ICAM-1 and ICAM-3 share a similar immunoglobulin-like structure and amino acid identity of about 48%, with the greatest homology observed in domains 2 and 3 [42], their differential pattern of expression and cellular distribution suggest a different functional role [42]. The interactions of ICAM-1 and ICAM-3 with lymphocyte function-associated antigen (LFA)-1 are integral to the normal functioning of the immune system [42]. ICAM-3 is expressed on resting leucocytes and is potentially the most important ligand for LFA-1 in the initiation of the immune response because the expression of ICAM-1 on resting leucocytes is low [17]. Although sICAM-3 binds to LFA-1 with an affinity approximately nine-times weaker than sICAM-1, sICAM-1 and sICAM-3 compete with each other for binding to LFA-1 [42]. As we did not find changes in sICAM-1 levels post interventions in this study, we speculate that the increase in sICAM-3 levels as a result of changes in exercise and/or diet behavior in this study may exhibit a "buffer" for the sICAM-1 function, potentially leading to down-regulating vascular endothelial inflammation. It is not fully understood whether the increase of sICAM-3 by cardio training and caloric reduction in prehypertensive and hypertensive subjects reflects a cardio-protective mechanism. Given the lack of knowledge in the vascular function of sICAM-3 and its implications as a vascular inflammatory biomarker, a follow-up investigation is necessary to examine its vascular action and interactions separate of or in conjunction with other better-known vascular endothelial markers such as sICAM-1.

Another relevant potential underlying pathway in hypertension, metabolic syndrome, dyslipidaemia, and abdominal obesity, is the dysregulation of the hypothalamic–pituitary–adrenal (HPA) axis leading to catecholamine activation of β-adrenergic receptors (β-ARs) [43]. This may lead to altered leukocyte/endothelial binding, endothelial injury with up-regulation of endothelial ICAM-1 expression and increase of inflammatory cytokines [44]. In this context, regular aerobic exercise has also been shown to enhance β-AR sensitivity in the context of age-related decline in adrenergic responsiveness, i.e., increase of total peripheral resistances, which is a relevant factor underlying hypertension, atherosclerosis, and vascular insufficiency [45,46].

This study has a number of limitations. First, a weakness of the experimental design of this study is the lack of healthy BP controls. Thus, we are unable to determine whether the inflammatory, adhesion, and prothrombotic factors measured were indeed elevated in our sample of individuals with hypertension and prehypertension as compared with healthy individuals, and whether the changes induced by diet and exercise in these factors are at the level of clinical benefits. Second, a randomized and controlled trial of 12-week intervention of health behavior change was proven challenging and resulted in modest group sizes, limiting statistical power. More importantly, few significant differences found among intervention groups led us to scrutinize the actual changes in exercise and diet behavior. In reality, in spite of our best efforts to avoid "cross-contamination" between health behaviors, participants naturally began modifying their exercise or diet behavior regardless of their intervention group assignment. Some participants assigned to wait-list control condition also began to change their health behavior. Although troubling for behavior intervention trials, this kind of behavior is not particularly surprising, as exercise and healthy diet behaviors tend to co-occur [47]. It was revealed also particularly challenging to prohibit study volunteers who exhibit "readiness" to change their health behavior from doing so to follow randomization to a wait-list control group in a trial such as this. Therefore, as aforementioned, we collapsed all groups into one sample and applied multivariate regression analyses to the whole sample in order to account for exercise and diet behavior changes in practice during the intervention period. Third, regarding the dietary intervention, we have to mention that we did not differ short supply chain (SSC) from long supply chain (LSC) food included in the DASH [48]. A recent cross-sectional study found that only individuals adhering to the Mediterranean diet with an SSC had a significantly reduced prevalence of metabolic syndrome compared to those with an LSC [48]. Further, recent studies have shown that inflammatory effects of food parameters exist with a high variability [49] due to either a different genetic pattern or to diverse genetic–environmental interactions, and potential interactions (synergism, antagonism) among food parameters. However, as previously proposed, such a "dietary inflammatory index" ought to be advanced further [49]. Another intervention group, diet alone, may have contributed to important additional information. Fourth, our study did not explore the role of gender in the potentially differing effects of exercise and/or diet on inflammatory or prothrombotic markers, which was beside the primary aim of the study and limited by a limited sample size. Future studies should investigate the effect of gender not only on the intervention effects but also such behavior changes.

In summary, regular exercise and caloric reduction in individuals at risk of essential hypertension may have differential effects on biomarkers of CVD risk which may have clinical implications for the prevention of atherothrombotic cardiovascular disease. Assessments of the actual behavioral changes above and beyond intervention group assignment appear to be important. Nonetheless, the evidence of beneficial effects of regular physical activity on CV health and prevention of CVD risk, including BP, lipid levels and glucose tolerance [50] needs to be highlighted.

Author Contributions: Conceptualization, S.H., K.J.C., C.L.R., R.v.K. and P.J.M.; methodology, E.-Y.N.W., S.H., K.L.W. and P.J.M.; software, E.-Y.N.W.; formal analysis, E.-Y.N.W., S.H. and R.v.K.; investigation, all authors; resources, S.H., R.v.K., E.-Y.N.W. and P.J.M.; data curation, K.L.W.; writing—original draft preparation, E.-Y.N.W.; writing—review and editing, all authors; visualization, E.-Y.N.W. and S.H.; supervision, E.-Y.N.W., S.H. and P.J.M.; project administration, E.-Y.N.W., S.H. and P.J.M.; funding acquisition, P.J.M. All authors have read and agreed to the published version of the manuscript.

Funding: This research was funded by NIH Grants HL44915 (to P.J.M.), in part by NIH grants HL57265-08, HL073355, and MO1RR-00827 (University of California San Diego General Clinical Research Center Grant), and P60 MD00220 (San Diego EXPORT Center Grant).

Acknowledgments: Special thanks to the dedicated personal trainers and staff at the Mission Valley YMCA and La Jolla YMCA. This work had been submitted posthumously for Karen Calfas whose scientific contribution to the field and public health impact she has made are greatly appreciated and honored.

Conflicts of Interest: The authors declare no conflict of interest.

References

1. Vasan, R.S.; Beiser, A.; Seshadri, S.; Larson, M.G.; Kannel, W.B.; D'Agostino, R.B.; Levy, D. Residual lifetime risk for developing hypertension in middle-aged women and men: The framingham heart study. *JAMA* **2002**, *287*, 1003–1010. [CrossRef] [PubMed]
2. Retta, T.M.; Randall, O.S. Hypertension and concomitant diseases: A guide for evidence-based therapy. *J. Natl. Med. Assoc.* **2004**, *96*, 450–460.
3. Goetzel, R.Z.; Long, S.R.; Ozminkowski, R.J.; Hawkins, K.; Wang, S.; Lynch, W. Health, absence, disability, and presenteeism cost estimates of certain physical and mental health conditions affecting U.S. employers. *J. Occup. Environ. Med.* **2004**, *46*, 398–412. [CrossRef] [PubMed]
4. DeSouza, C.A.; Dengel, D.R.; Macko, R.F.; Cox, K.; Seals, D.R. Elevated levels of circulation cell adhesion molecule in uncomplicated essential hypertension. *Am. J. Hypertens.* **1997**, *10*, 1335–1341. [CrossRef]
5. de Faria, A.P.; Ritter, A.M.; Sabbatini, A.R.; Corrêa, N.B.; Brunelli, V.; Modolo, R.; Moreno, H. Deregulation of soluble adhesion molecules in resistant hypertension and its role in cardiovascular remodeling. *Circ. J.* **2016**, *80*, 1196–1201. [CrossRef] [PubMed]
6. Komatsu, S.; Panes, J.; Russell, J.M.; Anderson, D.C.; Muzykantov, V.R.; Miyasaka, M.; Granger, D.N. Effects of chronic arterial hypertension on constitutive and induced intercellular adhesion molecule-1 expression in vivo. *Hypertension* **1997**, *29*, 683–689. [CrossRef]
7. Ross, R. Atherosclerosis—An inflammatory disease. *N. Engl. J. Med.* **1999**, *340*, 115–126. [CrossRef]
8. Raggi, P.; Genest, J.; Giles, J.T.; Rayner, K.J.; Dwivedi, G.; Beanlands, R.S.; Gupta, M. Role of inflammation in the pathogenesis of atherosclerosis and therapeutic interventions. *Atherosclerosis* **2018**, *276*, 98–108. [CrossRef]
9. Chae, C.U.; Lee, R.T.; Rifai, N. Blood pressure and inflammation in apparently healthy men. *Hypertension* **2001**, *38*, 399–403. [CrossRef]
10. Peeters, A.C.; Netea, M.G.; Janssen, M.C.; Kullberg, B.J.; Van der Meer, J.W.; Thien, T. Pro-inflammatory cytokines in patients with essential hypertension. *Eur. J. Clin. Invest.* **2001**, *31*, 31–36. [CrossRef]
11. Mirhafez, S.R.; Mohebati, M.; Feiz Disfani, M.; Saberi Karimian, M.; Ebrahimi, M.; Avan, A.; Eslami, S.; Pasdar, A.; Rooki, H.; Esmaeili, H.; et al. An imbalance in serum concentrations of inflammatory and anti-inflammatory cytokines in hypertension. *J. Am. Soc. Hypertens.* **2014**, *8*, 614–623. [CrossRef]
12. Ridker, P.M.; Buring, J.E.; Cook, N.R.; Rifai, N. C-reactive protein, the metabolic syndrome, and risk of incident cardiovascular events: An 8-year follow-up of 14719 initially healthy American women. *Circulation* **2003**, *107*, 391–397. [CrossRef] [PubMed]
13. Horvei, L.D.; Grimnes, G.; Hindberg, K.; Mathiesen, E.B.; Njølstad, I.; Wilsgaard, T.; Brox, J.; Braekkan, S.K.; Hansen, J.B. C-reactive protein, obesity, and the risk of arterial and venous thrombosis. *J. Thromb. Haemost.* **2016**, *14*, 1561–1571. [CrossRef] [PubMed]
14. Hashimoto, H.; Kitagawa, K.; Hougaku, H.; Etani, H.; Hori, M. Relationship between C-reactive protein and progression of early carotid atherosclerosis in hypertensive subjects. *Stroke* **2004**, *35*, 1625–1630. [CrossRef] [PubMed]
15. Schillaci, G.; Pirro, M.; Gemelli, F.; Pasqualini, L.; Vaudo, G.; Marchesi, S.; Siepi, D.; Bagaglia, F.; Mannarino, E. Increased C-reactive protein concentrations in never-treated hypertension: The role of systolic and pulse pressures. *J. Hypertens.* **2003**, *21*, 1841–1846. [CrossRef]
16. Ridker, P.M.; Hennekens, C.H.; Roitman-Johnson, B.; Buring, J.E.; Grodstein, F. Plasma concentration of soluble intercellular adhesion molecule 1 and risks of future myocardial infarction in apparently healthy men. *Lancet* **1998**, *351*, 88–92. [CrossRef]
17. Fawcett, J.; Holness, C.L.; Needham, L.A.; Turley, H.; Gatter, K.C.; Mason, D.Y.; Simmons, D.L. Molecular cloning of ICAM-3, a third ligand for LFA-1, constitutively expressed on resting leukocytes. *Nature* **1992**, *360*, 481–484. [CrossRef]
18. Whelton, S.P.; Chin, A.; Xin, X. Effect of aerobic exercise on blood pressure: A meta-analysis of randomized, controlled trials. *Ann. Intern. Med.* **2002**, *136*, 493–503. [CrossRef]
19. Chobanian, A.V.; Bakris, G.L.; Black, H.R.; Cushman, W.C.; Green, L.A.; Izzo, J.L., Jr.; Jones, D.W.; Materson, B.J.; Oparil, S.; Wright, J.T., Jr.; et al. Seventh report of the joint national committee on prevention, detection, evaluation, and treatment of high blood pressure. *Hypertension* **2003**, *42*, 1206–1252. [CrossRef]
20. Bacon, S.L.; Sherwood, A.; Hinderliter, A.; Blumenthal, J.A. Effects of exercise, diet and weight loss on high blood pressure. *Sports Med.* **2004**, *34*, 307–316. [CrossRef]

21. Lesniak, K.T.; Dubbert, P.M. Exercise and hypertension. *Curr. Opin. Cardiol.* **2001**, *16*, 356–359. [CrossRef] [PubMed]
22. Carroll, S.; Dudfield, M. What is the relationship between exercise and metabolic abnormalities? A review of the metabolic syndrome. *Sports Med.* **2004**, *34*, 371–418. [CrossRef] [PubMed]
23. Bremner, A.D. Antihypertensive medication and quality of life—Silent treatment of a silent killer? *Cardiovasc. Drugs. Ther.* **2002**, *16*. [CrossRef] [PubMed]
24. Nicklas, B.J.; You, T.; Pahor, M. Behavioural treatments for chronic systemic inflammation: Effects of dietary weight loss and exercise training. *CMAJ* **2005**, *172*, 1199–1209. [CrossRef] [PubMed]
25. Geffken, D.F.; Cushman, M.; Burke, G.L.; Polak, J.F.; Sakkinen, P.A.; Tracy, R.P. Association between physical activity and markers of inflammation in a healthy elderly population. *Am. J. Epidemiol.* **2001**, *153*, 242–250. [CrossRef]
26. Pischon, T.; Hankinson, S.E.; Hotamisligil, G.S.; Rifai, N.; Rimm, E.B. Leisure-time physical activity and reduced plasma levels of obesity-related inflammatory markers. *Obes. Res.* **2003**, *11*, 1055–1064. [CrossRef]
27. von Känel, R.; Hong, S.; Pung, M.A.; Mills, P.J. Association of blood pressure and fitness with levels of atherosclerotic risk markers pre-exercise and post-exercise. *Am. J. Hypertens.* **2007**, *20*, 670–675. [CrossRef]
28. DeSouza, C.A.; Jones, P.P.; Seals, D.R. Physical activity status and adverse age-related differences in coagulation and fibrinolytic factors in women. *Arterioscler. Thromb. Vasc. Biol.* **1998**, *18*, 362–368. [CrossRef]
29. Mills, P.J.; Hong, S.; Redwine, L.; Carter, S.M.; Chiu, A.; Ziegler, M.G.; Dimsdale, J.E.; Maisel, A.S. Physical fitness attenuates leukocyte-endothelial adhesion in response to acute exercise. *J. Appl. Physiol.* **2006**, *101*, 785–788. [CrossRef]
30. Hong, S.; Johnson, T.A.; Farag, N.H.; Guy, H.J.; Matthews, S.C.; Ziegler, M.G. Attenuation of T lymphocyte demargination and adhesion molecule expression in response to moderate exercise in fit versus non-fit individuals. *J. Appl. Physiol.* **2005**, *98*, 1057–1063. [CrossRef]
31. Godin, G.; Shephard, R.J. A simple method to assess exercise behavior in the community. *Can. J. Appl. Sport. Sci.* **1985**, *10*, 141–146. [PubMed]
32. Phillips, K.M.; Stewart, K.K.; Karanja, N.M.; Windhauser, M.M.; Champagne, C.M.; Swain, J.F.; Lin, P.H.; Evans, M.A. Validation of diet composition for the dietary approaches to stop hypertension trial. DASH collaborative research group. *J. Am. Diet. Assoc.* **1999**, *99*, S60–S68. [CrossRef]
33. Zimmerman, E.; Wylie-Rosset, J. Nutrition therapy for hypertension. *Curr. Diab. Report.* **2003**, *3*, 404–411. [CrossRef]
34. Expert Panel on the Identification, Evaluation, and Treatment of Overweight in Adults. Clinical guidelines on the identification, evaluation, and treatment of overweight and obesity in adults: Executive summary. *Am. J. Clin. Nutr.* **1998**, *68*, 899–917. [CrossRef] [PubMed]
35. Edwards, K.M.; Wilson, K.L.; Sadja, J.; Ziegler, M.G.; Mills, P.J. Effects on blood pressure and autonomic nervous system function of a 12-week exercise or exercise plus DASH-diet intervention in individuals with elevated blood pressure. *Acta Physiol. (Oxf.)* **2011**, *203*, 343–350. [CrossRef] [PubMed]
36. Sadja, J.; Tomfohr, L.; Jiménez, J.A.; Edwards, K.M.; Rock, C.L.; Calfas, K.; Mills, P.J. Higher physical fatigue predicts adherence to a 12-week exercise intervention in women with elevated blood pressure. *Health Psychol.* **2012**, *31*, 156–163. [CrossRef] [PubMed]
37. Mills, P.J.; Maisel, A.S.; Ziegler, M.G.; Dimsdale, J.E.; Carter, S.; Kennedy, B.; Woods, V.L., Jr. Peripheral blood mononuclear cell-endothelial adhesion in human hypertension following exercise. *J. Hypertens.* **2000**, *18*, 1801–1806. [CrossRef] [PubMed]
38. Chen, N.G.; Abbasi, F.; Lamendola, C.; McLaughlin, T.; Cooke, J.P.; Tsao, P.S.; Reaven, G.M. Mononuclear cell adherence to cultured endothelium is enhanced by hypertension and insulin resistance in healthy nondiabetic volunteers. *Circulation* **1999**, *100*, 940–943. [CrossRef]
39. Pedersen, B.K. IL-6 Signalling in exercise and disease. *Biochem. Soc. Trans.* **2007**, *35*, 1295–1297. [CrossRef]
40. Leeuwenberg, J.F.; Smeets, E.F.; Neefjes, J.J.; Shaffer, M.A.; Cinek, T.; Jeunhomme, T.M.; Ahern, T.J.; Buurman, W.A. E-selectin and intercellular adhesion Molecule-1 are released by activated human endothelial cells in vitro. *Immunology* **1992**, *77*, 543–549.
41. Rohde, L.E.; Lee, R.T.; Rivero, J.; Jamacochian, M.; Arroyo, L.H.; Briggs, W.; Rifai, N.; Libby, P.; Creager, M.A.; Ridker, P.M. Circulating cell adhesion molecules are correlated with ultrasound-based assessment of carotid atherosclerosis. *Arterioscler. Thromb. Vasc. Biol.* **1998**, *18*, 1765–1770. [CrossRef] [PubMed]

42. Woska, J.R., Jr.; Morelock, M.M.; Jeanfavre, D.D.; Caviness, G.O.; Bormann, B.J.; Rothlein, R. Molecular comparison of soluble intercellular adhesion molecule (SICAM)-1 and SICAM-3 binding to lymphocyte function-associated antigen. *J. Biol. Chem.* **1998**, *273*, 4725–4733. [CrossRef]
43. Ciccarelli, M.; Santulli, G.; Pascale, V.; Trimarco, B.; Iaccarino, G. Adrenergic receptors and metabolism: Role in development of cardiovascular disease. *Front. Physiol.* **2013**, *4*, 265. [CrossRef] [PubMed]
44. Schedlowski, M.; Hosch, W.; Oberbeck, R.; Benschop, R.; Jacobs, R.; Raab, H.; Schmidt, R. Catecholamines modulate human NK cell circulation and function via spleen-independent ß2-adrenergic mechanisms. *J. Immunol.* **1996**, *156*, 93–99. [PubMed]
45. Santulli, G.; Ciccarelli, M.; Trimarco, B.; Iaccarino, G. Physical activity ameliorates cardiovascular health in elderly subjects: The functional role of the β adrenergic system. *Front. Physiol.* **2013**, *4*, 20. [CrossRef] [PubMed]
46. Gambardella, J.; Morelli, M.B.; Wang, X.J.; Santulli, G. Pathophysiological mechanisms underlying the beneficial effects of physical activity in hypertension. *J. Clin. Hypertens. (Greenwich)* **2020**. [CrossRef]
47. Hong, S.; Bardwell, W.A.; Natarajan, L.; Flatt, S.W.; Rock, C.L.; Newman, V.A.; Madlensky, L.; Mills, P.J.; Dimsdale, J.E.; Thomson, C.A.; et al. Correlates of physical activity levels in breast cancer survivors participating in the women's healthy eating and living (WHEL) study. *Breast Cancer Res. Treat.* **2007**, *101*, 225–232. [CrossRef]
48. Santulli, G.; Pascale, V.; Finelli, R.; Visco, V.; Giannotti, R.; Massari, A.; Morisco, C.; Ciccarelli, M.; Illario, M.; Iaccarino, G.; et al. We are what we eat: Impact of food from short supply chain on metabolic syndrome. *J. Clin. Med.* **2019**, *8*, 2061. [CrossRef] [PubMed]
49. Gambardella, J.; Santulli, G. Integrating diet and inflammation to calculate cardiovascular risk. *Atherosclerosis* **2016**, *253*, 258–261. [CrossRef]
50. Grøntved, A.; Koivula, R.W.; Johansson, I.; Wennberg, P.; Østergaard, L.; Hallmans, G.; Renström, F.; Franks, P.W. Bicycling to work and primordial prevention of cardiovascular risk: A cohort study among swedish men and women. *J. Am. Heart Assoc.* **2016**, *5*, e004413. [CrossRef]

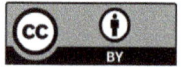

© 2020 by the authors. Licensee MDPI, Basel, Switzerland. This article is an open access article distributed under the terms and conditions of the Creative Commons Attribution (CC BY) license (http://creativecommons.org/licenses/by/4.0/).

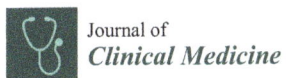

Article

Interleukin-1β Mediates Arterial Thrombus Formation via NET-Associated Tissue Factor

Luca Liberale [1,2], Erik W. Holy [3], Alexander Akhmedov [1], Nicole R. Bonetti [1,4], Fabian Nietlispach [3], Christian M. Matter [1,3], François Mach [5], Fabrizio Montecucco [2,6], Jürg H. Beer [1,4], Francesco Paneni [1,3,7], Frank Ruschitzka [3], Peter Libby [8], Thomas F. Lüscher [1,9] and Giovanni G. Camici [1,3,7,*]

1 Center for Molecular Cardiology, Schlieren Campus, University of Zurich, 8952 Schlieren, Switzerland; luca.liberale@uzh.ch (L.L.); alexander.akhmedov@uzh.ch (A.A.); nicole.bonetti@uzh.ch (N.R.B.); christian.matter@uzh.ch (C.M.M.); juerg-hans.beer@ksb.ch (J.H.B.); francesco.paneni@uzh.ch (F.P.); thomas.luescher@zhh.ch (T.F.L.)
2 First Clinic of Internal Medicine, Department of Internal Medicine, University of Genoa, 16132 Genoa, Italy; fabrizio.montecucco@unige.it
3 Department of Cardiology, University Hospital Zurich, 8091 Zurich, Switzerland; erik.holy@usz.ch (E.W.H.); fabian.nietlispach@usz.ch (F.N.); frank.ruschitzka@usz.ch (F.R.)
4 Department of Internal Medicine, Cantonal Hospital of Baden, 5404 Baden, Switzerland
5 Department of Cardiology, Hopital Universitaire de Geneve, 1206 Geneve, Switzerland; francois.mach@unige.ch
6 IRCCS Ospedale Policlinico San Martino Genoa—Italian Cardiovascular Network, 16132 Genoa, Italy
7 Department of Research and Education, University Hospital Zurich, 8001 Zurich, Switzerland
8 Division of Cardiovascular Medicine, Department of Medicine, Brigham and Women's Hospital, Harvard Medical School, 02115 Boston, MA, USA; plibby@bwh.harvard.edu
9 Royal Brompton and Harefield Hospitals and Imperial College, London SW3 6NP, UK
* Correspondence: Giovanni.camici@uzh.ch; Tel.: +41-44-635-64-68

Received: 4 November 2019; Accepted: 21 November 2019; Published: 26 November 2019

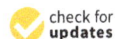

Abstract: CANTOS reported reduced secondary atherothrombotic events in patients with residual inflammatory risk treated with the inhibitory anti-IL-1β antibody, Canakinumab. Yet, mechanisms that underlie this benefit remain elusive. Recent work has implicated formation of neutrophil extracellular traps (NETosis) in arterial thrombosis. Hence, the present study explored the potential link between IL-1β, NETs, and tissue factor (TF)—the key trigger of the coagulation cascade—in atherothrombosis. To this end, ST-elevation myocardial infarction (STEMI) patients from the Swiss multicenter trial SPUM-ACS were retrospectively and randomly selected based on their CRP levels. In particular, 33 patients with STEMI and high C-reactive protein (CRP) levels (≥ 10 mg/L) and, 33 with STEMI and low CRP levels (≤ 4 mg/L) were investigated. High CRP patients displayed elevated circulating IL-1β, NETosis, and NET-associated TF plasma levels compared with low CRP ones. Additionally, analysis of patients stratified by circulating IL-1β levels yielded similar results. Moreover, NETosis and NET-associated TF plasma levels correlated positively in the whole population. In addition to the above, translational research experiments provided mechanistic confirmation for the clinical data identifying IL-1β as the initial trigger for the release of the pro-coagulant, NET-associated TF. In conclusion, blunted TF presentation by activated neutrophils undergoing NETosis may provide a mechanistic explanation to reduced secondary atherothrombotic events as observed in canakinumab-treated patients in CANTOS.

Keywords: IL-1β; Canakinumab; arterial thrombosis; tissue factor; neutrophil extracellular traps

1. Introduction

The Canakinumab Anti-inflammatory Thrombosis Outcomes Study (CANTOS) [1] affirmed in humans the inflammatory theory of atherosclerosis [2]. In CANTOS, over 10,000 post-myocardial infarction patients with residual inflammatory risk (defined as high-sensitivity C-reactive protein (hs-CRP) concentrations $\geq$ 2 mg/L) and treated with currently mandated concomitant cardiovascular (CV) therapy randomly received placebo or one of 3 doses of the interleukin (IL)-1β neutralizing antibody canakinumab. Canakinumab treatment reduced the primary composite endpoint (non-fatal myocardial infarction or stroke and cardiovascular death) by 15%, and blunted circulating levels of hsCRP and IL-6 by 35–40% without lowering atherogenic lipids [1]. Yet, the molecular mechanisms underlying this clinical benefit, particularly its thrombotic component, remain incompletely understood.

Occlusive arterial thrombus formation following plaque rupture or erosion causes most myocardial infarctions and many ischemic strokes [3]. Several experimental observations suggest a strong bidirectional link between inflammation, atherosclerosis and arterial thrombosis [4–8]. Indeed, inflammatory conditions favour atherothrombosis as reflected by increased plaque burden and CV event rates in patients with chronic inflammatory diseases [9]. Moreover, thrombosis itself can also induce and enhance inflammation thus setting the stage for a vicious cycle involving different pathways, and more prominently the tissue factor (TF)-thrombin axis [10]. Recent work has implicated neutrophil extracellular traps (NETs) in thrombosis by various mechanisms including presentation of tissue factor procoagulant activity [11–13]. Formation of NETs contributes to the host defence properties of neutrophils. Various infectious and non-infectious stimuli induce NETs which consist of extracellular strands of unwound DNA in complex with histones and proteins from neutrophil granules [13,14].

Hence, the present study explored the molecular mechanisms by which canakinumab reduces atherothrombotic events, as observed in CANTOS. To this end, we tested the hypothesis that IL-1β, NETosis, and TF-bearing NETs interrelate in a cohort of patients with ST-elevation myocardial infarction (STEMI) and different degree of systemic inflammation randomly selected from the Swiss SPUM-ACS trial (ClinicalTrials.gov number NCT01000701) [15]. To provide mechanistic explanations for these clinical findings, mouse experiments used a murine canakinumab-surrogate antibody (01BSUR) IL-1β to inhibit this cytokine in lipopolysaccharide (LPS)-treated mice before induction of arterial thrombosis by endothelial-specific photochemical injury.

2. Experimental Section

2.1. Patient Enrollment and Blood Sampling

The SPUM–ACS study (Special Program University Medicine–Acute Coronary Syndromes) is a prospective cohort study of consecutive acute coronary syndrome (ACS) patients hospitalized in different Swiss university hospitals registered in ClinicalTrials.gov (NCT01000701). Details of the study have been reported previously [15]. Briefly, patients with ACS undergoing coronary angiography were consecutively enrolled in four Swiss medical centres between December 2009 and October 2012. Exclusion criteria were severe physical disability, inability to give consent owing to dementia, and life expectancy of <1 year for non-cardiac reasons. Inclusion criteria were age $\geq$18 years, ST-segment elevation myocardial infarction (STEMI), non-ST-segment–elevation myocardial infarction, or unstable angina. The local ethics committees approved the study and all patients gave written informed consent in compliance with the Declaration of Helsinki as listed under ClinicalTrials.gov number NCT01000701.

STEMI patients were enrolled at the Andreas-Grüntzig-Catheterisation laboratory of the Department of Cardiology at the University Hospital Zurich, Switzerland, within 72 h after pain onset, and subdivided into two groups. Specifically, plasma samples of 33 STEMI patients with high circulating C-reactive protein (CRP) levels $\geq$ 10 mg/L and 33 STEMI patients with low CRP levels $\leq$ 4 mg/L and were analysed. Liver or kidney failure, active cancer, infections, or autoimmune disease were exclusion criteria. Blood was drawn from the arterial sheath into EDTA tubes at the time of diagnostic coronary angiography and centrifuged at 2700 g for 10 min at room temperature to obtain plasma, and frozen and stored in aliquots at −80 °C until serial measurement in the core laboratory (Department of Clinical Chemistry, University Hospital Zurich, Switzerland).

2.2. IL-1β Quantification in Human Plasma

Plasma levels of IL-1β were measured by high-sensitivity ELISA following the manufacturer's instructions (Quantikine® HSLB00D, R&D Systems, Minneapolis, MN). Plasma samples with an absorbance value below the lowest IL-1β concentration included in the standard curve (assessed in duplicates) were assigned an absorbance equal to that of the lowest point of the standard curve.

2.3. NETosis Assessment in Human and Murine Plasma

Quantification of circulating NET remnants such as myeloperoxidase (MPO)-DNA complexes by ELISA appears to be the current, most specific and objective assay to monitor NETosis in vivo [12,16,17]. As previously described [12,17], microtiter plates were coated with anti-MPO antibody (5 μg/mL, Cat No. 07-496, Merck, Darmstadt, Germany) overnight at 4 °C. After blocking with 1% BSA, the serum was added in combination with the peroxidase-conjugated anti-DNA monoclonal antibody (part of the commercial cell death detection kit; Roche, Basel, Switzerland) according to the manufacturer's instructions. After 2 h of incubation and accurate washing with PBS, the peroxidase substrate (ATBS) from the kit was added to each plate. The absorbance at 405 nm wavelength was measured after 40 min incubation in the dark, 490 nm was used as reference wavelength.

2.4. Tissue Factor-DNA Complexes Quantification in Human and Murine Plasma

To assess the NET contribution to circulating TF levels, we sought to quantify the fraction of TF associated with circulating DNA. This protocol adapted that used for MPO-DNA complex assessment to detect TF–DNA complexes. Briefly, microtiter plate was coated with either human or mouse TF capture antibody (parts of the commercial DuoSet® ELISA kits from R&D Systems, Cat No. DY2339 and DY3178-05, respectively) according to the manufacturer's instructions. After overnight incubation and blocking with 1% BSA, serum was added in combination with the peroxidase-conjugated anti-DNA monoclonal antibody (component No.2 of the commercial cell death detection kit from Roche, cat No. 11774425001) following the manufacturer's instructions. Validation experiments measured MPO-DNA and TF–DNA complexes in human plasma incubated with increasing concentration of LPS to stimulate NETosis (Supplemental Figure S1). Briefly, blood was collected in EDTA tubes (Vacutainer, BD Diagnostics) from a healthy donor and aliquoted in tubes containing increasing concentration of LPS dissolved in PBS (0–25 μg/mL) [18]. After 2 h, plasma was isolated by centrifugation at 2700 g for 15 min and MPO-DNA and TF–DNA complexes assessed as mentioned above (Supplemental Figure S1).

2.5. Animals

Experiments used 12-week-old male C57BL/6 wild-type mice (Charles-River Lab, Freiburg im Breisgau, Germany); all rodents were kept in a temperature-controlled animal facility under normal light/dark cycle with free access to food and water. All procedures were approved by the Committee for Animal Testing of the Canton of Zurich, Switzerland (ZH023/17). Animal experiments were performed conform to the Directive 2010/63/EU of the European Parliament and of the Council of 22 September 2010 on the protection of animals used for scientific purposes.

2.6. Monoclonal anti IL-1β Antibody

Dr. Hermann Gram (Novartis, Basel, Switzerland) kindly provided the highly specific canakinumab-surrogate anti-mouse IL-1β antibody 01BSUR. Since the human anti IL-1β antibody (i.e., canakinumab) does not neutralize the rodent antigen, experiments used this monoclonal anti-IL-1β antibody instead. Novartis used 01BSUR, a murine IgG2a/k isotype, in all parallel pre-clinical studies performed for the development of canakinumab [19,20].

2.7. Treatments and Arterial Thrombosis

As previously described [21], mice received 5 mg/kg lipopolysaccharide (LPS) (E. coli O111: B4, Sigma–Aldrich, St. Louis, MO, USA) by intraperitoneal (i.p.) injection 10 h before the laser-induced arterial thrombosis to trigger inflammation. Five hours after LPS administration and for the remaining 5 h before exposure to the thrombosis protocol, animals randomly received the murine canakinumab-surrogate antibody (01BSUR, 10 µg/g) or vehicle (i.e., NaCl 0.9%) via tail vein injection. The unique dose was chosen to reproduce the canakinumab concentration in sera from patients enrolled in the clinical trial CACZ885A2102 (NCT00487708), as previously described [20,22–25].

Ten hours after i.p. LPS injection and five hours after i.v. treatment with the canakinumab-surrogate antibody, mice underwent photochemical injury of the common carotid artery CCA as previously described (Figure 1A) [26–28]. Briefly, mice were anaesthetized using pentobarbital (87 mg/kg body weight); after midline neck incision, the right common carotid artery was exposed under an operating microscope. To induce photochemical injury of the endothelium, rose bengal (50 mg/kg body weight) was injected into the tail vein and the common carotid artery was exposed to a laser light beam (1.5 mW, 540 nm, Mellesgriot Inc., Carlsbad, CA, USA) at a distance of 6 cm for 60 min. Carotid blood flow and heart rate were monitored (Doppler flow probe carotid artery Transonic Systems Inc., 0.5 VB) until occlusion (flow ≤0.1 mL for 1 min) or for a maximum of 120 min, in case arterial thrombosis was not detected.

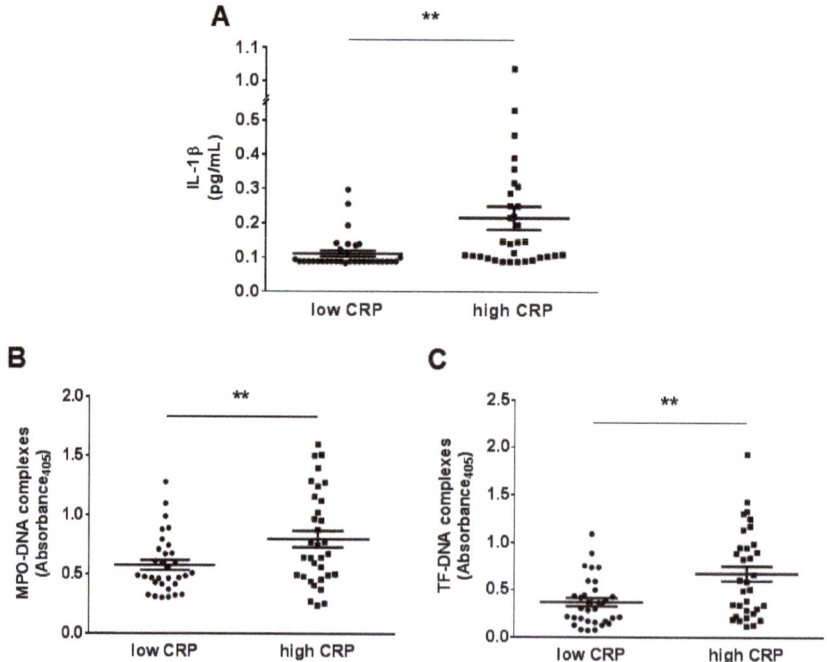

Figure 1. *Cont.*

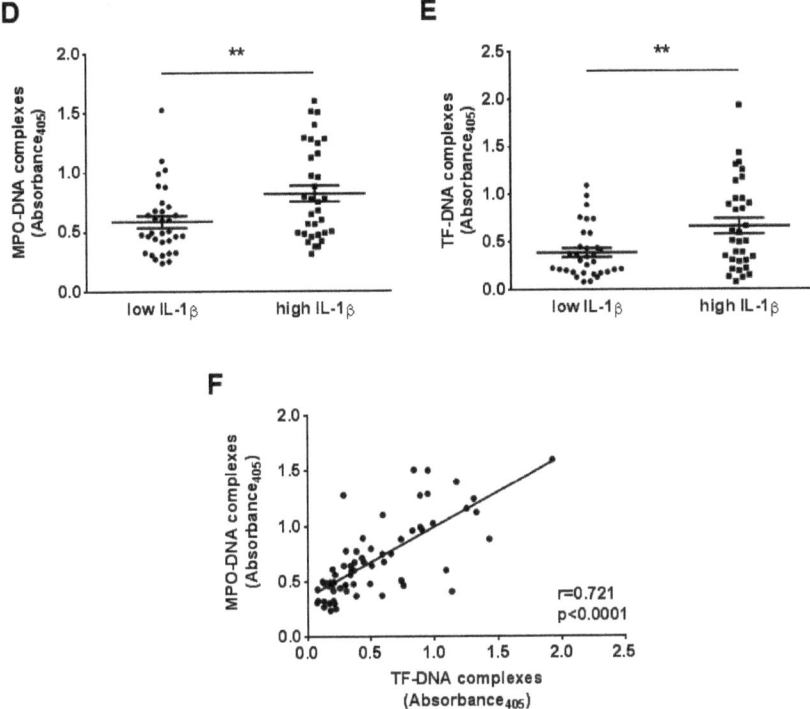

Figure 1. Levels of IL-1β, neutrophil extracellular traps (NETosis), NET-associated tissue factor and their relationships in patients with coronary disease. (**A**) STEMI patients with high systemic inflammation have higher IL-1β plasma levels than those with lower C-reactive protein (CRP) levels (n = 33). (**B**) Patients with STEMI and high CRP levels showed increased levels of NETosis assessed by plasma MPO-DNA complexes (n = 32–33) (**C**) Plasma tissue factor TF)-DNA complexes rose in patients with STEMI and high circulating CRP compared to less inflamed patients (n = 33). (**D–E**) Similarly, in patients categorized according to circulating IL-1β levels (above or below the median value of our cohort 0.1041 pg/mL), those with high levels of this cytokine also showed increased myeloperoxidase (MPO)-DNA and TF–DNA circulating complexes (n = 33) (**F**) A positive relationship was detectable among plasma IL-1β and MPO-DNA complexes in the whole cohort (n = 66). **$p < 0.01$. CRP = C reactive protein, IL-1β = interleukin-1β, MPO = myeloperoxidase, STEMI − ST-elevated myocardial infarction, TF = tissue factor.

2.8. Artery and Plasma Sampling for Tissue Factor Assessment

Aortas were collected after euthanasia and snap frozen in liquid nitrogen. They were subsequently homogenized in the lysis buffer (Tris 50 mM, NaCl 150 mM, EDTA 1 mM, NaF 1 mM, DTT 1 mM, aprotinin 10 mg/mL, leupeptin 10 mg/mL, Na3VO4 0.1 mM, phenylmethylsulfonyl fluoride (PMSF) 1 mM, and NP-40 0.5%); next, total protein concentration was determined by Bradford protein assay according to the manufacturer's recommendations (VWR Life Science AMRESCO, Solon, OH, USA). Blood was collected via intracardiac puncture and immediately mixed with EDTA. The EDTA-blood solution was then centrifuged for 15 min at 3000 g. Plasma was collected and snap-frozen in liquid nitrogen. TF protein measurement used a colorimetric enzyme-linked immunosorbent assay (ELISA) specific for the mouse protein (DY3178-05; R&D systems, Minneapolis, MN, USA) following the manufacturer's instructions. For aortas, TF concentration measured by ELISA was normalized to the total protein content of the sample. TF content was expressed as pg/mg of total protein.

2.9. Statistical Analysis

Data are expressed as mean ± SEM. All statistical analyses used GraphPad Prism 6 software (GraphPad Software, Inc, La Jolla, CA, USA). Data were analysed by one-way analysis of variance (ANOVA) with Bonferroni *post hoc* test for multiple comparisons or unpaired two-tailed Student's *t*-test as appropriate. Fisher's exact test was used for comparison of categorical data between study subjects, and Pearson's correlation analysis was used to test the correlation between two quantitative variables. A probability *p* value below 0.05 was considered as statistically significant.

3. Results

3.1. IL-1β levels, NETosis and TF–DNA Complexes Increase in STEMI Patients with High Systemic Inflammation

To explore the relationship between IL-1β, NETosis, and TF-bearing NETs we have retrospectively and randomly selected patients with STEMI and different degree of systemic inflammation (CRP ≤ 4 mg/L or ≥ 10 mg/L) from the Swiss SPUM-ACS trial. Then, IL-1β levels as well as circulating MPO-DNA and TF–DNA complexes were measured by ELISA and compared between the high CRP and low CRP groups.

66 STEMI patients (33 for each degree of inflammation group) with a median age of 66 years were enrolled. Table 1 reports a complete assessments of demographic and clinic characteristics of the whole cohort. As expected, patients were at high cardiovascular risk with 65.2% of them being active smokers, 50.0% suffering from hypertension and another 50% showing dyslipidaemia. Ongoing medical therapy at the time of angiography (i.e., anti-platelets, diuretic, anti-hypertensive or lipid-lowering drugs) is detailed in Table 1. Of importance, the two groups did not differ in blood pressure, BMI, smoking habits, comorbidities (i.e., dyslipidaemia and diabetes mellitus) or medications.

Table 1. Demographic and clinical characteristics of the study cohort.

	Whole Cohort (*n* = 66)	Low CRP * (*n* = 33)	High CRP (*n* = 33)	*p*
Demographic				
Age, years	66 ± 12	66 ± 12	65 ± 12	NS
Gender, m/f	46/20	23/10	23/10	NS
Clinical and biochemical				
Systolic BP [†], mmHg	130 ± 23	130 ± 26	123 ± 20	NS
Diastolic BP, mmHg	78±15	81±16	75±12	NS
BMI [‡], Kg/m^2	25.5±3.6	25.2±3.6	25.8±3.6	NS
Hypertension	33 (50.0%)	17 (51.5%)	16 (48.5%)	NS
Diabetes	9 (13.6%)	5 (15.2%)	4 (12.1%)	NS
Active smokers	43 (65.2%)	10 (30.0%)	18 (54.5%)	NS
Total-c [§], mmol/L	4.93±1.12	5.15±1.26	4.70±0.93	NS
HDL-c [‖], mmol/L	1.22±0.31	1.24±0.27	1.21±0.34	NS
LDL-c [#], mmol/L	3.31±1.13	3.57±1.23	3.07±0.97	NS
Dyslipidaemia	33 (50.0%)	17 (51.5%)	16 (48.5%)	NS
Medications				
Aspirin	17 (25.8%)	9 (27.3%)	8 (24.2%)	NS
Clopidogrel	2 (3.0%)	1 (3.0%)	1 (3.0%)	NS
ACE-I ** or ARBs [††]	17 (26.2%)	11 (33.3%)	6 (18.8%)	NS
β-blockers	10 (15.2%)	7 (21.2%)	3 (9.1%)	NS
Diuretics	6 (9.1%)	4 (12.1%)	2 (6.1%)	NS
Statins	12 (18.2%)	4 (12.1%)	8 (24.2%)	NS

* CRP: C reactive protein; [†] BP: blood pressure; [‡] BMI: body mass index; [§] Total-c: total cholesterol; [‖] HDL-c: high density lipoprotein cholesterol; [#] LDL-c: low density lipoprotein cholesterol; ** ACE-I: angiotensin converting enzyme inhibitors; [††] ARBs: angiotensin receptor blockers.

Circulating IL-1β levels increased significantly in STEMI patients with high CRP concentrations as compared to those with lower CRP (0.215 ± 0.034 vs. 0.111 ± 0.009 pg/mL; *p* < 0.01; Figure 1A).

Circulating plasma MPO-DNA complexes were also higher in the high CRP group compared to patients with low CRP (0.80 ± 0.07 vs. 0.58 ± 0.04; $p < 0.01$; Figure 1B). Furthermore, patients with STEMI and elevated CRP had statistical significantly higher levels of circulating TF–DNA complexes than those with low CRP levels as compared the less inflamed subjects (0.67 ± 0.08 vs. 0.37 ± 0.04; $p < 0.01$; Figure 1C). Categorization of patients according to circulating IL-1β levels (above or below its median value in the cohort: 0.1041 pg/mL) yielded similar results to those observed with lower and higher CRP cut-off points as defined above (0.821 ± 0.07 vs. 0.586 ± 0.05 for MPO-DNA and 0.66 ± 0.08 vs. 0.39 ± 0.05 for TF–DNA; $p < 0.01$ for both; Figure 1D–E). Moreover, a strong positive correlation was observed in the entire STEMI cohort between the NETosis marker MPO-DNA and NET-associated TF in plasma (r = 0.721; $p < 0.001$; Figure 1F).

3.2. IL-1β Neutralization Delays Arterial Thrombotic Occlusion In Vivo in LPS-Treated Mice

Murine thrombosis experiments sought to mimic an underlying inflammatory condition by administering LPS, as done previously [21]. Next, animals received the canakinumab-surrogate antibody (01BSUR, 10 µg/g) and underwent the thrombosis protocol (Figure 2A). This pre-treatment resembles the situation of recurrent events in CANTOS participants, who were stable at time of enrollment (≥ 30 d post qualifying event.). Compared to controls, inflamed mice treated with anti-IL-1β antibody showed a 50% increase in time to occlusion (24.9 ± 2.2 vs. 39.2 ± 2.3 min, $p < 0.001$, Figure 2B,C). The two study groups had comparable initial mean flow and heart rates (0.66 ± 0.05 vs. 0.67 ± 0.04 mL/min and 333 ± 15 vs. 354 ± 16 beats/min, respectively; Figure 2D,E).

3.3. Treatment with Canakinumab-Surrogate Anti-Mouse IL-1β Antibody Reduces Plasma Levels of Tissue Factor

To investigate the mechanisms that underlie the decreased thrombotic potential observed in canakinumab-surrogate treated mice, plasma and aortic lysates were analysed for TF levels, the key trigger of the extrinsic coagulation cascade. TF plasma levels decreased in mice treated with the anti-IL-1β antibody (37.07 ± 4.14 vs. 49.49 ± 3.17 pg/mL; Figure 3A) as compared to controls. On the other hand, TF levels in aortic extracts from the two treatment arms did not differ (1413 ± 101.8 vs. 1623 ± 130.8 pg/mg of protein; Figure 3B).

3.4. Anti-IL-1β Treatment Reduces NETosis and NET-Associated Tissue Factor Levels

Since arterial TF levels did not differ between treated and untreated animals, the current study focused on circulating protein as a possible mediator of the retarded thrombosis post IL-1β inhibition. Several cell types contribute to the circulating TF pool during arterial thrombosis. Indeed, NETs can promote thrombus formation by presenting active TF in the setting of myocardial infarction.[12] Animals treated with anti-IL-1β antibody have reduced levels of circulating MPO-DNA complexes (a marker of in vivo NETosis) after thrombus formation, as compared to vehicle-treated animals (0.082 ± 0.010 vs. 0.152 ± 0.024; $p < 0.05$; Figure 4A). To determine whether the reduced circulating TF levels observed in the treatment group related directly to the reduced NETosis, TF–DNA complexes were assessed in plasma from the two treatment arms. IL-1β inhibition significantly reduced levels of TF–DNA complexes after thrombus formation, as compared to control treatment (0.048 ± 0.012 vs. 0.099 ± 0.018; $p < 0.05$; Figure 4B). Blood cell counts did not differ in the two study subgroups (Table 2).

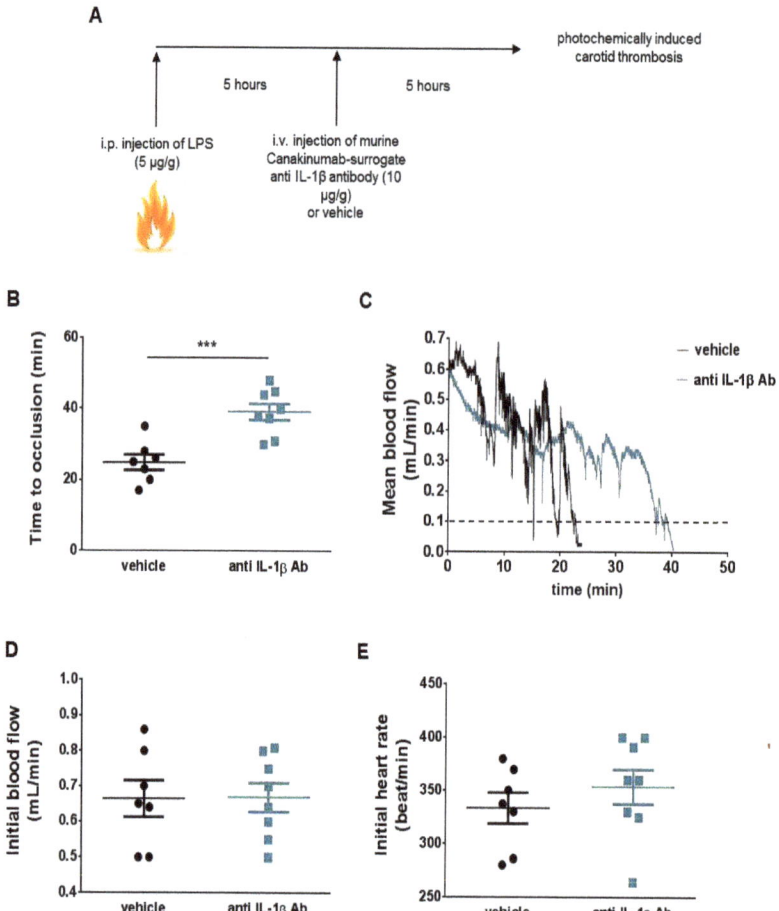

Figure 2. Anti-IL-1β antibody retards arterial thrombosis. (**A**) In an attempt to simulate the design of Canakinumab Anti-inflammatory Thrombosis Outcomes Study (CANTOS), which enrolled patients with residual inflammatory risk, animals received lipopolysaccharide (LPS) (5 µg/g, i.p) 10 h before undergoing photochemically induced carotid thrombosis. The anti-mouse IL-1β monoclonal antibody was administered to the animal intravenously via tail vein injection 5 h before thrombosis at a single dose of 10 µg/g, vehicle (i.e., NaCl 0.9%) was used as negative control. (**B**) Animals treated with monoclonal antibody against IL-1β (anti IL-1β Ab) showed increased time to occlusion as compared to vehicle-treated ones (n = 7–8). (**C**) Representative trace of mean blood flow until occlusion (mean flow ≤ 0.1 mL for 1 min) in the two study groups. (**D**,**E**) Baseline blood flow and heart rate did not differ among treated and untreated animals (n = 7–8). ***$p < 0.001$. IL-1β = interleukin-1β, LPS = lipopolysaccharide.

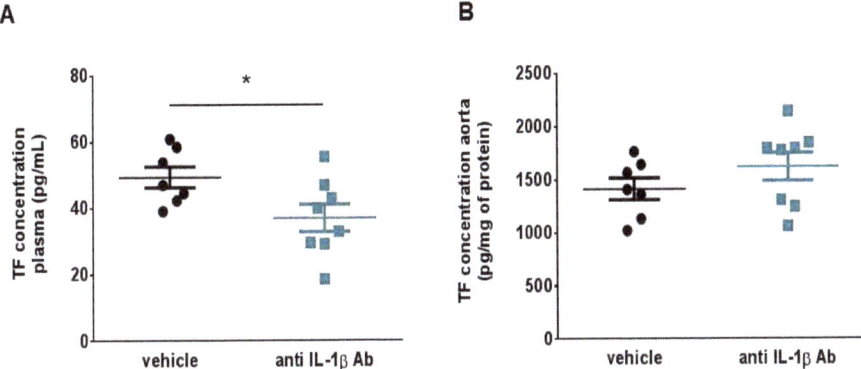

Figure 3. IL-1β blockade reduces different tissue factor pools in mice with arterial thrombosis. (**A**) Treatment with the canakinumab-surrogate antibody (anti IL-1β Ab) reduced plasma TF levels as assessed by ELISA ($n = 7$–8). (**B**) Treated and untreated animals showed no difference in terms of TF concentration in aorta lysates ($n = 7$). * $p < 0.05$. ELISA = enzyme-linked immunosorbent assay, IL-1β = interleukin-1β, TF = tissue factor.

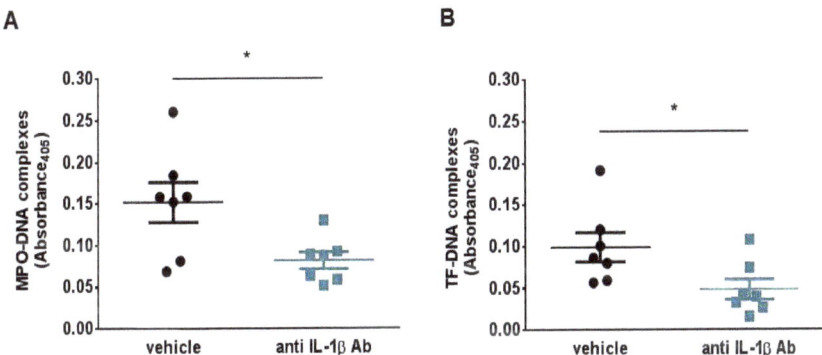

Figure 4. IL-1β blockade limits NETosis and NET-associate tissue factor levels. (**A**) Animal treated with the murine anti IL-1β antibody showed a significant reduction in the level of NETosis plasma marker MPO-DNA complexes ($n = 7$) (**B**) Levels of NET-associated TF fell after thrombosis in animals treated with the anti-IL-1β antibody as assessed by plasma TF–DNA complexes ($n = 7$). * $p < 0.05$. IL-1β = interleukin-1β, MPO = myeloperoxidase, NET = neutrophil extracellular trap, TF = tissue factor.

Table 2. Peripheral blood cell count.

	Vehicle	Anti IL *-1β	p
Total WBC [‡] (10^3/mm^3)	1.37 ± 0.13	1.38 ± 0.18	NS
Lymphocytes (%)	43.1 ± 5.2	32.3 ± 4.2	NS
Neutrophils (%)	51.4 ± 5.0	62.7 ± 4.2	NS
Monocytes (%)	5.5 ± 0.6	5.0 ± 0.7	NS
NLR [†]	1.5 ± 0.3	2.7 ± 0.7	NS
Platelets (10^3/mm^3)	297.6 ± 44.2	312.8 ± 28.8	NS

* IL: interleukin; [†] NLR: neutrophil to lymphocyte ratio; [‡] WBC: white blood cells.

4. Discussion

Ischaemic heart disease and stroke caused by atherothrombotic complications lead global causes of morbidity and mortality triggered by inflammatory bursts [29–31]. Recently, CANTOS established a causal role of inflammation in humans with previous ACS and residual inflammatory risk by showing reduced recurrent cardiovascular events after treatment with canakinumab (an anti-IL-1β antibody) [1]. The present study probed the potential mechanisms by which canakinumab may reduce thrombotic events.

This study tested the hypothesis that IL-1β influences NET formation and NETs' association with tissue factor (TF) the key trigger of the coagulation cascade in atherothrombosis. To assess the role of inflammation, ACS patients with different degree of systemic inflammation—so as to simulate the conditions observed in patients enrolled in CANTOS—were selected. In particular, 33 patients with STEMI and high C-reactive protein (CRP) levels (≥ 10 mg/L) and, 33 with STEMI and low CRP levels (≤ 4 mg/L), were investigated.

Patients were retrospectively and randomly selected from the Swiss multi-center trial SPUM-ACS (n = 1639, NCT01000701). The SPUM–ACS study (Special Program University Medicine–Acute Coronary Syndromes) is a prospective cohort study of consecutive acute coronary syndrome (ACS) patients hospitalized in different Swiss university hospitals. Details of the study have been reported previously [15]. Previous investigations have implicated NETs in coronary artery disease [14,32], and the present report correlates systemic inflammation and IL-1β with MPO-DNA complexes, currently considered an established assay for NETosis in vivo [16]. We further assessed circulating NETs-associated TF by measuring plasma TF–DNA complexes and documented their significant elevation in STEMI patients with high CRP plasma levels compared to those with lower CRP. Additionally, categorization of patients according to circulating IL-1β levels showed higher NETosis rate and levels of TF–DNA complexes in patients with higher levels of this cytokine. Moreover, the levels of NET-associated TF correlated with MPO-DNA circulating levels, a novel finding that indicates their strong interdependency. Stakos et al. recently reported NET-associated TF isolated from the culprit coronary artery of ACS patients [12]. Furthermore, these authors found that TF required the intact NET scaffold to be biologically active [12]. The relationship reported here between levels of systemic inflammation, IL-1β, NETosis and NET-associated TF production indicates a common regulating pathway and supports the hypothesis of TF arising from neutrophil undergoing NETosis, as a possible mediator of the benefits of canakinumab treatment.

Experimental data have long suggested a role for IL-1β in atherothrombosis [33,34]; indeed, IL-1β causes vascular smooth muscle cell dysfunction, activates endothelial cells and induces pro-coagulant and adhesion protein expression [35,36]. Furthermore, experimental and human atherosclerotic plaques contain IL-1β and its loss of function limits experimental atherosclerosis [37,38]. Similarly, CANTOS demonstrated that IL-1β blockade reduces recurrent myocardial infarction in human after ACS [1]. The current study sought to experimentally investigate the mechanisms of this effect and showed blunted thrombosis in inflamed mice treated with canakinumab surrogate to resemble the IL-1β-mediated inflammatory risk of patients enrolled in CANTOS.

Arterial thrombosis mediated by activation of platelets and TF causes most ACS [39]. Patients with CV risk factors as well as those with ACS have increased levels of TF [40–42]. Various cell types produce TF including endothelial cells, monocytes/macrophages and smooth muscle cells in response to different pro-inflammatory cytokines, among which IL-1β is one of the best-characterized [43–45]. In light of the above, we hypothesized that treatment with IL-1β antibody could reduce thrombus formation by targeting TF in vascular and/or circulating cells. IL-1β neutralization in mice reduced TF levels in plasma but not in arterial tissue, suggesting that in our experimental setting IL-1β inhibition primarily targets circulating TF.

As recently reported, activated neutrophils can contribute to blood-borne TF and thrombus formation by binding the injured endothelium [10,46]. Although neutrophils contain TF, either endogenous or acquired via microparticle internalization, questions remained on how these cells release it [10]. In 2012, Kambas et al [47]. reported that neutrophils can release large amounts of TF in the form of NETs. They further showed that NET-associated TF indeed derives from neutrophils, and that the thrombin eventually formed can activate platelets. The same authors reported a requirement for neutrophil priming with pro-inflammatory cytokines (i.e., IL-1β and TNF-α) for TF mRNA translation [47]. In line with the above, the current study found blunted NETosis (MPO-DNA complexes) in IL-1β-blocked animals after thrombus formation, thus underscoring the important role of IL-1β in priming neutrophils for NETosis during inflammatory conditions [48]. Next, we assessed whether blunted NETosis could account for the reduction in TF levels as seen in anti-IL-1β-treated animals by measuring TF–DNA complex in the plasma. Affirming our hypothesis, animals pretreated with IL-1β antibody showed significantly reduced NET-associated TF levels compared to controls. A possible role for IL-1β in NETosis induction has long been hypothesized [49] and recently confirmed in a publication by Meher et al [50]. Here, the authors report that IL-1β localizes within NETs in mice with experimental abdominal aortic aneurysms and that IL-1β blockade inhibits NETosis in isolated neutrophils [50]. They proposed a mechanism by which IL-1β–induced ceramide synthesis triggers the release of NETs by inducing nuclear Cer 16:0 synthesis, which permeabilizes the nuclear membrane and triggers NETosis. Accordingly, attenuation of NETosis can result from either inhibition of IL-1β signaling (IL-1 receptor antagonist treatment) or inhibition of ceramide synthases (fumonisin B1 treatment) [50]. Furthermore, we recently investigated IL-1 isoform association with NETs [51]. Curiously, we found that NET-associated cathepsin G degrades IL-1β to inactive fragments, but actually cleaves IL-1α to a more active form. The IL-1α isoform rather than IL-1β isoform accounts for activation of tissue factor expression and activity on human endothelial cells by NETs [51]. Thus, canakinumab might reduce thrombosis rate by blunting IL-1β-mediated NETosis synergistically with the reduction of other known IL-1β pro-thrombotic features such as its agonist role on platelets [52].

The current study has some limitations which merit consideration. First, patients enrolled in this clinical cohort had less use of CV medications at baseline than in CANTOS, as would be expected in a group that included individuals with a first MI, in contrast to the secondary prevention population in CANTOS. Animal experiments permit in-depth investigation of molecular mechanisms but do not necessarily faithfully replicate the clinical setting. CANTOS enrolled patients with a previous ACS with comorbidities and treated with many medications, conditions that do not apply to the rodents used in this study. Also, while CANTOS reported a reduction of secondary CV events, we here show a reduction of the thrombotic potential in the non-atherosclerotic mouse carotid arteries. Lastly, to mirror the pro-inflammatory state of the CANTOS cohort, we challenged mice with LPS to induce an inflammatory response. This intervention does not fully reproduce the low-grade inflammation observed in patients enrolled in CANTOS. Yet, low-dose LPS treatment is a well-established and reproducible method for experimental induction of inflammation that does not rely on altered metabolic conditions or genetic manipulations, unlike many other models (e.g., dyslipidaemia and obesity models, cytokine overexpressing animals), and thus avoids numerous variables in the experimental conditions. Furthermore, hsCRP—the inclusion criteria for the CANTOS trial—is not a reliable marker of inflammation in mice [53].

5. Conclusions

In conclusion, this study proposes reduced TF production by neutrophils undergoing NETosis as a novel mechanistic contributor to the reduction in CV events achieved by treatment with canakinumab in the CANTOS trial. The results affirm the tight interrelationship of inflammation with thrombosis, and point to processes and biomarkers that merit monitoring in further attempts to address residual cardiovascular risk with anti-inflammatory interventions.

Supplementary Materials: The following are available online at http://www.mdpi.com/2077-0383/8/12/2072/s1, Supplemental Figure S1. TF–DNA complex assay validation.

Author Contributions: L.L., P.L., F.P., T.F.L. and G.G.C. conceived the project and the experimental set-up; L.L., A.A. and N.R.B. performed experiments; C.M.M., F.Ma. and T.F.L. coordinated the enrollment of the patients

(SPUM-ACS study); L.L. and G.G.C. wrote the manuscript; E.W.H., F.N., J.H.B., F.Mo. and F.R. provided critical input for the set-up and analysis for the clinical part of the study; all authors critically reviewed the manuscript and contributed to discussion and interpretation of results.

Funding: The present work was supported by the Swiss National Science Foundation (to G.G.C. (310030_175546), T.F.L. (310030_166576) and the SPUM-ACS consortium (33CM30-124112 and 32473B_163271)), the Alfred and Annemarie von Sick Grants for Translational and Clinical Research Cardiology and Oncology to G.G.C. and the Foundation for Cardiovascular Research–Zurich Heart House. G.G.C. and F.P. are recipients of a H.H. Sheikh Khalifa bin Hamad Al Thani Foundation Assistant Professorship at the Faculty of Medicine. Dr. Libby has received funding from the National Heart, Lung, and Blood Institute (R01HL080472 and R01HL134892), the American Heart Association (18CSA34080399), and the RRM Charitable Fund.

Acknowledgments: We thank Hermann Gram from the Novartis Institutes for BioMedical Research for kindly supplying the anti-mouse IL-1β monoclonal antibody. We are grateful to the principal investigators of the SPUM-ACS study: Stephan Windecker, University of Bern, Peter Jüni, University of Bern, Nicholas Rodondi, MD, University of Lausanne, Switzerland. Furthermore, we acknowledge the diligent work of the independent clinical events committee for SPUM-ACS: Matthias Pfisterer, University of Basel (chair), Tiziano Moccetti, CardioCentro Lugano, Lukas Kappenberger, University of Lausanne, Switzerland. We also thank the local study nurses (Anika Adam and Christine Hager), the lab technicians, the central data monitors, the electronic data capturing system (2mt GmbH Ulm, Germany) and the members of the local catheter teams for their invaluable work.

Conflicts of Interest: T.F.L. and C.M.M. have been member of the Canakinumab advisory board of Novartis and have received honoraria as well as educational grants to the institution. P.L. is an unpaid consultant to, or involved in clinical trials for Amgen, AstraZeneca, Esperion Therapeutics, Ionis Pharmaceuticals, Kowa Pharmaceuticals, Novartis, Pfizer, Sanofi-Regeneron, and XBiotech, Inc. PL is a member of scientific advisory board for Amgen, Corvidia Therapeutics, DalCor Pharmaceuticals, IFM Therapeutics, Kowa Pharmaceuticals, Olatec Therapeutics, Medimmune, Novartis, and XBiotech, Inc. Libby's laboratory has received research funding in the last 2 years from Novartis. All other authors declare no conflict of interest.

References

1. Ridker, P.M.; Everett, B.M.; Thuren, T.; MacFadyen, J.G.; Chang, W.H.; Ballantyne, C.; Fonseca, F.; Nicolau, J.; Koenig, W.; Anker, S.D.; et al. Antiinflammatory Therapy with Canakinumab for Atherosclerotic Disease. *N. Engl. J. Med.* **2017**, *377*, 1119–1131. [CrossRef] [PubMed]
2. Libby, P. Inflammation in atherosclerosis. *Nature* **2002**, *420*, 868–874. [CrossRef] [PubMed]
3. Lippi, G.; Franchini, M.; Targher, G. Arterial thrombus formation in cardiovascular disease. *Nat. Rev. Cardiol.* **2011**, *8*, 502–512. [CrossRef] [PubMed]
4. Montecucco, F.; Liberale, L.; Bonaventura, A.; Vecchie, A.; Dallegri, F.; Carbone, F. The Role of Inflammation in Cardiovascular Outcome. *Curr. Atheroscler. Rep.* **2017**, *19*, 11. [CrossRef]
5. Hansson, G.K.; Libby, P.; Tabas, I. Inflammation and plaque vulnerability. *J. Intern. Med.* **2015**, *278*, 483–493. [CrossRef]
6. Libby, P.; Simon, D.I. Inflammation and thrombosis: The clot thickens. *Circulation* **2001**, *103*, 1718–1720. [CrossRef]
7. Jackson, S.P.; Darbousset, R.; Schoenwaelder, S.M. Thromboinflammation: Challenges of therapeutically targeting coagulation and other host defense mechanisms. *Blood* **2019**, *133*, 906–918. [CrossRef]
8. Casula, M.; Montecucco, F.; Bonaventura, A.; Liberale, L.; Vecchié, A.; Dallegri, F.; Carbone, F. Update on the role of Pentraxin 3 in atherosclerosis and cardiovascular diseases. *Vascul. Pharmacol.* **2017**, *99*, 1–12. [CrossRef]
9. Carbone, F.; Bonaventura, A.; Liberale, L.; Paolino, S.; Torre, F.; Dallegri, F.; Montecucco, F.; Cutolo, M. Atherosclerosis in Rheumatoid Arthritis: Promoters and Opponents. *Clin. Rev. Allergy Immunol.* **2018**, 1–14. [CrossRef]
10. Kambas, K.; Mitroulis, I.; Ritis, K. The emerging role of neutrophils in thrombosis-the journey of TF through NETs. *Front. Immunol.* **2012**, *3*, 385. [CrossRef]
11. Martinod, K.; Wagner, D.D. Thrombosis: Tangled up in NETs. *Blood* **2014**, *123*, 2768–2776. [CrossRef] [PubMed]
12. Stakos, D.A.; Kambas, K.; Konstantinidis, T.; Mitroulis, I.; Apostolidou, E.; Arelaki, S.; Tsironidou, V.; Giatromanolaki, A.; Skendros, P.; Konstantinides, S.; et al. Expression of functional tissue factor by neutrophil extracellular traps in culprit artery of acute myocardial infarction. *Eur. Heart. J.* **2015**, *36*, 1405–1414. [CrossRef] [PubMed]

13. Bonaventura, A.; Montecucco, F.; Dallegri, F.; Carbone, F.; Lüscher, T.F.; Camici, G.G.; Liberale, L. Novel findings in neutrophil biology and their impact on cardiovascular disease. *Cardiovasc. Res.* **2019**, *115*, 1266–1285. [CrossRef] [PubMed]
14. Bonaventura, A.; Liberale, L.; Carbone, F.; Vecchié, A.; Díaz-Cañestro, C.; Camici, G.; Montecucco, F.; Dallegri, F. The Pathophysiological Role of Neutrophil Extracellular Traps in Inflammatory Diseases. *Thromb. Haemost.* **2018**, *118*, 6–27. [CrossRef]
15. Weidmann, L.; Obeid, S.; Mach, F.; Shahin, M.; Yousif, N.; Denegri, A.; Muller, O.; Räber, L.; Matter, C.M.; Lüscher, T.F. Pre-existing treatment with aspirin or statins influences clinical presentation, infarct size and inflammation in patients with de novo acute coronary syndromes. *Int. J. Cardiol.* **2019**, *275*, 171–178. [CrossRef]
16. Masuda, S.; Nakazawa, D.; Shida, H.; Miyoshi, A.; Kusunoki, Y.; Tomaru, U.; Ishizu, A. NETosis markers: Quest for specific, objective, and quantitative markers. *Clin. Chim. Acta* **2016**, *459*, 89–93. [CrossRef]
17. Kessenbrock, K.; Krumbholz, M.; Schönermarck, U.; Back, W.; Gross, W.L.; Werb, Z.; Gröne, H.-J.; Brinkmann, V.E.; Jenne, D. Netting neutrophils in autoimmune small-vessel vasculitis. *Nat. Med.* **2009**, *15*, 623–625. [CrossRef]
18. Khan, M.A.; Farahvash, A.; Douda, D.N.; Licht, J.-C.; Grasemann, H.; Sweezey, N.; Palaniyar, N. JNK Activation Turns on LPS- and Gram-Negative Bacteria-Induced NADPH Oxidase-Dependent Suicidal NETosis. *Sci. Rep.* **2017**, *7*, 3409. [CrossRef]
19. European Medicines Evaluation Agency (EMEA). CHMP Assessment Report for Ilaris. Available online: http://www.ema.europa.eu/docs/en_GB/document_library/EPAR_-_Public_assessment_report/human/001109/WC500031679.pdf (accessed on 5 March 2019).
20. Osborn, O.; Brownell, S.E.; Sanchez-Alavez, M.; Salomon, D.; Gram, H.; Bartfai, T. Treatment with an Interleukin 1 beta antibody improves glycemic control in diet-induced obesity. *Cytokine* **2008**, *44*, 141–148. [CrossRef]
21. Gaul, D.S.; Weber, J.; Van Tits, L.J.; Sluka, S.; Pasterk, L.; Reiner, M.F.; Calatayud, N.; Lohmann, C.; Klingenberg, R.; Pahla, J.; et al. Loss of Sirt3 accelerates arterial thrombosis by increasing formation of neutrophil extracellular traps and plasma tissue factor activity. *Cardiovasc. Res.* **2018**, *114*, 1178–1188. [CrossRef]
22. Awan, Z.; Denis, M.; Roubtsova, A.; Essalmani, R.; Marcinkiewicz, J.; Awan, A.; Gram, H.; Seidah, N.G.; Genest, J. Reducing Vascular Calcification by Anti-IL-1beta Monoclonal Antibody in a Mouse Model of Familial Hypercholesterolemia. *Angiology* **2016**, *67*, 157–167. [CrossRef]
23. Liberale, L.; Diaz-Cañestro, C.; Bonetti, N.R.; Paneni, F.; Akhmedov, A.; Beer, J.H.; Montecucco, F.; Lüscher, T.F.; Camici, G.G. Post-ischaemic administration of the murine Canakinumab-surrogate antibody improves outcome in experimental stroke. *Eur. Heart J.* **2018**, *39*, 3511–3517. [CrossRef]
24. Chakraborty, A.; Tannenbaum, S.; Rordorf, C.; Lowe, P.J.; Floch, D.; Gram, H.; Roy, S. Pharmacokinetic and pharmacodynamic properties of canakinumab, a human anti-interleukin-1beta monoclonal antibody. *Clin. Pharmacokinet.* **2012**, *51*, e1–e18. [CrossRef]
25. Diaz-Canestro, C.; Reiner, M.F.; Bonetti, N.R.; Liberale, L.; Merlini, M.; Wüst, P.; Amstalden, H.; Briand-Schumacher, S.; Semerano, A.; Sessa, M.; et al. AP-1 (Activated Protein-1) Transcription Factor JunD Regulates Ischemia/Reperfusion Brain Damage via IL-1beta (Interleukin-1beta). *Stroke* **2019**, *50*, 469–477. [CrossRef]
26. Holy, E.W.; Akhmedov, A.; Speer, T.; Camici, G.G.; Zewinger, S.; Bonetti, N.; Tanner, F.C.; Beer, J.H.; Lüscher, T.F. Carbamylated Low-Density Lipoproteins Induce a Prothrombotic State Via LOX-1: Impact on Arterial Thrombus Formation In Vivo. *J. Am. Coll. Cardiol.* **2016**, *68*, 1664–1676. [CrossRef]
27. Breitenstein, A.; Stämpfli, S.F.; Reiner, M.F.; Shi, Y.; Keller, S.; Akhmedov, A.; Clerigué, A.S.; Spescha, R.D.; Beer, H.-J.; Lüscher, T.F.; et al. The MAP kinase JNK2 mediates cigarette smoke-induced arterial thrombosis. *Thromb. Haemost.* **2017**, *117*, 83–89.
28. Stampfli, S.F.; Akhmedov, A.; Gebhard, C.; Lohmann, C.; Holy, E.W.; Rozenberg, I.; Spescha, R.; Shi, Y.; Luscher, T.F.; Tanner, F.C.; et al. Aging induces endothelial dysfunction while sparing arterial thrombosis. *Arterioscler. Thromb. Vasc. Biol.* **2010**, *30*, 1960–1967. [CrossRef]
29. Organization, W.H. The Top 10 Causes of Death. Available online: http://www.who.int/news-room/fact-sheets/detail/the-top-10-causes-of-death (accessed on 5 March 2019).

30. Liberale, L.; Camici, G.G. The Role of Vascular Aging in Atherosclerotic Plaque Development and Vulnerability. *Curr. Pharm. Des.* **2019**, *25*, 3098–3111. [CrossRef]
31. Carbone, F.; Liberale, L.; Bonaventura, A.; Cea, M.; Montecucco, F. Targeting Inflammation in Primary Cardiovascular Prevention. *Curr. Pharm. Des.* **2016**, *22*, 5662–5675. [CrossRef]
32. Borissoff, J.I.; Joosen, I.A.; Versteylen, M.O.; Brill, A.; Fuchs, T.A.; Savchenko, A.S.; Gallant, M.; Martinod, K.; Cate, H.T.; Hofstra, L.; et al. Elevated levels of circulating DNA and chromatin are independently associated with severe coronary atherosclerosis and a prothrombotic state. *Arterioscler. Thromb. Vasc. Biol.* **2013**, *33*, 2032–2040. [CrossRef]
33. Libby, P. Interleukin-1 Beta as a Target for Atherosclerosis Therapy: Biological Basis of CANTOS and Beyond. *J. Am. Coll. Cardiol.* **2017**, *70*, 2278–2289. [CrossRef] [PubMed]
34. Fearon, W.F.; Fearon, D.T. Inflammation and cardiovascular disease: Role of the interleukin-1 receptor antagonist. *Circulation* **2008**, *117*, 2577–2579. [CrossRef] [PubMed]
35. Bevilacqua, M.P.; Pober, J.S.; Majeau, G.R.; Cotran, R.S.; Gimbrone, M.A., Jr. Interleukin 1 (IL-1) induces biosynthesis and cell surface expression of procoagulant activity in human vascular endothelial cells. *J. Exp. Med.* **1984**, *160*, 618–623. [CrossRef] [PubMed]
36. Bevilacqua, M.P.; Pober, J.S.; Wheeler, M.E.; Cotran, R.S.; Gimbrone, M.A., Jr. Interleukin 1 acts on cultured human vascular endothelium to increase the adhesion of polymorphonuclear leukocytes, monocytes, and related leukocyte cell lines. *J. Clin. Investig.* **1985**, *76*, 2003–2011. [CrossRef]
37. Galea, J.; Armstrong, J.; Gadsdon, P.; Holden, H.; Francis, S.E.; Holt, C.M. Interleukin-1 beta in coronary arteries of patients with ischemic heart disease. *Arterioscler. Thromb. Vasc. Biol.* **1996**, *16*, 1000–1006. [CrossRef]
38. Kirii, H.; Niwa, T.; Yamada, Y.; Wada, H.; Saito, K.; Iwakura, Y.; Asano, M.; Moriwaki, H.; Seishima, M. Lack of interleukin-1beta decreases the severity of atherosclerosis in ApoE-deficient mice. *Arterioscler. Thromb. Vasc. Biol.* **2003**, *23*, 656–660. [CrossRef]
39. Breitenstein, A.; Tanner, F.C.; Luscher, T.F. Tissue factor and cardiovascular disease: Quo vadis? *Circ. J.* **2010**, *74*, 3–12. [CrossRef]
40. Lim, H.S.; Blann, A.D.; Lip, G.Y. Soluble CD40 ligand, soluble P-selectin, interleukin-6, and tissue factor in diabetes mellitus: Relationships to cardiovascular disease and risk factor intervention. *Circulation* **2004**, *109*, 2524–2528. [CrossRef]
41. Sambola, A.; Osende, J.; Hathcock, J.; Degen, M.; Nemerson, Y.; Fuster, V.; Crandall, J.; Badimon, J.J. Role of risk factors in the modulation of tissue factor activity and blood thrombogenicity. *Circulation* **2003**, *107*, 973–977. [CrossRef]
42. Suefuji, H.; Ogawa, H.; Yasue, H.; Kaikita, K.; Soejima, H.; Motoyama, T.; Mizuno, Y.; Oshima, S.; Saito, T.; Tsuji, I.; et al. Increased plasma tissue factor levels in acute myocardial infarction. *Am. Heart J.* **1997**, *134*, 253–259. [CrossRef]
43. Puhlmann, M.; Weinreich, D.M.; Farma, J.M.; Carroll, N.M.; Turner, E.M.; Alexander, H.R., Jr. Interleukin-1beta induced vascular permeability is dependent on induction of endothelial tissue factor (TF) activity. *J. Transl. Med.* **2005**, *3*, 37. [CrossRef] [PubMed]
44. Osnes, L.T.; Westvik, A.B.; Joo, G.B.; Okkenhaug, C.; Kierulf, P. Inhibition of IL-1 induced tissue factor (TF) synthesis and procoagulant activity (PCA) in purified human monocytes by IL-4, IL-10 and IL-13. *Cytokine* **1996**, *8*, 822–827. [CrossRef] [PubMed]
45. Schecter, A.D.; Spirn, B.; Rossikhina, M.; Giesen, P.L.A.; Bogdanov, V.; Fallon, J.T.; Fisher, E.A.; Schnapp, L.M.; Nemerson, Y.; Taubman, M.B. Release of active tissue factor by human arterial smooth muscle cells. *Circ. Res.* **2000**, *87*, 126–132. [CrossRef] [PubMed]
46. Darbousset, R.; Thomas, G.M.; Mezouar, S.; Frere, C.; Bonier, R.; Mackman, N.; Renné, T.; Dignat-George, F.; Dubois, C.; Panicot-Dubois, L. Tissue factor-positive neutrophils bind to injured endothelial wall and initiate thrombus formation. *Blood* **2012**, *120*, 2133–2143. [CrossRef]
47. Kambas, K.; Mitroulis, I.; Apostolidou, E.; Girod, A.; Chrysanthopoulou, A.; Pneumatikos, I.; Skendros, P.; Kourtzelis, I.; Koffa, M.; Kotsianidis, I.; et al. Autophagy mediates the delivery of thrombogenic tissue factor to neutrophil extracellular traps in human sepsis. *PLoS ONE* **2012**, *7*, e45427. [CrossRef]
48. Keshari, R.S.; Jyoti, A.; Dubey, M.; Kothari, N.; Kohli, M.; Bogra, J.; Barthwal, M.K.; Dikshit, M. Cytokines induced neutrophil extracellular traps formation: Implication for the inflammatory disease condition. *PLoS ONE* **2012**, *7*, e48111. [CrossRef]

49. Mitroulis, I.; Kambas, K.; Chrysanthopoulou, A.; Skendros, P.; Apostolidou, E.; Kourtzelis, I.; Drosos, G.I.; Boumpas, D.T.; Ritis, K. Neutrophil extracellular trap formation is associated with IL-1beta and autophagy-related signaling in gout. *PLoS ONE* **2011**, *6*, e29318. [CrossRef]
50. Meher, A.K.; Spinosa, M.; Davis, J.P.; Pope, N.; Laubach, V.E.; Su, G.; Serbulea, V.; Leitinger, M.; Ailawadi, N.; Upchurch, G.R., Jr. Novel Role of IL (Interleukin)-1beta in Neutrophil Extracellular Trap Formation and Abdominal Aortic Aneurysms. *Arterioscler. Thromb. Vasc. Biol.* **2018**, *38*, 843–853. [CrossRef]
51. Folco, E.J.; Mawson, T.L.; Vromman, A.; Bernardes-Souza, B.; Franck, G.; Persson, O.; Nakamura, M.; Newton, G.; Luscinskas, F.W.; Libby, P. Neutrophil Extracellular Traps Induce Endothelial Cell Activation and Tissue Factor Production through Interleukin-1α and Cathepsin G. *Arterioscler. Thromb. Vasc. Biol.* **2018**, *38*, 1901–1912. [CrossRef]
52. Brown, G.T.; Narayanan, P.; Li, W.; Silverstein, R.L.; McIntyre, T.M. Lipopolysaccharide stimulates platelets through an IL-1beta autocrine loop. *J. Immunol.* **2013**, *191*, 5196–5203. [CrossRef]
53. Pepys, M.B.; Baltz, M.; Gomer, K.; Davies, A.J.; Doenhoff, M. Serum amyloid P-component is an acute-phase reactant in the mouse. *Nature* **1979**, *278*, 259–261. [CrossRef] [PubMed]

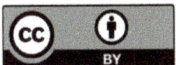

© 2019 by the authors. Licensee MDPI, Basel, Switzerland. This article is an open access article distributed under the terms and conditions of the Creative Commons Attribution (CC BY) license (http://creativecommons.org/licenses/by/4.0/).

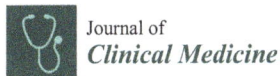

Article

Depressed Myocardial Energetic Efficiency Increases Risk of Incident Heart Failure: The Strong Heart Study

Maria-Angela Losi [1,2], Raffaele Izzo [1,2], Costantino Mancusi [1,2], Wenyu Wang [3], Mary J. Roman [4], Elisa T. Lee [5], Barbara V. Howard [6], Richard B. Devereux [4] and Giovanni de Simone [1,2,4,*]

1. Hypertension Research Center, University Federico II of Naples, I-80131 Naples, Italy
2. Department of Advanced Biomedical Sciences, University Federico II of Naples, I-80131 Naples, Italy
3. College of Public Health, University of Oklahoma Health Sciences Center, Oklahoma City, OK 73104, USA
4. Department of Medicine, Weill Cornell Medical College, New York, NY 10065, USA
5. Center for American Indian Health Research, University of Oklahoma Health Sciences Center, Oklahoma City, OK 73126, USA
6. Medstar Health Research Institute, and Georgetown-Howard Universities Center for Translational Sciences, Washington, DC 20057, USA
* Correspondence: simogi@unina.it; Tel.: +39-081-746-20-25

Received: 17 June 2019; Accepted: 16 July 2019; Published: 17 July 2019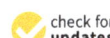

Abstract: An estimation of myocardial mechano-energetic efficiency (MEE) per unit of left ventricular (LV) mass (MEEi) can significantly predict composite cardiovascular (CV) events in treated hypertensive patients with normal ejection fraction (EF), after adjustment for LV hypertrophy (LVH). We have tested whether MEEi predicts incident heart failure (HF), after adjustment for LVH, in the population-based cohort of a "Strong Heart Study" (SHS) with normal EF. We included 1912 SHS participants (age 59 ± 8 years; 64% women) with preserved EF (≥50%) and without prevalent CV disease. MEE was estimated as the ratio of stroke work to the "double product" of heart rate times systolic blood pressure. MEEi was calculated as MEE/LV mass, and analyzed in quartiles. During a follow-up study of 9.2 ± 2.3 years, 126 participants developed HF (7%). HF was preceded by acute myocardial infarction (AMI) in 94 participants. A Kaplan-Meier plot, in quartiles of MEEi, demonstrated significant differences, substantially due to the deviation of the lowest quartile ($p < 0.0001$). Using AMI as a competing risk event, sequential models of Cox regression for incident HF (including significant confounders), demonstrated that low MEEi predicted incident HF not due to AMI ($p = 0.026$), after adjustment for significant effect of age, LVH, prolonged LV relaxation, diabetes, and smoking habits with negligible effects for sex, hypertension, antihypertensive therapy, obesity, and hyperlipemia. Low LV mechano-energetic efficiency per unit of LVM, is a predictor of incident, non-AMI related, HF in subjects with initially normal EF.

Keywords: left ventricular hypertrophy; heart failure with preserved ejection fraction; population study; stroke volume; heart rate; echocardiography

1. Introduction

Heart failure (HF) is predominantly a disease of the elderly, with nearly 50% of patients having preserved (p) left ventricular (LV) ejection fraction (EF) [1]. Although mechanisms for HFpEF remain incompletely understood, diastolic dysfunction, because it underlies myocardial hypertrophy and fibrosis, is thought to play a dominant role [2]. However, diastolic dysfunction also occurs in systolic HF (HFrEF) and is also common in elderly hypertensive individuals without HF [3]. Thus, abnormalities other than diastolic function are likely to be involved in HFpEF, especially in the presence of LV hypertrophy (LVH) [4].

There is evidence that pressure-overload LVH preserves EF as a measure of LV systolic function at the chamber level, even when contractility is reduced at the level of cardiomyocytes [5]. However, when paralleling the magnitude of LV chamber dimensions, even at normal values of LV systolic chamber function, important differences can occur in the magnitude of stroke volume (SV, i.e. LV pump performance), heart rate (HR), and blood pressure (BP) [6]. As a consequence, at a given EF, hemodynamic workload might differ substantially [6] and, in fact, SV is more predictive of incident HF than EF [7].

A new parameter of LV performance has been recently proposed as a surrogate measure of myocardial mechano-energetic efficiency (MEE), which is the ratio between produced external systolic work (stroke work, SW) and an estimate of myocardial oxygen consumption (MVO2) [8]. MEE per unit of LV mass (MEEi) has been demonstrated to predict composite adverse cardiovascular (CV) events in treated hypertensive patients after adjustment for LVH [9].

One unexplored issue is whether MEEi can also help explain incidence of HF, after adjustment for LVH, in the presence of initial normal EF in population studies. Accordingly, this analysis has been designed to assess whether MEEi can improve the identification of phenotypes at high risk of incident HF in members of the "Strong Heart Study" (SHS) cohort who were free of prevalent cardiovascular (CV) disease and initially had normal EF.

2. Methods

2.1. Participants

We analyzed data from the SHS, a population-based cohort study of CV risk factors and disease in American Indians. Detailed descriptions of the study design and methods have been previously reported [10]. At time of enrollment, a total of 4549 American Indian men and women, aged 45 to 74 years, from communities in Arizona, southwestern Oklahoma, and South and North Dakota participated in the first SHS examination, conducted from 1989 to 1991 (phase 1). The cohort was followed and re-examined twice and has been under continuous yearly surveillance for CV events. The second examination evaluated 89% of all surviving members of the original cohort, who also underwent standard Doppler echocardiography. Thus, the second SHS examination was used as baseline for the present analysis.

From the population of 2794 participants available for the analysis, we excluded 441 participants with prevalent CV (220 with a history of myocardial infarction or cardiac ischemic disease, 44 with a history of stroke and 177 with chronic heart failure) and 94 for low ejection fraction (i.e <50%), 14 because of serum triglycerides (>750 mg/dL), and 333 participants because of incomplete echocardiographic assessment. Thus, for the present study, we included 1912 SHS participants (age 59 ± 8 years; 64% women) with baseline preserved EF and without prevalent CV disease. Institutional review boards of the participating institutions and the participating tribes approved the study and submission of the manuscript.

2.2. Measurements and Definitions

The SHS used standard methodology and strict quality control at each clinical examination [11], which included a personal interview, physical examination with anthropometric and blood pressure measurement, and morning blood sample collection after a 12-hour fast. Exams were performed at local community settings and Indian Health Service clinics by trained study staff.

Arterial hypertension was defined as blood pressure ≥140/90 mmHg or current antihypertensive treatment. Obesity was classified as body mass index ≥30 kg/m^2. Diabetes was defined as fasting glucose ≥126 mg/dL or use of antidiabetic medication. Hyperlipemia was defined as total cholesterol

>200 mg/dL and/or triglyceridemic value >150 mg/dL. Smoking habits were defined as non-smoker, former smoker, and current smoker.

2.3. Echocardiography

Echocardiograms were performed using phased-array machines, with M-mode, two-dimensional, and Doppler capabilities, as previously reported [12]. Echocardiograms were evaluated in the Core Laboratory at the Weill Cornell Medical College in New York by expert readers blinded to the participant's clinical details, using a computerized review station (Digisonics, Inc., Houston, TX, USA) equipped with digitizing tablets and monitor screen overlays for calibration and performance of each needed measurement. Reproducibility of echocardiographic measures was tested in the Weill Cornell adult echocardiography laboratory in an ad hoc designed study [13].

LV internal dimensions and wall thickness were measured as end-diastole and end-systole, respectively, as previously reported [12]. Relative wall thickness, LV mass, and LV mass index (by normalization for height in m$^{2.7}$) were also estimated [6]. LVH was defined with LV mass index >47 g/m$^{2.7}$ for both sexes, a validated population-specific cut-point, maximizing the population risk attributable to LVH [14]. SV was calculated as the difference between LV end-diastolic and end-systolic volumes by the z-derived method [6,15]. EF was obtained by the ratio of SV to end-diastolic volume. Midwall fractional shortening was measured as previously described [16].

The ratio of early to late peak diastolic velocities (E/A ratio) was measured as previously described [17]. Based on previous analyses in the SHS, the E/A ratio was categorized as "normal" when it was between 0.6 and 1.5, in "prolonged relaxation" when it was <0.6 and in "restrictive physiology" when it was >1.5 [17].

To assess MEE, we estimated SW as the product of systolic BP times SV (mmHg × mL). Myocardial oxygen consumption (MVO2) could be estimated using the "double product" (DP) of systolic BP × heart rate [18]. Using this second method, MEE may be estimated in mL/s:

$$MEE = \frac{SW}{DP} \approx \frac{mmHg \times mL}{mmHg \times bpm} = \frac{mL}{bpm \times 60^{-1}} = \frac{mL}{s} \quad (1)$$

Because of the reportedly close dependence of MEE on LV mass, normalization for LV mass was done to estimate energetic expenditure per unit of myocardial mass (MEEi in mL/s/g) [9].

2.4. Outcome

CV events were recorded and adjudicated as previously reported using standardized criteria. [10]. The end-point of the present study was the first occurrence of HF, defined by the Framingham criteria for HF, as previously described [7]. Due to the potential interference with the analyzed outcome, occurrence of acute myocardial infarction (AMI) prior to HF was also censored for analysis as a competing risk event.

2.5. Statistical Analysis

Data were analyzed using IBM-SPSS-statistics (version 23.0; SPSS, New Jersey), and expressed as mean ± 1SD. MEEi was categorized in quartiles and analyzed in exploratory analyses, using linear contrast for trend analysis for age and Kendall's tau as a test for monotonic trends with categorical variables. Cumulative incidences of HF in quartiles of MEEi were analyzed using a Kaplan-Meier plot. Further analyses were focused on the lowest MEEi (corresponding to 25th percentile of the distribution).

We calculated hazard ratios and 95% confidence intervals (CI) of incident HF, using three sequential models of Cox regression. In the first Cox model, the outcome was analyzed in relation to LVH and patterns of E/A ratio, adjusting for age and sex. In the second model, low MEEi, hypertension and anti-hypertensive therapy (no/yes) were forced into the model. In the third model, obesity and diabetes were added to explore how the previous models could be changed by the co-presence of additional CV risk factors. Since the end-point of the present analysis, HF, can also be a consequence of a preceding AMI, a Cox regression was run using AMI preceding HF as a competing risk event. Thus, we censored AMI occurring before HF, in competition with the primary predictor, MEEi [19].

3. Results

Among 1912 SHS participants with normal EF and without prevalent CV disease included in this analysis, prevalence of arterial hypertension, obesity, and diabetes were 27, 51, and 40%, respectively.

Table 1 shows that while age was similar among quartiles of MEEi, the proportion of women was progressively lower with decreasing quartiles of MEEi, and concentric LV geometry and LVH were progressively higher (all p for trend <0.0001), paralleling the progressive increase in prevalent hypertension, obesity, and diabetes (all p for trend <0.0001). There was a significant trend for mitral E/A ratios of <0.6 to sharply increase in the lowest quartile of MEEi, whereas mitral E/A ratios of >1.5 progressively decreased with decreasing quartiles of MEEi (all p for trend <0.0001). Hyperlipemia and smoking habits were not different within quartiles of MEEi.

Table 1. Characteristics of quartiles of LV mass-normalized myocardial mechano-energetic efficiency (MEEi).

		Quartiles of Indexed Myocardial Mechano-Energetic Efficiency			
	Whole Population ($n = 1912$)	≥0.45 ($n = 478$)	0.40–0.44 ($n = 477$)	0.35–0.39 ($n = 479$)	≤0.34 ($n = 478$)
Age (years)	59 ± 8	59 ± 8	60 ± 8	59 ± 8	60 ± 8
Hypertension (%) [a]	27%	22%	25%	29%	34%
Proportion of women (%) [a]	64%	68%	69%	65%	55%
Concentric LV geometry (%) [a]	4%	0.2%	1%	2%	11%
LV Hypertrophy (%) [a]	23%	9%	18%	23%	40%
Mitral E/A ratio <0.6 (%) [a]	4.1	2.1	2.5	1.3	10.5
Mitral E/A ratio >1.5 (%) [a]	2.6	4.5	3.4	1.5	1.1
Obesity (%) [a]	51%	40%	51%	57%	58%
Diabetes (%) [a]	40%	25%	37%	41%	57%
Hyperlipemia (%)	58	57	55	59	62
Former smoker (%)	35	33	34	36	38
Current smoker	36	39	35	34	35

LV = left ventricular; [a] Kendall's τ-b: all $p < 0.0001$.

Although only patients with initially normal EF were included in this study, 12% of variability of EF was explained by MEEi, but the explained variability rises to 42% when LV systolic function was evaluated by midwall shortening.

During follow-up studies (median 9.9 years, inter-quartile range 9.3–10.4 years), 126 (7%) participants developed HF, 94 of them after AMI. A Kaplan-Meier cumulative hazard plot demonstrated a significant log-rank, substantially due to the marked deviation of the lowest quartiles of MEEi (Figure 1).

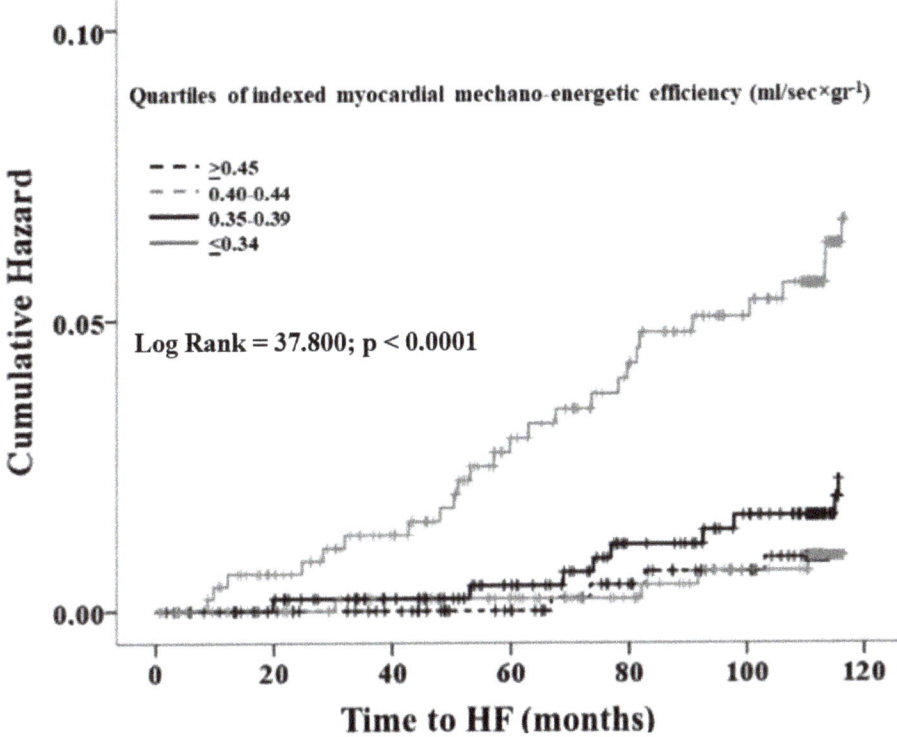

Figure 1. Cumulative hazard of incident heart failure (HF) for quartiles of myocardial mechano-energetic efficiency per unit of left ventricular mass (MEEi). Continuous grey line represents the lowest MEEi quartile.

As seen in Figure 1, we compared the lowest MEEi quartile (i.e. ≤0.34 mL × s^{-1} × g^{-1}) with all others, defined for convenience as "normal MEEi". Low MEEi was present in 47% of the subgroup, compared to 24% in the subgroup without incident HF ($p < 0.0001$). Table 2 shows sequential models of Cox regressions for incident HF. Low MEEi predicted incident HF after adjustment for LVH and prolonged relaxation. The impact of low MEEi was reduced after the inclusion of diabetes and smoking habits into the model.

The Cox models were also run using continuous variables for systolic blood pressure, body mass index, MEEi, and LV mass index instead of categories, without modifications, and compared to what has been reported in Table 2. Specifically, for each unit of increasing MEEi, there was a significant 2% reduction of hazard of incident-adverse CV events (hazard ratio (HR)= 0.02; 95% CI 0.002–0.347; $p < 0.006$).

A multicollinearity test was performed using all covariates of model 3 to calculate the variance inflation factor (VIF). The value of VIF was always <1.9, demonstrating optimal performance of the model and the low level of multicollinearity between LVH and low MEEi.

Table 2. Sequential models of proportional hazard analysis of incident heart failure (HF) in relation to low MEEi.

Predictors	Model 1			Model 2			Model 3		
	p	HR	95%CI	p	HR	95%CI	p	HR	95%CI
Age (years)	0.004	1.04	1.01–1.06	0.007	1.04	1.01–1.06	0.001	1.05	1.02–1.08
Female sex	0.666	0.93	0.62–1.38	0.846	0.96	0.63–1.46	0.833	1.05	0.68–1.61
LV Hypertrophy	<0.0001	2.51	1.70–3.73	0.001	2.01	1.37–3.10	0.004	1.89	1.23–2.91
E/A <0.6	<0.0001	3.72	1.99–6.98	0.002	2.85	1.48–5.51	0.004	2.60	1.35–5.05
E/A >1.5	0.612	0.60	0.08–4.33	0.629	0.61	0.09–4.43	0.800	0.77	0.11–5.60
Low MEEi				0.005	1.83	1.21–2.79	0.026	1.61	1.06–2.44
Hypertension				0.484	1.27	0.66–2.45	0.672	1.15	0.60–2.23
Anti-hypertensive therapy (y/n)				0.012	2.28	1.20–4.35	0.094	1.75	0.91–3.35
Diabetes							<0.0001	3.11	2.01–4.80
Obesity							0.191	0.76	0.50–1.15
Hyperlipemia							0.832	0.96	0.64–1.43
Former smoker							0.006	2.11	1.24–3.60
Current Smoker							0.003	2.38	1.35–4.17

LV = left ventricular; MEEi = indexed myocardial mechano-energetic efficiency; HR = hazard ratio.

4. Discussion

Our analysis demonstrates that in a population-based study with initially normal left ventricular ejection fraction (LVEF), reduced myocardial mechano-energetic efficiency for each g of myocardial mass is a strong predictor of incident HF after adjustment for LVH, prolonged relaxation, and associated CV risk factors, including hypertension, obesity, diabetes, and smoking habits. Our analysis merged CV risk factors with markers of preclinical CV disease. The causative effect of primary risk factors was largely offset by their direct effects on the CV system. The only risk factor that could not be fully offset by CV phenotype was diabetes, which in fact remains a potent risk factor for HF, even after adjustment for CV phenotype, as we have previously demonstrated [20].

In our analysis, we provided an estimation of myocardial energetic efficiency using a very simple method on the basis of a simple assumption, which has been already used in different circumstances [5,18], i.e., that MVO2 consumption mainly depends on developed pressure and frequency of contraction. More complex models of estimating myocardial oxygen consumption have been proposed, with strong rationale, but are likely less suitable for a clinical use [21].

4.1. The Conundrum of Development of HF

It is not surprising that a condition of low myocardial mechano-energetic efficiency per unit of myocardial mass significantly contributes to identifying a CV phenotype at risk of developing HF. The link between alterations of myocardial energy balance and HF should merit more attention, especially in the setting of HFpEF. Although we do not have follow-up echocardiograms to compare, we may postulate that incident HFpEF is frequent in our population sample, because our hazard analysis was controlled for incident, intercurrent AMI as a competing risk factor for incident HF, indirectly minimizing the chance that post-ischemic systolic HF could play a substantial role in our findings. Given the frustrating results related to the attempt to improve outcomes in HFpEF [22] and related to the insufficient understanding of its mechanisms, shifting the attention from hemodynamics and cardiac mechanics to the process of production and utilization of energy might be productive [23].

Although increased LV mass is in fact a critical marker of risk, considerable heterogeneity can be found, especially in the setting of HFpEF. In clinical trials and contemporary registries, approximately one-third to two-thirds of patients with HFpEF do not exhibit clear-cut LVH [24]. A proportion of HFpEF patients exhibit eccentric LVH rather than the more usual concentric pattern [24]. Even more intriguing is the evidence that approximately 50% of patients with HFpEF and normal LV mass do not have hypertension [24].

Furthermore, it is noteworthy that in this population with normal EF at baseline, MEEi could explain as much as 42% of midwall shortening variability, compared to the expected negligible correlation with ejection fraction. This finding is physiologically consistent with the assumption that LV systolic chamber function is only a very rough indicator of the status of myocardial mechanics.

Other pathogenetic mechanisms should be investigated.

4.2. Diastolic Dysfunction

Diastolic dysfunction is considered especially important in the context of HFpEF [24]. However, in echocardiographic sub-studies, one-third of patients randomized in controlled trials of HFpEF exhibited normal diastolic function, and a further 20% to 30% only had mild or grade 1 diastolic dysfunction [24]. In addition, a recent study of elderly subjects (age 67 to 90 years) without HF found that 96% of them had abnormal diastolic function, according to guideline-based definitions. In a condition in which diastolic dysfunction has been considered a definite pathophysiologic feature ("diastolic heart failure"), it is unclear whether the absence of diastolic dysfunction in HFpEF reflects a limitation of echocardiography, at least at the light of the present recommendations, or suggests pathophysiological mechanisms that are independent of diastolic function in a substantial proportion of patients. But, perhaps even more importantly, HF is always characterized by increased filling pressure (and therefore real diastolic dysfunction), no matter whether or not EF is reduced.

4.3. LV Production, Delivery, and Utilization of Energy

The evidence of impaired myocardial energy balance adds pathophysiological rationale to the strong effect of increased LV mass function as a marker of risk for HF. The index presented in this and in previous longitudinal analyses [9] allows a concentration of attention on physiological mechanisms more related to the production, delivery, and utilization of energy. While normal hearts mainly oxidize fatty acids to produce energy (ATP), hearts with stage B HF require a shift of production of energy (ATP) toward the most convenient glucose-pyruvate oxidation, a shift that implies adequate insulin sensitivity [25].

An important possible mechanism reducing myocardial efficiency is in fact insulin resistance [26]. The emerging evidence that this index is influenced by conditions of insulin resistance [25] is an indirect validation of our physiologic postulate. This is evident in the present and previous analyses in which diabetes exhibits a substantial importance as a predictor of HF, even more than hypertension (confirmed in the present analysis, as seen in Table 2). The progressive decline of MEEi with the increasing prevalence of diabetes and obesity was demonstrated previously in our Italian registry of hypertensive patients [9,25]. Insulin resistance, typical of type 2 diabetes, results in difficulty in the utilization of glucose [27], increasing reliance on fatty acid oxidation for up to 80–90% of acetyl CoA, at the expense of glucose and lactate oxidation [28]. This increase in fatty acid oxidation is the main determinant of the increased MVO2 at zero work, because of the lower oxygen efficiency for ATP synthesis using fatty acids as substrates [29].

Due to the above considerations and given the ethnic specificity of the SHS, and the particular high prevalence of diabetes and obesity, our findings are not necessarily generalizable and might need to be clarified in other populations with different genetic and environmental backgrounds, especially because algorithms for risk prediction might be substantially affected by prevalence and distribution of individual risk factors [30].

4.4. Final Considerations

Despite the strong association with incident HF, many unconsidered factors could have an impact on the progression of HF, potentially reducing the impact of baseline low myocardial mechano-energetic efficiency during follow-up. Among them, the control of diabetes or blood pressure during follow-up could have a significant impact on the progression of diastolic dysfunction and precipitation of HF. Further studies should help clarifying pathophysiological mechanisms linking myocardial mechano-energetic efficiency to diastolic dysfunction and control of blood pressure and diabetes.

5. Conclusions

This study demonstrated that depressed LV mechano-energetic efficiency per unit of LV mass, computed by using a simple approach comparing external work with the estimated oxygen consumption, is a powerful predictor of incident HF after adjustment for LVH and other confounders in an unselected population-based cohort of American Indians with normal baseline EF. Our results might serve as a hypothesis when testing for a better evaluation of pathophysiology of HFpEF.

Author Contributions: Conceptualization, M.A.L., R.I. and G.d.S.; Data curation, W.W., M.J.R., E.T.L., B.V.H. and R.B.D.; Formal analysis, M.A.L., R.I., C.M., R.B.D. and G.d.S.; Methodology, C.M., W.W., M.J.R., E.T.L., B.V.H. and R.B.D.; Validation C.M., W.W., M.J.R., E.T.L., B.V.H. and R.B.D.; Writing—original draft, M.A.L.; Writing—review & editing, M.A.L. and G.d.S

Funding: Dr R.I. received a grant from the University Federico II of Naples, Italy.

Conflicts of Interest: The authors declare no conflict of interest.

References

1. Vasan, R.S.; Larson, M.G.; Benjamin, E.J.; Evans, J.C.; Reiss, C.K.; Levy, D. Congestive heart failure in subjects with normal versus reduced left ventricular ejection fraction: prevalence and mortality in a population-based cohort. *J. Am. Coll. Cardiol.* **1999**, *33*, 1948–1955. [CrossRef]
2. Zile, M.R.; Brutsaert, D.L. New concepts in diastolic dysfunction and diastolic heart failure: Part II: causal mechanisms and treatment. *Circulation* **2002**, *105*, 1503–1508. [CrossRef] [PubMed]
3. Kitzman, D.W. Diastolic dysfunction in the elderly. Genesis and diagnostic and therapeutic implications. *Cardiol. Clin.* **2000**, *18*, 597–617. [CrossRef]
4. Kawaguchi, M.; Hay, I.; Fetics, B.; Kass, D.A. Combined ventricular systolic and arterial stiffening in patients with heart failure and preserved ejection fraction: implications for systolic and diastolic reserve limitations. *Circulation* **2003**, *107*, 714–720. [CrossRef] [PubMed]
5. Laine, H.; Katoh, C.; Luotolahti, M.; Kantola, I.; Jula, A.; Takala, T.O.; Ruotsalainen, U.; Iida, H.; Haaparanta, M.; Nuutila, P.; et al. Myocardial Oxygen Consumption Is Unchanged but Efficiency Is Reduced in Patients With Essential Hypertension and Left Ventricular Hypertrophy. *Circulation* **1999**, *100*, 2425–2430. [CrossRef]
6. de Simone, G.; Izzo, R.; Aurigemma, G.P.; De Marco, M.; Rozza, F.; Trimarco, V.; Stabile, E.; De Luca, N.; Trimarco, B. Cardiovascular risk in relation to a new classification of hypertensive left ventricular geometric abnormalities. *J. Hypertens.* **2015**, *33*, 745–754. [CrossRef] [PubMed]
7. De Marco, M.; Gerdts, E.; Mancusi, C.; Roman, M.J.; Lonnebakken, M.T.; Lee, E.T.; Howard, B.V.; Devereux, R.B.; de Simone, G. Influence of Left Ventricular Stroke Volume on Incident Heart Failure in a Population With Preserved Ejection Fraction (from the Strong Heart Study). *Am. J. Cardiol.* **2017**, *119*, 1047–1052. [CrossRef]
8. de Simone, G.; Chinali, M.; Galderisi, M.; Benincasa, M.; Girfoglio, D.; Botta, I.; D'Addeo, G.; de Divitiis, O. Myocardial mechano-energetic efficiency in hypertensive adults. *J. Hypertens.* **2009**, *27*, 650–655. [CrossRef]
9. de Simone, G.; Izzo, R.; Losi, M.A.; Stabile, E.; Rozza, F.; Canciello, G.; Mancusi, C.; Trimarco, V.; De Luca, N.; Trimarco, B. Depressed myocardial energetic efficiency is associated with increased cardiovascular risk in hypertensive left ventricular hypertrophy. *J. Hypertens.* **2016**, *34*, 1846–1853. [CrossRef]
10. Howard, B.V.; Lee, E.T.; Cowan, L.D.; Devereux, R.B.; Galloway, J.M.; Go, O.T.; Howard, W.J.; Rhoades, E.R.; Robbins, D.C.; Sievers, M.L.; et al. Rising Tide of Cardiovascular Disease in American Indians. *Circulation* **1999**, *99*, 2389–2395. [CrossRef]
11. Ferrara, L.A.; Capaldo, B.; Mancusi, C.; Lee, E.T.; Howard, B.V.; Devereux, R.B.; de Simone, G. Cardiometabolic risk in overweight subjects with or without relative fat-free mass deficiency: The Strong Heart Study. *Nutr. Metab. Cardiovasc. Dis.* **2014**, *24*, 271–276. [CrossRef] [PubMed]
12. Devereux, R.B.; Roman, M.J.; Liu, J.E.; Lee, E.T.; Wang, W.; Fabsitz, R.R.; Welty, T.K.; Howard, B.V. An appraisal of echocardiography as an epidemiological tool. The Strong Heart Study. *Ann. Epidemiol.* **2003**, *13*, 238–244. [CrossRef]
13. Palmieri, V.; Dahlof, B.; DeQuattro, V.; Sharpe, N.; Bella, J N.; de Simone, G.; Paranicas, M.; Fishman, D.; Devereux, R.B. Reliability of echocardiographic assessment of left ventricular structure and function: The PRESERVE study. Prospective Randomized Study Evaluating Regression of Ventricular Enlargement. *J. Am. Coll. Cardiol.* **1999**, *34*, 1625–1632. [CrossRef]
14. de Simone, G.; Kizer, J.R.; Chinali, M.; Roman, M.J.; Bella, J.N.; Best, L.G.; Lee, E.T.; Devereux, R.B. Strong Heart Study Investigators. Normalization for body size and population-attributable risk of left ventricular hypertrophy: The Strong Heart Study. *Am. J. Hypertens.* **2005**, *18*, 191–196. [CrossRef] [PubMed]
15. de Simone, G.; Devereux, R.B.; Ganau, A.; Hahn, R.T.; Saba, P.S.; Mureddu, G.F.; Roman, M.J.; Howard, B.V. Estimation of left ventricular chamber and stroke volume by limited M-mode echocardiography and validation by two-dimensional and Doppler echocardiography. *Am. J. Cardiol.* **1996**, *78*, 801–807. [CrossRef]
16. de Simone, G.; Devereux, R.B.; Koren, M.J.; Mensah, G.A.; Casale, P.N.; Laragh, J.H. Midwall left ventricular mechanics. An independent predictor of cardiovascular risk in arterial hypertension. *Circulation* **1996**, *93*, 259–265. [CrossRef] [PubMed]
17. Bella, J.N.; Palmieri, V.; Roman, M.J.; E Liu, J.; Welty, T.K.; Lee, E.T.; Fabsitz, R.R.; Howard, B.V.; Devereux, R.B. Mitral ratio of peak early to late diastolic filling velocity as a predictor of mortality in middle-aged and elderly adults: the Strong Heart Study. *Circulation* **2002**, *105*, 1928–1933. [CrossRef]

18. Vanoverschelde, J.L.; Wijns, W.; Essamri, B.; Bol, A.; Robert, A.; LaBar, D.; Cogneau, M.; Michel, C.; Melin, J.A. Hemodynamic and mechanical determinants of myocardial O_2 consumption in normal human heart: Effects of dobutamine. *Am. J. Physiol. Circ. Physiol.* **1993**, *265*, H1884–H1892. [CrossRef]
19. Losi, M.A.; Izzo, R.; De Marco, M.; Canciello, G.; Rapacciuolo, A.; Trimarco, V.; Stabile, E.; Rozza, F.; Esposito, G.; De Luca, N.; et al. Cardiovascular ultrasound exploration contributes to predict incident atrial fibrillation in arterial hypertension: The Campania Salute Network. *Int. J. Cardiol.* **2015**, *199*, 290–295. [CrossRef]
20. de Simone, G.; Devereux, R.B.; Roman, M.J.; Chinali, M.; Barac, A.; Panza, J.A.; Lee, E.T.; Galloway, J.M.; Howard, B.V. Does cardiovascular phenotype explain the association between diabetes and incident heart failure? The Strong Heart Study. *Nutr. Metab. Cardiovasc. Dis.* **2013**, *23*, 285–291. [CrossRef]
21. Devereux, R.B.; Bang, C.N.; Roman, M.J.; Palmieri, V.; Boman, K.; Gerdts, E.; Nieminen, M.S.; Papademetriou, V.; Wachtell, K.; Hille, D.A.; et al. Left Ventricular Wall Stress-Mass-Heart Rate Product and Cardiovascular Events in Treated Hypertensive Patients: LIFE Study. *Hypertension* **2015**, *66*, 945–953. [CrossRef] [PubMed]
22. Massie, B.M.; Carson, P.E.; McMurray, J.J.; Komajda, M.; McKelvie, R.; Zile, M.R.; Anderson, S.; Donovan, M.; Iverson, E.; Staiger, C.; et al. Irbesartan in Patients with Heart Failure and Preserved Ejection Fraction. *New Engl. J. Med.* **2008**, *359*, 2456–2467. [CrossRef] [PubMed]
23. Wende, A.R.; Brahma, M.K.; McGinnis, G.R.; Young, M.E. Metabolic Origins of Heart Failure. *JACC Basic Transl. Sci.* **2017**, *2*, 297–310. [CrossRef] [PubMed]
24. Lewis, G.A.; Schelbert, E.B.; Williams, S.G.; Cunnington, C.; Ahmed, F.; McDonagh, T.A.; Miller, C.A. Biological Phenotypes of Heart Failure With Preserved Ejection Fraction. *J. Am. Coll. Cardiol.* **2017**, *70*, 2186–2200. [CrossRef] [PubMed]
25. Mancusi, C.; Losi, M.A.; Izzo, R.; Canciello, G.; Manzi, M.V.; Sforza, A.; De Luca, N.; Trimarco, B.; de Simone, G. Effect of diabetes and metabolic syndrome on myocardial mechano-energetic efficiency in hypertensive patients. The Campania Salute Network. *J. Hum. Hypertens.* **2017**, *31*, 395–399. [CrossRef]
26. Kolwicz, S.C., Jr.; Purohit, S.; Tian, R. Cardiac metabolism and its interactions with contraction, growth, and survival of cardiomyocytes. *Circ. Res.* **2013**, *113*, 603–616. [CrossRef]
27. Ferrannini, E. Insulin Resistance versus Insulin Deficiency in Non-Insulin-Dependent Diabetes Mellitus: Problems and Prospects. *Endocr. Rev.* **1998**, *19*, 477–490. [CrossRef]
28. Aasum, E.; Hafstad, A.D.; Severson, D.L.; Larsen, T.S. Age-Dependent Changes in Metabolism, Contractile Function, and Ischemic Sensitivity in Hearts From db/db Mice. *Diabetes* **2003**, *52*, 434–441. [CrossRef]
29. Hinkle, P.C. P/O ratios of mitochondrial oxidative phosphorylation. *Biochim. Biophys. Acta* **2005**, *1706*, 1–11. [CrossRef]
30. Ferrario, M.M.; Chiodini, P.; E Chambless, L.; Cesana, G.; Vanuzzo, D.; Panico, S.; Sega, R.; Pilotto, L.; Palmieri, L.; Giampaoli, S. Prediction of coronary events in a low incidence population. Assessing accuracy of the CUORE Cohort Study prediction equation. *Int. J. Epidemiol.* **2005**, *34*, 413–421. [CrossRef]

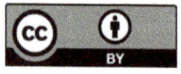

© 2019 by the authors. Licensee MDPI, Basel, Switzerland. This article is an open access article distributed under the terms and conditions of the Creative Commons Attribution (CC BY) license (http://creativecommons.org/licenses/by/4.0/).

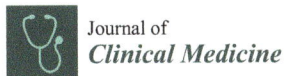

Review

Short-Term Therapies for Treatment of Acute and Advanced Heart Failure—Why so Few Drugs Available in Clinical Use, Why Even Fewer in the Pipeline?

Piero Pollesello [1,*], Tuvia Ben Gal [2], Dominique Bettex [3], Vladimir Cerny [4], Josep Comin-Colet [5], Alexandr A. Eremenko [6], Dimitrios Farmakis [7], Francesco Fedele [8], Cândida Fonseca [9], Veli-Pekka Harjola [10], Antoine Herpain [11], Matthias Heringlake [12], Leo Heunks [13], Trygve Husebye [14], Visnja Ivancan [15], Kristjan Karason [16], Sundeep Kaul [17], Jacek Kubica [18], Alexandre Mebazaa [19], Henning Mølgaard [20], John Parissis [21], Alexander Parkhomenko [22], Pentti Põder [23], Gerhard Pölzl [24], Bojan Vrtovec [25], Mehmet B. Yilmaz [26] and Zoltan Papp [27,28]

1. Critical Care, Orion Pharma, 02101 Espoo, Finland
2. Heart Failure Unit, Rabin Medical Center, Tel Aviv University, Petah Tikva 4941492d, Israel; bengalt@clalit.org.il
3. Institute of Anaesthesiology, University Hospital of Zurich, University of Zurich, 8091 Zurich, Switzerland; dominique.bettex@usz.ch
4. Department of Anesthesiology, Perioperative Medicine and Intensive Care, Masaryk Hospital, J.E. Purkinje University, 400 96 Usti nad Labem, Czech Republic; vladimir.cerny@fnhk.cz
5. Heart Diseases Institute, Hospital Universitari de Bellvitge, 08015 Barcelona, Spain; josepcomin@gmail.com
6. Department of Cardiac Intensive Care, Petrovskii National Research Centre of Surgery, Sechenov University, 119146 Moscow, Russia; aeremenko54@mail.ru
7. Department of Cardiology, Medical School, University of Cyprus, 1678 Nicosia, Cyprus; dimitrios_farmakis@yahoo.com
8. Department of Cardiovascular, Respiratory, Nephrology, Anesthesiology and Geriatric Sciences, 'La Sapienza' University of Rome, 00185 Rome, Italy; Francesco.Fedele@uniroma1.it
9. Heart Failure Clinic of S. Francisco Xavier Hospital, CHLO, 1449-005 Lisbon, Portugal; mcandidafonseca@gmail.com
10. Emergency Medicine, Department of Emergency Medicine and Services, Helsinki University Hospital, University of Helsinki, 00014 Helsinki, Finland; Veli-Pekka.Harjola@hus.fi
11. Department of Intensive Care, Experimental Laboratory of Intensive Care, Erasme Hospital, Université Libre de Bruxelles, 1050 Bruxelles, Belgium; Antoine.Herpain@erasme.ulb.ac.be
12. Department of Anesthesiology and Intensive Care Medicine, University of Lübeck, 23562 Lübeck, Germany; Matthias.Heringlake@uksh.de
13. Department of Intensive Care Medicine, Amsterdam UMC, Location VUmc 081 HV, The Netherlands; l.heunks@vumc.nl
14. Department of Cardiology, Oslo University Hospital Ullevaal, 0372 Oslo, Norway; tr-huse@online.no
15. Department of Anesthesiology, Reanimatology and Intensive Care, University Hospital Centre, 10000 Zagreb, Croatia; vivancan@kbc-zagreb.hr
16. Transplant Institute, Sahlgrenska University Hospital, 413 45 Gothenburg, Sweden; kristjan.karason@medfak.gu.se
17. Intensive Care Unit, National Health Service, Leeds LS2 9JT, UK; sunnykaul@aol.com
18. Department of Cardiology and Internal Medicine, Nicolaus Copernicus University, 87-100 Torun, Poland; jkubica@cm.umk.pl
19. Department of Anaesthesiology and Critical Care Medicine, AP-HP, Saint Louis and Lariboisière University Hospitals, Université de Paris and INSERM UMR-S 942-MASCOT, 75010 Paris, France; alexandre.mebazaa@aphp.fr
20. Department of Cardiology, Århus University Hospital, 8200 Århus, Denmark; hennmoel@rm.dk
21. Emergency Department, Attikon University Hospital, National and Kapodistrian University of Athens, 157 72 Athens, Greece; jparissis@yahoo.com

22 Emergency Cardiology Department, National Scientific Center M.D. Strazhesko Institute of Cardiology, 02000 Kiev, Ukraine; aparkhomenko@yahoo.com
23 Department of Cardiology, North Estonia Medical Center, 13419 Tallinn, Estonia; Pentti.Poder@regionaalhaigla.ee
24 Department of Internal Medicine III, Cardiology and Angiology, Medical University of Innsbruck, 6020 Innsbruck, Austria; gerhard.poelzl@tirol-kliniken.at
25 Advanced Heart Failure and Transplantation Center, Department of Cardiology, Ljubljana University Medical Center, SI-1000 Ljubljana, Slovenia; bojan.vrtovec@gmail.com
26 Department of Cardiology, Dokuz Eylul University Faculty of Medicine, 35340 Izmir, Turkey; cardioceptor@gmail.com
27 Division of Clinical Physiology, Department of Cardiology, Faculty of Medicine, University of Debrecen, H-4032 Debrecen, Hungary; pappz@med.unideb.hu
28 HAS-UD Vascular Biology and Myocardial Pathophysiology Research Group, Hungarian Academy of Sciences, 4001 Debrecen, Hungary
* Correspondence: piero.pollesello@orionpharma.com; Tel.: +35-85-0966-4191

Received: 3 October 2019; Accepted: 28 October 2019; Published: 1 November 2019

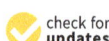

Abstract: Both acute and advanced heart failure are an increasing threat in term of survival, quality of life and socio-economical burdens. Paradoxically, the use of successful treatments for chronic heart failure can prolong life but—per definition—causes the rise in age of patients experiencing acute decompensations, since nothing at the moment helps avoiding an acute or final stage in the elderly population. To complicate the picture, acute heart failure syndromes are a collection of symptoms, signs and markers, with different aetiologies and different courses, also due to overlapping morbidities and to the plethora of chronic medications. The palette of cardio- and vasoactive drugs used in the hospitalization phase to stabilize the patient's hemodynamic is scarce and even scarcer is the evidence for the agents commonly used in the practice (e.g., catecholamines). The pipeline in this field is poor and the clinical development chronically unsuccessful. Recent set backs in expected clinical trials for new agents in acute heart failure (AHF) (omecamtiv, serelaxine, ularitide) left a field desolately empty, where only few drugs have been approved for clinical use, for example, levosimendan and nesiritide. In this consensus opinion paper, experts from 26 European countries (Austria, Belgium, Croatia, Cyprus, Czech Republic, Denmark, Estonia, Finland, France, Germany, Greece, Hungary, Israel, Italy, The Netherlands, Norway, Poland, Portugal, Russia, Slovenia, Spain, Sweden, Switzerland, Turkey, U.K. and Ukraine) analyse the situation in details also by help of artificial intelligence applied to bibliographic searches, try to distil some lesson-learned to avoid that future projects would make the same mistakes as in the past and recommend how to lead a successful development project in this field in dire need of new agents.

Keywords: acute heart failure; advanced heart failure; short-term hemodynamic therapy; regulatory clinical trials; clinical development; levosimendan

1. Introduction

Despite the availability of successful treatments for chronic heart failure (CHF), acute heart failure (AHF) and advanced heart failure (AdHF) still impose considerable and rising health burdens in their impact on life expectancy and quality of life of an increasingly elderly population and the associated social and economic burdens.

AHF and AdHF syndromes are a collection of symptoms, signs and markers with different aetiologies, different clinical courses and different cardiac reserve. The innately complex nature of these conditions is further exacerbated by the fact that they are preponderantly encountered in an elderly population with overlapping morbidities and a plethora of chronic medications including drugs for serious co-morbidities.

In an acute episode, when a patient decompensates despite optimal p.o. medications, intravenous cardio- and vasoactive drugs are used to stabilize the situation. However, the repertoire of such drugs is relatively narrow—diuretics, vasodilators and inotropes—and evidence for sustained benefit of these agents is often strikingly thin—demonstration of mortality and morbidity gains in the long term remain elusive. Disappointingly, the number of successful innovations in recent years has been small.

Recent experiences with an array of innovative cardio- and vasoactive drugs in acute heart failure were recently summarized in a review by Machaj et al. [1] (see Table 1 for studies on AHF).

Table 1. Recent large-scale regulatory Phase III trials testing novel therapies for acute heart failure. Data extracted from Machaj et al. [1].

Agent Name	Omecamtiv Mecarbil	Ularitide	Serelaxin	
Trial name	ATOMIC-AHF	TRUE-AHF	RELAX-AHF	RELAX-AHF-2
Registry number	NCT01300013	NCT01661634	NCT00520806	NCT01870778
Sample size	614 AHF patients	2.157 AHF patients	1.161 pts hospitalized for AHF	6.600 AHF patients
Outcomes	• failed to meet the primary endpoint of dyspnoea improvement • increased SET	• no significant differences in primary endpoints • significant dyspnea reduction in 83% of eligible patients	• VAS AUC scale dyspnea improvement • fewer deaths at day 180	• failed to meet primary endpoints (180-day cardiovascular death and worsening heart failure through day-5)
Observed adverse events	• no difference in adverse effect rate compared to placebo	• adverse effect on dyspnea in 17% of ineligible patients (prohibited intravenous medications)	• infrequent hypotensive events	• no serious adverse events

Abbreviations: AHF, acute heart failure; VAS AUC, visual analogue scale area under the curve.

These results follow a course that has become familiar in this area of cardiovascular medical research in recent years—ingenious and scientifically plausible novel agents show often considerable promise in pre-clinical evaluations; that promise is carried forward into Phase I trials in humans and sometimes into Phase 2 trials in patients but pivotal or definitive Phase 3 trials interventions disappoint expectations and deliver no evidence of benefit on the nominated primary endpoint(s) or on clinically-relevant outcomes such as longer-term survival. Other authors offer similar tabulations and reach similar conclusions [2,3]. In advanced heart failure (AdHF) a recent update on the field had a conspicuous focus on developments in transplantation medicine and mechanical ventricular assist devices but was strikingly silent on the topic of medical innovations [4].

In a commentary published in 2014 reasons were identified that have contributed to this frustrating state of affairs [5]. Five years on and with the situation in many ways no better, it seems timely to re-visit this issue and to ask if the latest crop of negative clinical trials would trigger a reform of heart failure-targeted clinical research. We consider a root-and-branch reform to be essential if we are to break out of the pattern intimated in Table 1 and reinvigorate a therapeutic pipeline that with few exceptions has been painfully threadbare and unproductive for several decades.

The main obstacles to progress already identified in that 2014 essay merit brief re-examination:

(1) The therapeutic field is complicated, the definitions of AHF and AdHF are not straightforward, with many aetiologies and various, often quickly evolving manifestations. Moreover, there is still a debate not only on the definition but also on the existence of some heart failure syndromes, for example, heart failure with mid-range ejection fraction [6] (HFmrEF). The combination of a broad-spectrum pathophysiology with vague definitions based on few parameters may preclude identifying meaningful group of patients benefitting of one particular drug instead of another.

(2) The barrier to new entrants is set very high by the fact that regulatory clinical trials in AHF are targeted at demonstrating a reduction in longer-term mortality from drugs intended to be used as short-term interventions. Most trials are configured to evaluate the candidate drug as an addition to standard-of-care medications—that makes it very difficult to demonstrate significant and meaningful increases in survival (or indeed in lesser outcomes such as relief of dyspnoea) [7,8]. Hence, in order to deliver convincing findings, regulatory studies need to be both large and lengthy, leading to erosion of patent life. Additional complications relate to the regulatory requirements of populous emerging markets. The need to undertake both pivotal (often international) clinical trials but increasingly also locally-conducted single-country trials to secure marketing approval in some large national markets implies a duplication of funding and other resources, all of which add to the total costs of development and weaken the business case.

(3) The use of many traditional therapies with low levels of evidence to keep patients alive and to overcome the acute decompensation (e.g., generic intravenous vasodilators, diuretics, inotropes and vasopressors) makes it very difficult for new entrants to demonstrate a persuasive risk-benefit profile when the regulatory clinical studies must be conducted versus a placebo group that mandates use of extensive "standard of care" (SoC) therapy.

All these factors may discourage the sort of ambitious investment that might produce durable innovation and progress; other therapeutic areas may appear less risky or more rewarding to pharmaceutical companies considering where to place their research and development (R&D) effort. From a commercially-focussed perspective heart failure in all its manifestations, including AHF and AdHF, is a complex condition in which "there can be no realistic expectation of a blockbuster.... and where it is wrong (both morally and commercially) to encourage hopes that such a drug is just around the corner [5]." As a corollary of this, the emergence of an era of personalized therapies implies both an opportunity and also an obligation to focus drug research in heart failure towards specific and precisely-defined sub-pathologies and to abandon, as irrational and futile, a search for a panacea.

With no substantive additions to the therapeutic repertoire in recent times and the world of medicine (and indeed the world in general) poised for unprecedented changes in the nature, scale and accessibility of data, the argument for a complete revision of the theory, philosophy and practice of research in heart failure drug design is, we suggest, compelling. One early casualty of such a revision may be the end of almost any reliance on left ventricular ejection fraction (LVEF) as a primary metric in the characterization of heart failure.

2. A Systematic Analysis of the Past 20 Years

In order to understand better the field of drug development in the acute and advanced presentation of heart failure in the latest 20 years we performed an artificial intelligence (AI)-mediated search for all regulatory trials of Phase 3 on new chemical entities (NCE) aimed to validate the benefits of drugs developed for short-term treatment of AHF (including the wording "acutely decompensated heart failure") and/or AdHF published after the year 2000. Clinical trials were searched using full-text search against studies' descriptions with the NCE and the therapy area names. Using semantic similarity, studies implying semantic similarity of less than 30% with "heart failure" were filtered out. Reports exhibiting excessive semantic similarity with "kidney disease" or "addiction" were penalized to filter out studies focused principally on these topics and only mentioning heart diseases in passing (this condition applied for example, for studies involving dopamine). Comparator classes, first posting date of the study and patient enrolment were added to the data set. Finally, the results were checked independently by two researchers for their consistency.

We identified 36 regulatory clinical trials in the past 20 years which were classified as Phase III (Figure 1). Those studies were aimed to test the hypothesis of clinical benefits of 16 different NCE (mainly exerting hemodynamic effects such as inotropy, vasodilation, diuresis), only few of which were finally approved in the U.S.A. or in Europe for use in AHF. By plotting the studies in chronological order, it can be seen that the density of Phase III trials publications has been consistently low in the past two decades (Figure 2). To be noticed is that, among the few trials in which the hypothesis was statistically proven, three (LIDO, RUSSLAN and REVIVE) tested the effect of levosimendan in AHF.

The total number of patients included in the 36 clinical trial was circa 38,000, notwithstanding that our search did not include either the Phase I and II trials or any Phase IV study. The fact that so many patients have been enrolled in this long series of inconclusive or negative studies should be considered of significance.

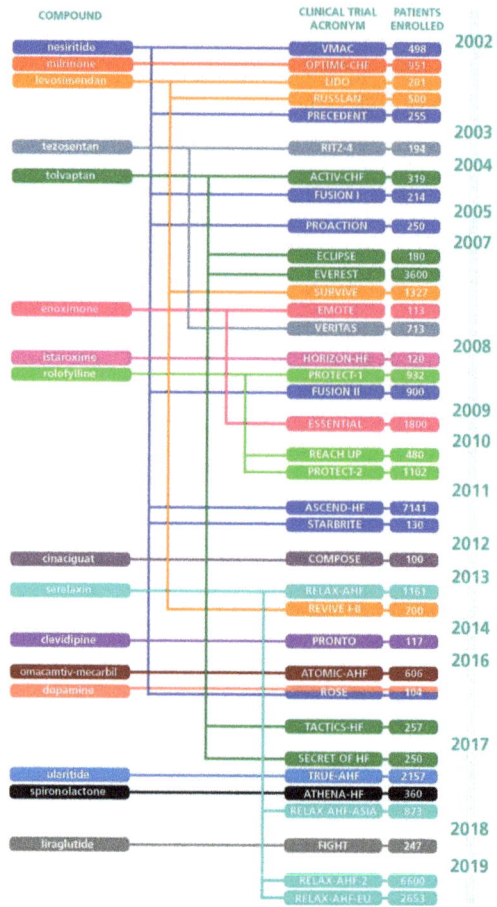

Figure 1. Regulatory clinical trials of Phase III for drugs meant for short-term treatment of acute heart failure (AHF) and/or advanced heart failure (AdHF), published in the past 20 years. For each study, the year of publication of the main report, the first author and the PMID are the following—VMAC, 2002, VMAC investigators, 11911755; OPTIME-CHF, 2002, Cuffe MS, 11911756; LIDO, 2002, Follath F, 12133653; RUSSLAN 2002 Moiseyev VS 12208222; PRECEDENT, 2002, Burger AJ, 12486437; RITZ-4, 2003, O'Connor CM, 12742280; ACTIV-CHF, 2004, M. Gheorghiade, 15113814; FUSION I, 2004, Yancy CW, 15342289; PROACTION, 2005, Peacock WF, 15915407; EVEREST, 2007, Konstam MA, 17384437; ECLIPSE, 2007, Udelison JE, published as abstract; SURVIVE, 2007, Mabazaa A, 17473298; EMOTE, 2007, Feldman AM, 17967591; VERITAS, 2007, McMurray JJ, 17986694; HORIZON-HF, 2008, Gheorghiade M, 18534276; PROTECT-1, 2008, Cotter G, 18926433; ESSENTIAL, 2009, Metra M, 19700774; FUSION II, 2008, Yancy CW, 19808265; REACH UP, 2010, Gottlieb SS, 20797594; PROTECT-2, 2010, Massie BM, 20925544; ASCEND-HF, 2011, O'Connor, 21732835; STARBRITE, 2011, Sha MR, 21807321; COMPOSE, 2012, Gheorghiade M, 22713287; RELAX-AHF, 2013, Teerlink JR, 23141816; REVIVE I-II, 2013, Packer M, 24621834; PRONTO, 2014, Peacock WF, 24655702; ATOMIC-AHF, 2016, Teerlink JR, 27012405; ROSE, 2016, Wan SH, 27512103; ROSE, 2016, Wan SH, 27512103; TACTICS-HF, 2016, Felker GM, 27654854; RELAX-AHF-ASIA, 2017, Sato N, 27825893; SECRET OF HF, 2017, Konstam MA, 28302292; TRUE-AHF, 2017, Packer M, 28402745; ATHENA-HF, 2017, Butler J, 28700781; FIGHT, 2018, Sharma A, 30120812; RELAX-AHF-EU, 2019, Maggioni AP, 30604559; RELAX-AHF-2, 2019, Metra M, 31433919.

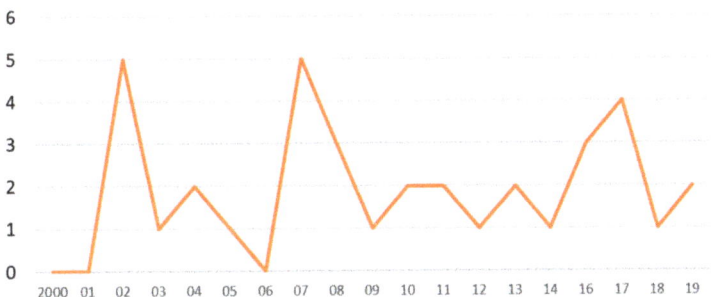

Figure 2. Amount of regulatory clinical trials of Phase III for drugs meant for short-term treatment of AHF and/or AdHF per year of publication in the period 2000–2019.

3. Also the Recent Clinical Trials have Disappointed

Before addressing these themes in more detail, it is appropriate to look briefly at some experiences in recent decades in the development of intravenous (i.v.) drug therapies.

Omecamtiv mecarbil binds with high affinity to the catalytic domain of myosin, increasing the number of myosin heads available to cross-link with actin. In theory, this augments cardiomyocyte contractility without increasing intracellular free ionic calcium or cardiomyocyte oxygen consumption [1]. In reality, the history of omecamtiv mecarbil might be seen rather as a demonstration that the pharma industry sometimes has a short memory. Candidate drugs which prolong the contractility transient were discontinued several decades ago because of their potential for harm in ischaemic conditions [9]. Omecamtiv mecarbil – at least at high plasma concentrations—shares some of these characteristics [10] and the ATOMIC-AHF trial produced a biomarker signal similar to that seen during myocardial infarction [11] (a higher median plasma troponin level) that might be related to cardiac ischemia described in an earlier Phase II trial [12]. The regulatory clinical programme for omecamtiv mecarbil in AHF has been halted. Insights on the safety and efficacy of oral omecamtiv mecarbil for chronic heart failure may be expected from the GALACTIC-HF study, due to complete in 2021.

Serelaxin is a recombinant form of the endogenous hormone relaxin-2 and exerts vasodilatory, anti-inflammatory and anti-fibrotic effects [13]. The RELAX-AHF trial produced evidence of lower incidence of worsening heart failure during hospitalization [14] but the later RELAX-AHF-2 trial, which unlike RELAX-AHF, was powered for mortality, found no impact on 180-day cardiovascular mortality and a numerical but not statistically significant effect on worsening heart failure [15]. The challenge of deciding which of these sets of findings is most relevant to the treatment of AHF patients is evident. Further illustrations of the complexities and challenges of assigning weight to the results of clinical trials is provided by the demonstration that patients in RELAX-AHF were substantially unrepresentative of patients with AHF in the United States, Latin America or Asia-Pacific [16] and by the report that the RELAX-AHF-EU trial, yielded results similar to and supportive of RELAX-AHF [17] in the context of open-label drug administration.

Ularitide, a synthetic form of the human natriuretic peptide urodilatin, exerts vasodilator, diuretic and natriuretic effects via the natriuretic peptide receptor/particulate guanylate cyclase/cyclic guanosine monophosphate pathway and displayed beneficial effects such as symptom relief and vasodilation in animal models of heart failure as well as early-phase clinical studies in heart failure patients, In a Phase 3 trial (TRUE-AHF) in patients with acute heart failure, however, short-term ularitide treatment did not affect a clinical composite end point or reduce long-term cardiovascular mortality despite various nominally favourable physiological effects (and without affecting cardiac troponin levels) [18].

The early promise of istaroxime, which promotes the activity of sarco(endo)plasmic reticulum Ca^{2+}-ATPase 2 (SERCA2) and thereby promotes expulsion of free intracellular ionic calcium through transmembrane sodium/calcium channels appears not to been sustained since the publication of the findings of the HORIZON study [19–21] and the results of the CUPID-HF study suggest that gene transfer of the SERCA2 gene is not yet a proven intervention [22].

Two studies of the nitroxyl (HNO) moiety (NCT01096043 and NCT10192325), commenced in 2010 appear to remain incomplete and unreported while evaluation of a follow-up molecule designated a BMS-986231 (previously CXL-1427) are in only preliminary stages [23]. The list of set-backs continues with tezosentan, nesiritide, tolvaptan, milrinone, enoximone, rolofylline, clevidipine, SLV320, cinaciguat, dopamine, liraglutide and high-dose spironolactone (see Figure 1).

4. Levosimendan—A Rare Case

Levosimendan, an inodilator that promotes contractility by binding to calcium saturated troponin C and vasodilatory and cardioprotective effects through the opening of adenosine triphosphate-dependent potassium (K_{ATP}) channels is one of few agents of recent decades to establish itself in the medical repertoire for AHF and AdHF for its sustained hemodynamic, neurohormonal and symptomatic effects [24,25]. This status rests on findings from a series of Phase II and III studies published in the early 2000s. Two large post-approval clinical trials (SURVIVE and REVIVE) did not substantiate an indication of long-term effects but both a meta-analysis involving data from more than 6000 patients and a real-world registry involving over 5000 patients (ALARM-HF) were strongly indicative of long term survival benefit [26,27] – at a minimum to the extent that levosimendan use has never been associated with increased mortality, whereas the use of adrenergic/calcium mobilizing inotropes such as dobutamine has. At this regard, it is worth reminding that several authors in the past recognized a correlation between the effects of cardiovascular drugs on intracellular calcium and on long-term survival in heart failure, to the advantage of drugs which do not elevate either calcium transient or mitochondrial calcium, such as levosimendan [28–30].

Finally, since no attenuation of the hemodynamic effect of levosimendan is apparent in patients treated with beta-blockers [31,32] – now a substantial proportion of the overall heart failure population – the drug has been favoured for use in such patients in the most recent edition of ESC guidelines [33].

Levosimendan has also been evaluated in randomized controlled trials in advanced heart failure (Levo-Rep (NCT01065194), LION-Heart (NCT01536132) and LAICA (NCT00988806)) [34–36]. Observations in those trials are indicative of clinical benefits including reduction in NT-pro-BNP levels and trends towards reductions in heart failure readmissions and heart failure-related mortality. Those trends were corroborated in metanalyses where statistically significant reductions in long-term mortality and re-hospitalization were demonstrated [37,38] and subsequently in the RELEVANT-HF study, in which the addition of intermittent levosimendan therapy at 3-4 week intervals was associated over the course of 6 months with a substantially lower percentage of days in hospital (2.8 ± 6.6% vs. 9.4 ± 8.2%; $p < 0.0001$) and in the cumulative number and length of HF-related admissions (both $p < 0.0001$ vs. control), plus a marked but non-significant improvement in 1-year survival free from death/need for implantation of a ventricular assist device or urgent transplantation (86% vs. 78%) [39].

5. Even the Established Drugs May Not "Work."

Very recently, at the European Society of Cardiology Congress, the GALACTIC trial reported that early intensive vasodilation using personalized high doses of nitrates, oral hydralazine and rapid up-titration of ACE inhibitors or angiotensin II receptor blockers did not improve 180-day mortality in a cohort of 781 acute heart failure patients [40]. This trial is notable, among other things, for the fact that short-term use of conventional "tried and tested" (and extremely cheap) vasodilators, administered in an intensive regime and at high dose was just as ineffectual at influencing longer-term mortality as novel agents such as ularitide and serelaxin. The inability to demonstrate survival benefit even from drugs that are established as part of the therapeutic armamentarium for AHF highlights some fundamental issues contributing to the paucity of new drug therapies in recent decades—for example, are we targeting the wrong pathological processes in our drug development programmes or are we privileging inappropriate endpoints in clinical trials and thus hampering the regulatory approval of useful new agents?

The general lack of evidence for an ongoing survival benefit from acute-phase treatments for AHF requires some reflection. While perhaps not fully subscribing to its philosophical outlook we find much to agree with in the views of McCullough [41], who has argued that AHF (and by extension AdHF) is a situation often long in the making and that to expect any therapy administered for ≤48 h to make a robust difference to survival or rehospitalization many months after the index admission is to misunderstand the pathophysiology of these conditions.

6. Where Next and How to Get There?

Readers looking for a way forward from this seeming impasse may find encouragement in a recent review by Triposkiadis and colleagues [42]. We consider that publication to be a most significant contribution to this arena of cardiovascular research for the manner in which it articulates and crystallizes lines of critical thinking that have been apparent for some years but which, through advances in technology, are now poised to transform both the conception of heart failure and its modes of treatment.

A central premise of this work is that describing heart failure in terms of LVEF, while useful in its time, has become counter-productive and increasingly is obscuring the pathophysiological realities of heart failure, with adverse consequences for the evolution of therapy [43,44]. We concur with Triposkiadis et al. [42] that heart failure is "a heterogeneous syndrome in which functional and structural biomarkers change dynamically during disease progression in a patient-specific fashion" and that the condition as a whole may usefully be portrayed as a spectrum in which, depending on their proximity within that spectrum, individual presentations may or may not have overlapping phenotypes and shared underlying pathologies. Features of heart failure identified by Triposkiadis et al. [42] as occurring across the heart failure spectrum include:

1. Bidirectional transitions of LVEF due to disease treatment and progression
2. Endothelial dysfunction, cardiomyocyte dysfunction and cardiomyocyte injury
3. Systolic and diastolic left ventricular dysfunction
4. Left atrial dysfunction
5. Myocardial fibrosis
6. Skeletal myopathy
7. Heart failure serum markers
8. Neurohumoral activation

From that starting position Triposkiadis et al. [42] advocate the development of a wholly new classification of heart failure based on ultra-detailed phenotyping of the sort now made possible by advances in biological technologies and computing. This process, illustrated in Figure 3, proves a basis both for the better application of existing therapies and to shape the development of new agents. Two pathways of stratification are identified by this reasoning – one is hypothesis-driven, based for example on disease aetiology or mechanism or shaped by known pharmacological pathways of action; the other is hypothesis-free approach driven by the modern capacity to acquire unprecedented volumes of phenotype data and to analyse that data at unprecedented speeds and granularity, so identifying characteristics (or "signatures") that differentiate sub-sets of patients with different heart failure phenotypes, different outcomes and different responses to various therapies.

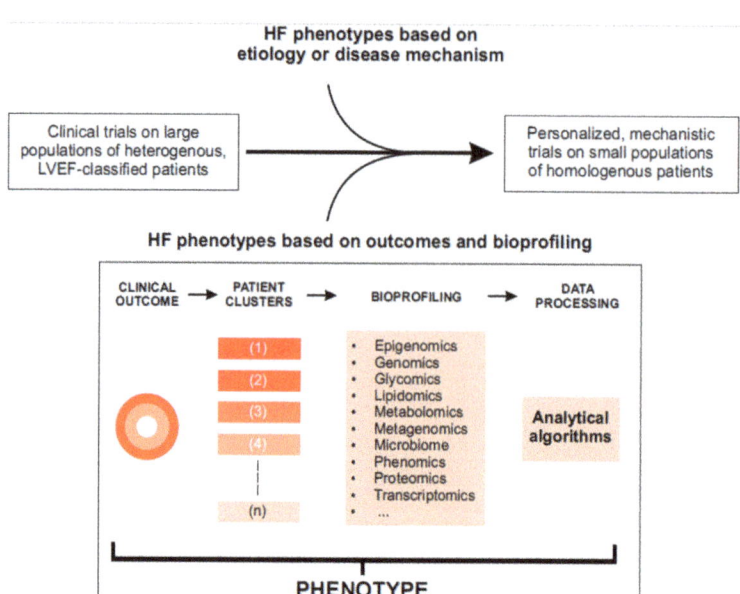

Figure 3. Advances in information and data-processing technology have created a base from which heart failure research can be re-configured towards highly defied phenotypes in ways that will facilitate both the optimal use of current therapies and the identification of new agents specifically tailored to a particular pathophysiology. See text for further discussion. Freely from Triposkiadis et al [42].

Finally, in order to stratify HF patients, it should be mandatory to consider systematically the functions of other organs such as lung, kidney, liver, brain, hematopoietic system and so on, as proposed recently [45].

7. Invasive versus Non-Invasive Monitoring

When comparing the measures suggested for the diagnosis of AHF in the most recent European guidelines [33] with previous versions, an obvious trend to avoid invasive diagnostic measures (like using a pulmonary artery catheter) in AHF can be noticed. It would be wrong to rely primarily on simple clinical signs for assessing the severity and the type of failure in AHF—its complex manifestations and haemodynamic profile cannot be adequately diagnosed and differentiated by bedside assessment. Additionally, not any single word within 85 pages of the guidelines can be found on monitoring the systemic oxygen consumption and delivery by determination of mixed or at least central venous oxygen saturation; despite heart failure is classically defined as the inability of the heart, to maintain an adequate oxygen supply to the tissues. One may argue that the lack of progress in clinical development of new agents for treatment of AHF may be also explained by the inappropriate diagnostic measures and monitoring modalities recommended by the current guidelines and that even the best drugs will fail if they are inappropriately used within the multiple manifestations of heart failure. We should also consider alternatives to the Swan Ganz catheter, as recently reviewed by a large panel of experts [46].

8. Will the Data Revolution Break the Logjam?

These proposals may be seen in the wider context of an explosion in personal data accessible for analysis and the rapidly evolving science of AI. Timely recent reviews of these themes have been published, identifying both the opportunities and the many challenges that these new technologies present [47–50]. As non-experts in those fields we are constrained in what we might say with authority about these developments but concur with Sim [49] on several aspects of the use of mobile data-reporting devices in health, including the observations that "Tracking and reporting data are a mean to an end not an end in itself" and that "Innovation in electronic sensing is in many ways outpacing the imagination for how these sensors can be used clinically." The second of those sentiments may be seen a warning to expect some developments in data acquisition to turn out to be diversions (or blind alleys) in the clinical context.

Beyond these thoughts is the much more significant challenge of sifting this unprecedented mass of data to identify signs, signals and biomarkers that are robust, reliable, meaningful and capable of being used to guide therapy. The work Deng and colleagues, who have advocated for pre-procedural gene expression profiles of peripheral blood mononuclear cells as indicative of longer-term survival prospects in patients with AdHF undergoing mechanical circulatory support, is an illustration of the immense and exciting potential in this area [51,52]. We are unreservedly positive for the longer-term prospects in this area but once more concur with the views of Sim [49] and others, about the challenges of successful implementation [53–55].

In the imminent era of Big Data as a day-to-day reality filtering the signal from the noise will be essential if clinicians are not to be simply overwhelmed by the volumes of information suddenly at their disposal. The USA alone is estimated to generate per annum 14 petabytes of data just from echocardiography results, a volume of material that defies exhaustive analysis by conventional methods [47]. Machine learning and AI may be central to the effective identification and analysis and orderly presentation of relevant data. Unsupervised machine learning (when computers are tasked to identify underlying relationships in a dataset) combined with 'pan-omic' analysis (i.e., genomics, proteomics, transcriptomics, metabolomics, etc.) from high throughput molecular profiling may provide a practical foundation for the sort of precision phenotyping aspired to by Triposkiadis et al. [42] and for 'hyper-local analytics' [47]. Deep learning, based on neural networks, is another aspect of the machine learning and AI revolution likely to find applications in cardiology [56,57].

The challenges of bringing machine learning and AI effectively into the practice of cardiology and more specifically into the management of heart failure are not to be underestimated (see Shameer et al. [47] and Johnson et al. [48] for excellent commentary on current methodologies and some of their pitfalls and limitations, including some observations on the cost barriers that may be encountered in acquiring biomedical data) but seem likely to be overcome within a short span of years. There are ample reasons for optimism in this area but confident prediction of what will become available and when and to what effect is beyond the powers of these authors.

9. Trials Design—Time for a Change?

Research into new therapies for AHF and AdHF in recent decades has come to resemble the definition of insanity ascribed to Einstein—doing the same thing over and over again and hoping for a different result. One emerging therapy after another is added to the SoC repertoire in a Phase 3 trial and in that context each in turn fails to meet the prespecified endpoints for meaningful efficacy.

We may have reached a stage where the broad-spectrum pathophysiology of HF, with different signs, symptoms and manifestations, different aetiologies and different patient co-morbidities, explored against a background of SoC medication, may preclude identifying meaningful incremental clinical benefits using traditional trial methodology.

One response to this situation may lie in the adoption of a composite clinical endpoint evaluated in a hierarchical manner. The methodology ensures that all trial participants contribute to the overall outcome analysis through one or more of the specified outcomes; this has helpful practical implications for the number of patients needed and the length of follow-up required to generate endpoint data. Highly affirmative initial results have emerged from the ATTR-ACT study, which used this methodology to evaluate tafamidis in transthyretin amyloid cardiomyopathy [58] and the LeoDOR study (NCT03437226) is currently using a similar approach to outcome assessment in AdHF patients receiving intermittent cycles of levosimendan therapy [59,60].

More radical ways forward may include the adoption of Bayesian adaptive trial design, which facilitates the study of multiple treatment approaches and therapies in multiple patient phenotypes within a single trial, while maintaining a reasonable sample size [61]. Another possibility is the adoption of the group-sequential multi-arm multi-stage (MAMS) trial. The relative strengths and limitations of these methods have been reviewed in detail [62,63]. Overarching these methods is the concept of the "platform" trial, a clinical study with a single master protocol in which multiple treatments are evaluated simultaneously. This offers flexibilities such as dropping treatments for futility or adding new treatments during the course of a trial. Platform trials have the attraction of being able to deliver robust results with fewer patients and less time than a traditional two-arm trial [64].

Some cautionary comments are appropriate at this point. These emergent trial methods may be attractive for their statistical and methodological properties but their implementation in practice can be very highly resource-intensive, even by usual standards and especially when they include biomarkers. Essential preparation for Bayesian adaptive platform trials includes extensive stakeholder consultations, in-depth statistical modelling and definition of both the best outcome measures and intra-study endpoints. Morrell et al. [65], Hague and colleagues [66] and Schiavone et al. [67] have recently offered some observations on the practicalities of conducting platform trials, based on first-hand experience and enquiry. One aspect of note is that "the biomarker-stratified trial has the effect of making staff in the trial office aware of specific patients in a unique way compared to non-stratified trials," despite anonymization" [65]. This represents a profound alteration to the human environment of clinical trials' conduct, which may be amplified by the emergence of 'decentralized' clinical trials that are conducted via mobile health or telemedicine platforms and involve virtual recruitment, delivery of trial products direct to the participants' homes and smartphone-assisted outcome assessment [49].

10. Some Views for the Future

The various trends and opportunities we have identified in this review outline a future for the development of treatments for acute or advanced heart failure perhaps very different from those of the past 20 years. Significantly, however, we might re-write that sentence to give an important different emphasis—*"The various trends and opportunities we have identified in this review outline a future for the treatment of acute or advanced heart failure perhaps very different from those of the past 20 years."* Readers will note that this second description emphasizes changes in the usage of drugs over the development of new drugs.

Our views in this regard are shaped by two notable recent publications [2,68], both of which have argued that what matters to patients who are hospitalized with a decompensation event is that they avoid further such hospitalizations and avoid the increase in mortality that occurs during the recovery phase. Viewed from that perspective the clinical stabilization achieved during the acute phase of hospital admission may be a secondary objective and to a substantial degree disconnected from the longer-term outcomes that patients prize. As Hamo and colleagues have pointed out [2], the physiological changes that lead to hospitalization take place days or weeks before hospitalization whereas the major adverse outcomes of death or rehospitalization mostly occur post-discharge. That temporal difference, combined with the now extensive evidence that acute-phase symptom relief with available therapies does not reliably improve long-term outcomes strongly suggests that either (a) relief of symptoms may be dissociated from central pathophysiological mechanisms; or (b) any pathophysiological pathway that is targeted by an acute-phase intervention is not going to be fully rectified by such short-term therapy. Conceivably both of these considerations may apply simultaneously.

Further, it is difficult to distinguish between patients suffering from the heart failure syndrome who still have cardiac reserve and respond to short-term therapy with stabilization and those who display a similar a clinical picture but show little benefit and poor outcome due to a totally worn out heart.

The need, as Hamo et al. [2] express it, to assign the right drug to the right patients at the right time to deliver meaningful benefit to AHF or AdHF patients is likely to be facilitated to a quite extraordinary degree by the developments in data acquisition and analysis we have acknowledged and the hyper-detailed phenotyping anticipated by Triposkiadis et al. [42]. That pathway of evolution in patient profiling might indeed provide insights and a firmer basis for the development of effective and successful new intravenous therapies. One possible outcome from this transformation is that the SoC repertoire that has dominated since the 1980s is finally superseded. The disappointing experience in clinical trials during the past 20 years of adding of new agents to SoC has created an impression that SoC rather than providing a foundation for further advances has acted as a glass ceiling through which newer agents struggle to break. With hyperdetailed insights into the pathophysiology of individual patients the way may finally be open to new agents precisely targeted to specific pathophysiological processes while the population-wide application of, say, ACE inhibitors and/or beta-blockers may come to be seen as too imprecise to be justifiable.

It is not less plausible, however, that the data revolution might re-shape clinical strategy around AHF and AdHF into a very different course in which an incident of decompensation is seen as a cue to intensify and optimise out-patient management with the express purpose of preventing future re-hospitalizations. We note in this context recent encouraging results using machine learning algorithms for the early detection of acute cardiac decompensation [69,70] or estimation of a patient's risk for early re-admission after an index event [71] plus descriptions of the use of machine learning and telemedicine to predict and monitor patients' treatment adherence [49,72]. Similar technologies might also be deployed to optimise the functioning and performance of specialist AdHF units such as that recently described by Kreusser and colleagues [73]. The success of the TIM-HF2 (NCT01878630) trial of telemedical interventional management in reducing unplanned cardiovascular hospital admissions and all-cause mortality is also highly pertinent in this context [74,75].

In such a scenario the emphasis in the development of overall effective medical therapy for AHF and AdHF may well be towards drugs that can be accommodated in the outpatient repertoire (and therefore probably given orally) rather than towards drugs (probably given parenterally) that are intended for the management of a decompensation crisis. Repurposing of existing agents, including drugs with no current cardiology indication, guided by new in-depth knowledge of pathophysiology is another possible line of development [76]. An ultimate goal for such a pathway would be to develop patient monitoring to such a degree of immediacy and accuracy ("ecological momentary assessment [49]") that decompensations are wholly avoided by prompt, appropriate clinical responses. Such a programme, if successfully implemented, might render the concept of "acute-phase intervention" substantially redundant by eliminating episodes of decompensation. A review of notable ongoing research in this area has recently appeared in this Journal [77].

As regards drug discovery and translational science in the field of acute cardiac care, the translational committee of the ESC-HFA issued some scientific bases [78] designed to pave the way towards the development of new agents but the preclinical field remains scarcely populated, with just some notable exceptions such as the calcium sensitizer/PDE inhibitor ORM-3819 [79,80].

11. Implications for Drug Development

Commercial and societal responses to this new world of ultra-detailed patient characterization and real-time monitoring must be considered. In an era of hyper-detailed patient profiling it may transpire that fitting the right drug to the right patient translates in practice to each new drug being appropriate for a small, even tiny, number of patients. "Heart failure" might be transformed into a myriad of orphan drug indications. The implications on the 'evidence based medicine' predilection for large trials is evident. The implications for commercial profitability and/or drug acquisition costs is even more prominent.

Some pertinent and sharply framed observations that have recently emerged on the possibility of a not-for-profit model of antibiotic development might conceivably also come to apply to drug design in heart failure [81]. We take no position on whether such a shift would be inherently a good or bad thing but certainly it would mark a profound departure from the current model of drug discovery and development. (See Dungen et al. [82] for another perspective on this issue.)

These financial pressures will not be confined to cardiology – medicine as a whole faces similar pressures and opportunities. To that extent we anticipate, therefore, that new arrangements for the funding of medical treatments will address these tensions—but we are not equipped to speculate about the form these new arrangements may take or any unintended consequences they may create.

12. Conclusions

Hospitalization for heart failure, whether as a presentation of AHF or a decompensation in the context of AdHF, results in a down-shift in the trajectory of the syndrome that is associated with worsening outcomes and patient quality of life and increased costs of care. Medical progress to address these challenges has substantially stalled in the past 20 years but advances in data technology and analytics, along with developments in clinical trials design now offer opportunities to re-envision heart failure as a complex pathophysiological continuum in ways that may help to bring a new generation of therapies into clinical use. Meanwhile it would be advisable for the clinicians to evaluate if the nearly total absence of evidence of benefit with some of the traditional i.v. drugs used in AHF and AdHF (such as the catecholamines or the phosphodiesterase inhibitors) warrants their elimination from routine use in favour of treatments where such evidence has been accrued (e.g., for levosimendan).

Author Contributions: P.P. sketched the working hypotheses of the review. P.P. and Z.P. guided, monitored and corrected the AI-driven search. All authors contributed to the discussion and approved the final version of the manuscript.

Acknowledgments: We thank Eemil Väisänen, Reaktor Group Oy, Helsinki, Finland, for invaluable help with setting up the AI-driven search and Shrestha Roy and Johanna Kuusisto, Orion Pharma Oyj, Espoo, Finland, for the graphic solutions. We acknowledge Hughes associates, Oxford, UK, for editorial assistance in the preparation of the manuscript.

Conflicts of Interest: The authors declare no conflict of interest. P.P. is full time employee of Orion Pharma, where levosimendan, one of the NCEs described in the text, was discovered and developed. In the latest 5 years, the other authors have received grants and speaker honoraria by Orion Pharma for investigator-initiated studies and educational lectures, respectively.

References

1. Machaj, F.; Dembowska, E.; Rosik, J.; Szostak, B.; Mazurek-Mochol, M.; Pawlik, A. New therapies for the treatment of heart failure: A summary of recent accomplishments. *Clin. Risk Manag.* **2019**, *15*, 147–155. [CrossRef] [PubMed]
2. Hamo, C.E.; Butler, J.; Gheorghiade, M.; Chioncel, O. The bumpy road to drug development for acute heart failure. *Eur. Heart J. Suppl.* **2016**, *18*, G19–G32. [CrossRef]
3. Tamargo, J.; Caballero, R.; Delpón, E. New drugs in preclinical and early stage clinical development in the treatment of heart failure. *Expert Opin. Investig. Drugs* **2019**, *28*, 51–71. [CrossRef] [PubMed]
4. Rame, J.E. Introduction to topical collection on updates in advanced heart failure. *Curr. Heart Fail. Rep.* **2019**. [CrossRef]
5. Pollesello, P. Drug discovery and development for acute heart failure drugs: Are expectations too high? *Int. J. Cardiol.* **2014**, *172*, 11–13. [CrossRef]
6. Farmakis, D.; Simitsis, P.; Bistola, V.; Triposkiadis, F.; Ikonomidis, I.; Katsanos, S.; Bakosis, G.; Hatziagelaki, E.; Lekakis, J.; Mebazaa, A.; et al. Acute heart failure with mid-range left ventricular ejection fraction: Clinical profile, in-hospital management, and short-term outcome. *Clin. Res. Cardiol.* **2017**, *106*, 359–368. [CrossRef]
7. Packer, M.; Colucci, W.; Fisher, L.; Massie, B.M.; Teerlink, J.R.; Young, J.; Padley, R.J.; Thakkar, R.; Delgado-Herrera, L.; Salon, J.; et al. Effect of levosimendan on the short-term clinical course of patients with acutely decompensated heart failure. *JACC Heart Fail.* **2013**, *1*, 103–111. [CrossRef]
8. Metra, M.; Teerlink, J.R.; Felker, G.M.; Greenberg, B.H.; Filippatos, G.; Ponikowski, P.; Teichman, S.L.; Unemori, E.; Voors, A.A.; Weatherley, B.D.; et al. Dyspnoea and worsening heart failure in patients with acute heart failure: results from the Pre-RELAX-AHF study. *Eur. J. Heart Fail.* **2010**, *12*, 1130–1139. [CrossRef]

9. Haikala, H.; Pollesello, P. Calcium sensitivity enhancers. *IDrugs* **2000**, *3*, 1199–1205.
10. Malik, F.I.; Hartman, J.J.; Elias, K.A.; Morgan, B.P.; Rodriguez, H.; Brejc, K.; Anderson, R.L.; Sueoka, S.H.; Lee, K.H.; Finer, J.T.; et al. Cardiac myosin activation: A potential therapeutic approach for systolic heart failure. *Science* **2011**, *331*, 1439–1443. [CrossRef]
11. Teerlink, J.R.; Felker, G.M.; McMurray, J.J.V.; Ponikowski, P.; Metra, M.; Filippatos, G.S.; Ezekowitz, J.A.; Dickstein, K.; Cleland, J.G.F.; Kim, J.B.; et al. Acute treatment with omecamtiv mecarbil to increase contractility in acute heart failure. *J. Am. Coll. Cardiol.* **2016**, *67*, 1444–1455. [CrossRef] [PubMed]
12. Cleland, J.G.; Teerlink, J.R.; Senior, R.; Nifontov, E.M.; McMurray, J.J.; Lang, C.C.; Tsyrlin, V.A.; Greenberg, B.H.; Mayet, J.; Francis, D.P.; et al. The effects of the cardiac myosin activator, omecamtiv mecarbil, on cardiac function in systolic heart failure: A double-blind, placebo-controlled, crossover, dose-ranging phase 2 trial. *Lancet* **2011**, *378*, 676–683. [CrossRef]
13. Gouda, P.; Ezekowitz, J.A. Update on the diagnosis and management of acute heart failure. *Curr. Opin. Cardiol.* **2019**, *34*, 202–206. [CrossRef] [PubMed]
14. Teerlink, J.R.; Cotter, G.; Davison, B.A.; Felker, G.M.; Filippatos, G.; Greenberg, B.H.; Ponikowski, P.; Unemori, E.; Voors, A.A.; Adams, K.F.; et al. Serelaxin, recombinant human relaxin-2, for treatment of acute heart failure (RELAX-AHF): A randomised, placebo-controlled trial. *Lancet* **2013**, *381*, 29–39. [CrossRef]
15. Metra, M.; Teerlink, J.R.; Cotter, G.; Davison, B.A.; Felker, G.M.; Filippatos, G.; Greenberg, B.H.; Pang, P.S.; Ponikowski, P.; Voors, A.A.; et al. Effects of serelaxin in patients with acute heart failure. *N. Engl. J. Med.* **2019**, *381*, 716–726. [CrossRef]
16. Wang, T.S.; Hellkamp, A.S.; Patel, C.B.; Ezekowitz, J.A.; Fonarow, G.C.; Hernandez, A.F. Representativeness of RELAX-AHF clinical trial population in acute heart failure. *Circ. Cardiovasc. Qual. Outcomes* **2014**, *7*, 259–268. [CrossRef]
17. Maggioni, A.P.; López-Sendón, J.; Nielsen, O.W.; Hallén, J.; Aalamian-Mattheis, M.; Wang, Y.; Ertl, G. Efficacy and safety of serelaxin when added to standard of care in patients with acute heart failure: Results from a PROBE study, RELAX-AHF-EU. *Eur. J. Heart Fail.* **2019**, *21*, 322–333. [CrossRef]
18. Packer, M.; O'Connor, C.; McMurray, J.J.V.; Wittes, J.; Abraham, W.T.; Anker, S.D.; Dickstein, K.; Filippatos, G.; Holcomb, R.; Krum, H.; et al. Effect of ularitide on cardiovascular mortality in acute heart failure. *N. Engl. J. Med.* **2017**, *376*, 1956–1964. [CrossRef]
19. Khan, H.; Metra, M.; Blair, J.E.A.; Vogel, M.; Harinstein, M.E.; Filippatos, G.S.; Sabbah, H.N.; Porchet, H.; Valentini, G.; Gheorghiade, M. Istaroxime, a first in class new chemical entity exhibiting SERCA-2 activation and Na–K-ATPase inhibition: A new promising treatment for acute heart failure syndromes? *Heart Fail. Rev.* **2009**, *14*, 277–287. [CrossRef]
20. Gheorghiade, M.; Blair, J.E.A.; Filippatos, G.S.; Macarie, C.; Ruzyllo, W.; Korewicki, J.; Bubenek-Turconi, S.I.; Ceracchi, M.; Bianchetti, M.; Carminati, P.; et al. Hemodynamic, echocardiographic, and neurohormonal effects of istaroxime, a novel intravenous inotropic and lusitropic agent. *J. Am. Coll. Cardiol.* **2008**, *51*, 2276–2285. [CrossRef]
21. NCT00616161, U.S. National Library of Medicine. Available online: https://clinicaltrials.gov/ct2/show/NCT00616161 (accessed on 6 September 2019).
22. Greenberg, B.; Butler, J.; Felker, G.M.; Ponikowski, P.; Voors, A.A.; Desai, A.S.; Barnard, D.; Bouchard, A.; Jaski, B.; Lyon, A.R.; et al. Calcium upregulation by percutaneous administration of gene therapy in patients with cardiac disease (CUPID 2): A randomised, multinational, double-blind, placebo-controlled, phase 2b trial. *Lancet* **2016**, *387*, 1178–1186. [CrossRef]
23. U.S. National Library of Medicine. Available online: https://clinicaltrials.gov (accessed on 1 September 2019).
24. Papp, Z.; Édes, I.; Fruhwald, S.; De Hert, SG.; Salmenperä, M.; Leppikangas, H.; Mebazaa, A.; Landoni, G.; Grossini, E.; Caimmi, P.; et al. Levosimendan: Molecular mechanisms and clinical implications: Consensus of experts on the mechanisms of action of levosimendan. *Int. J. Cardiol.* **2012**, *159*, 82–87. [CrossRef] [PubMed]
25. Farmakis, D.; Alvarez, J.; Gal, T.B.; Brito, D.; Fedele, F.; Fonseca, C.; Gordon, A.C.; Gotsman, I.; Grossini, E.; Guarracino, F.; et al. Levosimendan beyond inotropy and acute heart failure: Evidence of pleiotropic effects on the heart and other organs: An expert panel position paper. *Int. J. Cardiol.* **2016**, *222*, 303–312. [CrossRef] [PubMed]
26. Mebazaa, A.; Parissis, J.; Porcher, R.; Gayat, E.; Nikolaou, M.; Boas, F.V.; Delgado, J.F.; Follath, F. Short-term survival by treatment among patients hospitalized with acute heart failure: The global

ALARM-HF registry using propensity scoring methods. *Intensive Care Med.* **2011**, *37*, 290–301. [CrossRef] [PubMed]
27. Pollesello, P.; Parissis, J.; Kivikko, M.; Harjola, V.-P. Levosimendan meta-analyses: Is there a pattern in the effect on mortality? *Int. J. Cardiol.* **2016**, *209*, 77–83. [CrossRef] [PubMed]
28. Hasenfuss, G.; Pieske, B.; Castell, M.; Kretschmann, B.; Maier, L.S.; Just, H. Influence of the novel inotropic agent levosimendan on isometric tension and calcium cycling in failing human myocardium. *Circulation* **1998**, *98*, 2141–2147. [CrossRef] [PubMed]
29. Nagy, L.; Pollesello, P.; Papp, Z. Inotropes and inodilators for acute heart failure: Sarcomere active drugs in focus. *J. Cardiovasc. Pharmacol.* **2014**, *64*, 199–208. [CrossRef]
30. Pollesello, P.; Papp, Z.; Papp, J.G. Calcium sensitizers: What have we learned over the last 25 years? *Int. J. Cardiol.* **2016**, *203*, 543–548. [CrossRef]
31. Mebazaa, A.; Nieminen, M.S.; Filippatos, G.S.; Cleland, J.G.; Salon, J.E.; Thakkar, R.; Padley, R.J.; Huang, B.; Cohen-Solal, A. Levosimendan vs. dobutamine: Outcomes for acute heart failure patients on β-blockers in SURVIVE. *Eur. J. Heart Fail.* **2009**, *11*, 304–311. [CrossRef]
32. Bergh, C.-H.; Andersson, B.; Dahlström, U.; Forfang, K.; Kivikko, M.; Sarapohja, T.; Ullman, B.; Wikström, G. Intravenous levosimendan vs. dobutamine in acute decompensated heart failure patients on beta-blockers. *Eur. J. Heart Fail.* **2010**, *12*, 404–410. [CrossRef]
33. Ponikowski, P.; Voors, A.A.; Anker, S.D.; Bueno, H.; Cleland, J.G.F.; Coats, A.J.S.; Falk, V.; González-Juanatey, J.R.; Harjola, V.-P.; Jankowska, E.A.; et al. 2016 ESC Guidelines for the diagnosis and treatment of acute and chronic heart failure: The Task Force for the diagnosis and treatment of acute and chronic heart failure of the European Society of Cardiology (ESC) Developed with the special contribution of the Heart Failure Association (HFA) of the ESC. *Eur. Heart J.* **2016**, *37*, 2129–2200. [PubMed]
34. Altenberger, J.; Parissis, J.T.; Ulmer, H.; Poelzl, G.; LevoRep Investigators. Rationale and design of the multicentre randomized trial investigating the efficacy and safety of pulsed infusions of levosimendan in outpatients with advanced heart failure (LevoRep study). *Eur. J. Heart Fail.* **2010**, *12*, 186–192. [CrossRef] [PubMed]
35. Comín-Colet, J.; Manito, N.; Segovia-Cubero, J.; Delgado, J.; García Pinilla, J.M.; Almenar, L.; Crespo-Leiro, M.G.; Sionis, A.; Blasco, T.; Pascual-Figal, D.; et al. Efficacy and safety of intermittent intravenous outpatient administration of levosimendan in patients with advanced heart failure: The LION-HEART multicentre randomised trial: Levosimendan in advanced HF: The LION-HEART trial. *Eur. J. Heart Fail.* **2018**, *20*, 1128–1136. [CrossRef] [PubMed]
36. García-González, M.J.; LAICA Study Investigators. Efficacy and security of intermittent repeated levosimendan administration in patients with advanced heart failure: A randomized, double-blind, placebo controlled multicenter trial: LAICA study. In Proceedings of the European Society of Cardiology—Heart Failure Association Congress, Florence, Italy, 21 May 2016.
37. Silvetti, S.; Nieminen, M.S. Repeated or intermittent levosimendan treatment in advanced heart failure: An updated meta-analysis. *Int. J. Cardiol.* **2016**, *202*, 138–143. [CrossRef]
38. Silvetti, S.; Belletti, A.; Fontana, A.; Pollesello, P. Rehospitalization after intermittent levosimendan treatment in advanced heart failure patients: A meta-analysis of randomized trials: Repeated levosimendan in AdHF and rehospitalization. *ESC Heart Fail.* **2017**, *4*, 595–604. [CrossRef]
39. Oliva, F.; Perna, E.; Marini, M.; Nassiacos, D.; Cirò, A.; Malfatto, G.; Morandi, F.; Caico, I.; Perna, G.; Meloni, S.; et al. Scheduled intermittent inotropes for ambulatory advanced heart failure. The RELEVANT-HF multicentre collaboration. *Int. J. Cardiol.* **2018**, *272*, 255–259. [CrossRef]
40. Müller, C.E. GALACTIC—Goal-Directed AfterLoad Reduction in Acute Congestive Cardiac Decompensation. ESC Congress 2019, Paris, France. Hot Line Session 3. Available online: https://esc365.escardio.org/Congress/ESC-CONGRESS-2019/Hot-Line-Session-3/202174-galactic-goal-directed-afterload-reduction-in-acute-congestive-cardiac-decompensation-a-randomized-controlled-trial#video (accessed on 3 October 2019).
41. McCullough, P.A. How trialists and pharmaceutical sponsors have failed us by thinking that acute heart failure Is a 48-hour illness. *Am. J. Cardiol.* **2017**, *120*, 505–508. [CrossRef]
42. Triposkiadis, F.; Butler, J.; Abboud, F.M.; Armstrong, P.W.; Adamopoulos, S.; Atherton, J.J.; Backs, J.; Bauersachs, J.; Burkhoff, D.; Bonow, R.O.; et al. The continuous heart failure spectrum: Moving beyond an ejection fraction classification. *Eur. Heart. J.* **2019**, *40*, 2155–2163. [CrossRef]

43. Severino, P.; Mariani, M.V.; Fedele, F. Futility in cardiology: The need for a change in perspectives. *Eur. J. Heart Fail.* **2019**. [CrossRef]
44. Fedele, F.; Mancone, M.; Adamo, F.; Severino, P. Heart failure with preserved, mid-range, and reduced ejection fraction: The misleading definition of the new guidelines. *Cardiol. Rev.* **2017**, *25*, 4–5. [CrossRef]
45. Fedele, F.; Severino, P.; Calcagno, S.; Mancone, M. Heart failure: TNM-like classification. *J. Am. Coll. Cardiol.* **2014**, *63*, 1959–1960. [CrossRef] [PubMed]
46. De Backer, D.; Bakker, J.; Cecconi, M.; Hajjar, L.; Liu, D.W.; Lobo, S.; Monnet, X.; Morelli, A.; Myatra, S.N.; Perel, A.; et al. Alternatives to the Swan–Ganz catheter. *Intensive Care Med.* **2018**, *44*, 730–741. [CrossRef] [PubMed]
47. Shameer, K.; Johnson, K.W.; Glicksberg, B.S.; Dudley, J.T.; Sengupta, P.P. Machine learning in cardiovascular medicine: Are we there yet? *Heart* **2018**, *104*, 1156–1164. [CrossRef] [PubMed]
48. Johnson, K.W.; Torres Soto, J.; Glicksberg, B.S.; Shameer, K.; Miotto, R.; Ali, M.; Ashley, E.; Dudley, J.T. Artificial Intelligence in Cardiology. *J. Am. Coll. Cardiol.* **2018**, *71*, 2668–2679. [CrossRef] [PubMed]
49. Sim, I. Mobile Devices and Health. *N. Engl. J. Med.* **2019**, *381*, 956–968. [CrossRef]
50. Eurlings, C.G.M.J.; Boyne, J.J.; de Boer, R.A.; Brunner-La Rocca, H.P. Telemedicine in heart failure—more than nice to have? *Neth. Heart J.* **2019**, *27*, 5–15. [CrossRef]
51. Bondar, G.; Togashi, R.; Cadeiras, M.; Schaenman, J.; Cheng, R.K.; Masukawa, L.; Hai, J.; Bao, T.-M.; Chu, D.; Chang, E.; et al. Association between preoperative peripheral blood mononuclear cell gene expression profiles, early postoperative organ function recovery potential and long-term survival in advanced heart failure patients undergoing mechanical circulatory support. *PLoS ONE* **2017**, *12*, e0189420. [CrossRef]
52. Deng, M.C. A peripheral blood transcriptome biomarker test to diagnose functional recovery potential in advanced heart failure. *Biomark. Med.* **2018**, *12*, 619–635. [CrossRef]
53. Krittanawong, C.; Namath, A.; Lanfear, D.E.; Tang, W.H.W. Practical pharmacogenomic approaches to heart failure therapeutics. *Curr. Treat. Options Cardiovasc. Med.* **2016**, *18*, 60. [CrossRef]
54. Gensini, G.F.; Alderighi, C.; Rasoini, R.; Mazzanti, M.; Casolo, G. Value of telemonitoring and telemedicine in heart failure management. *Card. Fail. Rev.* **2017**, *3*, 116–121. [CrossRef]
55. Hemingway, H.; Asselbergs, F.W.; Danesh, J.; Dobson, R.; Maniadakis, N.; Maggioni, A.; van Thiel, G.J.M.; Cronin, M.; Brobert, G.; Vardas, P.; et al. Big data from electronic health records for early and late translational cardiovascular research: Challenges and potential. *Eur. Heart J.* **2018**, *39*, 1481–1495. [CrossRef] [PubMed]
56. Narula, S.; Shameer, K.; Salem Omar, A.M.; Dudley, J.T.; Sengupta, P.P. Machine-learning algorithms to automate morphological and functional assessments in 2D echocardiography. *J. Am. Coll. Cardiol.* **2016**, *68*, 2287–2295. [CrossRef] [PubMed]
57. Maragatham, G.; Devi, S. LSTM model for prediction of heart failure in big data. *J. Med. Syst.* **2019**, *43*, 111. [CrossRef] [PubMed]
58. Safety and Efficacy of Tafamidis in Patients with Transthyretin Cardimyopathy (ATTR-ACT). Available online: https://clinicaltrials.gov/ct2/show/results/NCT01994889?term=NCT01994889.&rank=1 (accessed on 11 September 2019).
59. Pölzl, G.; Allipour Birgani, S.; Comín-Colet, J.; Delgado, J.F.; Fedele, F.; García-Gonzáles, M.J.; Gustafsson, F.; Masip, J.; Papp, Z.; Störk, S.; et al. Repetitive levosimendan infusions for patients with advanced Chronic heart failure in the vulnerable post-discharge period: Rationale and design of the LeoDOR Trial. *Esc. Heart Fail.* **2019**, *6*, 174–181. [CrossRef] [PubMed]
60. Pölzl, G.; Altenberger, J.; Baholli, L.; Beltrán, P.; Borbély, A.; Comin-Colet, J.; Delgado, J.F.; Fedele, F.; Fontana, A.; Fruhwald, F.; et al. Repetitive use of levosimendan in advanced heart failure: Need for stronger evidence in a field in dire need of a useful therapy. *Int. J. Cardiol.* **2017**, *243*, 389–395. [CrossRef] [PubMed]
61. Collins, S.P.; Lindsell, C.J.; Pang, P.S.; Storrow, A.B.; Peacock, W.F.; Levy, P.; Rahbar, M.H.; Del Junco, D.; Gheorghiade, M.; Berry, D.A. Bayesian adaptive trial design in acute heart failure syndromes: Moving beyond the mega trial. *Am. Heart J.* **2012**, *164*, 138–145. [CrossRef] [PubMed]
62. Lin, J.; Bunn, V. Comparison of multi-arm multi-stage design and adaptive randomization in platform clinical trials. *Contemp. Clin. Trials* **2017**, *54*, 48–59. [CrossRef]
63. Wason, J.M.S.; Trippa, L. A comparison of Bayesian adaptive randomization and multi-stage designs for multi-arm clinical trials. *Stat. Med.* **2014**, *33*, 2206–2221. [CrossRef]
64. Saville, B.R.; Berry, S.M. Efficiencies of platform clinical trials: A vision of the future. *Clin. Trials* **2016**, *13*, 358–366. [CrossRef]

65. Morrell, L.; Hordern, J.; Brown, L.; Sydes, M.R.; Amos, C.L.; Kaplan, R.S.; Parmar, M.K.B.; Maughan, T.S. Mind the gap? The platform trial as a working environment. *Trials* **2019**, *20*, 297. [CrossRef]
66. Hague, D.; Townsend, S.; Masters, L.; Rauchenberger, M.; Van Looy, N.; Diaz-Montana, C.; Gannon, M.; James, N.; Maughan, T.; Parmar, M.K.B.; et al. Changing platforms without stopping the train: Experiences of data management and data management systems when adapting platform protocols by adding and closing comparisons. *Trials* **2019**, *20*, 294. [CrossRef] [PubMed]
67. Schiavone, F.; Bathia, R.; Letchemanan, K.; Masters, L.; Amos, C.; Bara, A.; Brown, L.; Gilson, C.; Pugh, C.; Atako, N.; et al. This is a platform alteration: A trial management perspective on the operational aspects of adaptive and platform and umbrella protocols. *Trials* **2019**, *20*, 264. [CrossRef] [PubMed]
68. Packer, M. Why are physicians so confused about acute heart failure? *N. Engl. J. Med.* **2019**, *381*, 776–777. [CrossRef] [PubMed]
69. Blecker, S.; Sontag, D.; Horwitz, L.I.; Kuperman, G.; Park, H.; Reyentovich, A.; Katz, S.D. Early identification of patients with acute decompensated heart failure. *J. Card. Fail.* **2018**, *24*, 357–362. [CrossRef]
70. Blecker, S.; Katz, S.D.; Horwitz, L.I.; Kuperman, G.; Park, H.; Gold, A.; Sontag, D. Comparison of approaches for heart failure case identification from electronic health record data. *JAMA Cardiol.* **2016**, *1*, 1014. [CrossRef]
71. Golas, S.B.; Shibahara, T.; Agboola, S.; Otaki, H.; Sato, J.; Nakae, T.; Hisamitsu, T.; Kojima, G.; Felsted, J.; Kakarmath, S.; et al. A machine learning model to predict the risk of 30-day readmissions in patients with heart failure: A retrospective analysis of electronic medical records data. *BMC Med. Inf. Decis. Mak.* **2018**, *18*, 44. [CrossRef]
72. Karanasiou, G.S.; Tripoliti, E.E.; Papadopoulos, T.G.; Kalatzis, F.G.; Goletsis, Y.; Naka, K.K.; Bechlioulis, A.; Errachid, A.; Fotiadis, D.I. Predicting adherence of patients with HF through machine learning techniques. *Healthc. Technol. Lett.* **2016**, *3*, 165–170. [CrossRef]
73. Kreusser, M.M.; Tschierschke, R.; Beckendorf, J.; Baxmann, T.; Frankenstein, L.; Dösch, A.O.; Schultz, J.-H.; Giannitsis, E.; Pleger, S.T.; Ruhparwar, A.; et al. The need for dedicated advanced heart failure units to optimize heart failure care: Impact of optimized advanced heart failure unit care on heart transplant outcome in high-risk patients: The need for dedicated AHFUs to optimize HF care. *ESC Heart Fail.* **2018**, *5*, 1108–1117. [CrossRef]
74. Koehler, F.; Koehler, K.; Deckwart, O.; Prescher, S.; Wegscheider, K.; Kirwan, B.-A.; Winkler, S.; Vettorazzi, E.; Bruch, L.; Oeff, M.; et al. Efficacy of telemedical interventional management in patients with heart failure (TIM-HF2): A randomised, controlled, parallel-group, unmasked trial. *Lancet* **2018**, *392*, 1047–1057. [CrossRef]
75. Möckel, M.; Koehler, K.; Anker, S.D.; Vollert, J.; Moeller, V.; Koehler, M.; Gehrig, S.; Wiemer, J.C.; Haehling, S.; Koehler, F. Biomarker guidance allows a more personalized allocation of patients for remote patient management in heart failure: Results from the TIM-HF2 trial. *Eur. J. Heart Fail.* **2019**. [CrossRef]
76. Matsumura, T.; Matsui, M.; Iwata, Y.; Asakura, M.; Saito, T.; Fujimura, H.; Sakoda, S. A Pilot Study of Tranilast for Cardiomyopathy of Muscular Dystrophy. *Intern. Med.* **2018**, *57*, 311–318. [CrossRef] [PubMed]
77. Andrès, E.; Talha, S.; Zulfiqar, A.-A.; Hajjam, M.; Ervé, S.; Hajjam, J.; Gény, B.; Hajjam El Hassani, A. Current research and new perspectives of telemedicine in chronic heart failure: Narrative review and points of interest for the clinician. *J. Clin. Med.* **2018**, *7*, 544. [CrossRef] [PubMed]
78. Maack, C.; Eschenhagen, T.; Hamdani, N.; Heinzel, F.R.; Lyon, A.R.; Manstein, D.J.; Metzger, J.; Papp, Z.; Tocchetti, C.G.; Yilmaz, M.B.; et al. Treatments targeting inotropy. *Eur. Heart J.* **2018**. [CrossRef] [PubMed]
79. Nagy, L.; Pollesello, P.; Haikala, H.; Végh, Á.; Sorsa, T.; Levijoki, J.; Szilágyi, S.; Édes, I.; Tóth, A.; Papp, Z.; et al. ORM-3819 promotes cardiac contractility through Ca2+ sensitization in combination with selective PDE III inhibition, a novel approach to inotropy. *Eur. J. Pharm.* **2016**, *775*, 120–129. [CrossRef] [PubMed]
80. Márton, Z.; Patariza, J.; Pollesello, P.; Varró, A.; Papp, J.G. The Novel inodilator ORM-3819 relaxes isolated porcine coronary arteries: Role of voltage-gated potassium channel activation. *J. Cardiovasc. Pharm.* **2019**, *74*, 218–224. [CrossRef] [PubMed]

81. Nielsen, T.B.; Brass, E.P.; Gilbert, D.N.; Bartlett, J.G.; Spellberg, B. Sustainable discovery and development of antibiotics—Is a nonprofit approach the future? *N. Engl. J. Med.* **2019**, *381*, 503–505. [CrossRef]
82. Dungen, H.-D.; Petroni, R.; Correale, M.; Coiro, S.; Monitillo, F.; Triggiani, M.; Leone, M.; Antohi, E.-L.; Ishihara, S.; Sarwar, C.M.S.; et al. A new educational program in heart failure drug development: The Brescia international master program. *J. Cardiovasc. Med.* **2018**, *19*, 411–421. [CrossRef]

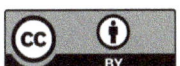 © 2019 by the authors. Licensee MDPI, Basel, Switzerland. This article is an open access article distributed under the terms and conditions of the Creative Commons Attribution (CC BY) license (http://creativecommons.org/licenses/by/4.0/).

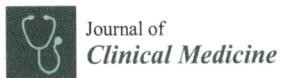

Review

The Vasoactive Mas Receptor in Essential Hypertension

Amalie L. Povlsen [1], Daniela Grimm [1,2,*], Markus Wehland [2], Manfred Infanger [2] and Marcus Krüger [2]

1. Department of Biomedicine, Aarhus University, Høegh-Guldbergsgade 10, 8000 Aarhus C, Denmark; amaliepovlsen@hotmail.com
2. Clinic for Plastic, Aesthetic and Hand Surgery, Otto von Guericke University, Leipziger Str. 44, 39120 Magdeburg, Germany; markus.wehland@med.ovgu.de (M.W.); manfred.infanger@med.ovgu.de (M.I.); marcus.krueger@med.ovgu.de (M.K.)
* Correspondence: dgg@biomed.au.dk; Tel.: +45-871-67693

Received: 19 December 2019; Accepted: 14 January 2020; Published: 18 January 2020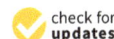

Abstract: The renin–angiotensin–aldosterone system (RAAS) has been studied extensively, and with the inclusion of novel components, it has become evident that the system is much more complex than originally anticipated. According to current knowledge, there are two main axes of the RAAS, which counteract each other in terms of vascular control: The classical vasoconstrictive axis, renin/angiotensin-converting enzyme/angiotensin II/angiotensin II receptor type 1 (AT_1R), and the opposing vasorelaxant axis, angiotensin-converting enzyme 2/angiotensin-(1-7)/Mas receptor (MasR). An abnormal activity within the system constitutes a hallmark in hypertension, which is a global health problem that predisposes cardiovascular and renal morbidities. In particular, essential hypertension predominates in the hypertensive population of more than 1.3 billion humans worldwide, and yet, the pathophysiology behind this multifactorial condition needs clarification. While commonly applied pharmacological strategies target the classical axis of the RAAS, discovery of the vasoprotective effects of the opposing, vasorelaxant axis has presented encouraging experimental evidence for a new potential direction in RAAS-targeted therapy based on the G protein-coupled MasR. In addition, the endogenous MasR agonist angiotensin-(1-7), peptide analogues, and related molecules have become the subject of recent studies within this field. Nevertheless, the clinical potential of MasR remains unclear due to indications of physiological-biased activities of the RAAS and interacting signaling pathways.

Keywords: hypertension; renin-angiotensin-aldosterone system; MasR; angiotensin-(1-7)

1. Introduction

Hypertension (HT) affects more than 1.3 billion individuals worldwide and is regarded a major risk factor for mortality and morbidity [1,2]. Extensive research confirms that HT is an independent risk factor for severe cardiovascular (CV) and renal events including myocardial infarction, heart failure, ischemic stroke, peripheral artery disease, and end-stage renal disease [3,4], and represents a major public health problem.

According to the guidelines of the European Society of Cardiology (ESC) and the European Society of Hypertension (ESH), HT is defined as an office systolic blood pressure (BP) ≥ 140 mmHg and/or diastolic BP of ≥ 90 mmHg [3]. This definition was generally accepted until 2017, where the guidelines of the American College of Cardiology (ACC) and the American Heart Association (AHA) lowered the threshold for diagnosis of HT to a systolic BP of ≥ 130 mmHg and/or a diastolic BP of ≥ 80 mmHg [4].

HT is considered a multifactorial disease that involves environmental and genetic factors, as well as lifestyle and risk-conferring behaviors [5,6]. It can be categorized as essential or secondary HT, of which essential HT accounts for about 95% of the hypertensive population, and refers to HT with no identifiable cause [3,7], while secondary HT accounts for 5–15% [3] and represents a complication to an identified cause, e.g., renovascular disease, endocrine disorders or drug association [3]. In comparison, proper and early intervention in secondary HT may help control BP in addition to treating the underlying cause [3], while the polygenic character of essential HT complicates treatment [8]. In addition, experimental research has suggested a link between HT and structural alterations in genes encoding separate components of the renin-angiotensin-aldosterone system (RAAS) [9,10], indicating that changes in the activity of RAAS-regulated genes may increase the risk of developing HT [8]. These findings suggest that HT is associated with a dysfunctional RAAS.

The RAAS has been studied extensively, and is known to play a pivotal role in BP control [11]. Among current treatment strategies, RAAS targeting is common and includes renin inhibitors, angiotensin-converting enzyme (ACE) inhibitors, angiotensin II type 1 receptor (AT_1R) antagonists (also known as angiotensin II receptor blockers, ARBs), mineralocorticoid receptor-antagonists and aldosterone synthase inhibitors, which all serve to block the RAAS at different loci [12,13]. In addition, diuretics, β-adrenoceptor antagonists and calcium channel blockers are drug classes that aid in lowering both BP and risk of CV events [3]. According to available data, the activity of the RAAS depends on a balance between the classical vasoconstrictive axis and the opposing vasorelaxant axis [14]. The latter is said to counteract the adverse effects mediated by AT_1R, which is linked to the pathophysiological actions of angiotensin II (Ang II) and to cardiovascular disease (CVD) [14]. The beneficial effects of the G-protein coupled Mas receptor (MasR) was originally associated with binding of endogenous Ang-(1-7). Yet, the discovery of novel agonists, e.g., CGEN-856S and AVE 0991, has extended the therapeutic potential of the RAAS, and furthermore, encouraging research data has led to the investigation of the potential of MasR-based drugs [15].

By illuminating various actions and interactions of MasR, related to vasculature and BP regulation, this review aims to examine the role of MasR in HT and to evaluate its potential as a target in antihypertensive drugs.

2. The Renin-Angiotensin-Aldosterone System (RAAS)

2.1. The Classical RAAS

Renin is considered the rate-limiting component of the RAAS, in which it is released in response to stimuli related to lowered BP, e.g., a decreased renal perfusion pressure, an increased sympathetic tone or a decreased delivery of sodium chloride to the macula densa [9]. Renin cleaves hepatic angiotensinogen into angiotensin I (Ang I), which is then converted into the main effector molecule, Ang II, by the angiotensin-converting enzyme (ACE) [13]. Ang II acts through G-protein coupled AT_1R to promote water and sodium retention, vasoconstriction, pro-inflammation, and adrenal secretion of aldosterone [13], which further synergistically accelerates renal sodium and water retention by stimulating the mineralocorticoid receptors [11]. In addition, the activation of mineralocorticoid receptors in extra-renal tissues, e.g., the heart and vessels, has been reported to promote endothelial dysfunction and tissue remodeling due to formation of reactive oxygen species (ROS) [12,13].

Ang II also binds to angiotensin II type 2 receptor (AT_2R) of the proximal tubule, cortical collecting ducts and resistance arteries, which promotes hypotensive and natriuretic effects, thus opposing the actions of AT_1R [15,16]. However, data suggest that AT_1R predominates in a physiological setting, due to the fact that experimental activation of AT_2R often requires pretreatment with ARBs, to prevent Ang II from binding AT_1R instead [16]. Local actions of Ang II thus depend on the combined net effect of AT_1R and AT_2R [17], and it seems likely that an abnormally high activity in the AT_1R predisposes to HT.

2.2. Extension of the RAAS

In the past few decades, extensive research on the RAAS has expanded our general understanding of the system, making it clear that it is much more complex than originally anticipated [15] and comprises various biologically active metabolites (Figure 1).

An alternate substrate for Ang II generation is Ang-(1-12), which serves as an upstream precursor for Ang I and Ang II [18]. Cleavage of Ang II by aminopeptidase A (APA) generates Ang-(2-8) (Ang III), which binds AT_1R to promote a pressor response similar to that of Ang II, but with a prominent role in the brain [19]. Specific APA inhibitors such as RB150 have thus been developed and are still being tested in animals [20]. Further cleavage of Ang III produces Ang-(3-8) (Ang IV), which binds AT_4R to promote vasodilation in cerebral and renal vascular beds, facilitating renal blood flow and sodium excretion [21].

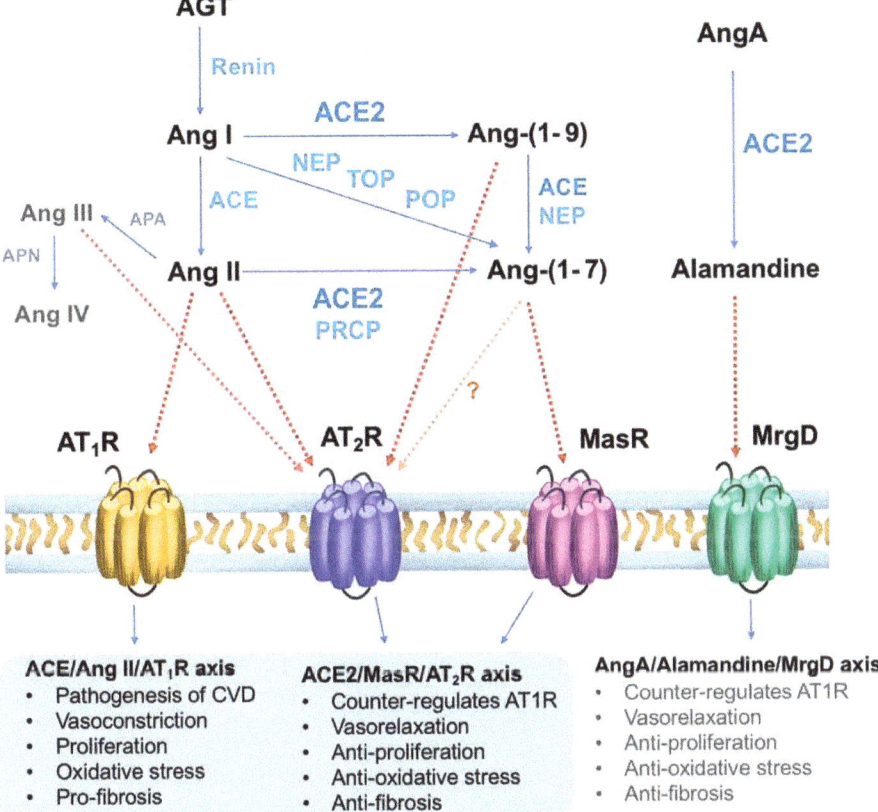

Figure 1. Schematic overview of the renin/ACE/Ang-II/AT_1R axis, ACE2/MasR/AT_2R axis and AngA/Alamandine-MrgD axis, modified from [22]. ACE, Angiotensin converting enzyme; AGT, angiotensinogen; Ang, angiotensin; APA, aminopeptidase A; APN, aminopeptidase N; AT_1R, angiotensin II type 1 receptor; AT_2R, angiotensin II type 2 receptor; MasR, Mas receptor; MrgD, Mas-related G-protein coupled receptor type D; NEP, neutral endopeptidase, POP, prolyloligopeptidase; PRCP, prolylcarboxypeptidase; TOP, thimet oligopeptidase.

Ang-(1-9) is another interesting metabolite due to its anti-hypertensive actions. It is generated from Ang I and induces AT_2R-mediated vasodilation, natriuresis, decreased CV remodeling and anti-proliferation [23]. In hypertensive models, Ang-(1-9) has been shown to ameliorate CV injury, while in clinical studies, it opposed CV remodeling in patients with HT and/or heart failure [24]. Evidence thus suggest a therapeutic potential of Ang-(1-9), but an in-depth evaluation is considered beyond the scope of this review.

Heptapeptide Ang-(1-7), which is a specific MasR agonist, plays a central role in the counterregulatory arm of the RAAS, ACE2/Ang-(1-7)/MasR. It can be generated by different enzymes, but with the most potent being ACE2 [25], which can produce Ang-(1-7) through hydrolysis of Ang II, or from Ang I with Ang-(1-9) as an intermediate step [15]. The former pathway is more favorable, due to ACE2's affinity to Ang II [17]. Ang-(1-7) only differs from Ang II in its lack of the C-terminal phenylalanine residue, and it was considered as a MasR agonist upon the discovery of a selective Ang-(1-7)-antagonist [26,27]. Ang-(1-7) exerts nitric oxide (NO)-dependent vasorelaxation via the MasR, which opposes the effects of AT_1R [26]. ACE2 and MasR are expressed in the same tissues, suggesting that Ang-(1-7) provides specific protection in these organs [25]. Yet, the relative role of different enzymes in the synthesis of Ang-(1-7) vary considerably, depending on cell type and tissue [28].

Furthermore, recent studies revealed interactions of Ang-(1-7) with other RAAS receptors, including AT_1R and AT_2R, suggesting that the actions of Ang-(1-7) rely on an interplay with the classical RAAS, and additionally depend on local expression levels of MasR, Ang-(1-7), Ang II, AT_1R and AT_2R [29].

Lastly, it should be mentioned that ACE2 converts angiotensin A into vasoactive alamandine, which is related to Ang-(1-7) and binds a Mas-related G-protein coupled type D receptor (MrgD) [30]. This constitutes an AngA/alamandine-MrgD pathway with similar properties to the ACE2/Ang-(1-7)/MasR axis [20]. The comparative difference is investigated in preclinical studies [31].

2.3. Blood Pressure Regulation by the RAAS

BP is a measure to describe the intravascular pressure generated by circulating blood, and it can be calculated from cardiac output (CO) and total peripheral resistance (TPR), in accordance with the law of Ohm [32]. Both CO and TPR, are affected by various mechanisms, including the RAAS, which is a vital regulator of homeostasis [25] and in particular of fluid volume, BP, electrolyte balance, and neuroendocrine functions [9].

According to the classical paradigm [15], sodium reabsorption is mediated by Ang II acting on renal sodium-hydrogen exchanger 3, while aldosterone acts on sodium-chloride cotransporter, ENaC, and renal outer medullary potassium channel [15]. Salt and water retention is triggered by hypovolemia, while potassium excretion is additionally stimulated by hyperkalemia [15]. As a consequence, BP is increased due to an expansion in the extracellular fluid volume. The RAAS-mediated pressor effect is further accelerated by an increase in sympathetic activity and a secretion of aldosterone and vasopressin [5,17]. With these mechanisms in consideration, the risk of developing essential HT is increased with a hyperactive RAAS. This theory is being supported by the successful treatment with RAAS blockers [9].

2.4. The Two Arms of the RAAS

The classical pathways leading to generation of angiotensin peptides have been described extensively, but the general understanding was challenged by the first description of Ang-(1-7) as an endogenous inhibitor of the RAAS [33]. This has led to a growing interest in characterizing counterregulatory components of the RAAS, while searching for novel targets in CVD therapy [12]. It is now believed that the RAAS consists of two distinct, opposing arms: ACE/Ang II/AT_1R and ACE2/Ang-(1-7)/MasR.

Overstimulation of the vasoconstrictive axis is associated with CVD, including HT and myocardial infarction with possible progression to heart failure [34]. The pathophysiology is associated with excessive vasoconstriction, fibrosis, endothelial dysfunction, tissue remodeling [34], and in particular with ROS formation by NADPH oxidase [35]. In addition, research has indicated that the detrimental effects are partially associated with a suppression of the counterregulatory arm of the RAAS, resulting in increased levels of Ang II and reduced levels of Ang-(1-7) [36]. Taken together, blocking the classical RAAS has served an effective the strategy in pharmacotherapy for decades.

On the other hand, the alternative vasorelaxant axis constitutes an intrinsically protective mechanism, associated with beneficial outcomes in CVD [25]. The actions of Ang-(1-7) were originally thought to be mediated exclusively through MasR. However, it has been demonstrated that Ang-(1-7) also binds to AT_2R and AT_1R, when present in higher levels [37,38]. In fact, it has been proposed that the AT_2R is responsible for the vasodepressor effects of Ang-(1-7) [38], while other studies suggest that Ang-(1-7) inhibits AT_1R in a non-competitive manner [31].

MasR is a biologically active peptide encoded by the *MAS1* gene, which was identified as a proto-oncogene, based on its ability to induce tumorigenicity in murine cells [26]. MasR is predominantly expressed in the brain and the testes, while moderate levels are found in the heart, kidney and vessels [39]. It has a similar structure to other G-protein coupled receptors (GPCRs) [40]. Human endothelium express MasR, through which Ang-(1-7) alters local redox balance and promotes vasodilation, oxidative stress reduction and antifibrosis [39]. Based on the observation that it triggered the release of vasopressin in a similar manner to Ang II, Ang-(1-7) was originally thought to be a selective MasR agonist [5,33]. The endothelial synthesis of Ang-(1-7) was first described by Santos et al. [41].

MasR was shown to constitutively couple to G_q-proteins and to promote ischemia-reperfusion in rats stimulated with synthetic peptide ligands [42]. Controversially, Ang-(1-7) does not induce G_q-related alternations, but rather acts through a non-G-protein mechanism to promote release of arachidonic acid, bradykinin and prostaglandins, while additionally activating endothelial nitric oxide synthase (eNOS) [42]. This was observed in spontaneously hypertensive rats (SHRs), in which the protective axis was blocked with an Ang-(1-7) antagonist, A-779, repealing the effects of Ang-(1-7) [35,43]. In a similar manner, this was observed in mice with ablation of the *MAS1* gene [39]. Yet, a study on human aortic endothelial cells suggested that Ang-(1-7) attenuates the classical RAAS through a mitogen-activated protein kinase cascade [35], while another proposed mechanism was that Ang-(1-7) inhibits Ang II-induced c-Src phosphorylation, which increases NO bioavailability and attenuates ROS formation [35]. Moreover, the ACE2/Ang-(1-7)/MasR axis could be a promising therapeutic option for diabetic patients since the activation of this axis through the use of cyclic Ang-(1-7) offered renoprotection in mice with type 2 diabetic nephropathy [44].

Taken together, these data indicate that distinct CV actions of Ang-(1-7) are mediated through MasR [15], but that this involves an interplay with other pathways of the RAAS. Furthermore, the effects of Ang-(1-7) seem to be affected by factors such as the presence of additional receptors and angiotensin peptides, local expression levels, and the general state of the tissue [17].

3. Novel MasR Agonists

In recent decades, the protective arm of the RAAS has been considered a promising approach in treatment of CVD, and different strategies are under investigation.

Based on the knowledge of ACE2, which is crucial in maintaining the balance between the opposing RAAS axes, a novel therapeutic strategy aims to increase endogenous levels of Ang-(1-7) by using ACE2 activators [45]. Alternatively, injection of endogenous alamandine has been shown to reduce BP and decrease post-ischemic reperfusion injury in SHRs [30], which is likely because of the morphological similarity between alamandine and Ang-(1-7). However, alamandine does not bind to MasR but to the MrgD receptor with similar properties [31]. Furthermore, alamandine has been compared with synthetic AVE 0991, which was the first orally active MasR agonist, in which organ protection was demonstrated as a dose-dependent vasorelaxation in aortic rings of SHRs [43]. This effect was absent in MasR deficient mice [46], and Faria-Silva et al. [47] further demonstrated how Ang-(1-7) and AVE 0991 both potentiate vasodilation in Wistar rats. The effects of AVE 0991 are multiple and quantitatively comparable to those of Ang-(1-7) [25]. In addition, blockage of AVE 0991 with Ang-(1-7) antagonists, A-779 and D-Pro⁷-Ang-(1-7), suggest that at least some of its actions are mediated through MasR [48]. So far, AVE 0991 has not yet been studied in humans [20].

Another strategy is the generation of metabolically stable Ang-(1-7) analogues [49,50] by encapsulating them with hydroxypropyl-β-cyclodextrin which protects the peptides from digestive enzymes, thus producing a feasible formulation for oral administration of Ang-(1-7) [50]. Another example is the peptidase-resistant thioether-bridged Ang-(1-7), which was shown to exert vasorelaxation in aortic rings of rats in addition to improving cardiac remodeling and endothelial function following myocardial infarction [51].

Advances in biotechnology have further enabled the discovery of novel agonists, such as CGEN-856 and CGEN-857 [28]. These were reported to display specificity for MasR, without binding neither to AT_1R nor to AT_2R. Vasoprotective effects of CGEN-856S were demonstrated in animals and included a dose-dependent vasodilation of precontracted aortic rings (maximal value 39.99 ± 5.03%) and vasorelaxation observed with infusion in SHRs [28].

Taken together, publications on novel MasR agonists report various beneficial properties of the receptor, while application of MasR-blockers, which abolish the actions of Ang-(1-7) and related peptides, additionally supports the theory that MasR improves endothelial function. Furthermore, genetic modification of animal models, e.g., Mas-deficient mice, emerged as a valuable tool in assessing actions and interactions of MasR, yielding an increasing body of evidence that reinforces the clinical potential of MasR in the management of HT.

4. Mas Receptor in the Management of Hypertension

Within the past decade, there seems to be an ongoing shift in the strategy of interfering with the activity of the RAAS [52]. Rather than blocking the classical pathway, as extensively done with the established drugs, an increasing body of evidence on the beneficial effects of MasR has encouraged researchers to exploit the potential of the ACE2/Ang-(1-7)/MasR axis in CV therapy [25,52]. This can be done using various Ang-(1-7) analogues and MasR agonists, as described (Table 1).

Notably, data on the competitive antagonism between Ang-(1-7) and Ang II for AT_1R has resulted in contrasting results and binding controversies, suggesting the possibility of pluridimensional receptor actions, which needs further clarifications. In order to identify the relevance of an AT_1R/Ang-(1-7) axis Galandrin et al. [29] studied the interactions of Ang-(1-7) and AT_1R by comparing Ang-(1-7)-mediated effects in phenylephrine-precontracted aortas in wild-type mice with those in AT_1R knockout mice. They found that Ang-(1-7) attenuated the contraction in wild type, but not in knockout or in the presence of AT_1R antagonist candesartan. The results demonstrated the possibility that Ang-(1-7) shows biased agonism for AT_1R, or even antagonism, independent of MasR. In a similar experimental setting with an Ang II-mediated aortic precontraction, Ang-(1-7) conversely potentiated the contraction through MasR and thus promoted the development of HT [29].

Taken together, these studies demonstrate biased actions of Ang-(1-7) and suggest that the effects mediated by the protective arm of the RAAS may depend on local interactions with the classical system [53]. Evidence of interactions between MasR and additional receptors, including bradykinin and endothelin receptors, further complicate the understanding of GPCR Mas [54,55], stressing the need for future studies to clarify how the relationship between MasR and Ang-(1-7) depends on e.g., cell type and local expression of other GPCRs. This could be crucial for developing future drugs targeting the MasR.

Table 1. Emerging potential drugs interacting with MasR.

Drug	Mechanism of Action	Effects on Blood Pressure	Status
AVE 0991	AT$_2$R/MasR agonist. Orally active nonpeptide drug.	AVE 0991 binding to bovine aortic endothelial cell membranes [43]. ACh-induced vasorelaxation in rats [47]. Potentiation of bradykinin through a Mas-mediated mechanism [48].	Preclinical studies
CGEN-856S CGEN-857	MasR agonist. Peptide drug.	Vasorelaxation in murine aortic rings [28]. Dose-dependent decrease in mean arterial pressure (MAP) in SHRs [28].	Preclinical studies
HPβCD-Ang-(1-7)	Stable Ang-(1-7) analogue. Hydroxypropyl-β-cyclodextrin protects Ang-(1-7) from digestive tract enzymes.	Chronic oral administration lowers BP in rats following ischemia-reperfusion injury [56].	Preclinical studies
Cyclic Ang-(1-7)	Peptidase resistant Ang-(1-7) analogue.	Improves endothelial function post-MI in male Sprague Dawley rats [51]. cAng-(1-7) improved peripheral endothelium-dependent vasodilation, as measured in isolated aortic rings [51].	Preclinical studies
RB150/QGC001	A central acting prodrug of the selective APA inhibitor, EC33. Orally available compound with the ability to cross the blood brain barrier.	Dose-dependent and long-lasting reduction in BP in rats, possibly following a specific blockage of the brain renin–angiotensin–aldosterone system [57].	Preclinical and phase II studies
Alamandine	Vasoactive peptide derivative of AngA with selective agonism on MrgD.	Central and peripheral BP reduction [20]. Diminishes reperfusion injury after ischemia [30].	Preclinical studies

5. Discussion

HT is a major risk factor for CV morbidity and mortality, and extensive research has been conducted to elucidate the pathophysiology of essential HT, which yet remains unclear [1]. Nevertheless, current data emphasizes that the NO-pathway plays a crucial role and that there is a distinct link between HT and a dysfunctional RAAS [9,10].

Within the past years, research in the field of antihypertensive therapy includes alternative RAAS pathways, novel mineralocorticoid receptor-antagonists, renin inhibitors and aldosterone synthesis inhibitors, peripheral noradrenergic inhibitors and gastrointestinal sodium modulators. This review particularly examined the clinical potential of MasR, which ameliorates CV injury by increasing levels of NO while reducing levels of ROS [35].

As demonstrated in animal-based studies, knowledge about the protective arm of the RAAS may pave the way for a new direction in treatment of HT, focusing on the endogenous protective mechanisms of the RAAS, rather than on the blockage of the classical system [52]. The potential of a new direction is reinforced by the positive CV effects of MasR agonists, such as AVE 0991, CGEN-856, or chemically modified Ang-(1-7). In preclinical studies it was shown that the nonpeptide compound AVE 0991 efficiently mimics the effects of Ang-(1-7) on the endothelium. The oral drug acts the stimulation of a specific, endothelial Ang-(1-7)-sensitive binding site causing kinin-mediated activation of endothelial NO synthase in bovine aortic endothelial cells [43]. Short-term Ang-(1-7) infusions significantly elevated the hypotensive effect of an intra-arterial ACh administration in normotensive rats [47]. A similar effect was seen with its analogue AVE 0991 [47]. The knowledge that Ang-(1-7) and its analogues improve endothelial function in vivo. opens new possibilities for the future treatment of CVD such as hypertension, and heart failure [47]. In addition, a synergistic effect of AVE 0991 and bradykinin on NO release was measured in normotensive rats. These findings show that AVE 0991 potentiates bradykinin through an Ang-converting enzyme–independent, NO-dependent receptor Mas-mediated mechanism. This effect may contribute to the improvement of endothelial function by AVE 0991 in vivo. [48].

Moreover, CGEN-856 and CGEN-857 revealed a high specificity for the Mas receptor, eliciting calcium influx in Chinese hamster ovary cells overexpressing Mas [28]. These peptides activate G protein–coupled receptors. CGEN-856S induced a NO- and Mas-dependent vasorelaxation in isolated aortic rings and decreased MAP in spontaneous hypertensive rats (SHRs) [28]. CGEN-856S is a novel Mas agonist with a therapeutic value, because it induces vasorelaxant, antihypertensive, and cardioprotective effects in SHRs [28]. There are similarities and differences among CGEN-856S, Ang-(1-7), and AVE 0991. CGEN-856S is apparently more stable than Ang-(1-7) and has no ACE-inhibitory activity. Due to its hydrophobicity, AVE 0991 is able to cross the blood-brain barrier and also shows central actions [28]. Some central effects of Ang-(1-7) are opposite to those evoked in the periphery. Therefore, it is important to study the possibility that some peripheral effects of AVE 0991 could be masked by its central actions. On the other hand, Ang-(1-7) is endogenous and has demonstrated well-characterized Mas-dependent actions [28].

Moreover, the inclusion of Ang-(1-7) into the oligosaccharide hydroxypropyl β-cyclodextrin (HPβCD) provided a stable oral analogue [56]. Long-term treatment with HPβCD/Ang-(1-7) in rats could attenuate the pathological remodeling process post-myocardial infarction (MI). This data indicated that Ang-(1-7) is acting beneficial in CVD [56].

In addition, a further compound is the stabilized, thioether-bridged analogue of Ang-(1-7) called cyclic Ang-(1-7), which was tested in a rat model of MI [51]. cAng-(1-7) lowered left ventricular end-diastolic pressure and improved endothelial function in rats. A recent paper showed that adding cAng-(1-7) to ACE-inhibitor therapy is beneficial to diabetic patients not completely responding to ACE-inhibitor therapy [44].

Another aspect to discuss is that a hyperactive brain renin angiotensin system (RAS) is involved in the development and maintenance of HT in several hypertensive animal models. In the murine brain, APA is involved in the conversion of Ang II to Ang III, an effector peptide of the brain RAS and responsible for vasopressin release [57]. RB150 is a prodrug of the specific and selective APA inhibitor EC33. Intravenously administered RB150 is crossing the blood-brain barrier, inhibits brain APA, and blocks central Ang III formation in rats [57]. These findings demonstrate an important role of brain APA as a candidate target for the treatment of HT. The authors suggest that RB150, a potent systemically active APA inhibitor, could be the prototype of a new class of antihypertensive agents for the treatment of certain forms of HT [57]. Targeting Ang III by inhibiting brain APA is now considered a novel treatment strategy in HT [58]. After crossing the blood-brain barrier RB150 generates two active molecules of EC33 that block brain APA activity. RB150 reduced blood pressure through inhibition of vasopressin release, which elevated diuresis. This is followed by a reduction in extracellular volume, a decrease in sympathetic tone, leading to a reduction of vascular resistances, and the improvement of the baroreflex function [58].

Today, RB150 received the new name firibastat by the World Health Organization. Phase Ia/Ib clinical trials demonstrated that firibastat is clinically and biologically well tolerated in healthy volunteers [58]. The clinical efficacy of firibastat in hypertensive patients was investigated in two phase II studies. Firibastat could represent the first drug of a novel class of antihypertensive drugs targeting the brain RAS [58].

New therapeutic approaches to prevent the activation of the brain neuromodulatory pathway may lead to improve heart failure (HF) are under investigation. The phase II study 'QUantum Genomics Incremental Dosing in Heart Failure - QUID-HF' (QUID-HF; ClinicalTrials.gov Identifier: NCT02780180) investigates safety and efficacy of the drug QGC001 (APA inhibitor and prodrug of EC33) vs. placebo in heart failure patients. Current phase III studies on HT with this drug are in the planning phase. Quantum Genomics announces positive FDA feedback on phase III program design of firibastat (QGC001) in resistant arterial hypertension.

Furthermore, ACE2 also converts Angiotensin A (AngA), a product of Ang II, into the peptide Alamandine, which interacts with the Mas-related G protein-coupled receptor D (MrgD) [20]. Alamandine decreased like AVE 0991 ventricular hypertrophy, reduced blood pressure and decreased reperfusion injury after ischemia in animal models [30,59–61].

The interactions of alamandine and Ang-(1-7) with the MrgD receptor demonstrate a potential role of this pathway in cardiovascular pathophysiology and diseases. This novel molecular pathway may play a key role in peripheral and central BP regulation and the process of cardiovascular remodelling.

Taken together, studies on Ang-(1-7) suggest the possibility of pluridimensional receptor actions, which depend on an interplay with additional pathways of the RAAS [53]. ACE2 and Ang-(1-7) counteract the adverse effects of RAS components (Figure 1) and have demonstrated protective effects on the vascular and cardiovascular system. Randomized clinical trials should be performed to study the effects of therapies targeting Ang-(1-7) and the Mas receptor. In addition, available data support the hypothesis that MasR acts to maintain endothelial function, as seen in MAS deficient mice or with application of MasR blockers [29].

6. Conclusions

It has become evident that the RAAS is more complex than originally anticipated and that an abnormally high activity within the system, for instance due to an imbalance between the counterregulatory axes, may contribute to the development of HT. In several preclinical studies, it has been demonstrated that amplification of the protective arm opposes the deleterious CV effects of the classical RAAS, by decreasing local tissue formation of ROS while stimulating the release of powerful locally acting vasodilators: NO, bradykinin and prostaglandins. Moreover, the pathophysiological consequences of the RAAS seem to depend on the balance obtained within the system, varying with changes in tissue condition and local expression levels of the signaling pathways. As a result of this, future studies on RAAS should focus less on a one peptide-one pathway approach, but on the evidence of tissue-specific pathways and on the local and systemic interactions of the RAAS. Furthermore, novel MasR agonists permit a new direction in RAAS-targeted therapy, and thus MasR shows a promising potential in future management of the global burden of HT, including the many associated comorbidities. Finally, this review emphasizes the need of studies to elucidate the signaling pathways of MasR, including the proposed cross-talks with additional RAAS components, and furthermore, the crucial need of clinical trials to confirm that the Mas-dependent pathway has a therapeutic effect in human essential HT. This requires demonstration of sufficient BP control and/or less adverse effects, in comparison with the use of classic RAAS inhibitors.

Author Contributions: Conceptualization, A.L.P. and D.G.; methodology, A.L.P.; validation, A.L.P., D.G., M.W. and M.K.; investigation, A.L.P.; resources, M.I.; writing—original draft preparation, A.L.P.; writing—review and editing, M.K., D.G. and M.W.; visualization, A.L.P.; supervision, D.G., M.K. and M.W. All authors have read and agreed to the published version of the manuscript.

Conflicts of Interest: The authors declare no conflict of interest.

References

1. Bloch, M.J. Worldwide prevalence of hypertension exceeds 1.3 billion. *J. Am. Soc. Hypertens.* **2016**, *10*, 753–754. [CrossRef] [PubMed]
2. Mills, K.T.; Bundy, J.D.; Kelly, T.N.; Reed, J.E.; Kearney, P.M.; Reynolds, K.; Chen, J.; He, J. Global disparities of hypertension prevalence and control: A systematic analysis of population-based studies from 90 countries. *Circulation* **2016**, *134*, 441–450. [CrossRef] [PubMed]
3. Williams, B.; Mancia, G.; Spiering, W.; Agabiti Rosei, E.; Azizi, M.; Burnier, M.; Clement, D.L.; Coca, A.; de Simone, G.; Dominiczak, A.; et al. 2018 ESC/ESH guidelines for the management of arterial hypertension. *Eur. Heart J.* **2018**, *39*, 3021–3104. [CrossRef] [PubMed]
4. Whelton, P.K.; Carey, R.M.; Aronow, W.S.; Casey, D.E., Jr.; Collins, K.J.; Dennison Himmelfarb, C.; DePalma, S.M.; Gidding, S.; Jamerson, K.A.; Jones, D.W.; et al. 2017 ACC/AHA/AAPA/ABC/ACPM/AGS/APhA/ASH/ASPC/NMA/PCNA Guideline for the Prevention, Detection, Evaluation, and Management of High Blood Pressure in Adults: Executive Summary: A Report of the American College of Cardiology/American Heart Association Task Force on Clinical Practice Guidelines. *Circulation* **2018**, *138*, e426–e483. [CrossRef] [PubMed]

5. Rossier, B.C.; Bochud, M.; Devuyst, O. The hypertension pandemic: An evolutionary perspective. *Physiology* **2017**, *32*, 112–125. [CrossRef] [PubMed]
6. Padmanabhan, S.; Caulfield, M.; Dominiczak, A.F. Genetic and molecular aspects of hypertension. *Circ. Res.* **2015**, *116*, 937–959. [CrossRef]
7. Carretero, O.A.; Oparil, S. Essential hypertension: Part II: Treatment. *Circulation* **2000**, *101*, 446–453. [CrossRef]
8. Wise, I.A.; Charchar, F.J. Epigenetic modifications in essential hypertension. *Int. J. Mol. Sci.* **2016**, *17*, 451. [CrossRef]
9. Drenjancevic-Peric, I.; Jelakovic, B.; Lombard, J.H.; Kunert, M.P.; Kibel, A.; Gros, M. High-salt diet and hypertension: Focus on the renin-angiotensin system. *Kidney Blood Press. Res.* **2011**, *34*, 1–11. [CrossRef]
10. Bogdarina, I.; Welham, S.; King, P.J.; Burns, S.P.; Clark, A.J. Epigenetic modification of the renin-angiotensin system in the fetal programming of hypertension. *Circ. Res.* **2007**, *100*, 520–526. [CrossRef]
11. Forrester, S.J.; Booz, G.W.; Sigmund, C.D.; Coffman, T.M.; Kawai, T.; Rizzo, V.; Scalia, R.; Eguchi, S. Angiotensin II signal transduction: An update on mechanisms of physiology and pathophysiology. *Physiol. Rev.* **2018**, *98*, 1627–1738. [CrossRef] [PubMed]
12. Oparil, S.; Schmieder, R.E. New approaches in the treatment of hypertension. *Circ. Res.* **2015**, *116*, 1074–1095. [CrossRef] [PubMed]
13. Mirabito Colafella, K.M.; Bovee, D.M.; Danser, A.H.J. The renin-angiotensin-aldosterone system and its therapeutic targets. *Exp. Eye Res.* **2019**, *186*, 107680. [CrossRef] [PubMed]
14. Te Riet, L.; van Esch, J.H.; Roks, A.J.; van den Meiracker, A.H.; Danser, A.H. Hypertension: Renin-angiotensin-aldosterone system alterations. *Circ. Res.* **2015**, *116*, 960–975. [CrossRef] [PubMed]
15. Seva Pessoa, B.; van der Lubbe, N.; Verdonk, K.; Roks, A.J.; Hoorn, E.J.; Danser, A.H. Key developments in renin-angiotensin-aldosterone system inhibition. *Nat. Rev. Nephrol.* **2013**, *9*, 26–36. [CrossRef] [PubMed]
16. Verdonk, K.; Danser, A.H.; van Esch, J.H. Angiotensin II type 2 receptor agonists: Where should they be applied? *Expert Opin. Investig. Drugs* **2012**, *21*, 501–513. [CrossRef] [PubMed]
17. Nehme, A.; Zouein, F.A.; Zayeri, Z.D.; Zibara, K. An update on the tissue renin angiotensin system and its role in physiology and pathology. *J. Cardiovasc. Dev. Dis.* **2019**, *6*, 14. [CrossRef]
18. Ahmad, S.; Varagic, J.; Groban, L.; Dell'Italia, L.J.; Nagata, S.; Kon, N.D.; Ferrario, C.M. Angiotensin-(1–12): A chymase-mediated cellular Angiotensin II substrate. *Curr. Hypertens. Rep.* **2014**, *16*, 429. [CrossRef]
19. Yugandhar, V.G.; Clark, M.A. Angiotensin III: A physiological relevant peptide of the renin angiotensin system. *Peptides* **2013**, *46*, 26–32. [CrossRef]
20. Stewart, M.H.; Lavie, C.J.; Ventura, H.O. Emerging therapy in hypertension. *Curr. Hypertens. Rep.* **2019**, *21*, 23. [CrossRef]
21. Smith, A.I.; Turner, A.J. What's new in the renin-angiotensin system? *Cell. Mol. Life Sci.* **2004**, *61*, 2675–2676. [CrossRef] [PubMed]
22. Gaspari, T.A.; Vinh, A.; Jones, E.S.; Widdop, R.E. Ganging up on Angiotensin II type 1 receptors in vascular remodeling. *Hypertension* **2012**, *60*, 17–19. [CrossRef] [PubMed]
23. Ocaranza, M.P.; Michea, L.; Chiong, M.; Lagos, C.F.; Lavandero, S.; Jalil, J.E. Recent insights and therapeutic perspectives of Angiotensin-(1–9) in the cardiovascular system. *Clin. Sci.* **2014**, *127*, 549–557. [CrossRef] [PubMed]
24. Ocaranza, M.P.; Moya, J.; Barrientos, V.; Alzamora, R.; Hevia, D.; Morales, C.; Pinto, M.; Escudero, N.; Garcia, L.; Novoa, U.; et al. Angiotensin-(1–9) reverses experimental hypertension and cardiovascular damage by inhibition of the angiotensin converting enzyme/ang ii axis. *J. Hypertens.* **2014**, *32*, 771–783. [CrossRef] [PubMed]
25. Ferreira, A.J.; Santos, R.A.; Bradford, C.N.; Mecca, A.P.; Sumners, C.; Katovich, M.J.; Raizada, M.K. Therapeutic implications of the vasoprotective axis of the renin-angiotensin system in cardiovascular diseases. *Hypertension* **2010**, *55*, 207–213. [CrossRef] [PubMed]
26. Bader, M.; Alenina, N.; Young, D.; Santos, R.A.S.; Touyz, R.M. The meaning of MAS. *Hypertension* **2018**, *72*, 1072–1075. [CrossRef] [PubMed]
27. Santos, R.A.; Campagnole-Santos, M.J.; Bara EHT, N.C.; Fontes, M.A.; Silva, L.C.; Neves, L.A.; Oliveira, D.R.; Caligiorne, S.M.; Rodrigues, A.R.; Gropen Junior, C.; et al. Characterization of a new angiotensin antagonist selective for Angiotensin-(1–7): Evidence that the actions of Angiotensin-(1–7) are mediated by specific angiotensin receptors. *Brain Res. Bull.* **1994**, *35*, 293–298. [CrossRef]

28. Savergnini, S.Q.; Beiman, M.; Lautner, R.Q.; de Paula-Carvalho, V.; Allahdadi, K.; Pessoa, D.C.; Costa-Fraga, F.P.; Fraga-Silva, R.A.; Cojocaru, G.; Cohen, Y.; et al. Vascular relaxation, antihypertensive effect, and cardioprotection of a novel peptide agonist of the MAS receptor. *Hypertension* **2010**, *56*, 112–120. [CrossRef]
29. Galandrin, S.; Denis, C.; Boularan, C.; Marie, J.; M'Kadmi, C.; Pilette, C.; Dubroca, C.; Nicaise, Y.; Seguelas, M.H.; N'Guyen, D.; et al. Cardioprotective Angiotensin-(1–7) peptide acts as a natural-biased ligand at the angiotensin II type 1 receptor. *Hypertension* **2016**, *68*, 1365–1374. [CrossRef]
30. Hrenak, J.; Paulis, L.; Simko, F. Angiotensin A/Alamandine/MrgD axis: Another clue to understanding cardiovascular pathophysiology. *Int. J. Mol. Sci.* **2016**, *17*, 1098. [CrossRef]
31. Qaradakhi, T.; Apostolopoulos, V.; Zulli, A. Angiotensin (1–7) and alamandine: Similarities and differences. *Pharmacol. Res.* **2016**, *111*, 820–826. [CrossRef] [PubMed]
32. Weber, M.A.; Schiffrin, E.L.; White, W.B.; Mann, S.; Lindholm, L.H.; Kenerson, J.G.; Flack, J.M.; Carter, B.L.; Materson, B.J.; Ram, C.V.; et al. Clinical practice guidelines for the management of hypertension in the community: A statement by the american society of hypertension and the international society of hypertension. *J. Clin. Hypertens.* **2014**, *16*, 14–26. [CrossRef] [PubMed]
33. Schiavone, M.T.; Santos, R.A.; Brosnihan, K.B.; Khosla, M.C.; Ferrario, C.M. Release of vasopressin from the rat hypothalamo-neurohypophysial system by Angiotensin-(1–7) heptapeptide. *Proc. Natl. Acad. Sci. USA* **1988**, *85*, 4095–4098. [CrossRef] [PubMed]
34. Wright, J.W.; Mizutani, S.; Harding, J.W. Pathways involved in the transition from hypertension to hypertrophy to heart failure. Treatment strategies. *Heart Fail. Rev.* **2008**, *13*, 367–375. [CrossRef]
35. Sampaio, W.O.; Henrique de Castro, C.; Santos, R.A.; Schiffrin, E.L.; Touyz, R.M. Angiotensin-(1–7) counterregulates Angiotensin II signaling in human endothelial cells. *Hypertension* **2007**, *50*, 1093–1098. [CrossRef]
36. Ferrario, C.M. ACE2: More of Ang-(1–7) or less Ang II? *Curr. Opin. Nephrol. Hypertens.* **2011**, *20*, 1–6. [CrossRef]
37. Villela, D.; Leonhardt, J.; Patel, N.; Joseph, J.; Kirsch, S.; Hallberg, A.; Unger, T.; Bader, M.; Santos, R.A.; Sumners, C.; et al. Angiotensin type 2 receptor (AT2R) and receptor mas: A complex liaison. *Clin. Sci.* **2015**, *128*, 227–234. [CrossRef]
38. Kostenis, E.; Milligan, G.; Christopoulos, A.; Sanchez-Ferrer, C.F.; Heringer-Walther, S.; Sexton, P.M.; Gembardt, F.; Kellett, E.; Martini, L.; Vanderheyden, P.; et al. G-protein-coupled receptor MAS is a physiological antagonist of the Angiotensin II type 1 receptor. *Circulation* **2005**, *111*, 1806–1813. [CrossRef]
39. Santos, R.A.S.; Sampaio, W.O.; Alzamora, A.C.; Motta-Santos, D.; Alenina, N.; Bader, M.; Campagnole-Santos, M.J. The ACE2/Angiotensin-(1–7)/MAS axis of the renin-angiotensin system: Focus on angiotensin-(1–7). *Physiol. Rev.* **2018**, *98*, 505–553. [CrossRef]
40. Young, D.; Waitches, G.; Birchmeier, C.; Fasano, O.; Wigler, M. Isolation and characterization of a new cellular oncogene encoding a protein with multiple potential transmembrane domains. *Cell* **1986**, *45*, 711–719. [CrossRef]
41. Santos, R.A.; Brosnihan, K.B.; Jacobsen, D.W.; DiCorleto, P.E.; Ferrario, C.M. Production of Angiotensin-(1–7) by human vascular endothelium. *Hypertension* **1992**, *19*, II56. [CrossRef] [PubMed]
42. Zhang, T.; Li, Z.; Dang, H.; Chen, R.; Liaw, C.; Tran, T.A.; Boatman, P.D.; Connolly, D.T.; Adams, J.W. Inhibition of mas g-protein signaling improves coronary blood flow, reduces myocardial infarct size, and provides long-term cardioprotection. *Am. J. Physiol. Heart Circ. Physiol.* **2012**, *302*, H299–H311. [CrossRef] [PubMed]
43. Wiemer, G.; Dobrucki, L.W.; Louka, F.R.; Malinski, T.; Heitsch, H. AVE 0991, a nonpeptide mimic of the effects of Angiotensin-(1–7) on the endothelium. *Hypertension* **2002**, *40*, 847–852. [CrossRef] [PubMed]
44. Cassis, P.; Locatelli, M.; Corna, D.; Villa, S.; Rottoli, D.; Cerullo, D.; Abbate, M.; Remuzzi, G.; Benigni, A.; Zoja, C. Addition of cyclic Angiotensin-(1–7) to angiotensin-converting enzyme inhibitor therapy has a positive add-on effect in experimental diabetic nephropathy. *Kidney Int.* **2019**, *96*, 906–917. [CrossRef]
45. Hernandez Prada, J.A.; Ferreira, A.J.; Katovich, M.J.; Shenoy, V.; Qi, Y.; Santos, R.A.; Castellano, R.K.; Lampkins, A.J.; Gubala, V.; Ostrov, D.A.; et al. Structure-based identification of small-molecule angiotensin-converting enzyme 2 activators as novel antihypertensive agents. *Hypertension* **2008**, *51*, 1312–1317. [CrossRef]

46. Lemos, V.S.; Silva, D.M.; Walther, T.; Alenina, N.; Bader, M.; Santos, R.A. The endothelium-dependent vasodilator effect of the nonpeptide Ang (1–7) mimic AVE 0991 is abolished in the aorta of Mas-knockout mice. *J. Cardiovasc. Pharmacol.* **2005**, *46*, 274–279. [CrossRef]
47. Faria-Silva, R.; Duarte, F.V.; Santos, R.A. Short-term Angiotensin (1–7) receptor mas stimulation improves endothelial function in normotensive rats. *Hypertension* **2005**, *46*, 948–952. [CrossRef]
48. Carvalho, M.B.; Duarte, F.V.; Faria-Silva, R.; Fauler, B.; da Mata Machado, L.T.; de Paula, R.D.; Campagnole-Santos, M.J.; Santos, R.A. Evidence for Mas-mediated bradykinin potentiation by the Angiotensin-(1–7) nonpeptide mimic AVE 0991 in normotensive rats. *Hypertension* **2007**, *50*, 762–767. [CrossRef]
49. Zhang, F.; Liu, J.; Li, S.F.; Song, J.X.; Ren, J.Y.; Chen, H. Angiotensin-(1–7): New perspectives in atherosclerosis treatment. *J. Geriatr. Cardiol.* **2015**, *12*, 676–682. [CrossRef]
50. Marques, F.D.; Ferreira, A.J.; Sinisterra, R.D.; Jacoby, B.A.; Sousa, F.B.; Caliari, M.V.; Silva, G.A.; Melo, M.B.; Nadu, A.P.; Souza, L.E.; et al. An oral formulation of Angiotensin-(1–7) produces cardioprotective effects in infarcted and isoproterenol-treated rats. *Hypertension* **2011**, *57*, 477–483. [CrossRef]
51. Durik, M.; van Veghel, R.; Kuipers, A.; Rink, R.; Haas Jimoh Akanbi, M.; Moll, G.; Danser, A.H.; Roks, A.J. The effect of the thioether-bridged, stabilized Angiotensin-(1–7) analogue cyclic Ang-(1–7) on cardiac remodeling and endothelial function in rats with myocardial infarction. *Int. J. Hypertens.* **2012**, *2012*, 536426. [CrossRef] [PubMed]
52. Santos, R.A. Angiotensin-(1–7). *Hypertension* **2014**, *63*, 1138–1147. [CrossRef] [PubMed]
53. Jiang, F.; Yang, J.; Zhang, Y.; Dong, M.; Wang, S.; Zhang, Q.; Liu, F.F.; Zhang, K.; Zhang, C. Angiotensin-converting enzyme 2 and Angiotensin 1–7: Novel therapeutic targets. *Nat. Rev. Cardiol.* **2014**, *11*, 413–426. [CrossRef] [PubMed]
54. Leonhardt, J.; Villela, D.C.; Teichmann, A.; Munter, L.M.; Mayer, M.C.; Mardahl, M.; Kirsch, S.; Namsolleck, P.; Lucht, K.; Benz, V.; et al. Evidence for heterodimerization and functional interaction of the Angiotensin type 2 receptor and the receptor mas. *Hypertension* **2017**, *69*, 1128–1135. [CrossRef] [PubMed]
55. Cerrato, B.D.; Carretero, O.A.; Janic, B.; Grecco, H.E.; Gironacci, M.M. Heteromerization between the bradykinin b2 receptor and the Angiotensin-(1–7) mas receptor: Functional consequences. *Hypertension* **2016**, *68*, 1039–1048. [CrossRef]
56. Marques, F.D.; Melo, M.B.; Souza, L.E.; Irigoyen, M.C.; Sinisterra, R.D.; de Sousa, F.B.; Savergnini, S.Q.; Braga, V.B.; Ferreira, A.J.; Santos, R.A. Beneficial effects of long-term administration of an oral formulation of Angiotensin-(1–7) in infarcted rats. *Int. J. Hypertens.* **2012**, *2012*, 795452. [CrossRef] [PubMed]
57. Fournie-Zaluski, M.C.; Fassot, C.; Valentin, B.; Djordjijevic, D.; Reaux-Le Goazigo, A.; Corvol, P.; Roques, B.P.; Llorens-Cortes, C. Brain renin-angiotensin system blockade by systemically active aminopeptidase a inhibitors: A potential treatment of salt-dependent hypertension. *Proc. Natl. Acad. Sci. USA* **2004**, *101*, 7775–7780. [CrossRef]
58. Llorens-Cortes, C.; Touyz, R.M. Evolution of a new class of antihypertensive drugs: Targeting the brain renin-angiotensin system. *Hypertension* **2020**, *75*, 6–15. [CrossRef]
59. Jesus, I.C.G.; Scalzo, S.; Alves, F.; Marques, K.; Rocha-Resende, C.; Bader, M.; Santos, R.A.S.; Guatimosim, S. Alamandine acts via MrgD to induce AMPK/NO activation against Ang II hypertrophy in cardiomyocytes. *Am. J. Physiol. Cell Physiol.* **2018**, *314*, C702–C711. [CrossRef]
60. Park, B.M.; Phuong, H.T.A.; Yu, L.; Kim, S.H. Alamandine protects the heart against reperfusion injury via the MrgD receptor. *Circ. J.* **2018**, *82*, 2584–2593. [CrossRef]
61. Liu, C.; Yang, C.X.; Chen, X.R.; Liu, B.X.; Li, Y.; Wang, X.Z.; Sun, W.; Li, P.; Kong, X.Q. Alamandine attenuates hypertension and cardiac hypertrophy in hypertensive rats. *Amino Acids* **2018**, *50*, 1071–1081. [CrossRef] [PubMed]

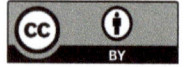

© 2020 by the authors. Licensee MDPI, Basel, Switzerland. This article is an open access article distributed under the terms and conditions of the Creative Commons Attribution (CC BY) license (http://creativecommons.org/licenses/by/4.0/).

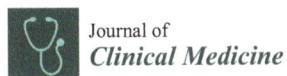

Article

Severity of Coronary Atherosclerosis and Risk of Diabetes Mellitus

Iginio Colaiori [1,†], Raffaele Izzo [2,†], Emanuele Barbato [2,*], Danilo Franco [2], Giuseppe Di Gioia [1,2], Antonio Rapacciuolo [2], Jozef Bartunek [1], Costantino Mancusi [2], Maria Angela Losi [2], Teresa Strisciuglio [2], Maria Virginia Manzi [2], Giovanni de Simone [2], Bruno Trimarco [2] and Carmine Morisco [2]

1 Cardiovascular Research Center Aalst OLV Hospital, 9300 Aalst, Belgium
2 Department of Advanced Biomedical Sciences, University of Naples Federico II, 80100 Napoli, Italy
* Correspondence: emanuele.barbato@unina.it; Tel.: +39(081)746-2253; Fax: +39(081)546-2256
† These authors equally contributed to the manuscript.

Received: 6 June 2019; Accepted: 19 July 2019; Published: 21 July 2019

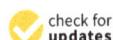

Abstract: Background: Cardio-vascular target organ damage predicts the onset of type 2 diabetes mellitus (DM) in hypertensive patients. Whether an increased incidence of DM is also in relation to the severity of coronary atherosclerosis is unknown. Objective: We evaluated the onset of DM in relation to the extent and severity of coronary atherosclerosis, using the SYNTAX (Synergy between Percutaneous Coronary Intervention with Taxus and Cardiac Surgery) score (SS), in patients with stable angina or acute coronary syndromes, referred for coronary angiography (CA). Methods: Non-diabetic patients that underwent CA for the first time were included, and the SS was computed. Predictors of DM onset in low, medium, and high SSs were investigated. Results: Five hundred and seventy patients were included, and the mean SS was 6.3 ± 7.6. During a median follow-up of 79 months (interquartile range (IQR): 67–94), 74 patients (13%) developed DM. The risk of DM onset was significantly higher in the patients with a medium or high SS (hazard ratio (HR)—95% confidence interval (CI): 16 (4–61), $p < 0.0001$; and 30 (9–105), $p < 0.0001$, vs low SS, respectively), even after adjustment for obesity, history of hypertension, impaired fasting glucose, and cardiovascular therapy. Conclusions: The severity and extent of the coronary atherosclerosis, evaluated by the SS, is a strong and independent predictor of the development of DM in patients, referred to CA.

Keywords: coronary artery disease; diabetes mellitus; atherosclerosis; coronary angiography

1. Introduction

Type 2 diabetes mellitus (DM) and cardiovascular (CV) disease are closely correlated. DM is associated with a two- to four-fold increased risk of coronary artery disease (CAD) and stroke [1]. On the other hand, CV diseases are the main causes of death and disability among patients with DM [2]. Furthermore, DM is associated with more extensive coronary atherosclerosis [3], and worse outcomes in acute coronary syndromes [4]. The association with coronary atherosclerosis spans from early stages of glucose intolerance to overt DM [5–7]. We previously demonstrated, in hypertensive patients, that uncontrolled blood pressure is associated with a two-fold increased risk of diabetes onset [8]. In addition, hypertension-mediated target organ damage (e.g., carotid atherosclerosis and left ventricular hypertrophy) is a significant predictor of DM onset, independently of the baseline metabolic profile, anti-hypertensive therapy, and other significant covariates [9]. Thus, a well-characterized phenotype of hypertensive patients, carrying features suggestive of a high atherosclerotic burden, places patients at a higher risk for developing DM during follow-up. However, at this time, there is no direct demonstration that atherosclerosis exposes patients to a higher risk of DM development with a dose-response pattern. Identifying patients with an increased risk of DM, in the setting of patients referred to Cat Labs for coronary angiography (CA), might be of paramount importance in terms of cardiovascular prevention [10]. Therefore, the early identification of individuals with established coronary artery disease at risk of type 2 DM could be further assessed for the severity of atherosclerosis, even before the clinical appearance of the disease, in order to promote the aggressive management of the metabolic profile in these patients.

Accordingly, we investigated whether the extension and severity of CAD diagnosed during CA might be predictive of the future onset of DM.

2. Research Design and Methods

2.1. Patients

We screened all of the consecutive patients who underwent CA at the Cardiovascular Center Aalst (Belgium), between 1 January 2009 and 31 December 2009. The exclusion criteria were as follows: previous coronary angiogram, history of myocardial infarction or coronary artery bypass graft, or the diagnosis of pre-existing diabetes. All patients signed informed consent for CA and for data collection before the procedure. During the index hospital admission for CA, the blood pressure (BP), heart rate (HR), body mass index (BMI), fasting glucose, glycated hemoglobin (HbA1c), lipid profile, and kidney function were routinely assessed for each patient. All of the patients underwent trans-thoracic echocardiogram (TTE), analyzed offline by one expert reader under the supervision of a senior consultant, using dedicated work-stations (Echo-PAC Clinical Workstation Software, GE Healthcare, Horten, Norway).

The SYNTAX (Synergy between Percutaneous Coronary Intervention with Taxus and Cardiac Surgery) score (SS) was calculated for all of the patients by two interventional cardiologists blinded to the baseline clinical characteristics, procedural data, and clinical outcomes. Each coronary lesion with more than a 50% diameter stenosis in vessels of at least 1.5 mm, by visual estimation, was scored separately using the SS algorithm from the related website [11]. To assess the intra-observer reproducibility, angiograms were re-analyzed by the same interventional cardiologist eight weeks after the first analysis. The investigator remained blinded to the results of the first analysis. After the first admission for CA (index procedure), patients were assessed for incidence of type 2 diabetes in all of the subsequent follow-up visits or laboratory exams at the Cardiovascular Center of Aalst. To standardize the follow-up (FU), we analyzed the ambulatory visits and laboratory data every 6 months, until the last FU.

2.2. Primary Endpoint

The primary endpoint of the study was the incidence of type 2 DM after index hospitalization. Diabetes was defined according to the 2018 American Diabetes Association (ADA) criteria, as follows: fasting plasma glucose of 126 mg/dL (7.0 m mol/L) or hemoglobin A1C of 6.5% (48 mmol/mol) [12]. To accurately date the first diagnosis of diabetes, we carefully checked on the initiation of anti-diabetic therapies, and on the laboratory data at the occasion of the outpatient clinic visit. The onset of diabetes was adjudicated based on the earliest evidence of ADA criteria at the follow-up.

2.3. Measurements and Definitions

Obesity was defined as a BMI of 30 kg/m^2. According to the ADA criteria, impaired fasting glucose (IFG) was considered when the fasting plasma glucose was between 101 and 125 mg/dL. The systolic and diastolic blood pressure (BP) was measured by standard aneroid sphygmomanometer after 5 min rest in the supine position. Three BP measurements were obtained in the sitting position, at 2 min intervals. The averages of these measurements were used for the analysis. Hypertension is defined as office systolic blood pressure (SBP) values of 140 mmHg, and/or diastolic BP (DBP) values of 90 mmHg, according to the European Society of Cardiology (ESC) guidelines [13]. We defined peripheral vascular disease (PVD) as disease documented by a vascular imaging study (including a Computed tomography (CT) scan, ultrasound, peripheral angiography, and magnetic resonance imaging (MRI) that was significant enough for the patient to be referred for elective vascular surgery or percutaneous intervention.

2.4. Statistical Analysis

The data were analyzed using IBM SPSS Statistics (version 25.0; SPSS, IBM, Armonk, NY, US), and expressed as mean ± 1 standard deviation (SD). The variables that were not normally distributed were log-transformed. The study population was divided into quartiles of SS. For the exploratory statistics, we considered the two lowest quartiles as low-risk SS (group 1); the third one, corresponding to the median of distribution, as moderate-risk SS (group 2); and the highest one, corresponding to the 75th percentile of the distribution, as high-risk SS (group 3). Analysis of variance (ANOVA) was used to compare the baseline characteristics of the three groups of patients according to SS. Under the assumption of increasing abnormalities from group 1 to group 3, polynomial linear and quadratic contrasts were used to estimate the trend. The χ^2 distribution was used to compare the categorical variables, with the Monte Carlo simulation in order to obtain exact p-values.

The incidence of diabetes in relation to the three groups of SS was assessed using three models of Cox regression analysis, as follows: (a) in the first model, age, gender, and metabolic profile were included; (b) in the second model, the echo parameters and classes of drugs were included; (c) in the third model, the dosages (low vs high dosages) of the statins (i.e., patients on rosuvastatine ≥20 mg/die or atorvastatine ≥40 mg/die were considered as high dosage) were included. A two-tailed p-value of <0.05 was used to reject the null hypothesis.

3. Results

3.1. Patients

Within the study period, 570 non-diabetic (mean age 65 ± 10 years; 69% males) patients fulfilled the inclusion and exclusion criteria, and were included in this analysis. Table 1 shows the demographic and clinical characteristics of the patients stratified by SS. In the patient population, the included SSs were as follows: SS low, 0 to ≤4; SS medium, >4 to ≤10; and SS high, >10. The patients in the high SS were older, and showed a lower heart rate and left ventricular ejection fraction. The basal fasting plasma glucose was found to be progressively higher among the patients with medium and high SS, while the lipid profile was more favorable in the medium SS. Table 2 shows the medical therapy at discharge from the index hospitalization. All four classes of medications considered in the analysis were prescribed more frequently in patients with a higher SS.

Table 1. Baseline demographic and clinical characteristics of participants stratified by SYNTAX score (SS).

	Low SS (n = 295)	Medium SS (n = 151)	High SS (n = 124)	p (for trend)
Age (years)	65.5 ± 10.4	63.9 ± 10.5	67.1 ± 10.3	0.045
Sex (male/female %)	68.8/31.2	72.8/27.2	74.2/25.8	NS
Smokers (%)	47.5	53.0	48.4	NS
Hypertensives (%)	67.5	76.8	75.8	NS
BMI (Kg/m^2)	27.1 ± 4.5	27.2 ± 4.3	27.3 ± 5.4	NS
Systolic BP (mmHg)	133.3 ± 22.0	128.8 ± 17.1	133.2 ± 19.4	NS
Diastolic BP (mmHg)	69.5 ± 11.4	69.3 ± 10.6	69.3 ± 11.3	NS
HR (bpm)	67.7 ± 12.2	66.9 ± 11.9	64.6 ± 8.7	0.048
Ejection Fraction (%)	67.9 ± 16.0	64.9 ± 14.0	61.6 ± 15.4	0.001
Fasting plasma glucose (mg/dL)	83.8 ± 13.2	85.6 ± 13.4	94.7 ± 13.5	0.0001
HbA1c (mmol/mol)	40.5 ± 8.7	40.4 ± 7.3	41.0 ± 7.5	NS
Total cholesterol (mg/dL)	172.6 ± 44.2	154.4 ± 36.6	156.0 ± 41.6	0.0001
LDL cholesterol (mg/dL)	91.8 ± 39.0	77.8 ± 31.4	81.1 ± 34.7	0.001
HDL cholesterol (mg/dL)	52.2 ± 16.8	51.0 ± 17.9	46.4 ± 14.5	0.01
Triacylglycerols (mg/dL)	147.3 ± 83.0	124.4 ± 67.4	146.1 ± 87.2	0.044

Table 1. *Cont.*

	Low SS (n = 295)	Medium SS (n = 151)	High SS (n = 124)	p (for trend)
GFR$_{EPI}$ (mL/min/1.73 m^2)	64.7 ± 28.3	70.5 ± 25.6	64.3 ± 24.8	NS
CRP (mg/L)	27.7 ± 77.1	15.9 ± 34.0	28.7 ± 67.5	NS
IFG (%)	12.5	15.2	36.3	0.0001

BMI = body mass index; BP = blood pressure; HR = heart rate; HbA1C = hemoglobin glycated A1C; LDL = low density lipoprotein; HDL = high density lipoprotein; GFR = glomerular filtration rate; CRP = C-reactive protein; IFG = impaired fasting glucose; NS = not significant.

Table 2. Classes of drugs prescribed at the discharge.

	Low SS (n = 295)	Medium SS (n = 151)	High SS (n = 124)	p
CCB (%)	2.7	8.6	14.5	<0.0001
β-blockers (%)	20.0	37.7	42.7	<0.0001
Statins (%)	39.0	76.8	83.9	<0.0001
Statins low dose (%)	32.5	58.3	64.5	<0.0001
Statins high dose (%)	6.5	18.5	19.4	<0.0001
Anti-RAS (%)	29.5	27.2	46.8	0.001

SS = SYNTAX score; CCB = calcium channel blockers; RAS = renin angiotensin system.

3.2. Follow-Up

During a median follow-up of 79 months (interquartile range (IQR): 67–94), 74 (13%) patients developed DM. The incidence of diabetes was significantly higher in the patients with a high SS (41%), than in patients with a medium (12%) and low SS (2%; p for trend < 0.0001; Figure 1). In the Cox regression analysis (Table 3), the predictors of DM onset during follow-up had higher baseline values of fasting plasma glucose (HR = 1.043; (95% CI 1.011–1.075); p < 0.008), medium SS (HR = 6.630; (95% CI 2.394–18.358); p < 0.0001), and high SS (HR = 14.789; (95% CI 5.796–37.737); p < 0.0001). The three curves (Figure 2) started to separate after 48–52 months from the index hospitalization, and further diverged after five years of follow-up. In the second Cox regression analysis performed by including the ejection fraction, heart rate, and the drugs prescribed (Table 4), the predictors of the new onset of DM were as follows: use of statins (HR = 6.953; (95% CI 1.618–29.880); p = 0.009), an anti-renin angiotensin system (RAS; HR = 3.338; (95% CI 1.917–5.812); p = 0.0001), medium SS (HR = 6.022; (95% CI 1.714–21.158); p = 0.005), and high SS (HR = 13.140; (95% CI 3.857–44.738); p < 0.0001) was further reinforced (Table 4). In the last model (Table 5), including the dosage of statins, the independent predictors of DM were a low dose of statins (HR = 8.631; (95% CI 2.017–36.931); p = 0.004), a high dose of statins (HR = 8.158; (95% CI 1.764–37.728); p = 0.007), anti-RAS (HR = 3.637; (95% CI 2.151–6.6.151); p < 0.0001), medium SS (HR = 3.505; (95% CI 1.274–9.644); p = 0.015), and high SS (HR = 8.906; (95% CI 3.404–23.296); p = 0.0001).

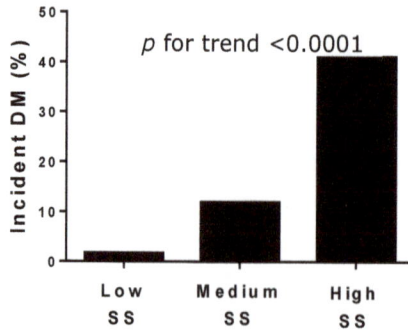

Figure 1. Rate of type 2 diabetes mellitus (DM) in the three SYNTAX score (SS) levels.

Table 3. Results of Cox regression, including the age, gender, and metabolic profile.

Predictors	Sig.	HR	95.0% CI	
			Lower	−Upper
Sex (1 male/2 female)	0.583	1.163	0.679	−1.993
Age (years)	0.085	1.026	0.996	−1.056
Fasting plasma glucose (mg/dL)	0.008	1.043	1.011	−1.075
LDL Cholesterol (mg/dL)	0.323	1.130	0.535	−2.385
IFG (y)	0.749	7.865	2.817	−21.959
Medium SS	0.000	6.630	2.304	−18.358
High SS	0.000	14.789	5.796	−37.737

Abbreviations as in Table 1. CI = confidence interval.

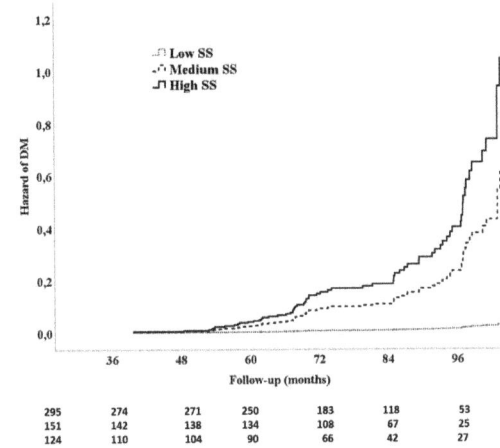

Figure 2. Cox regression time to event analysis for type 2 diabetes mellitus onset, in the function of the three SS levels.

Table 4. Results of Cox regression including ejection fraction, heart rate, and classes of drugs.

Predictors	Sig	HR	95.0% CI	
			Lower	−Upper
Ejection Fraction (%)	0.698	0.996	0.978	−1.015
HR (bpm)	0.128	1.021	0.994	−1.048
CCB (y)	0.549	0.215	0.643	−2.296
B-blockers (y)	0.416	1.223	0.753	−1.986
Statins (y)	0.009	6.953	1.618	−29.880
Anti RAS (y)	0.000	3.338	1.917	−5.812
Medium SS	0.005	6.022	1.714	−21.158
High SS	0.000	13.140	3.857	−44.768

Abbreviations as in Tables 1 and 2.

In patients who developed DM, no significant differences were detected in the incidence of major adverse cardiovascular events (i.e., death, myocardial infarction, or coronary revascularization) among the three SS subgroups ($p = 0.418$).

Table 5. Results of the COX regression, including the classes of drugs and statins dosage.

Predictors	Sig	HR	95.0% CI	
			Lower	Upper
CCB (y)	0.387	1.314	0.708	−2.440
B-blockers (y)	0.390	1.238	0.761	−2.013
Statins low dose (y)	0.004	8.631	2.017	−36.931
Statins high dose (y)	0.007	8.158	1.764	−37.728
Anti RAS (y)	0.0001	3.637	2.151	−6.151
Medium SS	0.015	3.505	1.274	−9.644
High SS	0.0001	8.906	3.404	−23.296

Abbreviations as in Tables 1 and 2.

4. Discussion

In non-diabetic patients, our study demonstrates, for the first time, a significant association between the severity and extent of coronary atherosclerosis, assessed by the SS, with the future development of type 2 DM. Compared with patients with low SS, those with medium or high values exhibited an 8-fold and 10-fold higher risk for developing type 2 DM during follow-up, an association that was independent of potential confounders, including initial metabolic profile, age, anthropometric and hemodynamic characteristics, and medications.

Vascular and Metabolic Disease

Our results parallel previous studies challenging the paradigm that type 2 DM normally precedes and portends to a higher risk of developing vascular atherosclerosis [14,15], although they provide direct evidence of this reverse temporal relation. Our results are consistent with findings in patients with essential hypertension, in whom both resistant hypertension [8] and left ventricular hypertrophy [9] precede the onset of type 2 DM. Our findings extend to patients with coronary artery disease (CAD), the evidence of this reverse temporal relation. We hypothesize that a possible vicious circle might be at the basis of this phenomenon. It is reasonable to speculate that the mechanisms relating atherosclerosis to the later onset of DM might be related to insulin resistance, rather than directly to a hyperglycaemic state. However, as the present study was not designed to explore the pathogenic mechanisms underlying the association between SS and the development of diabetes, the insulin sensitivity in our study population remained unexplored. Insulin resistance is a common pathogenic background for both DM and atherosclerosis [16,17]. Insulin resistance plays a mechanistic role, along with other risk factors, in the development of vascular damage and the occurrence of cardiovascular events (four) [18,19]. In particular, insulin resistance-mediated endothelial dysfunction (an early step of atherosclerosis) [20] has been proposed as a pathogenic mechanism of DM [21]. In turn, the presence of an extensive vascular atherosclerosis might facilitate the onset and maintenance of the insulin resistance state. This vicious circle can well explain how CV damage, instead of being a consequence, could progress, together with the development of DM.

Our results cannot exclude the possibility that sub-clinical DM was already present at the time of the index CA in patients who clinically manifested the disease during follow-up. As matter of fact, endothelial dysfunction precedes and predicts incident diabetes, supporting the hypothesis that vascular disease might precede pancreatic beta-cell failure, determining the shift from insulin resistance to diabetes [22]. Moreover, endothelial dysfunction and impaired nitric oxide-mediated vasodilatation have also been suggested to directly lead to reduced insulin delivery to skeletal muscles, resulting in peripheral insulin resistance and hyper-glycaemia [23].

It is of note that patients with medium or high SS manifested type 2 DM after a subclinical phase of nearly four years from the index CA. As SS was evaluated cross-sectionally, this study does not clarify whether the association between the magnitude of coronary atherosclerosis and the development of type 2 DM is a time-dependent or atherosclerotic-dependent phenomenon. However, the latter seems to play an important role, considering that the rate of DM increases with increasing the SS category (Figure 1).

The evidence that patients with more than a low SS have a much higher risk of incident type 2 DM is of clinical importance. It implies that these patients, in addition to their regular cardiovascular follow-up, require tailored management in terms of metabolic risk, including attention to pharmacological therapy. In particular, it has been demonstrated that a high-dose regimen with statins was associated with an increased risk of new-onset DM [24,25]. In keeping with these findings, we found that statin intake was significantly associated with more complex coronary artery disease, and was predictive of an increased rate of DM.

In terms of the choice of revascularization strategies, the knowledge of the higher risk of development of type 2 diabetes in patients with more than a low SS might favor surgical over percutaneous interventions, after taking into account the anatomical features of the CAD and the clinical conditions of the patient [26].

5. Conclusions

Our study demonstrates that the extension and severity of coronary atherosclerosis is a strong predictor of development of type 2 DM. This finding advocates the need for developing dedicated management strategies in patients with severe coronary artery disease, taking into account the risk of late metabolic impairment following the index coronary intervention.

Author Contributions: Conceptualization, I.C., R.I., C.M., and E.B.; methodology, E.B., M.A.L., J.B., and C.M.; validation, A.R., G.d.S., B.T., and J.B.; investigation, G.D.G., T.S., D.F., and M.V.M.; data curation, M.V.M., I.C., G.D.G., and T.S.; original draft preparation, I.C., R.I., C.M., and T.S.; writing (review and editing), I.C., D.F., R.I., and E.B.; supervision, A.R., B.T., C.M., E.B., and M.A.L.

Acknowledgments: T.S. and G.D.G. received a grant from the Cardiopath PhD program. R.I. and C.M. were recipients of University FEDERICO II financial support, annuity 2016.

Conflicts of Interest: The authors declare no conflict of interest.

References

1. Colhoun, H.M.; Betteridge, D.J.; Durrington, P.N.; Hitman, G.A.; Neil, H.A.; Livingstone, S.J.; Thomason, M.J.; Mackness, M.I.; Charlton-Menys, V.; Fuller, J.H.; et al. Primary prevention of cardiovascular disease with atorvastatin in type 2 diabetes in the Collaborative Atorvastatin Diabetes Study (CARDS): Multicentre randomised placebo-controlled trial. *Lancet* **2004**, *364*, 685–696. [CrossRef]
2. Wang, L.C.C.; Hess, C.N.; Hiatt, W.R.; Goldfine, A.B. Clinical Update: Cardiovascular Disease in Diabetes Mellitus: Atherosclerotic Cardiovascular Disease and Heart Failure in Type 2 Diabetes Mellitus Mechanisms, Management, and Clinical Considerations. *Circulation* **2016**, *133*, 2459–2502. [CrossRef] [PubMed]
3. Ryden, L.; Grant, P.J.; Anker, S.D.; Berne, C.; Cosentino, F.; Danchin, N.; Deaton, C.; Viigimaa, M.; Vlachopoulos, C.; Xuereb, R.G.; et al. Task Force on diabetes p-d, cardiovascular diseases of the European Society of C, European Association for the Study of D, ESC guidelines on diabetes, pre-diabetes, and cardiovascular diseases developed in collaboration with the EASD-summary. *Diabetes Vasc. Dis. Res.* **2014**, *11*, 133–173.
4. Deedwania, P.; Kosiborod, M.; Barrett, E.; Ceriello, A.; Isley, W.; Mazzone, T.; Raskin, P. American Heart Association Diabetes Committee of the Council on Nutrition PA, Metabolism: Hyperglycemia and acute coronary syndrome: A scientific statement from the American Heart Association Diabetes Committee of the Council on Nutrition, Physical Activity, and Metabolism. *Circulation* **2008**, *117*, 1610–1619. [PubMed]
5. Harris, M.I.; Klein, R.; Welborn, T.A.; Knuiman, M.W. Onset of NIDDM occurs at least 4-7 year before clinical diagnosis. *Diabetes Care* **1992**, *15*, 815–819. [CrossRef] [PubMed]

6. Hu, F.B.; Stampfer, M.J.; Haffner, S.M.; Solomon, C.G.; Willett, W.C.; Manson, J.E. Elevated risk of cardiovascular disease prior to clinical diagnosis of type 2 diabetes. *Diabetes Care* **2002**, *25*, 1129–1134. [CrossRef] [PubMed]
7. Acar, B.; Ozeke, O.; Karakurt, M.; Ozen, Y.; Ozbay, M.B.; Unal, S.; Karanfil, M.; Yayla, C.; Cay, S.; Maden, O.; et al. Association of Prediabetes with Higher Coronary Atherosclerotic Burden Among Patients with First Diagnosed Acute Coronary Syndrome. *Angiology* **2018**. [CrossRef]
8. Izzo, R.; Simone, G.; Chinali, M.; Iaccarino, G.; Trimarco, V.; Rozza, F.; Giudice, R.; Trimarco, B.; Luca, N. Insufficient control of blood pressure and incident diabetes. *Diabetes Care* **2009**, *32*, 845–850. [CrossRef]
9. Izzo, R.; Simone, G.; Trimarco, V.; Gerdts, E.; Giudice, R.; Vaccaro, O.; Luca, N.; Trimarco, B. Hypertensive target organ damage predicts incident diabetes mellitus. *Eur. Heart J.* **2013**, *34*, 3419–3426. [CrossRef]
10. Gillies, C.L.; Abrams, K.R.; Lambert, P.C.; Cooper, N.J.; Sutton, A.J.; Hsu, R.T.; Khunti, K. Pharmacological and lifestyle interventions to prevent or delay type 2 diabetes in people with impaired glucose tolerance: Systematic review and meta-analysis. *Bmj* **2007**, *334*, 299. [CrossRef]
11. Serruys, P.W.; Onuma, Y.; Garg, S.; Sarno, G.; Brand, M.; Kappetein, A.P.; Dyck, N.; Mack, M.; Holmes, D.; Feldman, T.; et al. Assessment of the SYNTAX score in the Syntax study. *EuroIntervention* **2009**, *5*, 50–56. [CrossRef] [PubMed]
12. American, D.A. Classification and Diagnosis of Diabetes: Standards of Medical Care in Diabetes-2018. *Diabetes Care* **2018**, *41*, S13–S27. [CrossRef] [PubMed]
13. Williams, B.; Mancia, G.; Spiering, W.; Agabiti, R.E.; Azizi, M.; Burnier, M.; Clement, D.L.; Coca, A.; Simone, G.; Dominiczak, A.; et al. ESC/ESH Guidelines for the management of arterial hypertension. *Eur. Heart J.* **2018**, *39*, 3021–3104. [CrossRef] [PubMed]
14. Gioia, D.G.; Scarsini, R.; Strisciuglio, T.; Biase, C.; Zivelonghi, C.; Franco, D.; Bruyne, B.; Ribichini, F.; Barbato, E. Correlation between Angiographic and Physiologic Evaluation of Coronary Artery Narrowings in Patients with Aortic Valve Stenosis. *Am. J. Cardiol.* **2017**, *120*, 106–110. [CrossRef] [PubMed]
15. Xaplanteris, P.; Ntalianis, A.; Bruyne, B.; Strisciuglio, T.; Pellicano, M.; Ciccarelli, G.; Milkas, A.; Barbato, E. Coronary lesion progression as assessed by fractional flow reserve (FFR) and angiography. *EuroIntervention* **2018**, *14*, 907–914. [CrossRef]
16. Olefsky, J.; Farquhar, J.W.; Reaven, G. Relationship between fasting plasma insulin level and resistance to insulin-mediated glucose uptake in normal and diabetic subjects. *Diabetes* **1973**, *22*, 507–513. [CrossRef] [PubMed]
17. Howard, G.; O'Leary, D.H.; Zaccaro, D.; Haffner, S.; Rewers, M.; Hamman, R.; Selby, J.V.; Saad, M.F.; Savage, P.; Bergman, R. Insulin sensitivity and atherosclerosis. The Insulin Resistance Atherosclerosis Study (IRAS) Investigators. *Circulation* **1996**, *93*, 1809–1817. [CrossRef]
18. Fournier, S.; Toth, G.G.; Bruyne, B.; Johnson, N.P.; Ciccarelli, G.; Xaplanteris, P.; Milkas, A.; Strisciuglio, T.; Bartunek, J.; Vanderheyden, M.; et al. Six-Year Follow-Up of Fractional Flow Reserve-Guided Versus Angiography-Guided Coronary Artery Bypass Graft Surgery. *Circ. Cardiovasc. Interv.* **2018**, *11*, e006368. [CrossRef]
19. Morisco, C.; Lembo, G.; Trimarco, B. Insulin resistance and cardiovascular risk: New insights from molecular and cellular biology. *Trends Cardiovasc. Med.* **2006**, *16*, 183–188. [CrossRef]
20. Carrizzo, A.; Izzo, C.; Oliveti, M.; Alfano, A.; Virtuoso, N.; Capunzo, M.; Pietro, P.; Calabrese, M.; Simone, E.; Sciarretta, S.; et al. The Main Determinants of Diabetes Mellitus Vascular Complications: Endothelial Dysfunction and Platelet Hyperaggregation. *Int. J. Mol. Sci.* **2018**, *19*, 2968. [CrossRef]
21. Tooke, J.E. Microvascular function in human diabetes. A physiological perspective. *Diabetes* **1995**, *44*, 721–726. [CrossRef]
22. Ferrannini, E. Insulin resistance versus insulin deficiency in non-insulin-dependent diabetes mellitus: Problems and prospects. *Endocr. Rev.* **1998**, *19*, 477–490. [CrossRef]
23. Balletshofer, B.M.; Rittig, K.; Enderle, M.D.; Volk, A.; Maerker, E.; Jacob, S.; Matthaei, S.; Rett, K. Haring HU: Endothelial dysfunction is detectable in young normotensive first-degree relatives of subjects with type 2 diabetes in association with insulin resistance. *Circulation* **2000**, *101*, 1780–1784. [CrossRef]

24. Preiss, D.; Seshasai, S.R.; Welsh, P.; Murphy, S.A.; Ho, J.E.; Waters, D.D.; DeMicco, D.A.; Barter, P.; Cannon, C.P.; Sabatine, M.S.; et al. Risk of incident diabetes with intensive-dose compared with moderate-dose statin therapy: A meta-analysis. *Jama* **2011**, *305*, 2556–2564. [CrossRef]
25. Izzo, R.; Simone, G.; Trimarco, V.; Giudice, R.; Marco, M.; Renzo, G.; Luca, N.; Trimarco, B. Primary prevention with statins and incident diabetes in hypertensive patients at high cardiovascular risk. *Nutr. Metab. Cardiovasc. Dis. NMCD* **2013**, *23*, 1101–1106. [CrossRef]
26. Farkouh, M.E.; Domanski, M.; Sleeper, L.A.; Siami, F.S.; Dangas, G.; Mack, M.; Yang, M.; Cohen, D.J.; Rosenberg, Y.; Solomon, S.D.; et al. Strategies for multivessel revascularization in patients with diabetes. *New Engl. J. Med.* **2012**, *367*, 2375–2384. [CrossRef]

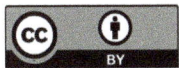 © 2019 by the authors. Licensee MDPI, Basel, Switzerland. This article is an open access article distributed under the terms and conditions of the Creative Commons Attribution (CC BY) license (http://creativecommons.org/licenses/by/4.0/).

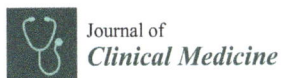

Article

Altered Metabolomic Profile in Patients with Peripheral Artery Disease

Ahmed Ismaeel [1], Marco E. Franco [2], Ramon Lavado [2], Evlampia Papoutsi [1], George P. Casale [3], Matthew Fuglestad [3], Constance J. Mietus [3], Gleb R. Haynatzki [4], Robert S. Smith [5], William T. Bohannon [5], Ian Sawicki [5], Iraklis I. Pipinos [3] and Panagiotis Koutakis [1,*]

1. Department of Nutrition, Food and Exercise Sciences, Florida State University, Tallahassee, FL 32306, USA
2. Department of Environmental Science, Baylor University, Waco, TX 76798, USA
3. Department of Surgery, University of Nebraska at Medical Center, Omaha, NE 68198, USA
4. Department of Biostatistics, University of Nebraska Medical Center, Omaha, NE 68198, USA
5. Department of Surgery, Baylor Scott and White Hospital, Temple, TX 76508, USA
* Correspondence: pkoutakis@fsu.edu; Tel.: +1-(850)-644-1829

Received: 24 August 2019; Accepted: 12 September 2019; Published: 14 September 2019

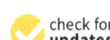

Abstract: Peripheral artery disease (PAD) is a common atherosclerotic disease characterized by narrowed or blocked arteries in the lower extremities. Circulating serum biomarkers can provide significant insight regarding the disease progression. Here, we explore the metabolomics signatures associated with different stages of PAD and investigate potential mechanisms of the disease. We compared the serum metabolites of a cohort of 26 PAD patients presenting with claudication and 26 PAD patients presenting with critical limb ischemia (CLI) to those of 26 non-PAD controls. A difference between the metabolite profiles of PAD patients from non-PAD controls was observed for several amino acids, acylcarnitines, ceramides, and cholesteryl esters. Furthermore, our data demonstrate that patients with CLI possess an altered metabolomic signature different from that of both claudicants and non-PAD controls. These findings provide new insight into the pathophysiology of PAD and may help develop future diagnostic procedures and therapies for PAD patients.

Keywords: peripheral artery disease (PAD); metabolomics; claudication; critical limb ischemia (CLI)

1. Introduction

Peripheral artery disease (PAD) is an atherosclerotic condition of the arteries supplying the lower extremities. PAD affects over 200 million people around the world, with an estimated prevalence of more than 20% for individuals over 80 years old [1,2]. The most common manifestation of symptomatic PAD is intermittent claudication (IC), a painful discomfort in the leg muscles during walking that produces gait dysfunction and severe functional limitation. A small subset of PAD patients (approximately 1.3%) present with critical limb ischemia (CLI), the more severe form of PAD, manifested by ischemic rest pain and tissue loss/gangrene [3,4]. Work from several groups, including our own, has demonstrated significant degenerative changes in all the tissues of the chronically ischemic legs of patients with PAD, including skin, muscles, nerves, and subcutaneous tissues [5,6]. These changes have been best studied in the skeletal muscle of the affected limbs [7–9] and demonstrate an acquired myopathy with significant metabolic components. The biochemical characteristics of this myopathy include mitochondrial dysfunction, accumulation of metabolic intermediates, increased oxidative damage, and cytokine upregulation [1,5,6,10–14]. These metabolic myopathic changes are present in the legs of both IC and CLI patients, with the myopathy of CLI being more severe than that of IC [15]. Beyond this ischemic myopathy, PAD is also directly associated with conditions like dyslipidemia, obesity or cachexia, diabetes, and insulin resistance, all of which involve dysregulation of metabolism and energy homeostasis [16,17].

Metabolomics, the study of small-molecule metabolites in biological systems [18,19], has been increasingly applied to cardiovascular disease, leading to recent discoveries in disease-specific biomarkers and their mechanistic implications [20]. Metabolomics can detect, quantify, and identify a number of intermediate compounds and end products of cellular metabolism in body fluids, tissues, and cells, thus providing a molecular phenotype that directly reflects biochemical activity [21,22]. This strategy can therefore be useful in identifying the signature profiles of patients at different stages of a disease, and has the potential of improving our understanding of the pathogenesis, diagnosis, risk-stratification, monitoring of disease progression, personalization of treatment [23], and monitoring of the response to different therapies [24].

The clinical application of metabolomics in the study of PAD has been thus far explored with two studies evaluating near-term mortality and arterial stiffness in PAD patients. The first study showed that the ^{1}H NMR metabolomic profiles of plasma lipid molecules are correlated with mortality in PAD patients [25]. Specifically, alterations in lipoprotein and phospholipid structures were the major chemical signals that were distinct between PAD patients who died in the near-term versus those PAD patients who did not. The second study demonstrated that tyrosine and oxidized low-density lipoprotein (oxLDL) are associated with arterial stiffness in PAD patients [26]. These two seminal studies point to the potential of metabolomic profiling for providing significant insight into the pathophysiology of PAD. With this study, we aimed to expand the metabolomic mapping of PAD and to compare the circulating metabolites of patients with IC, patients with CLI, and non-PAD controls.

2. Materials and Methods

2.1. Study Approval and Subjects

Twenty-six non-PAD controls, 26 patients with IC, and 26 patients with CLI were recruited by vascular surgeons at the University of Nebraska Medical Center (UNMC, 00707), the Veterans Affairs Nebraska-Western Iowa Medical Center, and Baylor Scott and White Hospital (BSWI, 160390) under approved IRB protocols. IC or CLI diagnoses were made after examination of medical history, a physical examination, measurement of the ankle-brachial index (ABI), and computerized or standard arteriography. All non-PAD controls had normal blood flow to their legs and were undergoing operations for manifestations other than PAD (Table 1). These patients also had no history of PAD symptoms, normal lower limb pulses, normal ABIs at rest and after stress, were sex-matched, and all led sedentary lifestyles.

2.2. Sample Collection and Preparation

Blood samples were obtained in the morning after an overnight fast. In total, 30 mL of blood was obtained from each patient and was immediately centrifuged for 10 minutes, 2000× g at 4 °C. Serum was aliquoted into separate polypropylene tubes and immediately stored at −80 °C. The Biocrates AbsoluteIDQ p400 HR kit (Biocrates Life Science AG, Innsbruck, Austria) was used to analyze 100 μL of serum from each patient. Compared to manual liquid chromatography-tandem mass spectrometry (LC-MS/MS) (Applied Biosystems/MDS Sciex., Foster City, CA, USA)) analysis and other technologies, the Biocrates kit allows for higher efficiency of separation, better limits of detection, decreased consumption of solvents, and absolute quantification of metabolites [27].

2.3. Targeted Identification and Quantification

The Biocrates AbsoluteIDQ p400 HR kit was used to measure more than 400 metabolites, including 21 amino acids, 21 biogenic amines, the sum of hexoses (as one metabolite, primarily glucose), 55 acylcarnitines, 18 diglycerides, 42 triglycerides, 24 lysophosphatidylcholines, 172 phosphatidylcholines, 31 sphingomyelins, 9 ceramides, and 14 cholesteryl esters. The complete list of metabolites assayed are provided in the Supplementary Material. Serum samples, blanks, calibration standards, and quality controls were prepared according to manual instructions. LC-MS/MS was used to analyze the amino acids and biogenic amines, and the remaining metabolites were analyzed by flow injection analysis (FIA) coupled with tandem mass spectrometry. All amino acids and biogenic amines were derivatized with phenylisothiocyanate. Metabolites were quantified using internal standards and multiple reactions monitoring (MRM). The samples were analyzed on a Thermo Scientific UltiMate 3000 Rapid Separation Quaternary HPLC System (Thermo Scientific, Madison, WI, USA), connected to a QExactive™ Focus Hybrid Quadrupole-Orbitrap™ Mass Spectrometer (Thermo Scientific, Waltham, MA, USA). The chromatographic column was obtained from Biocrates. Data first underwent a pre-processing step of peak integration to determine concentration based on calibration curves using Multiquant software (version 3.0, AB Sciex, Darmstadt, Germany). Following, data were uploaded into Biocrates MetIDQ software, and concentrations of FIA-monitored metabolites were calculated in MetIDQ. The experiment was also validated using the Biocrates software (version 5, MetIDQ, Biocrates, Innsbruck, Austria).

2.4. Phenylalanine/Tyrosine Ratio and Cholesteryl Esters CE (18:1)/CE (18:2)

We calculated the ratio of phenylalanine to tyrosine as a marker of inflammation [28] and the ratio of cholesteryl esters CE (18:1)/CE (18:2) as an indicator of the ratio of acyl-coenzyme A (CoA) cholesterol acyltransferase (ACAT), a pro-atherogenic enzyme, to serum lecithin cholesterol acyltransferase (LCAT), an anti-atherogenic enzyme that facilitates reverse cholesterol transport [29]. This relationship is based on the observation that CE (18:1) is the preferred fatty acid of ACAT, and CE (18:2) is preferred by LCAT. A higher (18:1) to (18:2) ratio is therefore believed to suggest higher ACAT activity [30,31].

2.5. Statistical Analyses

Baseline characteristics between non-PAD control, IC, and CLI subjects were compared using Chi-square and Fisher exact tests for categorical variables and analysis of variance (ANOVA) for continuous variables. One-way analysis of covariance (ANCOVA) was used for the rest of the analyses controlling for age, ABI, and diabetes mellitus. MetaboAnalyst 4.0 (www.metaboanalyst.ca) (version 4, McGill University, Montreal, QC, Canada) was used for statistical analysis of the metabolites' data, processed with normalization, scaling, and filtering [32].

A one-way analysis of covariance was used to identify differences between non-PAD control, IC, and CLI groups for all the metabolites adjusting for any significant covariates, followed by *post-hoc* analyses with Bonferroni correction. Pearson correlations were calculated to evaluate associations between the ABI and the metabolites. Discriminant function models were developed to classify patients as non-PAD control, IC, or CLI. First, discriminant analysis assumptions were verified, and the multivariate data were standardized to remove units and place each variable on the same scale. A stepwise selection procedure was used to analyze variable contribution [33]. This method uses both forward selection and backward elimination procedures to determine the contribution of parameters to the discriminatory power of the model. Further, after derivation of a discriminant model, the model was used to classify new observations. A full cross-validation procedure was executed to evaluate the model performance. Cross-validation is a standard multivariate statistical method used on small data sets, validating the model by assessing stability and determining how well it will perform on other data sets [33]. During training, the cross-validation technique rotates the membership of the metabolite, verifying that the results are not dependent on calibration versus validation group membership, thus ensuring that the model is not overfitting the data. All analyses were performed using SAS statistical software (version 9.3, SAS Institute Inc., Cary, NC, USA).

3. Results

3.1. Patient Demographics

The baseline demographic and clinical characteristics are presented in Table 1. As expected, IC and CLI patients had significantly lower ABI values than non-PAD control subjects (IC: 0.51 ± 0.18 vs. CLI: 0.18 ± 0.10 vs. non-PAD controls: 1.05 ± 0.05, $p < 0.001$). IC patients were younger than CLI patients ($p = 0.044$) and CLI patients had a higher ratio of diabetes mellitus ($p = 0.005$). No other differences were found among the different groups of subjects.

Table 1. Patient demographics at enrollment. Data are shown as mean ± standard deviation.

	Non-PAD Control (n = 26)	IC (n = 26)	CLI (n = 26)	p
Age (years)	63.2 ± 7.4	62.0 ± 7.3	67.6 ± 9.9 †	**0.044**
Male sex (%)	23 (88.50)	24 (92.3)	26 (100)	0.224
Body mass index	29.6 ± 6.5	27.1 ± 9.9	27.8 ± 5.6	0.476
ABI	1.05 ± 0.05	0.51 ± 0.18 *	0.18 ± 0.10 *,†	**<0.001**
Risk factors (%)				
Tobacco use				0.073
Current	10 (38.5)	14 (53.8)	6 (23.1)	
Never	9 (34.6)	3 (11.5)	6 (23.1)	
Former	7 (26.9)	9 (34.6)	14 (53.8)	
Hypertension	17 (65.4)	22 (84.6)	23 (88.5)	0.087
Diabetes mellitus	4 (15.4)	8 (30.8)	15 (57.7) *,†	**0.005**
Coronary Artery Disease	9 (34.6)	13 (50.0)	16 (61.5)	0.150
Obesity	9 (34.6)	7 (26.9)	6 (23.1)	0.642
Dyslipidemia	21 (80.8)	19 (73.1)	16 (61.5)	0.300

Note: The values presented in the column "*p*-value" represent the overall difference between the three groups; bold font indicates a significant difference between groups ($p < 0.05$); post-hoc differences in comparisons between individual groups are denoted below as: * = significant difference from non-PAD control, $p < 0.05$; † = significant difference from IC, $p < 0.05$.

3.2. Amino Acids

Nineteen amino acids were measured for all subjects, and the phenylalanine/tyrosine ratio was also calculated. The amino acids arginine, glutamine, proline, tryptophan, and tyrosine were significantly lower in CLI patients when compared to both IC patients and non-PAD controls (Table 2). In addition, levels of histidine and ornithine were significantly lower in both CLI and IC patients compared to non-PAD controls. The phenylalanine/tyrosine ratio was significantly higher in both CLI and IC patients compared to non-PAD controls (Table 2). No other differences were observed.

Table 2. Serum amino acids concentrations of the study subjects. Data are shown as mean ± standard error (µmol/L).

	Non-PAD Control (n = 26)	IC (n = 26)	CLI (n = 26)	p
Alanine	291.3 ± 23.1	356.1 ± 22.6 *	258.6 ± 24.0 †	**0.014**
Arginine	109.1 ± 5.3	117.4 ± 5.2	89.1 ± 5.5 *,†	**0.002**
Asparagine	31.7 ± 2.1	34.1 ± 2.0	30.5 ± 2.2	0.482
Citrulline	32.7 ± 3.6	37.5 ± 3.6	34.8 ± 3.8	0.626
Glutamine	580.5 ± 20.2	583.8 ± 19.8	495.3 ± 20.9 *,†	**0.007**
Glutamate	88.0 ± 5.9	65.7 ± 5.8 *	72.7 ± 6.2	**0.029**
Glycine	271.4 ± 20.1	298.6 ± 19.7	275.1 ± 20.9	0.575
Histidine	80.4 ± 2.7	73.0 ± 2.6 *	54.6 ± 2.8 *,†	**<0.001**
Leucine	199.5 ± 12.6	203.5 ± 12.4	177.6 ± 13.1	0.352
Lysine	146.2 ± 9.2	143.3 ± 8.9	121.9 ± 9.1	0.165
Methionine	30.8 ± 7.3	50.8 ± 7.2	30.4 ± 7.6	0.083
Ornithine	70.1 ± 3.9	60.7 ± 3.9 *	53.3 ± 4.2 *	**0.016**

Table 2. Cont.

	Non-PAD Control (n = 26)	IC (n = 26)	CLI (n = 26)	p
Phenylalanine	70.1 ± 3.7	69.7 ± 3.6	64.6 ± 3.9	0.567
Proline	207.2 ± 11.3	224.4 ± 11.9	158.9 ± 11.7 *,†	**0.001**
Serine	120.4 ± 4.9	117.7 ± 4.8	105.5 ± 5.1	0.116
Threonine	122.9 ± 8.3	121.6 ± 8.2	108.8 ± 8.6	0.473
Tryptophan	48.9 ± 3.1	53.6 ± 3.1	32.5 ± 3.2 *,†	**<0.001**
Tyrosine	62.7 ± 3.2	58.1 ± 3.2	46.6 ± 3.4 *,†	**0.006**
Valine	72.9 ± 5.1	80.6 ± 5.5	71.1 ± 5.3	0.376
Phenylalanine/Tyrosine	1.05 ± 0.06	1.25 ± 0.06 *	1.45 ± 0.07 *,†	**0.001**

Note: The values presented in the column "p-value" represent the overall difference between the three groups; bold font indicates a significant difference between groups ($p < 0.05$); post-hoc differences in comparisons between individual groups are denoted below as: * = significant difference from non-PAD control, $p < 0.05$; † = significant difference from IC, $p < 0.05$.

Of the amino acids, ABI was significantly correlated with histidine ($r = 0.463$, $p < 0.001$), ornithine ($r = 0.277$, $p = 0.017$), tryptophan ($r = 0.451$, $p < 0.001$), and the phenylalanine/tyrosine ratio ($r = -0.428$, $p < 0.001$).

3.3. Acylcarnitines, Hexoses, and Biogenic Amines

Acycarnitine was significantly lower in CLI patients compared to IC patients and non-PAD controls. Acylcarnitne was also associated with the ABI ($r = 0.378$, $p = 0.001$). In contrast, hydroxypropionylcarnitine, propionylcarnitine, and tiglylcarnitine were significantly higher in both the IC and CLI patients compared to non-PAD controls (Table 3). Of the biogenic amines, only putrescine was significantly different, higher in CLI patients compared to both IC patients and non-PAD controls (Table 4). No other differences were observed.

Table 3. Concentrations of serum acylcarnitines and hexoses of the study subjects. Data are shown as mean ± standard error (μmol/L).

	Non-PAD Control (n = 26)	IC (n = 26)	CLI (n = 26)	p
Acylcarnitine	43.5 ± 2.1	40.6 ± 2.1	31.1 ± 2.2 *,†	**0.001**
Acetyl-L-carnitine	8.7 ± 1.0	9.5 ± 1.1	9.6 ± 1.1	0.816
Propionylcarnitine	0.351 ± 0.038	0.391 ± 0.037	0.294 ± 0.039	0.221
Malonylcarnitine	0.006 ± 0.001	0.006 ± 0.001	0.007 ± 0.001	0.452
Hydroxypropionylcarnitine	0.040 ± 0.002	0.046 ± 0.002 *	0.047 ± 0.002 *	**0.003**
Propenoylcarnitine	0.017 ± 0.001	0.019 ± 0.001 *	0.019 ± 0.001 *	**0.050**
Butyrylcarnitine	0.169 ± 0.023	0.168 ± 0.023	0.153 ± 0.024	0.869
Hydroxybutyrylcarnitine	0.055 ± 0.015	0.093 ± 0.015	0.084 ± 0.016	0.189
Butenylcarnitine	0.030 ± 0.001	0.030 ± 0.001	0.029 ± 0.001	0.879
Isovalerylcarnitine	0.086 ± 0.01	0.092 ± 0.01	0.066 ± 0.01	0.189
Tiglylcarnitine	0.023 ± 0.01	0.025 ± 0.01 *	0.026 ± 0.01 *	**0.038**
Hexoses	5266 ± 489	6034 ± 479	5967 ± 508	0.476

Note: The values presented in the column "p-value" represent the overall difference between the three groups; bold font indicates a significant difference between groups ($p < 0.05$); post-hoc differences in comparisons between individual groups are denoted below as * = significant difference from non-PAD control, $p < 0.05$; † = significant difference from IC, $p < 0.05$.

Table 4. Concentrations of serum biogenic amines of the study subjects. Data are shown as mean ± standard error (µmol/L). ADMA: Asymmetric dimethyl arginine. SDMA: Symmetric dimethyl arginine. Met-SO: Methionine sulfoxide. t4-OH-Pro: Trans-4-hydroxyproline.

	Control (n = 26)	IC (n = 24)	CLI (n = 24)	p
ADMA	0.549 ± 0.03	0.543 ± 0.03	0.591 ± 0.03	0.544
SDMA	0.491 ± 0.05	0.530 ± 0.04	0.614 ± 0.05	0.249
Creatinine	92.8 ± 19.6	103.1 ± 19.5	139.1 ± 19.5	0.260
Kynurenine	2.03 ± 0.203	1.90 ± 0.199	2.42 ± 0.211	0.211
Met-SO	1.35 ± 0.847	3.47 ± 0.830	2.35 ± 0.880	0.198
Putrescine	0.011 ± 0.063	0.059 ± 0.062	0.328 ± 0.066 *,†	**0.003**
Serotonin	0.503 ± 0.107	0.793 ± 0.089	0.769 ± 0.114	0.096
Spermide	0.453 ± 0.137	0.312 ± 0.134	0.440 ± 0.142	0.716
t4-OH-Pro	11.0 ± 1.68	10.8 ± 1.65	10.4 ± 1.64	0.938
Taurine	86.7 ± 10.1	88.3 ± 12.3	65.6 ± 12.2	0.370

Note: The values presented in the column "p-value" represent the overall difference between the three groups; bold font indicates a significant difference between groups ($p < 0.05$); post-hoc differences in comparisons between individual groups are denoted below as: * = significant difference from non-PAD control, $p < 0.05$; † = significant difference from IC, $p < 0.05$.

3.4. Ceramides, Cholesteryl Esters, Sphingomyelins, Diglycerides, Triglycerides, and Phosphatidylcholines

Ceramides (Cer) (40:1), (41:1), and (42:1) were significantly lower in CLI patients compared to IC patients and non-PAD controls (Table 5). Cer (43:1) and (44:0) were significantly lower in both CLI and IC patients compared to non-PAD controls. Cholesteryl esters (CE) (16:0), (17:1), (18:2), (19:2), and (20:4) were significantly lower in CLI patients compared to IC patients and non-PAD controls (Table 6). Additionally, CE (17:0) was significantly lower in both CLI and IC patients compared to non-PAD controls, and the ratio of CE (18:1)/CE (18:2) was significantly higher in both CLI and IC patients compared to non-PAD controls. (Table 6). Finally, sphingomyelins, lysophosphatidylcholines, and phosphatidylcholines were all significantly lower in CLI patients compared to both IC patients and non-PAD controls (Table 6).

Table 5. Concentrations of serum ceramides of the study subjects. Data are shown as mean ± standard error (µmol/L).

	Control (n = 26)	IC (n = 24)	CLI (n = 24)	p
Cer (34:0)	0.054 ± 0.002	0.052 ± 0.002	0.045 ± 0.02 *	**0.038**
Cer (34:1)	0.174 ± 0.011	0.182 ± 0.011	0.168 ± 0.012	0.664
Cer (38:1)	0.136 ± 0.01	0.129 ± 0.01	0.114 ± 0.01	0.356
Cer (40:1)	0.702 ± 0.05	0.688 ± 0.04	0.508 ± 0.05 *,†	**0.014**
Cer (41:1)	0.550 ± 0.04	0.530 ± 0.04	0.312 ± 0.04 *,†	**0.001**
Cer (42:1)	2.16 ± 0.151	2.31 ± 0.148	1.35 ± 0.156 *,†	**<0.001**
Cer (42:2)	1.39 ± 0.083	1.46 ± 0.081	1.19 ± 0.086	0.094
Cer (43:1)	0.555 ± 0.030	0.466 ± 0.030 *	0.300 ± 0.032 *,†	**<0.001**
Cer (44:0)	0.286 ± 0.026	0.207 ± 0.025 *	0.202 ± 0.027 *	**0.048**

Note: The values presented in the column "p-value" represent the overall difference between the three groups; bold font indicates a significant difference between groups ($p < 0.05$); post-hoc differences in comparisons between individual groups are denoted below as: * = significant difference from non-PAD control, $p < 0.05$; † = significant difference from IC, $p < 0.05$.

Table 6. Concentrations of serum cholesteryl esters (CE), sphingomyelins, diglycerides, triglycerides, and phosphatidylcholines of the study subjects. Data are shown as mean ± standard error (µmol/L).

	Control (n = 26)	IC (n = 24)	CLI (n = 24)	p
CE (16:0)	168.9 ± 10.3	160.2 ± 10.1	106.8 ± 10.7 *,†	0.001
CE (16:1)	96.6 ± 14.9	103.6 ± 14.6	69.4 ± 15.5	0.281
CE (17:0)	10.9 ± 0.56	9.4 ± 0.55 *	7.2 ± 0.58 *,†	0.001
CE (17:1)	8.82 ± 0.76	8.45 ± 0.75	5.37 ± 0.79 *,†	0.007
CE (17:2)	0.94 ± 0.16	0.85 ± 0.15	0.49 ± 0.16	0.152
CE (18:1)	244 ± 55	422 ± 54	302 ± 58	0.067
CE (18:2)	3,015 ± 176	2,791 ± 172	1,870 ± 183 *,†	<0.001
CE (18:3)	119 ± 12.3	123.2 ± 12.0	83.8 ± 12.7	0.069
CE (19:2)	5.58 ± 0.64	5.82 ± 0.63	2.69 ± 0.66 *,†	0.001
CE (19:3)	0.92 ± 0.266	1.86 ± 0.26 *	0.49 ± 0.277 †	0.002
CE (20:4)	911 ± 70	892 ± 69	662 ± 73 *,†	0.041
CE (20:5)	91.9 ± 7.5	78.5 ± 7.4	59.7 ± 7.8 *	0.022
CE (22:5)	43.3 ± 2.5	46.2 ± 2.4	37.6 ± 2.6	0.069
CE (22:6)	91.3 ± 5.9	87.0 ± 5.8	71.4 ± 6.2	0.078
CE (18:1)/CE (18:2)	0.084 ± 0.02	0.169 ± 0.02 *	0.186 ± 0.02 *	0.008
Sphingomyelins	11.1 ± 0.49	10.8 ± 0.48	8.80 ± 0.51 *,†	0.007
Diglycerides	3.48 ± 0.34	4.47 ± 0.33 *	3.07 ± 0.348 †	0.014
Triglycerides	29.1 ± 3.91	40.1 ± 3.83	27.8 ± 4.06	0.055
Lysophosphatidylcholines	4.13 ± 0.24	4.44 ± 0.24	2.66 ± 0.25 *,†	0.001
Phosphatidylcholines	10.2 ± 0.65	12.2 ± 0.63 *	8.38 ± 0.67 *,†	0.001

Note: The values presented in the column "p-value" represent the overall difference between the three groups; bold font indicates a significant difference between groups (p < 0.05); post-hoc differences in comparisons between individual groups are denoted below as: * = significant difference from non-PAD control, p < 0.05; † = significant difference from IC, p < 0.05.

Of the ceramides, ABI was significantly associated with Cer (40:1) ($r = 0.505$, $p < 0.001$), Cer (41:1) ($r = 0.541$, $p < 0.001$), Cer (42:1) ($r = 0.488$, $p < 0.001$), and Cer (43:1) ($r = 0.638$, $p < 0.001$). Of the CEs, ABI was significantly associated with CE (16:0) ($r = 0.374$, $p = 0.001$), CE(17:0) ($r = 0.482$, $p < 0.001$), CE (17:1) ($r = 0.446$, $p < 0.001$), CE (18:2) ($r = 0.447$, $p < 0.001$), and CE (20:5) ($r = 0.459$, $p < 0.001$) (Table 7).

Table 7. Pearson correlation between ankle brachial index (ABI) and metabolites.

Metabolite/Metabolite Ratio	Pearson Correlation Coefficient (r)	Significance (p)
Acylcarnitine	0.378	0.001
Histidine	0.463	<0.001
Ornithine	0.277	0.017
Trytophan	0.451	<0.001
Phenylalanine/Tyrosine	−0.428	<0.001
Cer (40:1)	0.505	<0.001
Cer (41:1)	0.541	<0.001
Cer (42:1)	0.488	<0.001
Cer (43:1)	0.638	<0.001
CE (16:0)	0.374	0.001
CE (17:0)	0.482	<0.001
CE (17:1)	0.446	<0.001
CE (18:2)	0.447	<0.001
CE (20:5)	0.459	<0.001

3.5. Discriminant Function Analysis: Non-PAD Control vs. PAD and IC vs. CLI

The discriminant function analysis model was able to correctly classify the non-PAD control and PAD patients with a 93.6% accuracy. Using a cross-validation procedure to evaluate the discriminant model performance and stability also yielded an 87.2% accuracy in patient classification. Sensitivity and specificity are two basic quantities for measuring the accuracy of a diagnostic test. The sensitivity of a diagnostic test quantifies its ability to correctly identify non-PAD control subjects without the disease and is a measure of how well the test detects non-PAD control subjects. The sensitivity of the analysis was 73.1%. The specificity refers to the ability of a test to correctly identify subjects with PAD. The specificity of the analysis was 94.2%. Figure 1A represents the plot of the original discriminant function scores, and Equation (1) represents the unstandardized canonical discriminant function coefficients:

$$Di = -2.539 - 0.057(Carnitine) + 243.9(Hydroxypropionylcarnitine) \\ -449.2(Propionylcarnitine) + 1.36\left(\frac{Phenylalanine}{Tyrosine}\right) \\ +0.006(Alanine) - 0.020(Glutamate). \quad (1)$$

The discriminant function analysis model correctly classified the IC and CLI patients with a 90.4% accuracy. Using a cross-validation procedure to evaluate the discriminant model performance and stability also yielded an 84.6% accuracy in patient classification. For this model, the sensitivity (correctly identify IC patients) was 80.8%, and the specificity (correctly identify CLI patients) was 88.5%. Figure 1B represents the plot of the original discriminant function scores, and Equation (2) represents the unstandardized canonical discriminant function coefficients:

$$Di = -3.346 + 0.032(Histidine) + 5.83(Butyrylcarnitine) + 0.051(Tryptophan) \\ -0.865(Kynurenine). \quad (2)$$

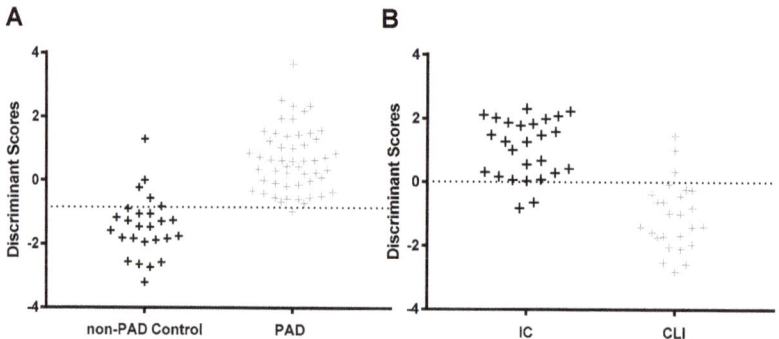

Figure 1. Discriminant function analysis model. Note: On the basis of metabolomic parameters, patient discriminant function scores can separate non-peripheral artery disease (PAD) control from PAD patients (**A**), and intermittent claudication (IC) patients from critical limb ischemia (CLI) patients (**B**).

4. Discussion

We conducted a broad metabolomic profiling of small molecules and lipids and compared metabolites between patients with IC, patients with CLI, and non-PAD controls. To our knowledge, this is the first example of metabolomics applied to evaluate patients in the two symptomatic categories of PAD versus controls. Compared to non-PAD controls, we found significant changes in the circulating levels of multiple metabolites in patients with CLI and patients with IC (Table 8). Our discriminant function analysis was able to correctly classify subjects into symptomatic PAD (both IC and CLI) vs. non-PAD controls, as well as IC vs. CLI groups, with a 93.6% and 87.2% accuracy, respectively. We found that a series of metabolites or metabolite ratios, including histidine, ornithine, phenylalanine/tyrosine, hydroxypropionyl-carnitine, propenoylcarnitine, tiglylcarnitine, Cer (43:1), Cer (44:0), CE (17:0), and CE (18:1)/CE (18:2), are significantly different in symptomatic PAD patients compared to non-PAD controls (Table 8). Several of these metabolites were also significantly correlated with the ABI, a test which may indicate PAD severity. These variables may therefore prove useful as diagnostic markers to identify PAD patients among a large population [34]. The measurement of some or a combination of these metabolites, although not currently common in most clinical laboratories, could become a much-needed, standard test for the early detection of PAD and may be incorporated into routine care cardiovascular risk prediction [35]. Additionally, the levels of a number of metabolites or metabolite ratios, including arginine, glutamine, proline, tryptophan, tyrosine, acylcarnitine, putrescine, Cer (40:1), Cer (41:1), Cer (42:1), CE (16:0), CE (17:1), CE (18:2), CE (19:2), CE (20:4), sphingomyelins, phosphatidylcholines, and lysophosphatidylcholines, were significantly different in CLI patients compared to IC patients and may prove to be valuable biomarkers for indicating which patients with IC are at higher risk of progressing to CLI. The moderate correlations between several of the ceramides and the ABI further support this. Notably, the strongest association between any of the metabolites with the ABI was that for Cer (43:1) ($r = 0.638$). It is possible that these metabolites alone or in combination can be used to produce a high-risk profile for PAD patients, allowing a personalized approach (more aggressive management, earlier intervention, and more frequent follow up for higher risk patients and less aggressive for lower risk patients) to providing care for PAD patients. The utility of such a profile should be tested in the near future as it may be able to direct the general care of PAD patients.

Table 8. List of altered metabolites in PAD.

Metabolite Class	Different in CLI	Higher/Lower	Different in PAD	Higher/Lower
Amino Acids	Arginine	↓	Histidine	↓
	Glutamine	↓	Ornithine	↓
	Proline	↓	Phenylalanine/tyrosine	↑
	Tryptophan	↓		
	Tyrosine	↓		
Acylcarnitines	Acylcarnitine	↓	Hydroxypropionyl-carnitine	↑
			Propenoylcarnitine	↑
			Tigylcarnitine	↑
Biogenic amines	Putrescine	↑		
Ceramides	Cer (40:1)	↓	Cer (43:1)	↓
	Cer (41:1)	↓	Cer (44:0)	↓
	Cer (42:1)	↓		
Cholesteryl esters, Sphingomyelin phosphatidyl-cholines	CE (16:0)	↓	CE (17:0)	↓
	CE (17:1)	↓	CE (18:1)/CE (18:2)	↑
	CE (18:2)	↓		
	CE (19:2)	↓		
	CE (20:4)	↓		
	Sphingomyelins	↓		
	Phosphatidyl-cholines	↓		
	Lysophosphatidyl-cholines	↓		

Note: "Different in CLI" are the metabolites or metabolite ratios that were significantly different between CLI patients and both IC patients and non-PAD controls. "Different in PAD" are the metabolites or metabolite ratios that were significantly different between both CLI and IC patients and non-PAD controls. ↑ represents higher and ↓ represents lower.

Several of the metabolite changes observed in this study in PAD patients are consistent with other reports from different pathologies. For example, serum levels of arginine were significantly reduced in CLI, which is consistent with several disorders linked to nitric oxide (NO) deficiency [36–38]. Likewise, ornithine, a byproduct of arginine, was reduced in both IC and CLI patients. Since NO is synthesized from L-arginine, lack of availability of this substrate is believed to be a factor that can lead to decreased plasma NO [36]. Impaired endothelial production of NO has been demonstrated in IC patients, and this may in fact be worse in patients with CLI [39]. Further, the ratio between serum levels of phenylalanine and tyrosine was elevated in PAD patients (both IC and CLI), and the phenylalanine/tyrosine ratio was inversely correlated with the ABI ($r = -0.428$). An elevated phenylalanine/tyrosine ratio has similarly been shown in different conditions associated with oxidative stress and inflammation, including acute brain ischemia [28]. This increased ratio may suggest diminished activity of the phenylalanine hydroxylase (PAH) enzyme by oxidation as well as tetrahydrobiopterin (BH4) deficiency, an essential cofactor of PAH [28]. Since BH4 is also a cofactor of nitric oxide synthase (NOS) and can be depleted by oxidative stress and inflammation, this ratio may also be indicative of NO dysregulation [39,40]

(Figure 2). Notably, oxidative stress and inflammation are hallmarks of PAD [41–44]. Several biomarkers of oxidative stress and inflammation, including malondyaldheide (MDA), 4-hydroxynonenale (4-HNE), isoprostanes, protein carbonyl groups, C-reactive protein (CRP), fibrinogen, tumor necrosis factor alpha (TNF-α), interferon-gamma (IFN-γ), monocyte chemoattractant protein-1 (MCP-1), and interleukin 6 (IL-6), have all been shown to be elevated in PAD patients in both circulation and skeletal muscle, and to increase with increasing disease stage [45].

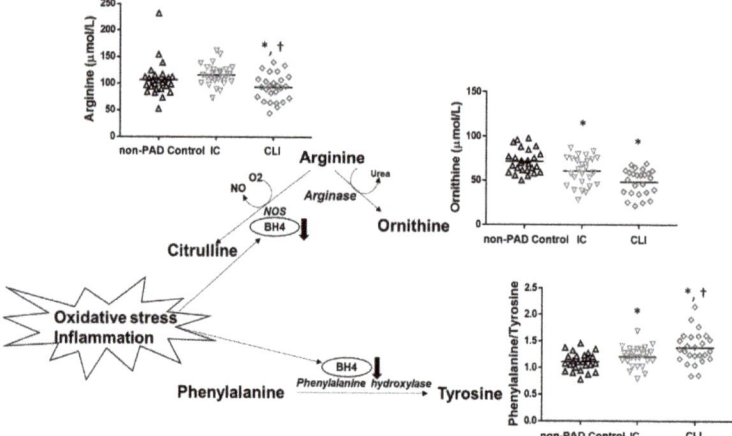

Figure 2. Potential mechanism (oxidative stress and inflammation) operating to produce decreased arginine and ornithine, increased phenylalanine to tyrosine ratio, and decreased nitric oxide bioavailability in PAD. Note: Tetrahydrobiopterin (BH4), an essential cofactor of nitric oxide synthase (NOS) and phenylalanine hydroxylase (PAH), is depleted by oxidative stress and inflammation. Therefore, reduced BH4 may explain the decreased turnover of phenylalanine to tyrosine observed in IC and CLI patients. Reduced BH4, as well as a lack of arginine availability, may play a role in impairing production of NO in PAD patients, leading to endothelial dysfunction. * denotes a significant difference from non-PAD controls and † denotes a significant difference from IC.

PAD patients also demonstrated significantly reduced levels of histidine, an amino acid with antioxidant and anti-inflammatory properties [46]. In vitro, histidine has been shown to blunt pro-inflammatory cytokine expression, and histidine supplementation has been used to control inflammation in obese patients with metabolic syndrome [47]. Patients with different conditions of enhanced oxidative stress, such as chronic kidney disease and coronary heart disease, have also been shown to have reduced levels of histidine [46,48], suggesting that depletion of histidine may indicate elevated oxidative stress, a condition that is well described in patients with IC and CLI [41,49,50].

CLI patients demonstrated further perturbations in amino acids not observed in IC patients that are also consistent with reports from other diseases and disorders. For example, reduced tryptophan levels have been associated with inflammation and immune activation, and have been shown to predict higher mortality in cardiovascular disease [51]. Specifically, reduced tryptophan may be due to accelerated conversion to kynurenine by indoleamine 2,3-dioxygenase (IDO1), which is activated by cytokines, such as tumor necrosis factor-alpha (TNF-α) and interferon gamma (IFN-γ) (Figure 3) [52]. Levels of kynurenine were also higher in CLI patients compared to both ICs and non-PAD controls, although differences were not significant statistically. In addition, glutamine levels were significantly lower in CLI patients. Reduced levels of glutamine are thought to be indicative of skeletal muscle catabolism [53]. Interestingly, CLI patients exhibit a severe myopathy that is characterized by myofiber degeneration, fibrosis, and muscle atrophy [49].

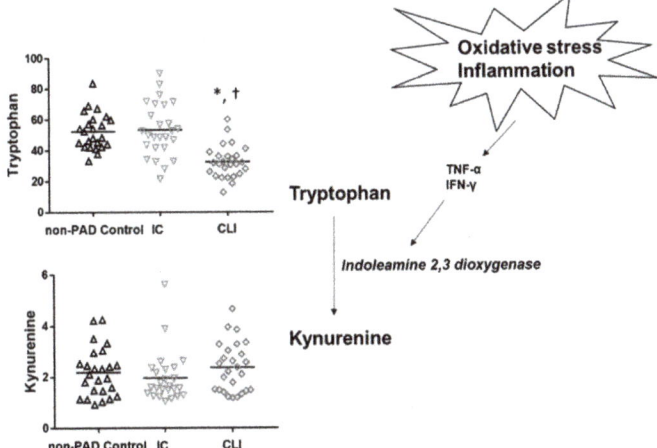

Figure 3. Potential mechanism (oxidative stress and inflammation) operating to produce decreased tryptophan levels in CLI. Note: Accelerated conversion of tryptophan to kynurenine is induced by inflammatory cytokines. Tryptophan is converted to kynurenine by the enzyme indoleamine 2,3 dioxygenase (IDO). IDO expression and activity are enhanced by tumor necrosis factor-alpha (TNF-α) and interferon-gamma (IFN-γ). Elevations in these cytokines may explain an increased conversion of tryptophan to kynurenine in CLI patients. * denotes a significant difference from non-PAD controls and † denotes a significant difference from IC.

Several carnitine esters and members of the acyl carnitines, including hydroxypropionylcarnitine, propionylcarnitine, and tiglylcarnitine, were significantly elevated in both IC and CLI patients compared to non-PAD controls. During the metabolism of amino acids, carbohydrates, and fatty acids, these substrates are converted to acyl-CoA intermediates for oxidation in the Krebs cycle. Under functional metabolism, carnitine buffers acyl-CoA by forming acylcarnitines. However, during metabolic stress, acyl-CoA is incompletely oxidized and accumulates, and transfer of the acyl group to carnitine thus leads to accumulation of acylcarnitine. Therefore, accumulation of acylcarnitines can be an indication of dysfunctional metabolism [54]. Early studies in IC patients showed that short-chain acylcarnitines accumulate in plasma, which is inversely correlated with exercise performance [55]. In skeletal muscle tissue from patients with unilateral claudication, acylcarnitine accumulation was specific only to the affected limb, and interestingly, accumulation of acylcarnitine was shown to be a better indicator of exercise performance than even the ABI [56].

In patients with more severe PAD, however, a reduction in total and acylcarnitine content has been shown [57]. This is consistent with our study, in which CLI patients also demonstrated reduced total acylcarnitine levels, which has been thought to suggest dysfunctional fatty acid β-oxidation [58,59]. Additionally, in our study there was a weak positive association between the ABI and total acylcarnitine ($r = 0.378$). The rate-limiting step in the β-oxidation of long-chain fatty acids is the conjugation of carnitine to fatty acyl coenzyme A (coA) by the enzyme carnitine palmitoyltransferase (CPT1) [60]. Since acylcarnitine levels remain constant and only levels of free carnitine are affected by factors, such as age and sex, low acylcarnitine levels may suggest metabolic alterations due to decreased levels of total carnitine, reduced CPT1 activity, or decreased availability of acyl-coA [59]. Consistent with a potentially dysfunctional fatty acid β-oxidation, muscle tissue from CLI patients demonstrates reduced expression of oxidative phosphorylation proteins, as well as lower mitochondrial respiratory capacity [15]. However, other carnitine esters, including hydroxypropionylcarnitine, propionylcarnitine, and tiglylcarnitine, were significantly elevated in both IC and CLI patients compared to non-PAD controls. Therefore, the role of carnitines in PAD warrants further exploration.

Sphingolipids are major components of cellular membranes, critical for the fluidity and architecture of the membrane. Sphingomyelins are a type of sphingolipid usually consisting of phosphocholine and ceramide. The metabolites of sphingolipids, such as ceramides, are important for regulating cell proliferation and survival, as well as the inflammatory responses [61]. In this study, levels of certain ceramides were markedly reduced in both IC and CLI patients. Further, CLI patients demonstrated reduced levels of sphingomyelins. Similar findings were reported for patients with sickle-cell disease, which is associated with a progressive vasculopathy, vascular occlusion, and endothelial dysfunction, all of which are pathophysiological aspects of PAD as well [39,62]. In contrast, however, other studies have shown that sphingomyelin and ceramides are independent risk factors for coronary heart disease and that higher levels are associated with atherosclerosis and the development of metabolic disease [63–66]. Future research is needed to clarify the alternations in sphingolipid metabolism in CLI patients. Phosphatidylcholine levels were lower in CLI patients, which is consistent with a study in patients with atherosclerosis, where reduced phosphatidylcholine levels were correlated with increased arterial stiffness, increased resting heart rate, and/or worsened endothelial function [67]. Interestingly, the hydrolysis of phosphatidylcholine to phosphatidic acid and choline is catalyzed by phospholipase D (PLD), and high PLD activity is associated with oxidative stress, inflammation, hypoxia, and atherosclerosis [68]. Finally, several cholesteryl ester species were lower in CLI patients as well. Of note, the ratio of cholesteryl ester CE (18:1)/CE (18:2) was significantly increased in both IC and CLI patients, which is consistent with findings in high fat diet-induced obese mice [29]. Since CE (18:1) is considered the preferred fatty acid of ACAT, this suggests higher ACAT activity, which is consistent with obesity and hypercholesterolemia [30].

Currently available options (risk factor management, medications, exercise therapy, and revascularization operations) for the management of PAD are limited. There are two medications, with only modest efficacy, approved for claudication, and operations are associated with considerable morbidity and poor durability [69,70]. PAD patients suffer from high rates of cardiovascular events, including stroke and myocardial infarction [71], and PAD also significantly impairs quality of life and leads to functional impairment and decline [72]. This highlights the importance of identifying novel targets for intervention for this population. In this study, we identified several metabolites that are altered in symptomatic PAD patients compared to non-PAD controls while also identifying a distinct metabolomic signature associated with only CLI [15].

One important limitation of this study is the sample size was relatively small. Thus, external validation from a larger sample could help add to the translational impact of the study results. Furthermore, while there is an emerging use of metabolomics in clinical settings, complexities and challenges, for example, related to testing strategies and quality control, limit its immediate clinical impact. Thus far, the field of metabolomics has primarily been limited to biomedical research and biomarker discovery; however, greater considerations must be taken into account for use as a clinical test. Therefore, this may also affect the translational impact of this study.

Another important point to note is the use of only serum may limit the generalizability of these findings to other fluids and tissues. Specifically, during centrifugation to separate serum from coagulated blood, platelets release proteins that include cytokines and metabolites into the serum [73]. Since anticoagulants are added before the removal of blood cells to obtain plasma, there may be differences between human plasma and serum metabolites. However, in a large study that compared metabolite concentrations between plasma and serum, although there were differences in the exact concentrations between blood matrices, the changes between groups were proportional and the correlation was high between plasma and serum [73]. This study also concluded that reproducibility was high in both plasma and serum and that either will lead to similar results in clinical studies (as long as the same matrix is used throughout), with serum potentially providing greater sensitivity in biomarker studies, thus supporting our use of serum in this study [73].

5. Conclusions

In conclusion, we identified a number of metabolites that are altered in PAD. To our knowledge, this is the first time that a complete metabolomic profiling comparing patients with different severities of PAD and non-PAD controls is presented. These data provide unique metabolomic fingerprints that may be helpful in screening for the presence of PAD, and may also be useful in risk-stratifying PAD patients and predicting their clinical outcomes. Further, these alterations provide insight into the disrupted pathways that underlie the pathophysiology of PAD and may contribute to a better understanding of the disease and to the development of novel therapeutic interventions for PAD patients.

Supplementary Materials: The following are available online at http://www.mdpi.com/2077-0383/8/9/1463/s1.

Author Contributions: A.I., M.E.F., R.L. and P.K. designed the study. M.F., R.S.S., W.T.B. and I.I.P. recruited the patients and collected the blood. I.I.P. was the Principal investigator of the clinical recruitment protocol. Metabolomics were performed and evaluated by R.L., P.K., G.P.C., E.P., I.S., C.J.M. Statistical analysis was performed and evaluated by G.R.H., A.I., and P.K., A.I., R.L., I.I.P. and P.K. wrote the manuscript and all authors contributed to the final version of the manuscript.

Funding: Research reported in this publication was supported by the National Institute on Aging of the National Institutes of Health under Award Numbers R01 AG034995, R01AG049868 and R01AG064420. The content is solely the responsibility of the authors and does not necessarily represent the official views of the National Institutes of Health. Additionally, the study was supported by the American Heart Association grant #17SDG33630088 and by the Charles and the Mary Heider Fund for Excellence in Vascular Surgery.

Acknowledgments: The authors would like to thank Alejandro Ramirez for technical support and to acknowledge the Baylor University Mass Spectrometry Center (Waco, Texas) for support during this work.

Conflicts of Interest: The authors declare no conflict of interest.

References

1. Criqui, M.H.; Aboyans, V. Epidemiology of peripheral artery disease. *Circ. Res.* **2015**, *116*, 1509–1526. [CrossRef] [PubMed]
2. Shu, J.; Santulli, G. Update on peripheral artery disease: Epidemiology and evidence-based facts. *Atherosclerosis* **2018**, *275*, 379–381. [CrossRef] [PubMed]
3. Gerhard-Herman, M.D.; Gornik, H.L.; Barrett, C.; Barshes, N.R.; Corriere, M.A.; Drachman, D.E.; Fleisher, L.A.; Fowkes, F.G.; Hamburg, N.M.; Kinlay, S.; et al. 2016 AHA/ACC Guideline on the Management of Patients With Lower Extremity Peripheral Artery Disease: Executive Summary: A Report of the American College of Cardiology/American Heart Association Task Force on Clinical Practice Guidelines. *Circulation* **2017**, *135*, e686–e725. [CrossRef] [PubMed]
4. Dua, A.; Lee, C.J. Epidemiology of Peripheral Arterial Disease and Critical Limb Ischemia. *Tech. Vasc. Interv. Radiol.* **2016**, *19*, 91–95. [CrossRef] [PubMed]
5. Pipinos, I.I.; Judge, A.R.; Selsby, J.T.; Zhu, Z.; Swanson, S.A.; Nella, A.A.; Dodd, S.L. The myopathy of peripheral arterial occlusive disease: Part 1. Functional and histomorphological changes and evidence for mitochondrial dysfunction. *Vasc. Endovascular Surg.* **2007**, *41*, 481–489. [CrossRef] [PubMed]
6. Pipinos, I.I.; Judge, A.R.; Selsby, J.T.; Zhu, Z.; Swanson, S.A.; Nella, A.A.; Dodd, S.L. The myopathy of peripheral arterial occlusive disease: Part 2. Oxidative stress, neuropathy, and shift in muscle fiber type. *Vasc. Endovascular Surg.* **2008**, *42*, 101–112. [CrossRef] [PubMed]
7. Brass, E.P.; Hiatt, W.R. Acquired skeletal muscle metabolic myopathy in atherosclerotic peripheral arterial disease. *Vasc. Med.* **2000**, *5*, 55–59. [CrossRef]
8. Rontoyanni, V.G.; Nunez Lopez, O.; Fankhauser, G.T.; Cheema, Z.F.; Rasmussen, B.B.; Porter, C. Mitochondrial Bioenergetics in the Metabolic Myopathy Accompanying Peripheral Artery Disease. *Front. Physiol.* **2017**, *8*, 141. [CrossRef]
9. Brass, E.P. Skeletal muscle metabolism as a target for drug therapy in peripheral arterial disease. *Vasc. Med.* **1996**, *1*, 55–59. [CrossRef]
10. Gardner, A.W.; Killewich, L.A.; Katzel, L.I.; Womack, C.J.; Montgomery, P.S.; Otis, R.B.; Fonong, T. Relationship between free-living daily physical activity and peripheral circulation in patients with intermittent claudication. *Angiology* **1999**, *50*, 289–297. [CrossRef]

11. Gardner, A.W.; Montgomery, P.S.; Scott, K.J.; Afaq, A.; Blevins, S.M. Patterns of ambulatory activity in subjects with and without intermittent claudication. *J. Vasc. Surg.* **2007**, *46*, 1208–1214. [CrossRef] [PubMed]
12. Myers, S.A.; Johanning, J.M.; Stergiou, N.; Lynch, T.G.; Longo, G.M.; Pipinos, I.I. Claudication distances and the Walking Impairment Questionnaire best describe the ambulatory limitations in patients with symptomatic peripheral arterial disease. *J. Vasc. Surg.* **2008**, *47*, 550–555. [CrossRef] [PubMed]
13. McDermott, M.M.; Ferrucci, L.; Guralnik, J.; Tian, L.; Liu, K.; Hoff, F.; Liao, Y.; Criqui, M.H. Pathophysiological changes in calf muscle predict mobility loss at 2-year follow-up in men and women with peripheral arterial disease. *Circulation* **2009**, *120*, 1048–1055. [CrossRef] [PubMed]
14. McDermott, M.M.; Guralnik, J.M.; Ferrucci, L.; Tian, L.; Pearce, W.H.; Hoff, F.; Liu, K.; Liao, Y.; Criqui, M.H. Physical activity, walking exercise, and calf skeletal muscle characteristics in patients with peripheral arterial disease. *J. Vasc. Surg.* **2007**, *46*, 87–93. [CrossRef] [PubMed]
15. Ryan, T.E.; Yamaguchi, D.J.; Schmidt, C.A.; Zeczycki, T.N.; Shaikh, S.R.; Brophy, P.; Green, T.D.; Tarpey, M.D.; Karnekar, R.; Goldberg, E.J.; et al. Extensive skeletal muscle cell mitochondriopathy distinguishes critical limb ischemia patients from claudicants. *JCI Insight* **2018**, *3*. [CrossRef] [PubMed]
16. Shammas, N.W. Epidemiology, classification, and modifiable risk factors of peripheral arterial disease. *Vasc. Health Risk Manag.* **2007**, *3*, 229–234. [CrossRef]
17. Selvin, E.; Erlinger, T.P. Prevalence of and risk factors for peripheral arterial disease in the United States: Results from the National Health and Nutrition Examination Survey, 1999–2000. *Circulation* **2004**, *110*, 738–743. [CrossRef]
18. Garcia-Fontana, B.; Morales-Santana, S.; Diaz Navarro, C.; Rozas-Moreno, P.; Genilloud, O.; Vicente Perez, F.; Perez del Palacio, J.; Munoz-Torres, M. Metabolomic profile related to cardiovascular disease in patients with type 2 diabetes mellitus: A pilot study. *Talanta* **2016**, *148*, 135–143. [CrossRef]
19. Trabado, S.; Al-Salameh, A.; Croixmarie, V.; Masson, P.; Corruble, E.; Feve, B.; Colle, R.; Ripoll, L.; Walther, B.; Boursier-Neyret, C.; et al. The human plasma-metabolome: Reference values in 800 French healthy volunteers; impact of cholesterol, gender and age. *PLoS ONE* **2017**, *12*, e0173615. [CrossRef]
20. Shah, S.H.; Kraus, W.E.; Newgard, C.B. Metabolomic profiling for the identification of novel biomarkers and mechanisms related to common cardiovascular diseases: Form and function. *Circulation* **2012**, *126*, 1110–1120. [CrossRef]
21. Fiehn, O.; Kopka, J.; Dormann, P.; Altmann, T.; Trethewey, R.N.; Willmitzer, L. Metabolite profiling for plant functional genomics. *Nat. Biotechnol.* **2000**, *18*, 1157–1161. [CrossRef] [PubMed]
22. Liu, X.; Xu, G. Recent advances in using mass spectrometry for mitochondrial metabolomics and lipidomics—A review. *Anal. Chim. Acta* **2018**, *1037*, 3–12. [CrossRef] [PubMed]
23. Dona, A.C.; Coffey, S.; Figtree, G. Translational and emerging clinical applications of metabolomics in cardiovascular disease diagnosis and treatment. *Eur. J. Prev. Cardiol.* **2016**, *23*, 1578–1589. [CrossRef] [PubMed]
24. Puchades-Carrasco, L.; Pineda-Lucena, A. Metabolomics Applications in Precision Medicine: An Oncological Perspective. *Curr. Top. Med. Chem.* **2017**, *17*, 2740–2751. [CrossRef] [PubMed]
25. Huang, C.C.; McDermott, M.M.; Liu, K.; Kuo, C.H.; Wang, S.Y.; Tao, H.; Tseng, Y.J. Plasma metabolomic profiles predict near-term death among individuals with lower extremity peripheral arterial disease. *J. Vasc. Surg.* **2013**, *58*, 989–996.e1. [CrossRef] [PubMed]
26. Zagura, M.; Kals, J.; Kilk, K.; Serg, M.; Kampus, P.; Eha, J.; Soomets, U.; Zilmer, M. Metabolomic signature of arterial stiffness in male patients with peripheral arterial disease. *Hypertens Res.* **2015**, *38*, 840–846. [CrossRef]
27. Saleem, F.; Bouatra, S.; Guo, A.C.; Psychogios, N.; Mandal, R.; Dunn, S.M.; Ametaj, B.N.; Wishart, D.S. The bovine ruminal fluid metabolome. *Metabolomics* **2013**, *9*, 360–378. [CrossRef]
28. Ormstad, H.; Verkerk, R.; Sandvik, L. Serum Phenylalanine, Tyrosine, and their Ratio in Acute Ischemic Stroke: On the Trail of a Biomarker? *J. Mol. Neurosci.* **2016**, *58*, 102–108. [CrossRef]
29. Eisinger, K.; Liebisch, G.; Schmitz, G.; Aslanidis, C.; Krautbauer, S.; Buechler, C. Lipidomic analysis of serum from high fat diet induced obese mice. *Int. J. Mol. Sci.* **2014**, *15*, 2991–3002. [CrossRef]
30. Roberts, C.K.; Liang, K.; Barnard, R.J.; Kim, C.H.; Vaziri, N.D. HMG-CoA reductase, cholesterol 7alpha-hydroxylase, LDL receptor, SR-B1, and ACAT in diet-induced syndrome X. *Kidney Int.* **2004**, *66*, 1503–1511. [CrossRef]

31. Lee, R.G.; Kelley, K.L.; Sawyer, J.K.; Farese, R.V., Jr.; Parks, J.S.; Rudel, L.L. Plasma cholesteryl esters provided by lecithin:cholesterol acyltransferase and acyl-coenzyme a:cholesterol acyltransferase 2 have opposite atherosclerotic potential. *Circ. Res.* **2004**, *95*, 998–1004. [CrossRef] [PubMed]
32. Xia, J.; Wishart, D.S. Web-based inference of biological patterns, functions and pathways from metabolomic data using MetaboAnalyst. *Nat. Protoc.* **2011**, *6*, 743. [CrossRef] [PubMed]
33. Hastie, T.; Tibshirani, R.; Friedman, J.H. *The Elements of Statistical Learning: Data Mining, Inference, and Prediction*, 2nd ed.; Springer: New York, NY, USA, 2009.
34. Krishna, S.M.; Moxon, J.V.; Golledge, J. A review of the pathophysiology and potential biomarkers for peripheral artery disease. *Int. J. Mol. Sci.* **2015**, *16*, 11294–11322. [CrossRef] [PubMed]
35. Joosten, M.M.; Pai, J.K.; Bertoia, M.L.; Gansevoort, R.T.; Bakker, S.J.; Cooke, J.P.; Rimm, E.B.; Mukamal, K.J. beta2-microglobulin, cystatin C, and creatinine and risk of symptomatic peripheral artery disease. *J. Am. Heart Assoc.* **2014**, *3*. [CrossRef] [PubMed]
36. Hess, S.; Baker, G.; Gyenes, G.; Tsuyuki, R.; Newman, S.; Le Melledo, J.M. Decreased serum L-arginine and L-citrulline levels in major depression. *Psychopharmacology (Berl.)* **2017**, *234*, 3241–3247. [CrossRef] [PubMed]
37. Morris, C.R.; Poljakovic, M.; Lavrisha, L.; Machado, L.; Kuypers, F.A.; Morris, S.M., Jr. Decreased arginine bioavailability and increased serum arginase activity in asthma. *Am. J. Respir. Crit. Care Med.* **2004**, *170*, 148–153. [CrossRef] [PubMed]
38. Kayanoki, Y.; Kawata, S.; Yamasaki, E.; Kiso, S.; Inoue, S.; Tamura, S.; Taniguchi, N.; Matsuzawa, Y. Reduced nitric oxide production by L-arginine deficiency in lysinuric protein intolerance exacerbates intravascular coagulation. *Metab. Clin. Exp.* **1999**, *48*, 1136–1140. [CrossRef]
39. Ismaeel, A.; Brumberg, R.S.; Kirk, J.S.; Papoutsi, E.; Farmer, P.J.; Bohannon, W.T.; Smith, R.S.; Eidson, J.L.; Sawicki, I.; Koutakis, P. Oxidative Stress and Arterial Dysfunction in Peripheral Artery Disease. *Antioxidants* **2018**, *7*, 145. [CrossRef]
40. Barbato, J.E.; Tzeng, E. Nitric oxide and arterial disease. *J. Vasc. Surg.* **2004**, *40*, 187–193. [CrossRef]
41. Koutakis, P.; Ismaeel, A.; Farmer, P.; Purcell, S.; Smith, R.S.; Eidson, J.L.; Bohannon, W.T. Oxidative stress and antioxidant treatment in patients with peripheral artery disease. *Physiol. Rep.* **2018**, *6*, e13650. [CrossRef]
42. Brevetti, G.; Giugliano, G.; Brevetti, L.; Hiatt, W.R. Inflammation in peripheral artery disease. *Circulation* **2010**, *122*, 1862–1875. [CrossRef] [PubMed]
43. Ozaki, Y.; Imanishi, T.; Akasaka, T. Inflammatory Biomarkers in Peripheral Artery Disease: Diagnosis, Prognosis, and Therapeutic Challenges. *Curr. Med. Chem.* **2015**, *22*, 2744–2753. [CrossRef]
44. Signorelli, S.S.; Anzaldi, M.; Fiore, V. Inflammation in peripheral arterial disease (PAD). *Curr. Pharm. Des.* **2012**, *18*, 4350–4357. [CrossRef] [PubMed]
45. Signorelli, S.S.; Scuto, S.; Marino, E.; Xourafa, A.; Gaudio, A. Oxidative Stress in Peripheral Arterial Disease (PAD) Mechanism and Biomarkers. *Antioxidants* **2019**, *8*, 367. [CrossRef] [PubMed]
46. Yu, B.; Li, A.H.; Muzny, D.; Veeraraghavan, N.; de Vries, P.S.; Bis, J.C.; Musani, S.K.; Alexander, D.; Morrison, A.C.; Franco, O.H.; et al. Association of Rare Loss-Of-Function Alleles in HAL, Serum Histidine: Levels and Incident Coronary Heart Disease. *Circ. Cardiovasc. Genet.* **2015**, *8*, 351–355. [CrossRef]
47. Feng, R.N.; Niu, Y.C.; Sun, X.W.; Li, Q.; Zhao, C.; Wang, C.; Guo, F.C.; Sun, C.H.; Li, Y. Histidine supplementation improves insulin resistance through suppressed inflammation in obese women with the metabolic syndrome: A randomised controlled trial. *Diabetologia* **2013**, *56*, 985–994. [CrossRef] [PubMed]
48. Watanabe, M.; Suliman, M.E.; Qureshi, A.R.; Garcia-Lopez, E.; Barany, P.; Heimburger, O.; Stenvinkel, P.; Lindholm, B. Consequences of low plasma histidine in chronic kidney disease patients: Associations with inflammation, oxidative stress, and mortality. *Am. J. Clin. Nutr.* **2008**, *87*, 1860–1866. [CrossRef] [PubMed]
49. Weiss, D.J.; Casale, G.P.; Koutakis, P.; Nella, A.A.; Swanson, S.A.; Zhu, Z.; Miserlis, D.; Johanning, J.M.; Pipinos, I.I. Oxidative damage and myofiber degeneration in the gastrocnemius of patients with peripheral arterial disease. *J. Transl. Med.* **2013**, *11*, 230. [CrossRef] [PubMed]
50. Koutakis, P.; Weiss, D.J.; Miserlis, D.; Shostrom, V.K.; Papoutsi, E.; Ha, D.M.; Carpenter, L.A.; McComb, R.D.; Casale, G.P.; Pipinos, I.I. Oxidative damage in the gastrocnemius of patients with peripheral artery disease is myofiber type selective. *Redox. Biol.* **2014**, *2*, 921–928. [CrossRef]
51. Murr, C.; Grammer, T.B.; Kleber, M.E.; Meinitzer, A.; Marz, W.; Fuchs, D. Low serum tryptophan predicts higher mortality in cardiovascular disease. *Eur. J. Clin. Investig.* **2015**, *45*, 247–254. [CrossRef]

52. Schrocksnadel, K.; Wirleitner, B.; Winkler, C.; Fuchs, D. Monitoring tryptophan metabolism in chronic immune activation. *Clin. Chim. Acta* **2006**, *364*, 82–90. [CrossRef] [PubMed]
53. Kinscherf, R.; Hack, V.; Fischbach, T.; Friedmann, B.; Weiss, C.; Edler, L.; Bartsch, P.; Droge, W. Low plasma glutamine in combination with high glutamate levels indicate risk for loss of body cell mass in healthy individuals: The effect of N-acetyl-cysteine. *J. Mol. Med.* **1996**, *74*, 393–400. [CrossRef] [PubMed]
54. Bieber, L.L. Carnitine. *Annu. Rev. Biochem.* **1988**, *57*, 261–283. [CrossRef] [PubMed]
55. Hiatt, W.R.; Nawaz, D.; Brass, E.P. Carnitine metabolism during exercise in patients with peripheral vascular disease. *J. Appl. Physiol.* **1987**, *62*, 2383–2387. [CrossRef] [PubMed]
56. Hiatt, W.R.; Wolfel, E.E.; Regensteiner, J.G.; Brass, E.P. Skeletal muscle carnitine metabolism in patients with unilateral peripheral arterial disease. *J. Appl. Physiol.* **1992**, *73*, 346–353. [CrossRef] [PubMed]
57. Brevetti, G.; Angelini, C.; Rosa, M.; Carrozzo, R.; Perna, S.; Corsi, M.; Matarazzo, A.; Marcialis, A. Muscle carnitine deficiency in patients with severe peripheral vascular disease. *Circulation* **1991**, *84*, 1490–1495. [CrossRef] [PubMed]
58. Saiki, S.; Hatano, T.; Fujimaki, M.; Ishikawa, K.I.; Mori, A.; Oji, Y.; Okuzumi, A.; Fukuhara, T.; Koinuma, T.; Imamichi, Y.; et al. Decreased long-chain acylcarnitines from insufficient beta-oxidation as potential early diagnostic markers for Parkinson's disease. *Sci. Rep.* **2017**, *7*, 7328. [CrossRef]
59. Miyagawa, T.; Miyadera, H.; Tanaka, S.; Kawashima, M.; Shimada, M.; Honda, Y.; Tokunaga, K.; Honda, M. Abnormally low serum acylcarnitine levels in narcolepsy patients. *Sleep* **2011**, *34*, 349–353A. [CrossRef]
60. McGarry, J.D.; Brown, N.F. The mitochondrial carnitine palmitoyltransferase system. From concept to molecular analysis. *Eur. J. Biochem.* **1997**, *244*, 1–14. [CrossRef]
61. Presa, N.; Gomez-Larrauri, A.; Rivera, I.G.; Ordonez, M.; Trueba, M.; Gomez-Munoz, A. Regulation of cell migration and inflammation by ceramide 1-phosphate. *Biochim. Biophys. Acta* **2016**, *1861*, 402–409. [CrossRef]
62. Aslan, M.; Kirac, E.; Kaya, S.; Ozcan, F.; Salim, O.; Kupesiz, O.A. Decreased Serum Levels of Sphingomyelins and Ceramides in Sickle Cell Disease Patients. *Lipids* **2018**, *53*, 313–322. [CrossRef] [PubMed]
63. Jiang, X.C.; Paultre, F.; Pearson, T.A.; Reed, R.G.; Francis, C.K.; Lin, M.; Berglund, L.; Tall, A.R. Plasma sphingomyelin level as a risk factor for coronary artery disease. *Arterioscl. Throm. Vas.* **2000**, *20*, 2614–2618. [CrossRef] [PubMed]
64. Nelson, J.; Jiang, X.C.; Tabas, I.; Tall, A.; Shea, S. Plasma sphingomyelin and subclinical atherosclerosis: Findings from the multi-ethnic study of atherosclerosis. *Am. J. Epidemiol.* **2006**, *163*, 903–912. [CrossRef] [PubMed]
65. Hanamatsu, H.; Ohnishi, S.; Sakai, S.; Yuyama, K.; Mitsutake, S.; Takeda, H.; Hashino, S.; Igarashi, Y. Altered levels of serum sphingomyelin and ceramide containing distinct acyl chains in young obese adults. *Nutr. Diabetes* **2014**, *4*, e141. [CrossRef] [PubMed]
66. Holland, W.L.; Summers, S.A. Sphingolipids, insulin resistance, and metabolic disease: New insights from in vivo manipulation of sphingolipid metabolism. *Endocr. Rev.* **2008**, *29*, 381–402. [CrossRef] [PubMed]
67. Paapstel, K.; Kals, J.; Eha, J.; Tootsi, K.; Ottas, A.; Piir, A.; Jakobson, M.; Lieberg, J.; Zilmer, M. Inverse relations of serum phosphatidylcholines and lysophosphatidylcholines with vascular damage and heart rate in patients with atherosclerosis. *Nutr. Metab. Cardiovasc. Dis.* **2018**, *28*, 44–52. [CrossRef] [PubMed]
68. Tappia, P.S.; Dent, M.R.; Dhalla, N.S. Oxidative stress and redox regulation of phospholipase D in myocardial disease. *Free Radic. Biol. Med.* **2006**, *41*, 349–361. [CrossRef]
69. Roset, P.N. Systematic review of the efficacy of cilostazol, naftidrofuryl oxalate and pentoxifylline for the treatment of intermittent claudication (Br J Surg 2012; 99: 1630–1638). *Br. J. Surg.* **2013**, *100*, 1838. [CrossRef]
70. Nowygrod, R.; Egorova, N.; Greco, G.; Anderson, P.; Gelijns, A.; Moskowitz, A.; McKinsey, J.; Morrissey, N.; Kent, K.C. Trends, complications, and mortality in peripheral vascular surgery. *J. Vasc. Surg.* **2006**, *43*, 205–216. [CrossRef]
71. Steg, P.G.; Bhatt, D.L.; Wilson, P.W.; D'Agostino, R., Sr.; Ohman, E.M.; Rother, J.; Liau, C.S.; Hirsch, A.T.; Mas, J.L.; Ikeda, Y.; et al. One-year cardiovascular event rates in outpatients with atherothrombosis. *JAMA* **2007**, *297*, 1197–1206. [CrossRef]

72. McDermott, M.M. Functional impairment in peripheral artery disease and how to improve it in 2013. *Curr. Cardiol. Rep.* **2013**, *15*, 347. [CrossRef] [PubMed]
73. Yu, Z.H.; Kastenmuller, G.; He, Y.; Belcredi, P.; Moller, G.; Prehn, C.; Mendes, J.; Wahl, S.; Roemisch-Margl, W.; Ceglarek, U.; et al. Differences between Human Plasma and Serum Metabolite Profiles. *PLoS ONE* **2011**, *6*. [CrossRef] [PubMed]

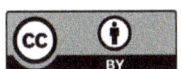

© 2019 by the authors. Licensee MDPI, Basel, Switzerland. This article is an open access article distributed under the terms and conditions of the Creative Commons Attribution (CC BY) license (http://creativecommons.org/licenses/by/4.0/).

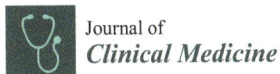

Article

Angiopoietins, Vascular Endothelial Growth Factors and Secretory Phospholipase A_2 in Ischemic and Non-Ischemic Heart Failure

Gilda Varricchi [1,2,3,4,*], **Stefania Loffredo** [1,2,3,4,*], **Leonardo Bencivenga** [1,5], **Anne Lise Ferrara** [1,2,3], **Giuseppina Gambino** [1], **Nicola Ferrara** [1], **Amato de Paulis** [1,2,3], **Gianni Marone** [1,2,3,4] **and Giuseppe Rengo** [1,6]

1. Department of Translational Medical Sciences, University of Naples Federico II, 80100 Naples, Italy; leonardobencivenga@gmail.com (L.B.); Anneliseferrara@gmail.com (A.L.F.); pina.gambino@gmail.com (G.G.); nicferra@unina.it (N.F.); depaulis@unina.it (A.d.P.); marone@unina.it (G.M.); giuseppe.rengo@unina.it (G.R.)
2. Center for Basic and Clinical Immunology Research (CISI), University of Naples Federico II, 80100 Naples, Italy
3. World Allergy Organization (WAO), Center of Excellence, 80100 Naples, Italy
4. Institute of Experimental Endocrinology and Oncology "G. Salvatore" (IEOS), National Research Council (CNR), 80100 Naples, Italy
5. Department of Advanced Biomedical Sciences, University of Naples Federico II, 80100 Naples, Italy
6. Istituti Clinici Scientifici Maugeri SpA Società Benefit, Via Bagni Vecchi, 1, 82037 Telese BN, Italy
* Correspondence: gildanet@gmail.com (G.V.); stefanialoffredo@hotmail.com (S.L.)

Received: 1 June 2020; Accepted: 17 June 2020; Published: 19 June 2020

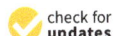

Abstract: Heart failure (HF) is a growing public health burden, with high prevalence and mortality rates. In contrast to ischemic heart failure (IHF), the diagnosis of non-ischemic heart failure (NIHF) is established in the absence of coronary artery disease. Angiopoietins (ANGPTs), vascular endothelial growth factors (VEGFs) and secretory phospholipases A_2 (sPLA$_2$s) are proinflammatory mediators and key regulators of endothelial cells. In the present manuscript, we analyze the plasma concentrations of angiogenic (ANGPT1, ANGPT2, VEGF-A) and lymphangiogenic (VEGF-C, VEGF-D) factors and the plasma activity of sPLA$_2$ in patients with IHF and NIHF compared to healthy controls. The concentrations of ANGPT1, ANGPT2 and their ratio significantly differed between HF patients and healthy controls. Similarly, plasma levels of VEGF-D and sPLA$_2$ activity were higher in HF as compared to controls. Concentrations of ANGPT2 and the ANGPT2/ANGPT1 ratio (an index of vascular permeability) were increased in NIHF patients. VEGF-A and VEGF-C concentrations did not differ among the three examined groups. Interestingly, VEGF-D was selectively increased in IFH patients compared to controls. Plasma activity of sPLA$_2$ was increased in IHF and NIHF patients compared to controls. Our results indicate that several regulators of vascular permeability and smoldering inflammation are specifically altered in IHF and NIHF patients. Studies involving larger cohorts of these patients will be necessary to demonstrate the clinical implications of our findings.

Keywords: angiopoietins; heart failure; VEGFs; sPLA$_2$; IHF; NIHF

1. Introduction

Heart failure (HF) represents a growing public health burden with an estimated prevalence in Europe and United States ranging from 0.4% to 2% [1]. Based on left ventricle ejection fraction (EF), HF recognizes three different classes: HF with a reduced EF (HFrEF with an EF < 40%); HF with a mild-range EF (HFmEF with an EF between 40% and 49%), and HF with a preserved EF

(HFpEF with an EF ≥ 50%) [2]. Although classification systems for HF causes are largely debated, within HFrEF ischemic heart disease represents the most common cause of myocardial injury and ventricular dysfunction, leading in a significant percentage of cases to post-ischemic heart failure (IHF). Non-ischemic HF (NIHF), which accounts for less than 50% of HFrEF cases, comprises all the remaining heterogeneous HF etiologies ranging from valvular diseases to toxic damage, up to metabolic conditions and genetic cardiomyopathies [3]. In a significant percentage (≅ 30%) of HF patients, the etiology remains undetermined, and the syndrome is referred to as "idiopathic HF" [4]. Identification of these diverse etiologies may be obtained through a complex diagnostic workup, frequently without a relevant therapeutic implication. Neurohormonal and inflammatory activation are widely recognized as playing a pivotal role in HF onset and progression, irrespective of etiology [5]. Despite advances in management and therapies, the prognosis in HF patients remains poor, thus a deeper knowledge of the molecular mechanisms involved in the complex HF pathophysiology are needed for the identification of novel therapeutic targets and biomarkers to stratify prognosis and drive decision-making processes [6]. To this aim, several investigations have focused their attention on inflammatory and neurohormonal molecules.

The angiopoietin (ANGPT) family is an important group of factors, specific for vascular endothelium, whose functions are mediated through two tyrosine kinase receptors, Tie1 and Tie2 [7]. The ANGPT-Tie ligand-receptor system exerts a key role in regulating vascular integrity [8,9]. Beside their roles in the modulation of angiogenesis [10,11] and lymphangiogenesis [12,13], ANGPTs also regulate inflammation in several disorders, including cardiovascular diseases [9,14,15]. Angiopoietin-1 (ANGPT1), produced by peri-endothelial mural cells (pericytes) [16] and immune cells [17,18], is a potent agonist of Tie2 receptor on endothelial cells [11,19]. ANGPT1 is an anti-inflammatory molecule [20] that maintains vascular integrity [21,22]. ANGPT2, stored in Weibel–Palade bodies in endothelial cells [23], is rapidly released in response to various stimuli [24]. ANGPT2 is considered a pro-inflammatory molecule [25,26] and inhibits ANGPT1/Tie2 interaction [10,27], resulting in vascular instability and leakage [26].

Elevated ANGPT2 levels have been found in patients with acute coronary syndrome [28,29], hypertension [30,31], congestive heart failure [32] and congenital heart failure [33]. ANGPT2 has been proposed as a prognostic biomarker of adverse cardiovascular events in myocardial infarction [34] and after percutaneous coronary intervention (PCI) [35,36]. In contrast, ANGPT1 plays a protective role in rodent models of vascular injuries [37,38].

The vascular endothelial growth factor (VEGF) family includes VEGF-A, VEGF-B, VEGF-C, and VEGF-D [39]. VEGFs and their receptors on blood and lymphatic endothelial cells play intricate roles in initiating and promoting inflammatory and tumor angiogenesis [40]. VEGF-A, the most potent proangiogenic factor [41], was first identified for its permeabilizing activity and named vascular permeability factor (VPF) [42]. VEGF-A and VEGF-B are key regulators of systemic and cardiac angiogenesis [39,43,44]. VEGF-C and VEGF-D are the most important modulators of inflammatory and tumor lymphangiogenesis [45,46]. Several studies have found elevated levels of circulating VEGF-A in patients with myocardial infarction [28,47–50]. By contrast, the roles of VEGF-A [32] VEGF-C and VEGF-D in HF remain unclear or totally unexplored.

Phospholipases A_2 (PLA$_2$) hydrolyze the fatty acids from membrane phospholipids releasing arachidonic acid and lysophospholipids [51–54]. Secreted or extracellular PLA$_2$ (sPLA$_2$) modulate vascular permeability [55] and activate inflammatory cells [53,56,57]. Circulating levels of sPLA$_2$ predict coronary events in patients with coronary artery disease [58] and in apparently healthy men and women [59]. Serum sPLA$_2$ levels also predict long-term mortality for HF after myocardial infarction [60]. Intima of coronary atherosclerotic lesions of patients with angina or myocardial infarction express sPLA$_2$ [61] and elevated serum levels of sPLA$_2$ increase the risk of early atherosclerosis [62].

While some studies are available on ANGPTs, VEGF isoforms, and sPLA$_2$ involvement in ischemic heart disease, very little is known in the clinical setting of IHF and, to the best of our knowledge, no data are available in NIHF. Thus, the aim of the present study is to evaluate the circulating levels of ANGPTs, VEGFs, and sPLA$_2$ activity in HF patients, particularly comparing the ischemic and non-ischemic etiologies.

2. Materials and Methods

2.1. Study Population

Patients with systolic HF were enrolled at the Department of Translational Medical Sciences of the University of Naples Federico II. Inclusion criteria were: age ≥ 18 years, diagnosis of HF from at least six months [2], left ventricular ejection fraction (LVEF) ≤ 45%, stable clinical condition during the month prior to inclusion, and an optimal guideline-based pharmacotherapy from at least three months, if not contraindicated. Exclusion criteria were represented by chronic obstructive pulmonary disease (COPD), diabetes mellitus (DM), immune disorders (rheumatoid arthritis, systemic lupus erythematosus, systemic sclerosis, Sjögren syndrome, vasculitis, psoriatic arthritis, dermatomyositis, ankylosing spondylitis), malignancies (also past), severe obesity as assessed through a body mass index (BMI) more than 32 kg/m^2, dialysis-dependent kidney failure, acute coronary syndromes and/or coronary revascularization in the previous 6 months, and an inability to provide informed consent. The control group was represented by subjects without HF and in accordance with the exclusion criteria. All patients underwent medical history evaluation and collection of demographic/clinical data, including age, gender, BMI, cardiovascular risk factors, and comorbidities. Clinical examination, transthoracic echocardiography, and serum BNP determination were performed at the time of the enrolment. The HF population was subsequently divided into two groups based on the HF etiology: ischemic HF (IHF) or non-ischemic HF (NIHF). Ischemic etiology was established based on either previous documented myocardial infarction and/or significant coronary artery disease with indication of cardiac revascularization. This study was approved by the Ethics Committee of the University of Naples Federico II (protocol number 124/17). All participants were carefully informed and signed a written consent to participate in the study.

2.2. Blood Sampling

Blood was collected during routine diagnostic procedures, scheduled in the course of hospital access for the determination of the main blood parameters (blood counts, biochemical. and coagulation profile), and the remaining plasma sample was labeled with a code that was documented into a data sheet. As mentioned above, blood samples were collected in patients under stable clinical conditions, strictly verifying all inclusion and exclusion criteria. The samples were collected by means of a clean venipuncture and minimal stasis using sodium citrate 3.2% as anticoagulant. After centrifugation (2000 g for 20 min at 22 °C), the plasma was divided into aliquots and stored at −80 °C until used. Technicians who performed the assays were blinded to the patients' history.

2.3. Assays of ANGPTs and VEGFs

Plasma levels of ANGPT1, ANGPT2, VEGF-A, VEGF-C, and VEGF-D were measured using commercially available ELISA kits (R&D System, Minneapolis, MN, USA) according to the manufacturer's instructions. The ELISA sensitivity was 156.25–10,000 pg/mL for ANGPT1, 31.1–4000 pg/mL for ANGPT2, 31.1–2000 pg/mL for VEGF-A, 62.5–4000 pg/mL for VEGF-C, and 31.3–2000 pg/mL for VEGF-D.

2.4. Assay of Phospholipase A$_2$ Activity

PLA$_2$ activity in the plasma of patients and healthy controls was measured by Life Technologies EnzChek (Milan, Italy) phospholipase A$_2$ assay. Briefly, a PLA$_2$ substrate cocktail consisting of 7-hydroxycoumarinyl-arachidonate (0.3 mM), 7-hydroxycoumarinyl-linolenate (0.3 mM), hydroxycoumarinyl 6-heptenoate (0.3 mM), dioleoylphosphatidylcholine (DOPC) (10 mM), and dioleoylphosphatidylglycerol (DOPG) (10 mM) was prepared in ethanol. Liposomes were formed by gradually adding 77 μL substrate/lipid cocktail to 10 mL of PLA$_2$ buffer (50 mM Tris–HCl, 100 mM NaCl, 1 mM CaCl$_2$) while stirring rapidly over 1 min using a magnetic stirrer. Fluorescence (excitation at 360 nm and emission at 460 nm) was measured and specific activity [relative fluorescent units (RFU)/mL] for each sample was calculated. Plasma (50 µL) was added to 96-well plates, and PLA_2 activity was evaluated by adding 50 µL of substrate cocktail.

2.5. Statistical Analysis

The sample size was determined by the primary outcome, which was defined through a comparison of ANGPT2 plasma levels between HF patients and healthy controls in a 1:1 ratio. Assuming an alpha error equal to 5% and a statistical power equal to 80%, considering the mean concentrations of ANGPT2 to be approximately 500 pg/mL in healthy individuals, according to previous evidence [32], a minimum of 70 patients (35 per group) are necessary to capture as significant a 40% difference in ANGPT2 plasma concentration between controls and HF patients. Data were analyzed with the GraphPad Prism 7 software package. Data were tested for normality using a D'Agostino-Pearson normality test. If normality was not rejected at the 0.05 significance level, we used parametric tests. Otherwise, for not-normally distributed data we used nonparametric tests. Statistical analysis was performed using a Student's *t*-test or one-way ANOVA and Bonferroni's multiple comparison test, as indicated in the figure legends. Correlations between two variables were assessed by Spearman's rank correlation analysis and reported as coefficients of correlation (*r*). Plasma concentrations of VEGFs and ANGPTs and activity of $sPLA_2$ are shown as the median (horizontal black line), the 25th and 75th percentiles (boxes), and the 5th and 95th percentiles (whiskers) of HF, NIHF, and IHF patients and controls. Statistically significant differences were accepted when the *p*-value was ≤0.05.

3. Results

3.1. Clinical and Demographic Characteristics of Overall Population

Table 1 summarizes the demographic and clinical characteristics of patients with IHF, NIHF, and matched healthy controls. The overall study population comprised 43 patients suffering from HF and 42 healthy donors, carefully selected according to inclusion/exclusion criteria. Patients with HF were divided into two groups based on HF etiology [3]: 19 with IHF and 25 with NIHF. Both HF groups were homogeneous in age, gender, BNP levels and LVEF. As expected, IHF and NIHF showed higher BNP levels and lower LVEFs compared to healthy controls (Table 1).

Table 1. Demographic and clinical characteristics of patients with ischemic heart failure (IHF) or non-ischemic heart failure (NIHF) and healthy controls.

Characteristics	Healthy Controls (N = 42)	IHF (N = 19)	NIHF (N = 25)
Age-median years (range)	75.5 (46–98)	77 (54–87)	65 (45–87)
Gender male-no. (%)	16 (38.1)	12 (63.1)	16 (64)
BMI (kg/m^2)	25.2 ± 4.1	25.4 ± 3.0	25.5 ± 4.2
Caucasian (%)	100	100	100
BNP (pg/mL)	50.6 ± 32.0	1025.8 ± 733.3 *	968.6 ± 802.2 *
Leukocytes (×10^3/mm^3)	7.2 ± 2.5	8.6 ± 4.1	7.9 ± 3.0
GFR (mL/min)	71.2 ± 23.3	48.5 ± 24.3	69.6 ± 32.4
LVEF (%)	61.6 ± 5.8	34.3 ± 6.9 *	34.6 ± 7.4 *

Data are expressed as the mean ± standard deviation of the mean (BMI, BNP, Leukocytes, GFR, LVEF) or median value (Age). IHF: ischemic heart failure; NIHF: non-ischemic heart failure; BNP: B-type natriuretic peptide; GFR: glomerular filtration rate (assessed through CKD-EPI equation); LVEF: left ventricular ejection fraction. * $p < 0.01$ when compared to healthy controls analyzed by one-way ANOVA and Bonferroni's multiple comparison test.

3.2. Plasma Concentrations of ANGPT1, ANGPT2, VEGF-A, VEGF-C, VEGF-D and PLA_2 Activity in Healthy Controls and HF Patients

As shown in Figure 1, lower concentrations of ANGPT1 and higher levels of ANGPT2 and ANGPT2/ANGPT1 ratios were detected in subjects suffering from HF compared to healthy controls. No differences were observed in plasma concentrations of VEGF-A and VEGF-C in the two groups (Figure 2). Otherwise, HF patients presented higher concentrations of VEGF-D compared to controls. Moreover, HF was associated with higher PLA_2 activity (Figure 3).

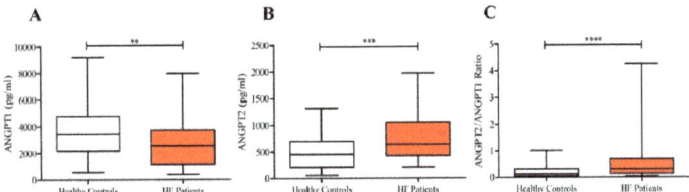

Figure 1. (**A**) Plasma concentrations of angiopoietin-1 (ANGPT1) in heart failure (HF) patients and in healthy controls; (**B**) Plasma concentrations of ANGPT2 in HF patients and in healthy controls; (**C**) ANGPT2/ANGPT1 ratio in HF patients and in healthy controls. Data are shown as the median (horizontal block line), the 25th and 75th percentiles (boxes), and the 5th and 95th percentiles (whiskers) (statistical analysis was performed by a Student's *t*-test). ** $p < 0.01$; *** $p < 0.001$; **** $p < 0.0001$.

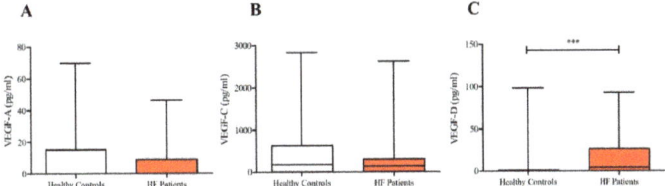

Figure 2. (**A**) Plasma concentrations of vascular endothelial growth factor-A (VEGF-A) in heart failure (HF) patients and in healthy controls; (**B**) plasma concentrations of VEGF-C in HF patients and in healthy controls; (**C**) plasma concentrations of VEGF-D in HF patients and in healthy controls. Data are shown as the median (horizontal block line), the 25th and 75th percentiles (boxes), and the 5th and 95th percentiles (whiskers) (statistical analysis was performed by a Student's *t*-test). *** $p < 0.001$.

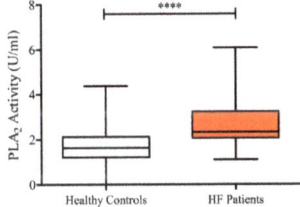

Figure 3. Plasma concentrations of sPLA$_2$ activity in HF patients and in healthy controls. Data are shown as the median (horizontal block line), the 25th and 75th percentiles (boxes), and the 5th and 95th percentiles (whiskers) (statistical analysis was performed by a Student's *t*-test). **** $p < 0.0001$.

3.3. Plasma Concentrations of ANGPT1, ANGPT2 and Their Ratio in Patients With IHF and NIHF

The concentrations of ANGPT1 were significantly reduced in NIHF compared to controls (Figure 4A). By contrast, the plasma concentrations of ANGPT2 were selectively increased only in NIHF compared to healthy donors (Figure 4B). Similarly, the ANGPT2/ANGPT1 ratio, a parameter of vascular permeability [63], was also increased only in NIHF patients compared to controls (Figure 4C). Importantly, no difference emerged between IHF group and healthy controls in the ANGPT2/ANGPT1 ratio, whereas there was a significant difference between the ANGPT2/ANGPT1 ratio in NIHF vs. IHF (Figure 4C). There were no differences in ANGPT1 or ANGPT2 between male and female values in both controls and patients. Moreover, the age of patients and the concentrations of the different mediators examined did not correlate.

3.4. Plasma Concentrations of VEGF-A, VEGF-C, and VEGF-C in Patients with IHF and NIHF

VEGF-A is a powerful permeability [42] and angiogenic mediator [41]. Elevated concentrations of VEGF-A have been found in patients with acute myocardial ischemia [28,47–50]. By contrast, the role of

VEGF-A in chronic heart failure remains unclear [32]. We found that the mean plasma concentrations of VEGF-A were essentially similar in patients with different types of HF and controls (Figure 5A).

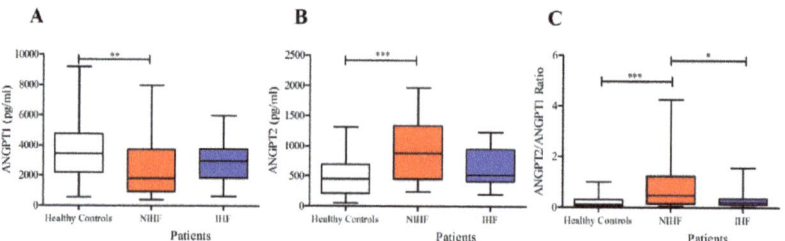

Figure 4. (**A**) Plasma concentrations of angiopoietin-1 (ANGPT1) in ischemic (IHF) and non-ischemic (NIHF) patients, and in healthy controls; (**B**) plasma concentrations of ANGPT2 in IHF and NIHF patients, and in healthy controls; (**C**) ANGPT2/ANGPT1 ratio in IHF and NIHF patients, and in healthy controls. Data are shown as the median (horizontal block line), the 25th and 75th percentiles (boxes), and the 5th and 95th percentiles (whiskers) (statistical analysis was performed by one-way ANOVA and Bonferroni's multiple comparison test). * $p < 0.05$; ** $p < 0.01$; *** $p < 0.001$.

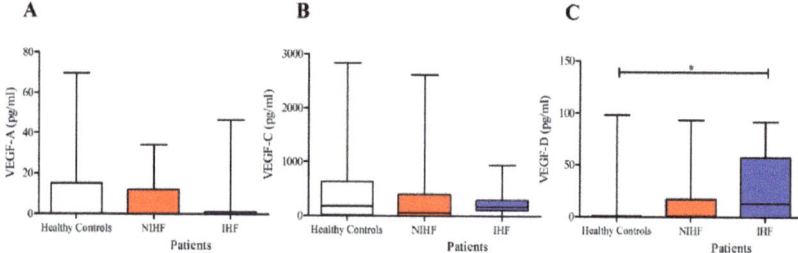

Figure 5. (**A**) Plasma concentrations of VEGF-A in IHF and NIHF patients and in healthy controls; (**B**) plasma concentrations of VEGF-C in IHF and NIHF patients and in healthy controls; (**C**) plasma concentrations of VEGF-D in IHF and NIHF patients and in healthy controls. Data are shown as the median (horizontal block line), the 25th and 75th percentiles (boxes), and the 5th and 95th percentiles (whiskers) (statistical analysis was performed by one-way ANOVA and Bonferroni's multiple comparison test). * $p < 0.05$

VEGF-C and VEGF-D are known to play a major role as lymphangiogenic factors acting on VEGF receptor 3 (VEGFR3) on lymphatic endothelial cells (LECs) [64,65]. More recently, it has been shown that these factors are produced by human cardiac mast cells [43] and, under certain circumstances, can exert a protective effect in cardiovascular disorders [66,67]. In addition, it has been demonstrated that VEGF-C and VEGF-D can exert different effects [45]. The mean plasma concentrations of VEGF-C did not differ in patients with different HF types and controls (Figure 5B). In contrast, the plasma concentrations of VEGF-D were increased in IHF patients compared to healthy controls (Figure 5C). There were no differences in VEGF-A, VEGF-C, and VEGF-D concentrations between male and female values in either controls and patients. Moreover, the age of patients and the concentrations of VEGFs examined did not correlate.

3.5. Plasma Concentrations of sPLA$_2$ Activity in Patients With IHF and NIHF

sPLA$_2$ modulates vascular permeability [55] and promotes inflammation [52,53,56]. Circulating sPLA$_2$ levels increase the risk of early atherosclerosis [62] and predict long-term mortality of HF after myocardial infarction [60]. Figure 6 shows that plasma activity of sPLA$_2$ activity was significantly increased in both groups of HF patients compared to healthy controls. There was no differences in sPLA$_2$ activity between male and female values in both controls and patients. Moreover, the age of patients and the concentration of sPLA$_2$ activity did not correlate.

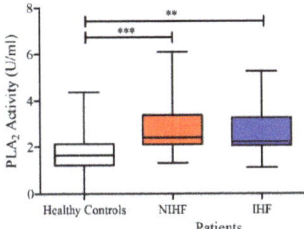

Figure 6. Plasma concentrations of sPLA$_2$ activity in IHF and NIHF patients and in healthy controls. Data are shown as the median (horizontal block line), the 25th and 75th percentiles (boxes), and the 5th and 95th percentiles (whiskers) (statistical analysis was performed by one-way ANOVA and Bonferroni's multiple comparison test). ** $p < 0.01$; *** $p < 0.001$.

3.6. Correlations between ANGPT1 or ANGPT2 Plasma Concentrations and sPLA$_2$ Activity in Patients with IHF and NIHF

As shown in Figure 7, there was an inverse correlation between plasma concentrations of ANGPT2 and ANGPT1 (Figure 7A) and sPLA$_2$ activity and ANGPT1 (Figure 7B) in NIHF patients. Furthermore, a positive correlation between PLA$_2$ activity and ANGPT2 was detected in NIHF (Figure 7C). No correlation was observed between sPLA$_2$ activity and the ANGPT2/ANGPT1 ratio in NIHF.

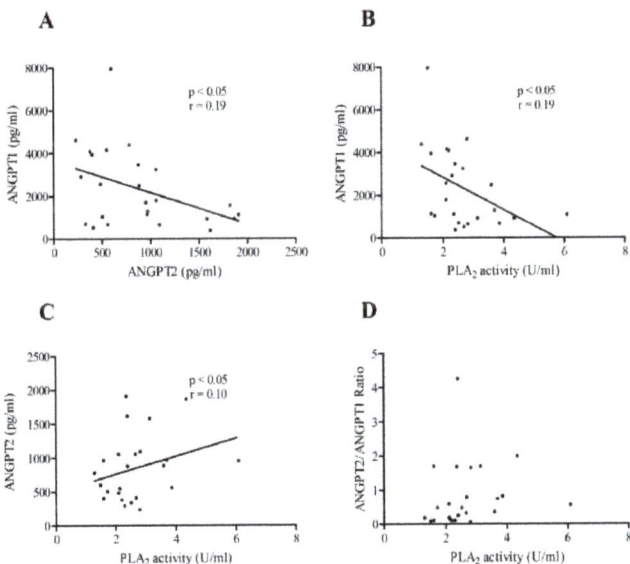

Figure 7. (**A**) Correlations between the plasma concentrations of ANGPT2 and ANGPT1 in NIHF patients; (**B**) correlation between circulating sPLA$_2$ activity and the concentration of ANGPT1 in NIHF patients; (**C**) correlation between the plasma concentration of sPLA$_2$ activity and ANGPT2 in NIHF patients; (**D**) correlation between the plasma concentration of sPLA$_2$ activity and the ANGPT2/ANGPT1 ratio in NIHF patients. Spearman's correlation coefficients (r) were calculated and are shown in the panels.

Contrariwise, no correlations were observed among the plasma concentrations of ANGPT1 and BNP, ANGPT2 and BNP, and sPLA$_2$ activity and BNP in NIHF patients. Similarly, no correlations were found between plasma concentrations of ANGPT1, ANGPT2, and sPLA$_2$ activity vs. LVEF in patients with IHF or NIHR.

4. Discussion

To the best of our knowledge, this is the first study reporting significant and distinct alterations of plasma concentrations from three different classes of proinflammatory mediators that are essential for vascular development, integrity and remodeling (i.e., angiopoietins, VEGFs, and secretory phospholipase A$_2$) in patients with two forms of HF (i.e., ischemic and non-ischemic).

ANGPTs bind to and activate the Tie2 receptor on endothelial cells [9,27]. ANGPT1, produced by periendothelial mural cells [16] acts as a vascular stabilizer by affecting the connections between endothelial cells and the cytoskeleton [68]. In contrast, ANGPT2, produced by blood endothelial cells [23], is rapidly released from Wiebel–Palade bodies in response to various stimuli [24]. ANGPT2 also binds to Tie2 [27] and antagonizes ANGPT1-mediated Tie2 phosphorylation, thereby inducing vascular instability and leakage [25,26,69]. In addition, ANGPT2 is an important permeability [63,70] and proinflammatory mediator [16].

Elevated circulating levels of ANGPT2 have been reported in acute coronary syndromes [28,29], and this mediator has been proposed as a negative prognostic marker after myocardial infarction [34] and PCI [35,36]. ANGPT2 is associated with a greater risk of cardiovascular mortality in the general population [71], as well as with higher mortality in patients suffering from myocardial infarction and cardiogenic shock [29,72]. A recent report demonstrates that ANGPT2 is highly expressed in endothelial cells at the border of the infarct area after ischemic injury in mice [15]. In the remodeling phase after myocardial infarction, endothelial- and macrophage-derived ANGPT2 promotes abnormal vascular remodeling and exacerbates inflammation. In contrast, ANGPT1 plays a protective role in preclinical models of vascular injury [37,38] and exerts anti-inflammatory effects [20].

Our study shows that HF is associated with reduced ANGPT1 plasma concentrations, increased ANGPT2 levels, and an increased ANGPT2/ANGPT1 ratio as compared with healthy controls. Of importance, different alterations of ANGPT1 and ANGPT2 expression have been detected in patients with IHF and NIHF. For instance, plasma levels of ANGPT1 are significantly decreased only in NIHF, but not in IHF patients compared to controls. Contrarywise, circulating levels of ANGPT2 are increased in NIHF, but not in IHF patients compared to healthy donors. Moreover, the ANGPT2/ANGPT1 ratio, an index of vascular permeability [63], was exclusively increased only in NIHF patients.

We did not find a correlation between plasma concentrations of ANGPT1 or ANGPT2 and BNP in either IHF or NIHF patients. In contrast, a recent study reported a significant correlation between serum concentrations of ANGPT2 and NT-proBNP in more than 200 patients that had undergone diagnostic cardiac catheterization [73]. Several explanations can justify these apparently different results. The latter study included patients with (54%) or without coronary artery disease, as well as with comorbidities (e.g., diabetes, hypertension) that may have influenced the results. In our study, the population of IHF and NIHF participants was selectively included, and patients with comorbidities were not selected. Although the two examined cohorts were rather small, the patients examined in our study were very homogeneous for the principal clinical and demographic features.

Our results may have clinical implications for patients suffering from HF. First, if confirmed in larger cohorts, the evaluation of plasma concentrations of ANGPT1, ANGPT2, and their ratio may be useful in the identification of different pathophysiological patterns underlying ischemic and non-ischemic HF. Second, the unique role of the ANGPTs/Tie2 signaling pathway in vascular stability suggests that it could serve as a target for therapeutic intervention in diseases whose pathophysiology comprises the alteration of vascular integrity [27], such as HF. Recently, it has been demonstrated that ANGPT2 inhibition, through an anti-ANGPT2 blocking antibody, substantially alleviated autoimmune inflammation [70]. Importantly, specific ANGPT2 deletion or the use of an anti-ANGPT2 antibody markedly reduced cardiac hypoxia, proinflammatory macrophage polarization, adverse vascular remodeling, and the consequent progression of HF after myocardial infarction in mice [15]. The results of the latter study contribute to elucidating the roles of ANGPT2 in the pathogenesis of post-ischemic cardiovascular remodeling. Finally, these fascinating experimental results designate ANGPT2 as a promising therapeutic target to prevent/ameliorate HF.

VEGF-A is a powerful permeability factor [42] and a potent proangiogenic and proinflammatory mediator [41,74]. Although several clinical studies have found elevated circulating levels of VEGF-A in myocardial infarction [28,47–50], the role of this mediator in HF still remains poorly elucidated. Our results show that, differently from acute vascular injuries, plasma levels of VEGF-A are not altered in the overall HF population or in either IHF or NIHF patients. Thus, our results suggest that this mediator could play different roles in an acute vs. chronic setting of myocardial ischemia.

VEGF-C and VEGF-D are major lymphangiogenic factors produced by human macrophages [52,75] and cardiac mast cells [43]. In a mouse model of HF, VEGF-C and VEGF-D were upregulated in the early stages of disease, with levels returning afterwards to baseline [76]. Levels of VEGF-C have been reported as elevated in patients with ischemic or non-ischemic cardiomyopathy [77]. An increased level of VEGF-D was found in an animal model of ischemic cardiomyopathy [78] as well as in human atherosclerotic lesions [79]. Recent evidence indicates that lymphangiogenesis [66] and VEGF-C improve cardiac functions after experimental myocardial infarction [80]. Our results indicate that the plasma concentrations of VEGF-C were similar in patients with HF (IHF and NIHF) and controls. Interestingly, the circulating concentrations of VEGF-D were increased in HF patients compared to controls, but significant differences were exclusively detected in IHF patients. The differential alterations of VEGF-C and VEGF-D in these patients is intriguing but not surprising. In fact, recent evidence demonstrates that VEGF-C and VEGF-D can differently modulate the immune system [45]. The possible role of VEGF-D in HF patients deserves further investigations.

PLA_2 activity was found increased in plasma from both groups of HF patients compared to healthy controls. PLA_2 modulates endothelial cell migration and vascular permeability in vitro and in humans [53,55–57,81]. Previous studies have demonstrated that circulating levels of $sPLA_2$ predict coronary events in patients with coronary artery disease [58], as well as in apparently healthy men and women [59]. Moreover, serum $sPLA_2$ levels also predicts readmission for HF after myocardial infarction [60]. More recently, elevated circulatory levels of $sPLA_2$ were associated with risk of early atherosclerosis [62]. Our study is, to our knowledge, the first to demonstrate that high plasma concentrations of PLA_2 activity can be found in HF patients, both with an ischemic and non-ischemic etiology.

Along with the epidemiologic transition of global population, the pathophysiology of HF has changed over time. According to the Framingham Heart Study, hypertension represented the most frequently associated condition in HF patients, irrespective of LVEF [82]. It is widely recognized that coronary heart disease represents the predominant cause of HFrEF [83]. Coronary stenosis-dependent cardiomyocyte hypoxia, through inadequate oxygen supply to metabolic needs and leading to ventricular dysfunction, may be the result of both acute and chronic cardiac ischemia. Indeed, in acute coronary syndromes, a sudden drop in myocardial perfusion rapidly determines cardiomyocyte injury. In the setting of chronic ischemia there is often an imbalance between coronary blood flow and augmented demand due to progressive atherosclerosis, especially under stress. This leads over time to hibernation, stunning, and secondary myocardial remodeling, resulting in reduced cardiac output [84].

NIHF pathophysiology is more heterogeneous due to several etiologic factors that are sometimes concurrent. The most relevant causes of NIHF are represented by primary valvular diseases, arterial hypertension, microbial cardiomyopathy, DM, toxic agents (drugs or alcohol), and genetic cardiomyopathies. Once all the listed factors have been excluded, idiopathic HF is the resulting diagnosis [85]. In NIHF there is a primary injury in the cardiomyocyte structure and function that manifests in cell apoptosis and a consequent substitution with fribotic tissue, without alteration in coronary flow.

However, independently from ischemic or non-ischemic etiology, all patients suffering from systolic HF present reduction of LVEF, maladaptive LV remodeling, and similar clinical presentations including dyspnea and hydro-saline retention. Our results identify an HF-dependent impact on the expression levels of several vascular permeability and inflammatory mediators, with different patterns in the clinical setting of NIHF and IHF that potentially reflect the above-mentioned pathophysiological differences.

Several immune cells produce sPLA$_2$ [86–88], ANGPTs [15,17,18,24,70,89], VEGF-A [43,52,74,90], and VEGF-C/VEGF-D [52,74,91]. In this study, we did not address the issue of the contribution of different cells to the increased plasma levels of these powerful inflammatory mediators observed in patients with IHF or NIHF. ANGPT2 appears to be a potential therapeutic option in experimental heart failure [15]. Future studies with the aim of identifying the cellular sources of these powerful mediators could lead to the identification of novel and selective therapeutic targets in IHF and NIHF patients.

The limited number of subjects enrolled represented the main limitation of the present investigation. However, it is important to point out that in order to identify specific differences between NIHF and IHF the study protocol included stringent exclusion criteria to reduce potential interference with the inflammatory and angiogenic patterns explored in the study. Indeed, very common comorbidities such as COPD, DM, immune disorders, malignancies, and severe obesity were excluded from the study. As a consequence, the patients examined were very homogeneous, but rather small. The results of this preliminary study will have to be extended in a future multicenter trial examining larger cohorts of IHF and NIHF patients.

5. Conclusions

In the present study we demonstrated that the ANGPT system is selectively modulated in NIHF patients, with an increased ANGPT2/ANGPT1 ratio compared to IHF and controls, whereas VEGF-D was exclusively augmented in IHF patients. In contrast, sPLA2 activity was increased in both IHF and NIHF patients compared to healthy controls. To the best of our knowledge this represents the first evidence reporting that several regulators of vascular permeability and inflammation is specifically altered in patients with IHF and NIHF, paving the way for the identification of new molecular mechanisms underlying HF pathophysiology and novel therapeutic targets.

Author Contributions: Conceptualization, G.V., S.L., G.M., and G.R.; methodology, S.L., L.B., G.G., and G.R.; software, S.L. and A.L.F.; validation, G.V., G.M., and G.R.; formal analysis, G.V., S.L., L.B., and A.L.F.; investigation, G.V., S.L., and A.L.F.; resources, G.M.; data curation, G.V., S.L., L.B., A.L.F., and G.R.; writing—original draft preparation, G.V., S.L., L.B., and G.M.; writing—review and editing, G.V., S.L., N.F., A.d.P., G.M., and G.R.; supervision, G.V., S.L., G.M., and G.R.; project administration, G.V., S.L., G.M., and G.R.; funding acquisition, G.M. All authors have read and agreed to the published version of the manuscript.

Funding: This work was supported in part by grants from the CISI-Lab Project (University of Naples Federico II), TIMING Project (Regione Campania), and Campania Bioscience.

Acknowledgments: The authors apologize to the many researchers who contributed importantly to this field and whose works were not cited because of space and citation restrictions. Leonardo Bencivenga has been supported by a research grant provided by the Cardiopath PhD program. The authors thank Gjada Criscuolo for a critical reading of the manuscript.

Conflicts of Interest: All authors declare no conflicts of interest.

Abbreviations

ACE	angiotensin-converting enzyme
ANGPT	angiopoietin
ARB	angiotensin receptor blocker
BMI	body mass index
BNP	B-type natriuretic peptide
COPD	chronic obstructive pulmonary disease
DM	diabetes mellitus

DOPC	dioleoylphosphatidylcholine
DOPG	dioleoyphosphatidylglycerol
EF	ejection fraction
GFR	glomerular filtration rate
HF	heart failure
IHF	ischemic heart failure
LVEF	left ventricular ejection fraction
NIHF	non-ischemic heart failure
PLA$_2$	phospholipase A$_2$
VEGF	vascular endothelial growth factor
VEGFR	vascular endothelial growth factor receptor

References

1. Hershberger, R.E.; Hedges, D.J.; Morales, A. Dilated cardiomyopathy: The complexity of a diverse genetic architecture. *Nat. Rev. Cardiol.* **2013**, *10*, 531–547. [CrossRef] [PubMed]
2. Ponikowski, P.; Voors, A.A.; Anker, S.D.; Bueno, H.; Cleland, J.G.F.; Coats, A.J.S.; Falk, V.; Gonzalez-Juanatey, J.R.; Harjola, V.P.; Jankowska, E.A.; et al. 2016 ESC Guidelines for the diagnosis and treatment of acute and chronic heart failure: The Task Force for the diagnosis and treatment of acute and chronic heart failure of the European Society of Cardiology (ESC) Developed with the special contribution of the Heart Failure Association (HFA) of the ESC. *Eur. Heart J.* **2016**, *37*, 2129–2200. [PubMed]
3. McNally, E.M.; Mestroni, L. Dilated cardiomyopathy: Genetic determinants and mechanisms. *Circ. Res.* **2017**, *121*, 731–748. [CrossRef] [PubMed]
4. Bozkurt, B.; Colvin, M.; Cook, J.; Cooper, L.T.; Deswal, A.; Fonarow, G.C.; Francis, G.S.; Lenihan, D.; Lewis, E.F.; McNamara, D.M.; et al. Current diagnostic and treatment strategies for specific dilated cardiomyopathies: A scientific statement from the american heart association. *Circulation* **2016**, *134*, e579–e646. [CrossRef] [PubMed]
5. Hartupee, J.; Mann, D.L. Neurohormonal activation in heart failure with reduced ejection fraction. *Nat. Rev. Cardiol.* **2017**, *14*, 30–38. [CrossRef]
6. Braunwald, E. Biomarkers in heart failure. *N. Engl. J. Med.* **2008**, *358*, 2148–2159. [CrossRef]
7. Wang, Q.; Zhao, Z.; Zhang, X.; Lu, C.; Ren, S.; Li, S.; Guo, J.; Liao, P.; Jiang, B.; Zheng, Y. Identifying microRNAs and their editing sites in Macaca mulatta. *Cells* **2019**, *8*, 682. [CrossRef]
8. Fiedler, U.; Augustin, H.G. Angiopoietins: A link between angiogenesis and inflammation. *Trends Immunol.* **2006**, *27*, 552–558. [CrossRef]
9. Akwii, R.G.; Sajib, M.S.; Zahra, F.T.; Mikelis, C.M. Role of Angiopoietin-2 in vascular physiology and pathophysiology. *Cells* **2019**, *8*, 471. [CrossRef]
10. Maisonpierre, P.C.; Suri, C.; Jones, P.F.; Bartunkova, S.; Wiegand, S.J.; Radziejewski, C.; Compton, D.; McClain, J.; Aldrich, T.H.; Papadopoulos, N.; et al. Angiopoietin-2, a natural antagonist for Tie2 that disrupts in vivo angiogenesis. *Science* **1997**, *277*, 55–60. [CrossRef]
11. Suri, C.; Jones, P.F.; Patan, S.; Bartunkova, S.; Maisonpierre, P.C.; Davis, S.; Sato, T.N.; Yancopoulos, G.D. Requisite role of angiopoietin-1, a ligand for the TIE2 receptor, during embryonic angiogenesis. *Cell* **1996**, *87*, 1171–1180. [CrossRef]
12. Fagiani, E.; Lorentz, P.; Kopfstein, L.; Christofori, G. Angiopoietin-1 and -2 exert antagonistic functions in tumor angiogenesis, yet both induce lymphangiogenesis. *Cancer Res.* **2011**, *71*, 5717–5727. [CrossRef] [PubMed]
13. Schulz, P.; Fischer, C.; Detjen, K.M.; Rieke, S.; Hilfenhaus, G.; von Marschall, Z.; Bohmig, M.; Koch, I.; Kehrberger, J.; Hauff, P.; et al. Angiopoietin-2 drives lymphatic metastasis of pancreatic cancer. *FASEB J.* **2011**, *25*, 3325–3335. [CrossRef] [PubMed]
14. Eklund, L.; Kangas, J.; Saharinen, P. Angiopoietin-Tie signalling in the cardiovascular and lymphatic systems. *Clin. Sci. (Lond.)* **2017**, *131*, 87–103. [CrossRef] [PubMed]
15. Lee, S.J.; Lee, C.K.; Kang, S.; Park, I.; Kim, Y.H.; Kim, S.K.; Hong, S.P.; Bae, H.; He, Y.; Kubota, Y.; et al. Angiopoietin-2 exacerbates cardiac hypoxia and inflammation after myocardial infarction. *J. Clin. Investig.* **2018**, *128*, 5018–5033. [CrossRef]
16. Daneman, R.; Zhou, L.; Kebede, A.A.; Barres, B.A. Pericytes are required for blood-brain barrier integrity during embryogenesis. *Nature* **2010**, *468*, 562–566. [CrossRef]

17. Prevete, N.; Staiano, R.I.; Granata, F.; Detoraki, A.; Necchi, V.; Ricci, V.; Triggiani, M.; De Paulis, A.; Marone, G.; Genovese, A. Expression and function of Angiopoietins and their tie receptors in human basophils and mast cells. *J. Biol. Regul. Homeost. Agents* **2013**, *27*, 827–839.
18. Fang, H.Y.; Hughes, R.; Murdoch, C.; Coffelt, S.B.; Biswas, S.K.; Harris, A.L.; Johnson, R.S.; Imityaz, H.Z.; Simon, M.C.; Fredlund, E.; et al. Hypoxia-inducible factors 1 and 2 are important transcriptional effectors in primary macrophages experiencing hypoxia. *Blood* **2009**, *114*, 844–859. [CrossRef]
19. Davis, S.; Aldrich, T.H.; Jones, P.F.; Acheson, A.; Compton, D.L.; Jain, V.; Ryan, T.E.; Bruno, J.; Radziejewski, C.; Maisonpierre, P.C.; et al. Isolation of angiopoietin-1, a ligand for the TIE2 receptor, by secretion-trap expression cloning. *Cell* **1996**, *87*, 1161–1169. [CrossRef]
20. Gamble, J.R.; Drew, J.; Trezise, L.; Underwood, A.; Parsons, M.; Kasminkas, L.; Rudge, J.; Yancopoulos, G.; Vadas, M.A. Angiopoietin-1 is an antipermeability and anti-inflammatory agent in vitro and targets cell junctions. *Circ. Res.* **2000**, *87*, 603–607. [CrossRef]
21. Jeansson, M.; Gawlik, A.; Anderson, G.; Li, C.; Kerjaschki, D.; Henkelman, M.; Quaggin, S.E. Angiopoietin-1 is essential in mouse vasculature during development and in response to injury. *J. Clin. Investig.* **2011**, *121*, 2278–2289. [CrossRef] [PubMed]
22. Thurston, G.; Rudge, J.S.; Ioffe, E.; Zhou, H.; Ross, L.; Croll, S.D.; Glazer, N.; Holash, J.; McDonald, D.M.; Yancopoulos, G.D. Angiopoietin-1 protects the adult vasculature against plasma leakage. *Nat. Med.* **2000**, *6*, 460–463. [CrossRef]
23. Gehling, U.M.; Ergun, S.; Schumacher, U.; Wagener, C.; Pantel, K.; Otte, M.; Schuch, G.; Schafhausen, P.; Mende, T.; Kilic, N.; et al. In vitro differentiation of endothelial cells from AC133-positive progenitor cells. *Blood* **2000**, *95*, 3106–3112. [CrossRef] [PubMed]
24. Fiedler, U.; Scharpfenecker, M.; Koidl, S.; Hegen, A.; Grunow, V.; Schmidt, J.M.; Kriz, W.; Thurston, G.; Augustin, H.G. The Tie-2 ligand angiopoietin-2 is stored in and rapidly released upon stimulation from endothelial cell Weibel-Palade bodies. *Blood* **2004**, *103*, 4150–4156. [CrossRef] [PubMed]
25. Fiedler, U.; Reiss, Y.; Scharpfenecker, M.; Grunow, V.; Koidl, S.; Thurston, G.; Gale, N.W.; Witzenrath, M.; Rosseau, S.; Suttorp, N.; et al. Angiopoietin-2 sensitizes endothelial cells to TNF-alpha and has a crucial role in the induction of inflammation. *Nat. Med.* **2006**, *12*, 235–239. [CrossRef]
26. Roviezzo, F.; Tsigkos, S.; Kotanidou, A.; Bucci, M.; Brancaleone, V.; Cirino, G.; Papapetropoulos, A. Angiopoietin-2 causes inflammation in vivo by promoting vascular leakage. *J. Pharmacol. Exp. Ther.* **2005**, *314*, 738–744. [CrossRef]
27. Saharinen, P.; Eklund, L.; Alitalo, K. Therapeutic targeting of the angiopoietin-TIE pathway. *Nat. Rev. Drug Discov.* **2017**, *16*, 635–661. [CrossRef]
28. Lee, K.W.; Lip, G.Y.; Blann, A.D. Plasma angiopoietin-1, angiopoietin-2, angiopoietin receptor tie-2, and vascular endothelial growth factor levels in acute coronary syndromes. *Circulation* **2004**, *110*, 2355–2360. [CrossRef]
29. Poss, J.; Fuernau, G.; Denks, D.; Desch, S.; Eitel, I.; de Waha, S.; Link, A.; Schuler, G.; Adams, V.; Bohm, M.; et al. Angiopoietin-2 in acute myocardial infarction complicated by cardiogenic shock—A biomarker substudy of the IABP-SHOCK II-Trial. *Eur. J. Heart Fail.* **2015**, *17*, 1152–1160. [CrossRef]
30. Patel, J.V.; Lim, H.S.; Varughese, G.I.; Hughes, E.A.; Lip, G.Y. Angiopoietin-2 levels as a biomarker of cardiovascular risk in patients with hypertension. *Ann. Med.* **2008**, *40*, 215–222. [CrossRef]
31. David, S.; Kumpers, P.; Lukasz, A.; Kielstein, J.T.; Haller, H.; Fliser, D. Circulating angiopoietin-2 in essential hypertension: Relation to atherosclerosis, vascular inflammation, and treatment with olmesartan/pravastatin. *J. Hypertens.* **2009**, *27*, 1641–1647. [CrossRef] [PubMed]
32. Chong, A.Y.; Caine, G.J.; Freestone, B.; Blann, A.D.; Lip, G.Y. Plasma angiopoietin-1, angiopoietin-2, and angiopoietin receptor tie-2 levels in congestive heart failure. *J. Am. Coll. Cardiol.* **2004**, *43*, 423–428. [CrossRef] [PubMed]
33. Lukasz, A.; Beutel, G.; Kumpers, P.; Denecke, A.; Westhoff-Bleck, M.; Schieffer, B.; Bauersachs, J.; Kielstein, J.T.; Tutarel, O. Angiopoietin-2 in adults with congenital heart disease and heart failure. *PLoS ONE* **2013**, *8*, e66861. [CrossRef] [PubMed]
34. Iribarren, C.; Phelps, B.H.; Darbinian, J.A.; McCluskey, E.R.; Quesenberry, C.P.; Hytopoulos, E.; Vogelman, J.H.; Orentreich, N. Circulating angiopoietins-1 and -2, angiopoietin receptor Tie-2 and vascular endothelial growth factor-A as biomarkers of acute myocardial infarction: A prospective nested case-control study. *BMC Cardiovasc. Disord.* **2011**, *11*, 31. [CrossRef] [PubMed]

35. Jian, W.; Li, L.; Wei, X.M.; Wu, C.Q.; Gui, C. Prognostic value of angiopoietin-2 for patients with coronary heart disease after elective PCI. *Medicine (Baltimore)* **2019**, *98*, e14216. [CrossRef]
36. Zeng, Z.Y.; Gui, C.; Li, L.; Wei, X.M. Effects of percutaneous coronary intervention on serum Angiopoietin-2 in patients with coronary heart disease. *Chin. Med. J. (Engl.)* **2016**, *129*, 631–635. [CrossRef]
37. Moxon, J.V.; Trollope, A.F.; Dewdney, B.; de Hollander, C.; Nastasi, D.R.; Maguire, J.M.; Golledge, J. The effect of angiopoietin-1 upregulation on the outcome of acute ischaemic stroke in rodent models: A meta-analysis. *J. Cereb. Blood Flow Metab.* **2019**, *39*, 2343–2354. [CrossRef]
38. Chiang, W.C.; Huang, Y.C.; Fu, T.I.; Chen, P.M.; Chang, F.C.; Lai, C.F.; Wu, V.C.; Lin, S.L.; Chen, Y.M. Angiopoietin 1 influences ischemic reperfusion renal injury via modulating endothelium survival and regeneration. *Mol. Med.* **2019**, *25*, 5. [CrossRef]
39. Varricchi, G.; Loffredo, S.; Galdiero, M.R.; Marone, G.; Cristinziano, L.; Granata, F.; Marone, G. Innate effector cells in angiogenesis and lymphangiogenesis. *Curr. Opin. Immunol.* **2018**, *53*, 152–160. [CrossRef]
40. Varricchi, G.; de Paulis, A.; Marone, G.; Galli, S.J. Future Needs in Mast Cell Biology. *Int. J. Mol. Sci.* **2019**, *20*, 4397. [CrossRef]
41. Sammarco, G.; Varricchi, G.; Ferraro, V.; Ammendola, M.; De Fazio, M.; Altomare, D.F.; Luposella, M.; Maltese, L.; Curro, G.; Marone, G.; et al. Mast cells, angiogenesis and lymphangiogenesis in human gastric cancer. *Int. J. Mol. Sci.* **2019**, *20*, 2106. [CrossRef] [PubMed]
42. Senger, D.R.; Galli, S.J.; Dvorak, A.M.; Perruzzi, C.A.; Harvey, V.S.; Dvorak, H.F. Tumor cells secrete a vascular permeability factor that promotes accumulation of ascites fluid. *Science* **1983**, *219*, 983–985. [CrossRef] [PubMed]
43. Varricchi, G.; Loffredo, S.; Borriello, F.; Pecoraro, A.; Rivellese, F.; Genovese, A.; Spadaro, G.; Marone, G. Superantigenic activation of human cardiac mast cells. *Int. J. Mol. Sci.* **2019**, *20*, 1828. [CrossRef] [PubMed]
44. Varricchi, G.; Pecoraro, A.; Marone, G.; Criscuolo, G.; Spadaro, G.; Genovese, A.; Marone, G. Thymic stromal lymphopoietin isoforms, inflammatory disorders, and cancer. *Front. Immunol.* **2018**, *9*, 1595. [CrossRef] [PubMed]
45. Fankhauser, M.; Broggi, M.A.S.; Potin, L.; Bordry, N.; Jeanbart, L.; Lund, A.W.; Da Costa, E.; Hauert, S.; Rincon-Restrepo, M.; Tremblay, C.; et al. Tumor lymphangiogenesis promotes T cell infiltration and potentiates immunotherapy in melanoma. *Sci. Transl. Med.* **2017**, *9*, eaal4712. [CrossRef] [PubMed]
46. Stacker, S.A.; Williams, S.P.; Karnezis, T.; Shayan, R.; Fox, S.B.; Achen, M.G. Lymphangiogenesis and lymphatic vessel remodelling in cancer. *Nat. Rev. Cancer* **2014**, *14*, 159–172. [CrossRef]
47. Heeschen, C.; Dimmeler, S.; Hamm, C.W.; Boersma, E.; Zeiher, A.M.; Simoons, M.L.; Investigators, C. Prognostic significance of angiogenic growth factor serum levels in patients with acute coronary syndromes. *Circulation* **2003**, *107*, 524–530. [CrossRef]
48. Hojo, Y.; Ikeda, U.; Zhu, Y.; Okada, M.; Ueno, S.; Arakawa, H.; Fujikawa, H.; Katsuki, T.; Shimada, K. Expression of vascular endothelial growth factor in patients with acute myocardial infarction. *J. Am. Coll. Cardiol.* **2000**, *35*, 968–973. [CrossRef]
49. Kawamoto, A.; Kawata, H.; Akai, Y.; Katsuyama, Y.; Takase, E.; Sasaki, Y.; Tsujimura, S.; Sakaguchi, Y.; Iwano, M.; Fujimoto, S.; et al. Serum levels of VEGF and basic FGF in the subacute phase of myocardial infarction. *Int. J. Cardiol.* **1998**, *67*, 47–54. [CrossRef]
50. Kranz, A.; Rau, C.; Kochs, M.; Waltenberger, J. Elevation of vascular endothelial growth factor-A serum levels following acute myocardial infarction. Evidence for its origin and functional significance. *J. Mol. Cell. Cardiol.* **2000**, *32*, 65–72. [CrossRef] [PubMed]
51. Dennis, E.A.; Cao, J.; Hsu, Y.H.; Magrioti, V.; Kokotos, G. Phospholipase A2 enzymes: Physical structure, biological function, disease implication, chemical inhibition, and therapeutic intervention. *Chem. Rev.* **2011**, *111*, 6130–6185. [CrossRef] [PubMed]
52. Granata, F.; Staiano, R.I.; Loffredo, S.; Petraroli, A.; Genovese, A.; Marone, G.; Triggiani, M. The role of mast cell-derived secreted phospholipases A2 in respiratory allergy. *Biochimie* **2010**, *92*, 588–593. [CrossRef] [PubMed]
53. Loffredo, S.; Ferrara, A.L.; Bova, M.; Borriello, F.; Suffritti, C.; Veszeli, N.; Petraroli, A.; Galdiero, M.R.; Varricchi, G.; Granata, F.; et al. Secreted phospholipases A2 in hereditary angioedema with C1-inhibitor deficiency. *Front. Immunol.* **2018**, *9*, 1721. [CrossRef] [PubMed]
54. Murakami, M.; Lambeau, G. Emerging roles of secreted phospholipase A(2) enzymes: An update. *Biochimie* **2013**, *95*, 43–50. [CrossRef] [PubMed]

55. Rizzo, M.T.; Nguyen, E.; Aldo-Benson, M.; Lambeau, G. Secreted phospholipase A(2) induces vascular endothelial cell migration. *Blood* **2000**, *96*, 3809–3815. [CrossRef]
56. Loffredo, S.; Marone, G. Hereditary angioedema: The plasma contact system out of control: Comment. *J. Thromb. Haemost.* **2018**, *16*, 2347–2348. [CrossRef] [PubMed]
57. Lambeau, G.; Gelb, M.H. Biochemistry and physiology of mammalian secreted phospholipases A2. *Ann. Rev. Biochem.* **2008**, *77*, 495–520. [CrossRef] [PubMed]
58. Kugiyama, K.; Ota, Y.; Takazoe, K.; Moriyama, Y.; Kawano, H.; Miyao, Y.; Sakamoto, T.; Soejima, H.; Ogawa, H.; Doi, H.; et al. Circulating levels of secretory type II phospholipase A(2) predict coronary events in patients with coronary artery disease. *Circulation* **1999**, *100*, 1280–1284. [CrossRef] [PubMed]
59. Boekholdt, S.M.; Keller, T.T.; Wareham, N.J.; Luben, R.; Bingham, S.A.; Day, N.E.; Sandhu, M.S.; Jukema, J.W.; Kastelein, J.J.; Hack, C.E.; et al. Serum levels of type II secretory phospholipase A2 and the risk of future coronary artery disease in apparently healthy men and women: The EPIC-Norfolk prospective population study. *Arterioscler. Thromb. Vasc. Biol.* **2005**, *25*, 839–846. [CrossRef]
60. Xin, H.; Chen, Z.Y.; Lv, X.B.; Liu, S.; Lian, Z.X.; Cai, S.L. Serum secretory phospholipase A2-IIa (sPLA2-IIA) levels in patients surviving acute myocardial infarction. *Eur. Rev. Med. Pharmacol. Sci.* **2013**, *17*, 999–1004.
61. Nijmeijer, R.; Meuwissen, M.; Krijnen, P.A.; van der Wal, A.; Piek, J.J.; Visser, C.A.; Hack, C.E.; Niessen, H.W. Secretory type II phospholipase A2 in culprit coronary lesions is associated with myocardial infarction. *Eur. J. Clin. Investig.* **2008**, *38*, 205–210. [CrossRef]
62. Sun, C.Q.; Zhong, C.Y.; Sun, W.W.; Xiao, H.; Zhu, P.; Lin, Y.Z.; Zhang, C.L.; Gao, H.; Song, Z.Y. Elevated Type II secretory phospholipase A2 increases the risk of early atherosclerosis in patients with newly diagnosed metabolic syndrome. *Sci. Rep.* **2016**, *6*, 34929. [CrossRef]
63. Loffredo, S.; Bova, M.; Suffritti, C.; Borriello, F.; Zanichelli, A.; Petraroli, A.; Varricchi, G.; Triggiani, M.; Cicardi, M.; Marone, G. Elevated plasma levels of vascular permeability factors in C1 inhibitor-deficient hereditary angioedema. *Allergy* **2016**, *71*, 989–996. [CrossRef]
64. Randolph, G.J.; Ivanov, S.; Zinselmeyer, B.H.; Scallan, J.P. The lymphatic system: Integral roles in immunity. *Ann. Rev. Immunol.* **2017**, *35*, 31–52. [CrossRef] [PubMed]
65. Zheng, W.; Aspelund, A.; Alitalo, K. Lymphangiogenic factors, mechanisms, and applications. *J. Clin. Investig.* **2014**, *124*, 878–887. [CrossRef] [PubMed]
66. Henri, O.; Pouehe, C.; Houssari, M.; Galas, L.; Nicol, L.; Edwards-Levy, F.; Henry, J.P.; Dumesnil, A.; Boukhalfa, I.; Banquet, S.; et al. Selective stimulation of cardiac lymphangiogenesis reduces myocardial edema and fibrosis leading to improved cardiac function following myocardial infarction. *Circulation* **2016**, *133*, 1484–1497. [CrossRef] [PubMed]
67. Shimizu, Y.; Polavarapu, R.; Eskla, K.L.; Pantner, Y.; Nicholson, C.K.; Ishii, M.; Brunnhoelzl, D.; Mauria, R.; Husain, A.; Naqvi, N.; et al. Impact of Lymphangiogenesis on cardiac remodeling after ischemia and reperfusion injury. *J. Am. Heart Assoc.* **2018**, *7*, e009565. [CrossRef]
68. Karaman, S.; Leppanen, V.M.; Alitalo, K. Vascular endothelial growth factor signaling in development and disease. *Development* **2018**, *145*, dev.151019. [CrossRef]
69. Park, J.S.; Kim, I.K.; Han, S.; Park, I.; Kim, C.; Bae, J.; Oh, S.J.; Lee, S.; Kim, J.H.; Woo, D.C.; et al. Normalization of tumor vessels by Tie2 activation and Ang2 inhibition enhances drug delivery and produces a favorable tumor microenvironment. *Cancer Cell* **2016**, *30*, 953–967. [CrossRef]
70. Li, Z.; Korhonen, E.A.; Merlini, A.; Strauss, J.; Wihuri, E.; Nurmi, H.; Antila, S.; Paech, J.; Deutsch, U.; Engelhardt, B.; et al. Angiopoietin-2 blockade ameliorates autoimmune neuroinflammation by inhibiting leukocyte recruitment into the CNS. *J. Clin. Investig.* **2020**, *130*, 1977–1990. [CrossRef]
71. Lorbeer, R.; Baumeister, S.E.; Dorr, M.; Nauck, M.; Grotevendt, A.; Volzke, H.; Vasan, R.S.; Wallaschofski, H.; Lieb, W. Circulating angiopoietin-2, its soluble receptor Tie-2, and mortality in the general population. *Eur. J. Heart Fail.* **2013**, *15*, 1327–1334. [CrossRef] [PubMed]
72. Link, A.; Poss, J.; Rbah, R.; Barth, C.; Feth, L.; Selejan, S.; Bohm, M. Circulating angiopoietins and cardiovascular mortality in cardiogenic shock. *Eur. Heart J.* **2013**, *34*, 1651–1662. [CrossRef] [PubMed]
73. Jian, W.; Mo, C.H.; Yang, G.L.; Li, L.; Gui, C. Angiopoietin-2 provides no incremental predictive value for the presence of obstructive coronary artery disease over N-terminal pro-brain natriuretic peptide. *J. Clin. Lab. Anal.* **2019**, *33*, e22972. [CrossRef] [PubMed]

74. Detoraki, A.; Staiano, R.I.; Granata, F.; Giannattasio, G.; Prevete, N.; de Paulis, A.; Ribatti, D.; Genovese, A.; Triggiani, M.; Marone, G. Vascular endothelial growth factors synthesized by human lung mast cells exert angiogenic effects. *J. Allergy Clin. Immunol.* **2009**, *123*, 1142–1149.e5. [CrossRef]
75. Staiano, R.I.; Loffredo, S.; Borriello, F.; Iannotti, F.A.; Piscitelli, F.; Orlando, P.; Secondo, A.; Granata, F.; Lepore, M.T.; Fiorelli, A.; et al. Human lung-resident macrophages express CB1 and CB2 receptors whose activation inhibits the release of angiogenic and lymphangiogenic factors. *J. Leukoc. Biol.* **2016**, *99*, 531–540. [CrossRef]
76. Huusko, J.; Lottonen, L.; Merentie, M.; Gurzeler, E.; Anisimov, A.; Miyanohara, A.; Alitalo, K.; Tavi, P.; Yla-Herttuala, S. AAV9-mediated VEGF-B gene transfer improves systolic function in progressive left ventricular hypertrophy. *Mol. Ther.* **2012**, *20*, 2212–2221. [CrossRef]
77. Abraham, D.; Hofbauer, R.; Schafer, R.; Blumer, R.; Paulus, P.; Miksovsky, A.; Traxler, H.; Kocher, A.; Aharinejad, S. Selective downregulation of VEGF-A(165), VEGF-R(1), and decreased capillary density in patients with dilative but not ischemic cardiomyopathy. *Circ. Res.* **2000**, *87*, 644–647. [CrossRef]
78. Park, J.H.; Yoon, J.Y.; Ko, S.M.; Jin, S.A.; Kim, J.H.; Cho, C.H.; Kim, J.M.; Lee, J.H.; Choi, S.W.; Seong, I.W.; et al. Endothelial progenitor cell transplantation decreases lymphangiogenesis and adverse myocardial remodeling in a mouse model of acute myocardial infarction. *Exp. Mol. Med.* **2011**, *43*, 479–485. [CrossRef]
79. Rutanen, J.; Leppanen, P.; Tuomisto, T.T.; Rissanen, T.T.; Hiltunen, M.O.; Vajanto, I.; Niemi, M.; Hakkinen, T.; Karkola, K.; Stacker, S.A.; et al. Vascular endothelial growth factor-D expression in human atherosclerotic lesions. *Cardiovasc. Res.* **2003**, *59*, 971–979. [CrossRef]
80. Klotz, L.; Norman, S.; Vieira, J.M.; Masters, M.; Rohling, M.; Dube, K.N.; Bollini, S.; Matsuzaki, F.; Carr, C.A.; Riley, P.R. Cardiac lymphatics are heterogeneous in origin and respond to injury. *Nature* **2015**, *522*, 62–67. [CrossRef]
81. David, S.; Kumpers, P.; Hellpap, J.; Horn, R.; Leitolf, H.; Haller, H.; Kielstein, J.T. Angiopoietin 2 and cardiovascular disease in dialysis and kidney transplantation. *Am. J. Kidney Dis.* **2009**, *53*, 770–778. [CrossRef] [PubMed]
82. McKee, P.A.; Castelli, W.P.; McNamara, P.M.; Kannel, W.B. The natural history of congestive heart failure: The Framingham study. *N. Engl. J. Med.* **1971**, *285*, 1441–1446. [CrossRef] [PubMed]
83. Sacks, D.; Baxter, B.; Campbell, B.C.V.; Carpenter, J.S.; Cognard, C.; Dippel, D.; Eesa, M.; Fischer, U.; Hausegger, K.; Hirsch, J.A.; et al. Multisociety consensus quality improvement revised consensus statement for endovascular therapy of acute ischemic stroke. *Int. J. Stroke* **2018**, *13*, 612–632. [CrossRef] [PubMed]
84. Albakri, A. Clinical and Medical Investigations Ischemic heart failure: A review of clinical status and meta-analysis of diagnosis and clinical management methods. *Clin. Med. Investig.* **2018**, *3*, 2–15.
85. Balmforth, C.; Simpson, J.; Shen, L.; Jhund, P.S.; Lefkowitz, M.; Rizkala, A.R.; Rouleau, J.L.; Shi, V.; Solomon, S.D.; Swedberg, K.; et al. Outcomes and effect of treatment according to etiology in HFrEF: An analysis of PARADIGM-HF. *JACC Heart Fail.* **2019**, *7*, 457–465. [CrossRef] [PubMed]
86. Hallstrand, T.S.; Lai, Y.; Hooper, K.A.; Oslund, R.C.; Altemeier, W.A.; Matute-Bello, G.; Gelb, M.H. Endogenous secreted phospholipase A2 group X regulates cysteinyl leukotrienes synthesis by human eosinophils. *J. Allergy Clin. Immunol.* **2016**, *137*, 268–277.e8. [CrossRef]
87. Murakami, M.; Yamamoto, K.; Miki, Y.; Murase, R.; Sato, H.; Taketomi, Y. The roles of the secreted phospholipase A2 gene family in immunology. *Adv. Immunol.* **2016**, *132*, 91–134.
88. Triggiani, M.; Giannattasio, G.; Calabrese, C.; Loffredo, S.; Granata, F.; Fiorello, A.; Santini, M.; Gelb, M.H.; Marone, G. Lung mast cells are a source of secreted phospholipases A2. *J. Allergy Clin. Immunol.* **2009**, *124*, 558–565.e1-3. [CrossRef]
89. Marone, G.; Borriello, F.; Varricchi, G.; Genovese, A.; Granata, F. Basophils: Historical reflections and perspectives. *Chem. Immunol. Allergy* **2014**, *100*, 172–192.
90. Loffredo, S.; Staiano, R.I.; Granata, F.; Genovese, A.; Marone, G. Immune cells as a source and target of angiogenic and lymphangiogenic factors. *Chem. Immunol. Allergy* **2014**, *99*, 15–36.
91. Varricchi, G.; Marone, G. Mast cells: Fascinating but still elusive after 140 years from their discovery. *Int. J. Mol. Sci.* **2020**, *21*, 464. [CrossRef]

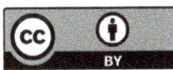

© 2020 by the authors. Licensee MDPI, Basel, Switzerland. This article is an open access article distributed under the terms and conditions of the Creative Commons Attribution (CC BY) license (http://creativecommons.org/licenses/by/4.0/).

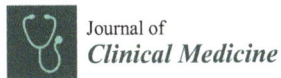

Review

Statin-Related Myotoxicity: A Comprehensive Review of Pharmacokinetic, Pharmacogenomic and Muscle Components

Richard Myles Turner * and Munir Pirmohamed

Department of Molecular and Clinical Pharmacology, Institute of Translational Medicine, University of Liverpool, Liverpool L69 3GL, UK; munirp@liverpool.ac.uk
* Correspondence: Richard.Turner@liverpool.ac.uk

Received: 7 November 2019; Accepted: 18 December 2019; Published: 20 December 2019

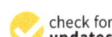

Abstract: Statins are a cornerstone in the pharmacological prevention of cardiovascular disease. Although generally well tolerated, a small subset of patients experience statin-related myotoxicity (SRM). SRM is heterogeneous in presentation; phenotypes include the relatively more common myalgias, infrequent myopathies, and rare rhabdomyolysis. Very rarely, statins induce an anti-HMGCR positive immune-mediated necrotizing myopathy. Diagnosing SRM in clinical practice can be challenging, particularly for mild SRM that is frequently due to alternative aetiologies and the nocebo effect. Nevertheless, SRM can directly harm patients and lead to statin discontinuation/non-adherence, which increases the risk of cardiovascular events. Several factors increase systemic statin exposure and predispose to SRM, including advanced age, concomitant medications, and the nonsynonymous variant, rs4149056, in SLCO1B1, which encodes the hepatic sinusoidal transporter, OATP1B1. Increased exposure of skeletal muscle to statins increases the risk of mitochondrial dysfunction, calcium signalling disruption, reduced prenylation, atrogin-1 mediated atrophy and pro-apoptotic signalling. Rare variants in several metabolic myopathy genes including CACNA1S, CPT2, LPIN1, PYGM and RYR1 increase myopathy/rhabdomyolysis risk following statin exposure. The immune system is implicated in both conventional statin intolerance/myotoxicity via LILRB5 rs12975366, and a strong association exists between HLA-DRB1*11:01 and anti-HMGCR positive myopathy. Epigenetic factors (miR-499-5p, miR-145) have also been implicated in statin myotoxicity. SRM remains a challenge to the safe and effective use of statins, although consensus strategies to manage SRM have been proposed. Further research is required, including stringent phenotyping of mild SRM through N-of-1 trials coupled to systems pharmacology omics- approaches to identify novel risk factors and provide mechanistic insight.

Keywords: statin; pharmacogenomics; muscle toxicity; mitochondria; prenylation; immune system

1. Introduction

Statins are oral hypolipidaemic drugs and amongst the most widely prescribed medications worldwide [1]; in the United Kingdom (UK) alone, ~7 million patients take a statin [2]. The first agent, mevastatin (ML-236B), was identified from *Penicillium citrinum* [3], but was never marketed due to adverse effects. Lovastatin (LVT), isolated from *Aspergillus terreus*, received its marketing authorisation in 1987 and was the first statin approved [4]. LVT also naturally occurs in certain foodstuffs including red yeast rice [5] and oyster mushrooms [6].

Statins are the first line hypolipidaemic drug class for managing cardiovascular (CV) disease (CVD), although ezetimibe, fibrates, bile acid sequestrants, and parenteral proprotein convertase subtilisin/kexin type 9 (PSCK9) inhibitors are also used in specific situations. In the UK, atorvastatin (ATV) 20 mg and 80 mg daily are the current first line guideline-recommended statins for primary and secondary CVD prevention, respectively [7]. However, due to historic prescribing, simvastatin (SVT) remains the most commonly prescribed statin in the UK, followed by ATV [8].

Statins competitively inhibit 3-hydroxy-3-methylglutaryl-Coenzyme A reductase (HMGCR), the rate limiting enzyme for *de novo* cholesterol synthesis in the mevalonate pathway (Figure 1). In response, a compensatory upregulation in hepatic low-density lipoprotein (LDL) receptor cell surface expression occurs [9], leading to a reduction in circulating LDL cholesterol (LDL-C) by ~30–63%, depending on statin and dose. Statins also reduce triglycerides (~20–40%) and raise high-density lipoprotein-cholesterol (HDL-C) (~5%) to a modest extent [10]. Large meta-analyses of statin randomized controlled trials (RCTs) have concluded that each 1 mmol/L reduction in LDL-C with statin therapy is associated with a 22% reduction in the rate of major CV events (coronary deaths, myocardial infarctions, strokes and coronary revascularisations) [11].

Beyond lowering cholesterol, statins have been associated with a range of beneficial pleiotropic effects including anti-inflammatory, antioxidant and immunomodulatory effects, inhibition of platelet activation, regulation of pyroptosis, and increased plaque stability [12–14]. For example, statins mediate a dose-dependent decrease in C-reactive protein [15], may impact renal function [16,17], and attenuate postpartum cardiovascular dysfunction in a rat preeclampsia model [18]. The mechanisms underlying these effects are incompletely understood. However, decreases in other products of the mevalonate pathway following statin-mediated HMGCR inhibition, including isoprenoid intermediates, dolichols, heme A and coenzyme Q_{10} (CoQ_{10},) (Figure 1), are thought to play a role [12].

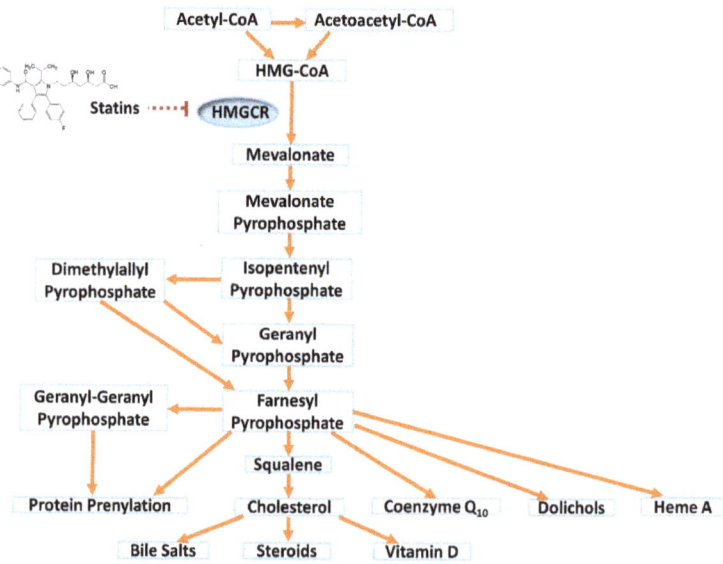

Figure 1. Statin inhibition of the mevalonate pathway.

Seven statins are currently licensed: ATV, fluvastatin (FVT), LVT, pitavastatin (PIT), pravastatin (PVT), rosuvastatin (RVT), and SVT. Statins can be sub-divided into: (i) those administered as the therapeutically inactive lactone (LVT, SVT) versus those administered as active acid statin (ATV, FVT, PVT, PIT, RVT); (ii) those that undergo extensive metabolism by the phase I cytochrome P450 (CYP) system (ATV, FVT, LVT, SVT) versus those excreted predominantly unchanged (PIT, PVT, RVT), and (iii) of the extensively metabolised statins, those primarily biotransformed by CYP3A4/5 (ATV, LVT, SVT) or CYP2C9 (FVT). Table 1 provides an overview of the different statins.

Table 1. Pharmacokinetic properties of the different statins.

Drug Property	Atorvastatin	Cerivastatin	Fluvastatin	Lovastatin	Pitavastatin	Pravastatin	Rosuvastatin	Simvastatin
Year approved	1996	1997 to 2001	1993	1987	2009	1991	2003	1991
Generic available	Yes	No	Yes	Yes	No	Yes	No	Yes
Daily dose (mg)	10–80	0.2–0.3	20–80	10–80	1–4	10–80	5–40	10–40
Equipotent dose (mg)	20	-	>80	80	4	80	5	40
Marketed drug form	Acid	Acid	Acid	Lactone	Acid	Acid	Acid	Lactone
log P (N-octanol/H$_2$O partition coefficient)	1.11 (lipophilic)	1.70 (lipophilic)	1.27 (lipophilic)	1.70 (lipophilic)	1.49 (lipophilic)	−0.84 (hydrophilic)	−0.33 (hydrophilic)	1.60 (lipophilic)
Oral absorption (%)	30	>98	98	31	80	37	50	65–85
Bioavailability (%)	14	60	29	<5	51	17	20	5
Effect of food on bioavailability	Decrease	No effect	Decrease	Increase	No effect	Decrease	No effect	No effect
Time to C$_{max}$ (hours)	1–2	2–3	2.5–3	2	1	1–1.5	3–5	1–4
Protein binding (%)	≥98	>99	98	>95	>99	~50	88	95
Volume of distribution	381 L	0.3 L/Kg	25	-	148 L	0.5 L/Kg	134 L	233 L
Extent of metabolism	High	High	High	High	Low	Low	Low	High
CYPs that metabolise statin acid form	CYP3A CYP2C8 †	CYP2C8 CYP3A	CYP2C9 CYP2C8 † CYP3A †	CYP3A	CYP2C9 CYP2C8 †	CYP2C9 CYP3A †	CYP2C9 CYP2C19 † CYP3A † CYP3A	CYP3A CYP2C8 †
CYPs that metabolise statin lactone form acid form	CYP3A	CYP3A	CYP3A	CYP3A	CYP3A CYP2D6 †	Not known	CYP2C9 † CYP2D6 †	CYP3A
UGTs involved in lactonization of statin acid form	UGT1A1 UGT1A3 UGT2B7	UGT1A3	Not known	UGT1A1 UGT1A3	UGT1A3 UGT2B7	None identified	UGT1A1 UGT1A3	None identified
Transporters for parent statin	OATP1B1, BCRP, MRP1, 2, 4, NTCP, P-gp, OATP1A2, 1B3, 2B1	OATP1B1, BCRP	OATP1B1, 1B3, 2B1, BCRP	OATP1B1, P-gp	OATP1B1, 1B3, BCRP, MRP2, NTCP, P-gp	OATP1B1, 1B3, 2B1, BSEP, BCRP, MRP2, P-gp; OAT3 in renal elimination	OATP1B1, BCRP, BSEP, MRP1, 2, 4, 5, P-gp, OATP1A2, 1B3, 2B1, NTCP; OAT3 in renal elimination	BCRP, P-gp (SVT acid: OATP1B1)
Metabolites formed	2-OH ATV, 4-OH ATV, ATV L, 2-OH ATV L, 4-OH ATV L	M-1 acid, M-23 acid, CVT L, M-1 L, M-23 L	5-OH FVT, 6-OH FVT, N-desopropyl FVT, FVT L	LVT acid, 6-OH LVT acid	PIT L	6-epi PVT, 3α-OH PVT, PVT L, 3α-OH PVT L	N-desmethyl RVT, RVT L	SVT acid, 3′,5′-dihydrodiol, 6′-exomethylene & 3-OH acid metabolites
Elimination t$_{1/2}$ (h)	14	2–3	3	2–5	12	1–3	19	2–3
Faecal excretion (%)	98	70	90	83	79	70	90	60
Renal excretion (%)	<2	30	5	10	15	20	10–28	13
References	[19–25]	[19,25–28]	[22,25,29]	[19,22,25,30,31]	[19,22,25,32,33]	[22,25,34–38]	[19,22,24,25,39–44]	[19,22,25,45–48]

ATV = atorvastatin; BCRP = breast cancer resistance protein; BSEP = bile salt export pump; CVT = cerivastatin; CYP = cytochrome P450; FVT = fluvastatin; L = lactone; LVT = lovastatin; M-1 = demethylation cerivastatin metabolite; M-23 = hydroxylation cerivastatin metabolite; MRP = multidrug resistance-associated protein; NTCP = sodium-taurocholate co-transporting polypeptide; OATP = organic anion-transporting polypeptide; -OH = hydroxy; P-gp = P-glycoprotein; PIT = pitavastatin; PVT = pravastatin; RVT = rosuvastatin; SVT = simvastatin; UGT = uridine 5′-diphospho-glucuronosyltransferase. † = denotes enzymes with a minor contribution to the known statin metabolism. Drug-metabolising adult CYP3A consists of CYP3A4 and variable CYP3A5 expression, dependent on CYP3A5 genotype. The underlined transporters are considered particularly important to the disposition of the statin.

There is notable interindividual variability in response to statin therapy with patients experiencing variable cholesterol lowering efficacy, recurrent CV events [1,15], and a 45-fold variation in statin plasma concentrations [49]. Importantly, a small subset of patients experience statin adverse drug reactions (ADRs), including statin-related myotoxicity (SRM), new-onset diabetes mellitus [50], and elevated liver transaminases [51,52]. Adverse effects on energy levels and exertional fatigue [53] and reduced exercise capacity [54] have been reported, but not confirmed [55]. Similarly, there have been post-marketing case reports of statin-induced memory loss and confusion, although overall, statins are not currently thought to cause cognitive dysfunction [56,57].

It is important to study SRM because, firstly, it can directly harm patients [58,59]. Secondly, despite the unequivocal CVD benefit of statins, statin discontinuation and non-adherence rates are high; ~43% of primary prevention and ~24% of secondary prevention patients become statin non-adherent after a median of ~24 months [60]. Muscle pain increases the likelihood of statin non-adherence and discontinuation [61] which, importantly, increases the risk of major CV events and mortality [62,63].

2. SRM Definitions

SRM is heterogeneous in presentation (Figure 2) and so case definitions vary between studies. Therefore, a recent effort has standardised nomenclature and classified SRM into seven distinct phenotypic categories [64]:

SRM 0 represents asymptomatic elevations in serum creatine kinase (CK) < 4 × the upper limit of normal (ULN);

SRM 1 and 2 are common myalgias (aches, cramps and/or weakness) with no (SRM 1) or minor CK elevations (< 4 × ULN, SRM 2);

SRM 3 represents increasingly infrequent myopathy with CK > 4 × but < 10 × ULN;

SRM 4 is severe myopathy with CK > 10 × but < 50 × ULN;

SRM 5 constitutes rare but potentially life-threatening rhabdomyolysis with either CK > 10 × ULN, muscle symptoms and renal impairment, or CK > 50 × ULN, and;

SRM 6 consists of very rare anti-HMGCR positive immune-mediated necrotizing myopathy, which persists despite statin cessation [64].

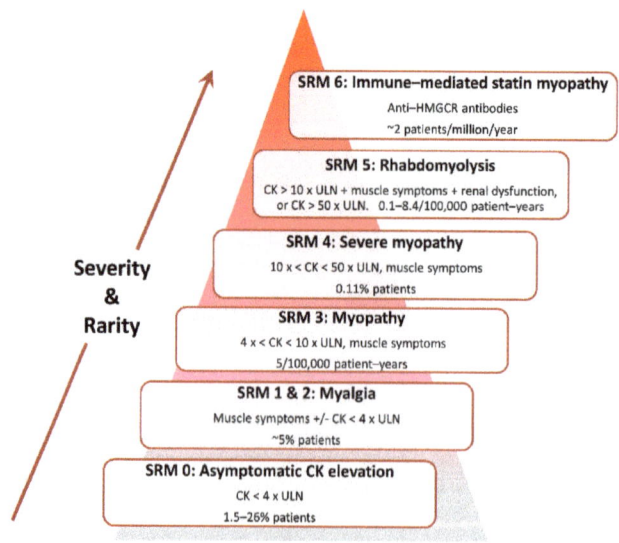

Figure 2. Classification of statin-related myotoxicity phenotypes.

Classification and estimated frequencies are based on Alfirevic et al., 2014 [64], except the myalgia frequency which is from Parker et al., 2013 [65].

Whilst these categories will standardise research, they are perhaps less meaningful as diagnostic criteria in clinical practice. The National Lipid Association (NLA) defines statin intolerance as the "inability to tolerate at least two statins: one statin at the lowest starting daily dose and another statin at any daily dose, due to either objectionable symptoms (real or perceived) or abnormal laboratory determinations, which are temporally related to statin treatment and reversible upon statin discontinuation [66]." The European Atherosclerosis Society (EAS) states "the assessment of statin-associated muscle symptoms includes the nature of muscle symptoms, increased CK levels and their temporal association with initiation of therapy with statin, and statin therapy suspension and re-challenge [67]."

3. SRM Clinical Presentation

SRM constitutes the most commonly reported statin adverse event, comprising approximately two-thirds of all adverse events [68]. The most common muscular symptoms are pain, heaviness, stiffness and cramps with or without subjective weakness [58,69]. Symptoms involving leg muscles (thighs, calves) are most frequent, although back, neck, shoulder and generalised muscular symptoms have also been described [58,69]. Tendonitis-associated pain has been reported [58]. Approximately 40% of patients with SRM note a potential trigger; most commonly, unusual physical exertion or a new medication [58]. Muscular pains are intermittent in three quarters of SRM patients, and constant in one quarter [58].

SRM is most common during the first year of treatment [70] with a median time to onset of one month [51]; over 80% of patients report not experiencing similar symptoms before statin treatment [58]. The muscular symptoms in the majority of SRM cases (~70–80%) are sufficiently intense to disrupt everyday activities [58,69]; this includes statin persistence and so, can present as MACE. The rarer severe myopathies and rhabdomyolysis can directly lead to hospitalisation.

4. SRM Frequency

Amongst licensed statins, the frequency of SRM appears highest with SVT, followed by ATV, and is lowest with FVT [58]. However, the true incidence of SRM is uncertain, occurring in 1.5–5% of participants in RCTs (relative to placebo groups) [71], compared to ~10–33% in observational studies [61,72]. This variability is potentially attributable to a range of factors, including different myotoxicity definitions and follow up procedures, lead-in periods, inclusion of different patient groups, and treatment blinding [73]. There is consensus that statins increase the risk of severe myopathy and rhabdomyolysis [50]. Of note, cerivastatin (CVT) was voluntarily withdrawn in 2001 because of 52 cases of fatal rhabdomyolysis [74]. However, the variability in reported SRM rates has sparked significant disagreement and controversy over the underlying benefit-risk profile of statins, particularly in patients at the lower end of the CVD risk spectrum [75].

The greater difficulty lies in determining the aetiology of the commoner milder musculoskeletal symptoms, and in particular, whether they are attributable to a statin and/or concurrent condition(s) (e.g., viral illnesses). On the one hand, the frequency of muscle-related adverse events did not differ between patients on ATV 10 mg daily or placebo in the large double-blind ASCOT-LLA RCT ($n = 10,180$), but became significantly more common in patients taking ATV 10 mg daily (1.26% per annum) compared to placebo (1.00% per annum) in the subsequent open label non-blinded extension phase [76]. This observation was attributed to the nocebo effect. On the other hand, a six-month double-blind RCT conducted in 420 healthy volunteers administered ATV 80 mg daily or placebo found increased myalgia amongst the subjects on ATV compared to the placebo group (9.4% vs. 4.6%, respectively, $p = 0.05$) [65]. Moreover, N-of-1 (single-patient) placebo-controlled trials involving patients with a history of SRM have reported that ~30–40% experience subsequent muscle-related events only on statin and not placebo [77,78]. This suggests that the muscle symptoms experienced by a third of symptomatic patients are likely statin-induced, whilst the remainder are probably not. The challenge is how to distinguish patients with true SRM from those with myalgia due to other causes.

5. SRM Pathogenesis

Several SRM risk factors have been identified and mechanisms proposed, but there is not yet a unified pathophysiological understanding. Nevertheless, two inter-dependent mechanisms are implicated: 1. increased statin systemic exposure due to clinical and pharmacogenomic factors, which increase skeletal muscle exposure, and 2. intracellular skeletal myocyte entry and disruption of muscle function (Figure 3).

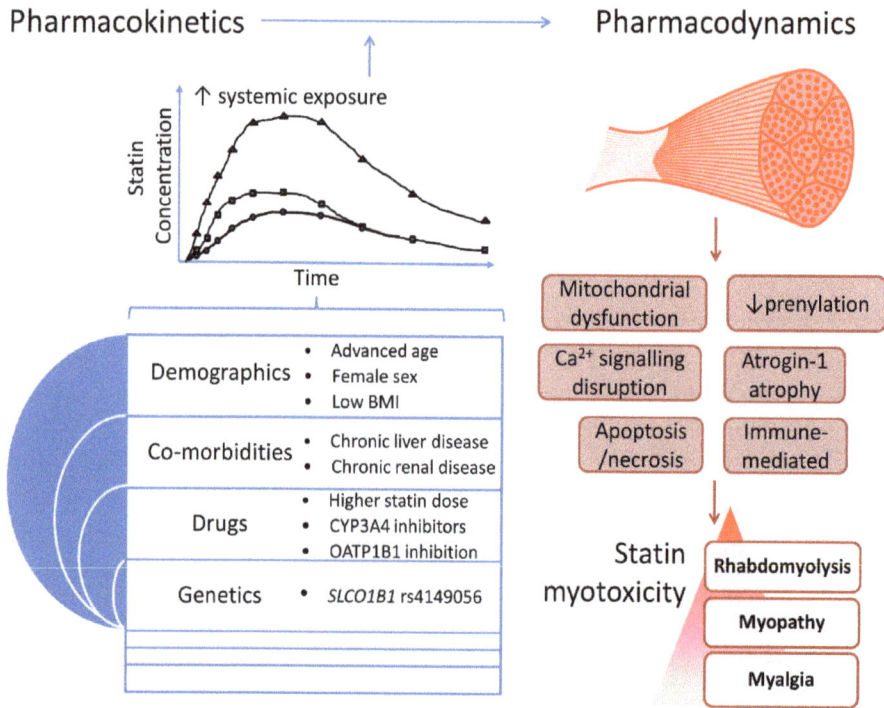

Figure 3. An integrated overview of processes implicated in statin myotoxicity.

6. Factors Associated with Statin Pharmacokinetics and Myotoxicity

The absorption, distribution, metabolism and elimination (ADME) pharmacokinetic (PK) characteristics of the different statins are listed in Table 1. Multiple clinical and pharmacogenomic factors have been associated with statin PK, and a subset also with SRM. These are reviewed below, with particular focus placed on the pharmacogenomic associations.

6.1. Clinical Factors

The clinical factors associated with statin PK and SRM are listed in Supporting Information Table S1, and Table 2, respectively. Several, but not all, identified clinical risk factors for SRM are associated with increased statin exposure (Table 2). Increasing dose increases statin exposure. Increasing age correlates with modestly greater statin exposure, except for FVT and RVT [29,43]. Women generally have modestly higher exposure to most statins, except for RVT and ATV. Whilst there is no difference in mean RVT exposure between genders [79], women have modestly lower circulating ATV levels compared to men [21], attributable to higher hydroxylation metabolism. Patients of Asian ancestry have an approximate 1.5–1.9-fold increase in median RVT exposure compared to Caucasian patients [80], and so the US Food & Drug Administration (FDA) recommends that Asian patients start with just 5 mg RVT daily [43]. All statins are predominantly excreted in faeces and so hepatic impairment can result in several fold increased exposure to several statins (e.g., ATV, FVT) [21,29], although the influence on RVT is more modest [81]. The association between alcoholism and SRM [82] may be partially mediated by alcohol-induced hepatic impairment and reduced body mass leading to increased statin exposure, although alcohol itself also causes myopathy [83]. Renal impairment is only associated with increased statin exposure for statins that are at least 10% renally excreted, with little impact on ATV or FVT [21,84]. Thus, the maximum effect of renal impairment is a 3-fold increase in RVT exposure [43]. Importantly, increasing dose, older age, female sex, low body mass index (BMI), liver disease and renal impairment have all been associated with SRM [64].

Table 2. Clinical risk factors of statin-related myotoxicity.

Category	Risk Factor	Reference
Demographics		
	Advanced age (>80 years old)	[51,82]
	Female gender	[51,85]
	Low body mass index	[73,82]
Ethnicity		
	Black African	[70]
	Caribbean	
Co-morbidities		
	Alcohol abuse	[82]
	Chronic kidney disease	[51,82,86,87]
	Chronic liver disease	[70,88]
	Diabetes mellitus	[88,89]
	Hypertension	[90]
	Hypothyroidism	[88]
	Vitamin D deficiency	[91–93]
Personal/family factors		
	Physical exercise	[58,94,95]
	Personal or family history of muscle pain	[58]
Diet		
	Grapefruit juice (CYP3A inhibition)	[96]
Drugs		
	Higher statin dose	[70,73,97]
	Corticosteroids	[88]
	CYP3A inhibitors (particularly for ATV, LVT, SVT)—e.g., amiodarone, ciclosporin, clarithromycin, erythromycin, protease inhibitors (e.g., indinavir, ritonavir)	[98–104]
	CYP2C9 inhibitors [†] (for FVT)—e.g., fluconazole	[105]
	OATP1B1 inhibition—e.g., gemfibrozil, ciclosporin	[99]

Adapted from Alfirevic et al., 2014 [64]. [†] = in renal transplant patients and limited to the subgroup carrying CYP2C9* 2 or * 3.

6.2. Pharmacogenomic Factors that Affect Statin Pharmacokinetics

A broad overview of the major enzymes and transporters generally involved in statin disposition is provided in Figure 4. Multiple genes alter statin PK, as summarised in Supporting Information Table S2; key genes are *CYPs*, *UGTs* (uridine 5′-diphospho-glucuronosyltransferases), *SLCO1B1* (solute carrier organic anion transporter family member 1B1) and the efflux transporters *ABCB1* (adenosine triphosphate (ATP)-binding cassette subfamily B member 1) and *ABCG2*, which are reviewed below. Table 3 lists studies that have investigated SRM pharmacogenomics. Overall, of the statin PK genes investigated, only *SLCO1B1* rs4149056 has been consistently associated with SRM.

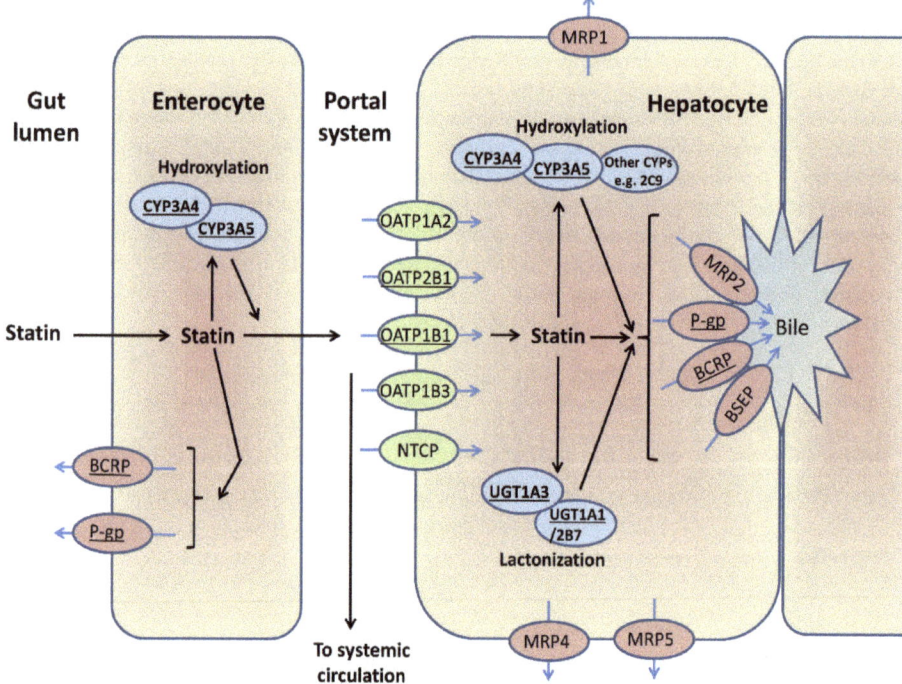

Figure 4. A general schema for statin disposition.

This figure shows the enzymes and transporters that can be involved in the first pass metabolism of different statins [19,24,38,106–108]. ATV, LVT, and SVT are hydroxylated by CYP3A4/5, and FVT by CYP2C9. Statin lactonization is mediated by UDP-glucuronosyltransferases. OATP1B1 is central to the hepatic uptake of statins, although other transporters can be involved. BCRP and/or P-gp are important in the intestinal and biliary efflux of statins, alongside other transporters. The major enzymes/transporters discussed further in this review are underlined.

Table 3. Pharmacogenomic investigations of statin-related myotoxicity.

Study	Design	Genes	Variants	Statin	N	Endpoint	Main Results
Statin Pharmacokinetics							
Bai 2019 [109]	Co, CG			RVT	758	Muscle symptoms +/− ↑CK	-OR 1.74 (95% CI 1.18–2.57), $p = 0.0052$ -No associations for ABCB1, ABCG2, CYP2C9, SLCO1B3 -GATM—see 'Muscle-related' section below
Carr 2019 [110]	GWAS, then MA		rs4149056 (521T > C, p.V174A)	SVT, CVT, ATV (+ others)	7764	CK > 10 × ULN or rhabdomyolysis	-all statins: OR 2.99 (95% CI 2.34–3.82), $p = 2.63 \times 10^{-18}$ -SVT: OR 5.91 (95% CI 4.10–8.51), $p = 1.46 \times 10^{-21}$ -ATV: no clear associations
Carr 2013 [89]	CC, CG	SLCO1B1		SVT, ATV (+ others)	448	Stop statin & CK > 4 × ULN	-all statins: OR 2.08 (95% CI 1.35–3.23), $p = 0.005$ -SVT: OR 2.13 (95% CI 1.29–3.54), $p = 0.014$ -COQ2—see 'Muscle-related' section below
Floyd 2019 [111]	MA, WES			SVT, CVT, ATV (+ others)	2552	Muscle symptoms & CK > 4 × ULN	-No genome-wide significant associations -rs4149056 in non-fibrate users secondary analysis: 4.01-fold ↑ risk (95% CI 2.61–6.17), $p = 5.46 \times 10^{-11}$
Danik 2013 [112]	RCT, CG			RVT	4404	Myalgia	No association detected
de Keyser 2014 [113]	Co, CG			SVT, ATV	1939	Statin dose decrease or switch	-SVT: HR 1.74 (95% CI 1.05–2.88), $p = 0.033$ -ATV > 20 mg: HR 3.26 (95% CI 1.47–7.35), $p = 0.004$ -No associations for SVT or ATV in replication set
Link 2008 [86]	CC, GWAS			SVT	175	CK > 3 × ULN & 5 × baseline, plus ↑ ALT	-SVT 80 mg: OR 4.5 (95% CI 2.6–7.7) -STV 40mg: OR 2.6 (95% CI 1.3–5.0), $p = 0.004$
Puccetti 2010 [114]	CC, CG			ATV, RVT	76	Muscular intolerance (muscle symptoms or ↑CK or ↑LFTs)	-ATV: OR 2.7 (95% CI 1.3–4.9), $p < 0.001$ -RVT: no association -COQ2—see 'Muscle-related' section below
Marciante 2011 [115]	CC, CGs & GWAS			CVT	917	Muscle symptoms & CK > 10 × ULN	-OR 1.89 (95% CI 1.40–2.56), $p = 3.62 \times 10^{-5}$ -No associations for CYP2C8, UGT1A1/1A3 -RYR2—see 'Muscle-related' section below
Voora 2009 [85]	RCT, CG			ATV, SVT, PVT	452	Stop statin, myalgia, or CK > 3 × ULN	-OR 1.7 (95% CI 1.04–2.8), $p = 0.03$. -Risk highest in patients on SVT. -No apparent association for PVT
Xiang 2018 [116]	MA, CG			SVT, CVT, RVT, ATV, PVT	11,008	Multiple-myalgia to rhabdomyolysis	-No associations for CYP2C8, 2C9, 2D6, 3A4 -SVT: OR 2.35 (95% CI 1.08–5.12), $p = 0.032$ -CVT: OR 1.95 (95% CI 1.47–2.57), $p < 0.001$ -RVT: OR 1.69 (95% CI 1.07–2.67), $p = 0.024$ -ATV or PVT: no associations
Elam 2017 [69]	CC, CG	SLCO2B1	rs12422149	SVT, ATV, RVT	19	Statin myalgia confirmed by re-challenge	↑ myalgia with rs4149056 variant allele ($p = 0.039$) ↑ myalgia with rs12422149 variant allele ($p = 0.001$) -RYR2—see 'Muscle-related' section below

Table 3. Cont.

Study	Design	Genes	Variants	Statin	N	Endpoint	Main Results
Statin Pharmacokinetics							
Ferrari 2014 [117]	CC, CG	SLCO1B1, ABCB1	rs4149056, rs2306283, 1236C > T, 3435C > T, 1236C > T,	ATV, RVT, SVT	66	CK > 3 × ULN, irrespective of symptoms	-rs4149056: OR 8.5 (95% CI 1.7–42.3), $p = 0.001$ -rs2306283: OR 0.3 (95% CI 0.06–0.91), $p = 0.022$ -ABCB1: OR 4.5 (95% CI 1.4–14.7), $p = 0.001$ -No association for ABCG2
Fiegenbaum 2005 [118]	Co, CG	ABCB1	2677G > A/T, 3435C > T	SVT	116	Myalgia	-↑ endpoint risk with ABCB1 variants ($p < 0.05$) -No associations with CYP3A4, 3A5
Hoenig 2011 [119]	Co, CG	ABCB1, SLCO1B1	3435C > T, rs4149056	ATV	117	Myalgia Adverse reactions	↑ risk carrying T compared to C allele ($p = 0.043$) -rs4149056: OR 2.3 (95% CI 1.03–4.98), $p = 0.043$
Mirosevic Skvrce 2015 [120]	CC, CG	ABCG2	rs2231142	ATV	130	Adverse reactions (61.7% myotoxicity); myalgia to rhabdomyolysis	-rs2231142: OR 2.75 (95% CI 1.10–6.87), $p = 0.03$ -No association for CYP3A4*22
Mirosevic Skvrce 2013 [105]	CC, CG	ABCG2, CYP2C9	rs2231142, *2, *3	FVT	104	Adverse reactions in renal transplant patients (90.4% myotoxicity); Statin dose decrease or switch	-rs2231142: OR 4.89 (95% CI 1.42–16.89) -*2 or *3 carriers: OR 2.44 (95% CI 1.05–5.71), $p = 0.037$ -↑ risk of endpoint in CYP2C9*2 or *3 carriers on a CYP2C9 drug inhibitor: OR 6.59, $p = 0.027$
Becker 2010 [121]	Co, CG	CYP3A4	*1B	SVT, ATV	1239		-SVT/ATV: HR 0.46 (95% CI 0.24–0.90), $p = 0.023$ -SVT only: HR 0.47 (95% CI 0.23–0.96), $p = 0.039$ -No association for ABCB1
Frudakis 2007 [122]	CC, CG	CYP2D6	*4	ATV, SVT	263	Stop statin due to muscle events	-ATV: OR 2.5 (95% CI 1.5–4.4), $p = 0.001$ -SVT: OR 1.7 (95% CI 0.9–3.2), $p = 0.067$
Mulder 2001 [123]	Co, CG	CYP2D6	*3, *4, *5, *2xN	SVT	88	Stop statin	↑ risk with CYP2D6 variants (RR = 4.7); a gene-dose trend
Wilke 2005 [124]	CC, CG	CYP3A4/5	3A4*1B, 3A5*3	ATV	137	Myalgia	No main associations detected
Zuccaro 2007 [125]	CC, CG	CYPs	Several	ATV, SVT, PVT (+ others)	100	Muscle symptoms +/- ↑CK	No associations for CYP2C9, 2D6, 3A5
Muscle-related							
Bai 2019 [109]	Co, CG	GATM	rs9806699	RVT	758	Muscle symptoms +/- ↑CK	OR 0.62 (95% CI 0.41–0.94), $p = 0.024$
Mangravite 2013 [126]	deQTL CG CCs	GATM	rs9806699 rs1719247	SVT	4413	Muscle symptoms & CK > 3 × ULN	-rs1719247 in LD with top deQTL, rs9806699: $r^2 = 0.76$ -MA: OR 0.60 (95% CI 0.45–0.81), $p = 6.0 \times 10^{-4}$
Carr 2013 [89]	CC, CG	COQ2	rs4693075	SVT, ATV (+ others)	448	Stop statin & CK > 4 × ULN	COQ2 rs4693075: no associations
Oh 2007 [127]	CC, CG	COQ2	rs6535454 rs4693075	ATV, RVT (+ others)	291	Muscle symptoms + stop statin or CK > 3 × ULN	-rs6535454: OR 2.42 (95% CI 0.99–5.89), $p = 0.047$ -rs4693075: OR 2.33 (95% CI 1.13–4.81), $p = 0.019$

Table 3. Cont.

Study	Design	Genes	Variants	Statin	N	Endpoint	Main Results
Muscle-related							
Puccetti 2010 [114]	CC, CG	COQ2	rs4693075	ATV, RVT	76	Muscular intolerance (muscle symptoms or ↑CK or ↑LFTs)	-RVT: OR 2.6 (95% CI 1.7–4.4), $p < 0.001$ -↑ risk of muscular symptoms and ↑CK with ATV: OR 3.1 (95% CI 1.9–6.4), $p < 0.001$
Ruano 2011 [128]	CC, CG	COQ2 ATP2B1 DMPK CPT2	rs4693570 rs17381194 rs672348 Several	ATV, SVT, RVT (+ others)	793	Myalgia	-COQ2 rs4693570 ($p = 0.000041$) or ATP2B1 rs17381194 ($p = 0.00079$) associated with ↑ risk. -DMPK rs672348 ($p = 0.0016$) associated with ↓ risk.
Vladutiu 2006 [129]	CC, CG	PYGM AMPD1	R49X, G204S Q12X, P48L, K287I	ATV, CVT, LVT, SVT	358	Muscle symptoms; CK ↑ reported	Overall, a fourfold ↑ in the number of mutant alleles (AMPD1 > CPT2/PYGM) in cases vs. statin-tolerant controls.
Tsivgoulis 2006 [130]	CRs, CG	DMPK NR3C4	CTG repeats CAG repeats	PVT, ATV, SVT	4	Muscle symptoms or fatigue & CK ↑	-1 case of each of type 1 myotonic dystrophy (DMPK), glycogen storage disease V (muscle histochemical diagnosis), mitochondrial myopathy (muscle biopsy & biochemical diagnosis), and Kennedy disease (NR3C4) diagnosed after starting statin and becoming symptomatic
Echaniz-Laguna 2010 [131]	Co, CG	NR3C4 PHKA1	CAG repeats Not specified	SVT, PVT, ATV (+ others)	52	Abnormal EMG & pathological analysis, if muscle features last > 3 months after statin ceased	-5 patients diagnosed with paraneoplastic polymyositis, Kennedy disease (NR3C4), glycogen storage disease IX (PHKA1), motor neuron disease, and necrotic myopathy of uncertain aetiology
Knoblauch 2010 [132]	CS, CG	CNBP	CCTG repeat	ATV, SVT (+ others)	3	Muscle symptoms that last after statin ceased +/- ↑CK	-All 3 cases diagnosed with type II myotonic dystrophy after becoming symptomatic after starting statin treatment
Voermans 2005 [133]	CR, CG	GAA	IVS1-13T > G 525del T	SVT	1	Muscle symptoms & CK ↑	-1 case of a compound heterozygote for glycogen storage disease II diagnosed after becoming symptomatic on SVT
Zeharia 2008 [134]	CC, CG	LPIN1	sequenced	Unknown	20	Myopathy with ↑CK	In 2 of 6 cases, exonic nucleotide substitutions thought harmful were found, vs. 0 in 14 statin-tolerant controls.
Vladutiu 2011 [135]	CC, CG	RYR1	34 mutations	Not specified	493	Muscle symptoms-often last post statin, +/- ↑CK	RYR1 mutations in 3 of 197 severe & 1 of 163 mild statin myopathies, vs. 0 of 133 statin-tolerant controls.
Isackson 2018 [136]	WES	RYR1 CACNA1S	Pathogenic variants	ATV, RVT, SVT (+ others)	126	Muscle symptoms & CK > 5 × ULN	12 of 76 (16%) of SRM patients had probably pathogenic variants in RYR1 or CACNA1S, which was 4-fold higher than in statin-tolerant controls.
Elam 2017 [69]	CC, CG	RYR2	rs2819742	SVT, ATV, RVT	19	Statin myalgia confirmed by re-challenge	-↑ myalgia with rs2819742 variant allele ($p = 0.016$) -No associations with GATM, COQ2, HTR3B, HTR7
Marciante 2011 [115]	CC, CGs & GWAS	RYR2	rs2819742	CVT	917	Muscle symptoms & CK > 10 × ULN	OR 0.48 (95% CI 0.36–0.63), $p = 1.74 \times 10^{-7}$

Table 3. Cont.

Study	Design	Genes	Variants	Statin	N	Endpoint	Main Results
Immune-system related							
Limaye 2015 [137]	Co, CG	HLA-DRB1*11	Typing to 'two-digit' resolution	Not specified	207	Anti-HMGCR antibodies in patients with idiopathic inflammatory myositis or immune-mediated necrotizing myopathy	-Anti-HMGCR antibodies in 19 of 207 myopathy cases -HLA-DRB1*11 more frequent in myopathy patients positive vs. negative for anti-HMGCR antibodies: OR 56.1 (95% CI 5.0–7739), $p = 0.001$ -3 anti-HMGCR positive myopathy patients had high resolution typing and all carried HLA-DRB1*11:01
Mammen 2012 [138]	CC, HLA typing	HLA-DRB1*11 DQA DQB	Typing resolution: -Intermediate; -High in DR11 Intermediate resolution	Not specified	733	Anti-HMGCR antibodies in patients with myositis/myopathy	-OR for HLA-DRB1*11:01 in anti-HMGCR myopathy patients vs. controls: ~24.5 ($p = 3.2 \times 10^{-10}$) and ~56.5 ($p = 3.1 \times 10^{-6}$) in white & black ethnicities, respectively -HLA-DQA1 and DQB6 less frequent in white anti-HMGCR positive patients than controls ($p = 5.5 \times 10^{-4}, 2.1 \times 10^{-5}$)
Siddiqui 2017 [139]	Co, CG	LILRB5	rs12975366	SVT, RVT (+ others)	1034	-1. Non-adherence & ↑CK -2. Statin intolerant & switched ≥ 2 other statins	-1: OR 1.81 (95% CI 1.34–2.45) -2: OR 1.36 (95% CI 1.07–1.73)
Pain perception							
Ruano 2007 [140]	CC, CG	HTR3B HTR7	rs2276307 rs1935349	ATV, SVT, PVT	195	Myalgia	-↑risk for rs2276307 ($p = 0.007$) & rs1935349 ($p = 0.026$) -No associations for HTR1D, 2A, 2C, 3A, 5A, 6, SLC6A4
Other							
Isackson 2011 [141]	GWAS	EYS	rs1337512, rs9342288, rs3857532	ATV (+ others)	399	Muscle symptoms-often last post therapy, +/- ↑CK	EYS SNPs conferred ↑ risk ($p = 0.0003$–0.0008), but did not survive multiple testing correction for GWAS.

CC = case-control study; CG = candidate gene; CI = confidence interval; CK = creatine kinase; Co = cohort study; CR = case report; CS = case series; deQTL = differential expression quantitative trait loci; GWAS = genome-wide association study; HR = hazard ratio; MA = meta-analysis; OR = odds ratio; RCT = randomized controlled trial; WES = whole-exome sequencing. Studies are ordered to preferentially group those that investigated the same gene(s) together.

6.2.1. CYP Phase 1 Hydroxylation

Metabolism is responsible for the clearance of 70% of the top 200 used drugs [142], a subset of 12 of the 57 putatively functional CYPs within the human *CYP* superfamily carry out 75% of drug biotransformations [143], and CYP3A metabolises the largest number of different drugs [142]. ATV, LVT and SVT are themselves extensively metabolised by CYP3A, with greater contributions from CYP3A4 than CYP3A5 [144]. Although no common missense variants are known for *CYP3A4*, the intronic variant, rs35599367 (*22, 522-191C > T), is associated with reduced *CYP3A4* hepatic mRNA and enzymatic activity [145]. *CYP3A4*22* increases the formation of non-functional CYP3A4 alternate splice variants with partial intron six retention, specifically in human liver but not small intestine [146]. *CYP3A4*22* is present with a minor allele frequency (MAF) of ~5% in Europeans, but is low/rare (~1%) in African and Asian populations [147]. *CYP3A4*22* is associated with reduced ATV hydroxylation [148] and ethnicity-restricted increases in SVT/SVT acid concentrations [48]. Although nuclear receptors are highly conserved [149], a single nucleotide polymorphism (SNP) within peroxisome proliferator-activated receptor-α (*PPARA*), rs4253728, has also been associated with reduced human hepatic CYP3A4 protein levels [148] and reduced metabolism of ATV [148] and likely SVT [150].

*CYP3A5*3* is a loss of function allele defined by rs776746 (6986G > A), which introduces a cryptic mRNA splice site resulting in a non-functional truncated protein [151], and has MAFs of ~18%, 69% and 94% in African, Asian and European populations, respectively [147], indicating allelic reversal. *CYP3A5*3/*3* has been associated with increased SVT and ATV L exposures [152,153].

Increased exposures to LVT [154,155] and SVT [156] have been tentatively reported in association with *CYP2D6* reduction/loss-of-function alleles (e.g., *5, *10, *14). However, in vitro studies have not identified LVT/SVT as CYP2D6 substrates [47,157,158], which puts these *CYP2D6*-LVT/SVT associations into doubt. Carrying *CYP2C9*3* has been associated with increased exposures to FVT and PIT, but not RVT or SVT (Table S2). *CYP2C9*2* was not associated with FVT exposure [159]. *CYP2C9*2* and *3 are both reduction-of-function nonsynonymous variants that reduce xenobiotic metabolism by ~30–40% and ~80–90%, respectively [160]. The MAF of *CYP2C9*3* is 7%, 4% and rare in Caucasian, Asian, and African populations, respectively.

Variants in *CYP3A4/5* and *CYP2D6* have been inconsistently associated with SRM or statin tolerability in some candidate gene studies [121–123] but not others [85,118,125]. Carrying *CYP2C9*2* or *3 may increase the risk of FVT adverse events (mainly myotoxicity), particularly when also receiving a CYP2C9 drug inhibitor [105]. However, all patients in this FVT study were renal transplant recipients [105], and so the generalisability of these findings remains unknown. None of these genes have yet been identified in SRM genome-wide association studies (GWAS) [86,115,141]. Thus, whilst *CYP* genetic variants are linked to altered statin exposure, their relationship with SRM remains uncertain.

6.2.2. UGT1A3 Phase 2 Glucuronidation

The UGT family is involved in phase II drug metabolism and consists of subfamilies UGT1A, UGT2A and UGT2B [161]. UGTs catalyse glucuronidation, typically transforming small lipophilic molecules into more hydrophilic metabolites, which are easier to excrete. Statin lactonization can occur either non-enzymatically at low intestinal pH [162], conceivably via a coenzyme A-dependent process [163], or via an unstable acyl glucuronide intermediate that undergoes spontaneous cyclization to a lactone analyte [164]. Statin lactone species are considered more myotoxic than their acid counterparts [165]. Depending on the statin, UGT1A3, 1A1 and UGT2B7 can be involved in acyl glucuronidation [19]. However, UGT1A3 has been consistently shown to have the highest in vitro statin lactonization rates [19]. *UGT1A3*2* is associated with increased UGT1A3 hepatocyte protein expression and *2/*2 volunteers have higher exposures of both ATV lactone and 2-hydroxy ATV lactone [161,166]. The common low expression *UGT1A1* dinucleotide tandem repeat promoter polymorphism, *28, has been associated with both *decreased* area under the ATV lactone concentration-time curve (AUC) [167] and *increased* lactonization [161]; this discrepancy is likely attributable to the extensive linkage disequilibrium within the UGT1A locus—for example, between *UGT1A1*28* and *UGT1A3*2* [161].

UGT1A1/1A3 variants have been sequenced to investigate CVT myotoxicity, but no association was identified [115]. To date, they have not been included in SRM candidate gene studies, nor identified in SRM GWAS.

6.2.3. SLCO1B1 Influx Transporter

SLCO1B1, located on chromosome 12p12.2, encodes organic anion-transporting polypeptide 1B1 (OATP1B1), which is a major hepatocyte-specific sinusoidal influx xenobiotic transporter. The nonsynonymous SNP, rs4149056 (521T > C, p.V174A), in exon five results in decreased intrinsic OATP1B1 transport activity [168]. The rs4149056 MAF is approximately 1%, 8% and 16% in African, Asian and European populations, respectively [147]. Importantly, rs4149056 521CC homozygosity has been associated with increases in statin AUC of 286% (LVT acid) [169], 221% (SVT acid) [170], 208% (PIT) [171], 144% (ATV) [172], 91% PVT [173], and 65% (RVT) [172]. However, rs4149056 has not been associated with FVT [173] or parent LVT [169] and SVT exposures [170].

Importantly, rs4149056 was identified in a seminal GWAS to be strongly associated with myopathy in 85 cases compared to 90 controls, all of whom were on SVT 80mg daily [86]. The odds ratio (OR) for myopathy in 521CC versus 521TT patients was 16.9 (95% confidence interval (CI) 4.7, 61.1), and a gene-dose trend was evident with an OR of 4.5 (95% CI 2.6–7.7) per C allele [86]. In patients on 40 mg SVT daily, the myopathy relative risk remained but was halved to ~2.6 (95% CI 1.3–5.0) per C allele, in keeping with a dose-related ADR [86]. This association between SVT myopathy and rs4149056 has been replicated [89,174] and confirmed in recent large meta-analyses [110,116]. Furthermore, rs4149056 has also been linked to milder adverse outcomes encompassing myalgia, prescription reductions and/or minor biochemical (e.g., CK) elevations indicative of SVT intolerance [69,85,113,175].

In adsition to SVT, historical cases of CVT-related rhabdomyolysis have been associated with rs4149056 [115]. Furthermore, a recent whole-exome sequencing endeavour reported that *SLCO1B1* rs4149056 is associated with statin myopathy (mainly SVT or CVT cases), which reached multiple testing significance when limited to patients not on a fibrate; however, no novel rare coding signals were detected [111]. Intriguingly, *SLCO1B1* rs4149056 has been recently associated with RVT myotoxicity (a composite of myalgias to rhabdomyolysis) in Han Chinese patients [109,176], although it was not previously associated with myalgias in patients of European descent receiving RVT [112]. A recent meta-analysis, largely including these studies, further suggested an association between rs4149056 and RVT myotoxicity [116]. Given the increased RVT exposure reported in Asian compared to Caucasian patients, which is partially but not completed explained by *ABCG2* rs2231142 (see Section 6.2.4) [80], Asian patients are perhaps more sensitive to further *SLCO1B1*-mediated increases in RVT exposure.

Overall, it has been suggested that rs4149056 might be relevant for severe myopathy (e.g., CK > 10 × ULN) due to several statins, with an effect size likely greatest for SVT (or LVT) and lowest for FVT, based upon the degree to which the rs4149056 minor C allele increases exposure to each statin [110]. Nevertheless, rs4149056 has not yet been clearly associated with PVT myotoxicity [85,116], and whilst an association between rs4149056 and ATV myotoxicity has been suggested [85,113] or reported [114], several other studies found no evidence [89,110,116,174,176–178]. Reasons for ongoing uncertainty regarding the role of rs4149056 in ATV myotoxicity include fewer ATV cases in studies (especially cases on high dose ATV) [89] and ATV appears less intrinsically myotoxic than SVT [165], as well as the impact of rs4149056 on exposure being smaller for ATV than SVT acid [172]. The latter is plausibly because ATV utilises OATP1B3, 2B1 and 1A2, as well as OATP1B1, for hepatocyte uptake [25].

In summary, the influence of rs4149056 on myotoxicity risk is clear for SVT, but incompletely resolved for the other licensed statins. Importantly, the FDA revised the SVT product label to reduce SVT 80 mg use because of the elevated myotoxicity risk [179]. Furthermore, the Clinical Pharmacogenetics Implementation Consortium (CPIC) guidelines recommend a lower SVT starting dose or an alternative statin, alongside consideration of routine CK surveillance, in patients already known to carry at least one 521C allele [180]. The Dutch Pharmacogenetic Working Group (DPWG) has published guidance for *SLCO1B1* rs4149056 and both SVT and ATV [181]. The DPWG SVT guideline first line recommendation is an alternate statin in 521C carriers, whilst the ATV guidance only recommends an alternate statin in 521C carriers with additional SRM clinical risk factors [181].

6.2.4. ABCB1 and ABCG2 Efflux Transporters

ABCB1 and *ABCG2* are both members of the superfamily of ATP-binding cassette (ABC) transporters and encode the efflux transporters P-glycoprotein (P-gp) and breast cancer resistance protein (BCRP), respectively. Both P-gp and BCRP are located in the apical (luminal) membrane of enterocytes and the canalicular membrane of hepatocytes, as well as other locations including the blood–brain barrier [182] and placenta [183,184]; they have broad substrate specificity.

ABCB1 has three common SNPs, rs1128503 (1236T-C, synonymous), rs2032582 (missense, 2677T-G) and rs1045642 (synonymous, 3435T-C); TTT homozygotes have ~55–60% increased exposure to both ATV and SVT acid [185]. The *ABCB1* T alleles have been associated with symptom-independent elevated CK levels [117] and muscle symptoms [118,119] in some candidate gene studies, but not with prescribing changes suggestive of statin intolerance [121], nor in SRM GWAS [110,115].

The nonsynonymous *ABCG2* SNP, rs2231142 (421C > A, p.Q141K), has MAFs of 1%, 10–29% and 9% in African, Asian, and European populations, respectively [147]. The 421AA genotype has been associated with a 2.4-fold increased exposure to RVT, ~2-fold increased exposures to ATV, FVT, and SVT, but no increased exposures to PIT or PVT [108]. Interestingly, carrying rs2231142 421A has been associated with an increased risk of myotoxicity with ATV [120], and in renal transplant recipients receiving FVT [105]. Both of these studies were small case control candidate gene studies and have not been confirmed in GWAS, although SRM GWAS analyses have included relatively few FVT cases to date [86,110,111,115].

6.3. Drug–Statin Interactions

Drug–statin interactions are common, can lead to several fold increases in statin exposure, and are established SRM risk factors. Ciclosporin is a potent inhibitor of CYP3A4 [186] and several transporters including OATP1B1, OATP1B3, OATP1B2, ABCG2, and P-gp [99,187], and universally increases systemic exposure of all statins (Table S1). Gemfibrozil and its glucuronide metabolite inhibit CYP2C8 and OATP1B1 and increase statin acid levels (except FVT). Importantly, ciclosporin and gemfibrozil are strongly associated with SRM [99]. CYP3A inhibitors (e.g., amiodarone, itraconazole, clarithromycin) consistently increase the systemic exposure of the CYP3A-metabolised statins (ATV, LVT, SVT) and are significant SRM risk factors [98,99]. Similarly, grapefruit juice, which inhibits CYP3A, has been linked to SVT rhabdomyolysis [96]. The novel cytomegalovirus viral terminase inhibitor, letermovir, increased ATV AUC by over 200%, attributable to inhibition of OATP1B1/3 and CYP3A, and is expected to increase exposure to other statins too [188]. Several antiretroviral drugs increase statin exposure through inhibition of CYP3A and/or OATP1B1, including protease inhibitors (e.g., lopinavir, saquinavir, tipranavir) and pharmacokinetic enhancers (e.g., ritonavir, cobicistat) [189]. As stated above, CYP2C9 inhibitors (e.g., fluconazole) may interact with *CYP2C9*2* or **3* carriage to increase FVT myotoxicity [105]. Beyond PK interactions, other drugs themselves linked with myotoxicity, including corticosteroids and colchicine, may also augment the risk of SRM [88,190]. In recognition of the importance of these interactions, specific recommendations for the management of clinically significant statin–drug interactions have been published [190].

7. Statin Uptake into Skeletal Muscle

Elevated systemic statin exposure plausibly increases intra-myocyte statin concentrations. Statin myocyte entry is likely facilitated by transporters, with statins being substrates for several sarcolemmal transporters. These include OATP2B1, multidrug resistance-associated protein (MRP) 1, MRP4, MRP5 and MCT4 (monocarboxylate transporter-4) [24,191]. Interestingly, the minor allele of the *SLCO2B1* nonsynonymous variant, rs12422149 (935G > A, p.R312Q), has been associated with increased SVT acid plasma clearance in population PK modelling [150], and with statin (mainly SVT) myalgia in a small candidate gene study (n = 19) [69]; both of these findings are potentially consistent with increased statin muscle uptake. It is also noteworthy that lipophilic statins (ATV, SVT) preferentially accumulate in skeletal muscle relative to hydrophilic statins (PVT, RVT) [192], which may help explain the greater myotoxicity of lipophilic statins [165]. The tissue distribution of transporters may also partially account for the lack of statin cardiomyotoxicity [191].

8. Statin-Induced Myocyte Dysfunction

Several mechanisms of myotoxicity have been proposed, as outlined below. Studies that investigated the role of muscle-related gene variants in SRM are detailed in Table 3.

8.1. Exercise

Physical exercise has been reported to trigger and exacerbate SRM [58]. Following the Boston marathon, runners taking a statin had higher CK rises than runners not on a statin [193]. Interestingly, increasing age was associated with higher CK elevations after the marathon only in those on a statin [193]. In professional athletes with hypercholesterolaemia, only 20% could tolerate a statin long term despite re-challenges with alternate statins and doses [194]. Thus, exercise and statins together can potentiate muscle adverse events [195]. Nevertheless, a systematic review has reported that the literature is inconsistent on whether statins objectively reduce exercise capacity and performance [55]. Interestingly, whilst the circulating levels of three muscle-specific microRNAs (miR-1, miR-133a, miR-206) increased after running a marathon irrespective of statin use, the circulating level of a fourth muscle microRNA, miR-499-5p, only increased 24 h after the marathon in runners taking a statin [196]. Follow-up studies in cultured C2C12 myotubes confirmed that extracellular miR-499-5p increases only when carbachol-induced muscle contraction is combined with statin exposure [196]. These observations suggest a role for epigenetics in statin-potentiated muscle injury, and suggest a biomarker for identifying patients with exercise-exacerbated SRM. Nevertheless, this biomarker requires replication. Lastly, these microRNA observations are from marathon runners and not necessarily applicable to more common, moderate exercise. Intriguingly, it has been suggested by some rodent studies that graduated exercise training can improve muscle tolerance to statin exposure [197,198]. Therefore, the findings that exercise to different degrees may either exacerbate or protect against SRM suggests that further work is required in this area to provide patients with clear advice on what to do in terms of exercise and statin use.

8.2. Pre-Existing Neuromuscular Disorders

Statin therapy can adversely interact with underlying neuromuscular disorders to exacerbate symptoms in patients with diagnosed disorders, or unmask previously asymptomatic disorders [199]. Clinical conditions exacerbated or unmasked by statin exposure include myasthenia gravis, dermato/polymyositis, inclusion body myositis, motor neuron disease, and MELAS (mitochondrial encephalopathy, lactic acidosis, and stroke-like episodes) [200–202]. MELAS is a rare mitochondrial disease generally associated with mutations in *MT-TL1* (mitochondrially encoded tRNA leucine 1, also known as *TRNL1*) and reported patients adversely affected by statin exposure had the *MT-TL1* A3243G mutation [201,202]. In such cases, symptoms (muscle-related or otherwise) often persist after statin cessation [129,203], which is an indication for further investigations in those patients not already known to have a neuromuscular disorder.

Patients with untreated hypothyroidism, which causes hypercholesterolaemia and hypothyroid myopathy, are at an increased risk of SRM. This SRM can resolve following statin discontinuation, or persist until thyroid hormone replacement [204,205].

Several metabolic myopathies have been associated with SRM, and often, patients were asymptomatic and unaware of the myopathy before starting statin treatment [130]. It is thought that these conditions increase susceptibility to SRM through reducing the ability of skeletal muscle to compensate to statin-induced myotoxic effects. Metabolic myopathies with an identified genetic mutation that has subsequently been found in patients presenting with SRM include: adenosine monophosphate deaminase (*AMPD1*) deficiency (formerly myoadenylate deaminase deficiency) [129], carnitine palmitoyltransferase 2 (*CPT2*) deficiency [129], glycogen storage diseases II (Pompe disease; *GAA* deficiency) [133], V (McArdle disease, *PYGM* deficiency) [129] and IX (muscle phosphorylase b kinase (*PHKA1*) deficiency) [131], malignant hyperthermia (*RYR1*, *CACNA1S*) [135,136], recurrent childhood myoglobinuria (*LPIN1* mutation) [134], and type I (*DMPK*) [130] and II (*CNBP*) [132] myotonic dystrophy. In addition, immune-mediated rippling muscle disease presenting after statin exposure has been reported [206], and mitochondrial myopathies presenting as rhabdomyolysis have been unmasked following statin treatment, although mitochondrial genetic mutations were not identified in these cases [130,207].

By way of example, the carrier frequency for McArdle disease was 12-fold higher in a cohort of patients with lipid lowering (predominantly statin)-induced myopathy, compared to general population controls [129]. One patient that developed muscular complaints *only* after CVT was homozygous for *PYGM* 49XX, a genotype of McArdle disease [129]. McArdle disease is an autosomal recessive disease due to complete deficiency of myophosphorylase (PYGM) activity. Myophosphorylase is a cytoplasmic enzyme involved in glycogenolysis; myophosphorylase deficiency limits muscle oxidative phosphorylation most likely due to impaired substrate delivery to mitochondria [208]. The roles of other select myopathy genes (*CPT2*, *RYR1*, *CACNA1S*) are covered in more detail in the relevant sections below. Overall, a background of carrying variants or incomplete penetrance of metabolic myopathies appears to sensitive individuals to statin myotoxicity.

8.3. Mitochondrial Impairment

An important role for mitochondrial impairment in SRM is indicated by the case reports [130,202,207] and series [129] that identified underlying mitochondrial dysfunction in patients with (non-resolving) SRM. For example, CPT2 is located within the mitochondrial inner membrane and undertakes oxidation of long-chain fatty acids in mitochondria alongside CPT1. The carrier frequency of *CPT2* variants associated with CPT2 deficiency was higher in SRM patients compared to controls [129]. CPT2 deficiency is an autosomal recessive disorder and a patient with genetically confirmed CP2 deficiency (113LL) was also identified in this study. This patient did have pre-existing symptoms, exacerbated by CVT [129]. Importantly, in vitro transcriptomic analysis has demonstrated that *CPT2* is amongst the top 1% of genes whose mRNA levels are perturbed by 75 drugs (including statins) that can cause rhabdomyolysis [209].

In vitro studies have demonstrated that the statin lactone species are markedly more myotoxic than statin acids, and SVT lactone and FVT lactone are more myotoxic than ATV lactone and PVT lactone [165]. Following ATV re-challenge, patients with previous SRM had higher systemic exposures to ATV lactone and 4-hydroxy ATV lactone (plus increased 2-hydroxy and 4-hydroxy ATV metabolite levels) compared to healthy controls [210]. Lactones have been shown to strongly inhibit (up to 84%) mitochondrial complex III and reduce respiratory capacity within in vitro myoblasts [192]. Furthermore, Q_0 of complex III was identified in silico to be an off-target binding site for statin lactones (but not statin acids) [192]. These observations were verified in muscle biopsies from SRM patients, in which complex III enzyme activity was reduced by 18% [192]. Interestingly, CVT lactone showed the greatest degree of complex III inhibition [192], in keeping with its pronounced rhabdomyolysis risk [74]. In contrast, a recent study in healthy male volunteers found no major differences in mitochondrial respiratory capacity after two weeks of daily SVT (80 mg) or PVT (40 mg). However, this study did find a trend for increased sensitivity to the complex I-linked substrate, glutamate, after SVT treatment, which might be an early indicator of adverse effects on skeletal muscle [211]. Moreover in primary human skeletal muscle cells (myotubes), SVT has been shown to impair respiration at mitochondrial complex I, increase mitochondrial oxidative stress through generation of reactive oxygen species (mitochondrial superoxide and hydrogen peroxide), and result in myotube apoptosis [212]. Other studies have reported that statin exposure does not affect the mitochondrial membrane potential [192,213,214], and so statins are unlikely to act as a mitochondrial uncoupler. Lastly, a recent in vitro study has reported that CVT-induced muscle mitochondrial dysfunction is associated with decreased intracellular miR-145 and increased pro-apoptotic gene expression (*APAF1*, *CASP10*); enforced miR-145 expression reduced the apoptotic cell population. However, this study was in a rhabdomyosarcoma cell line and requires replication [215].

Overall, the evidence strongly supports mitochondrial dysfunction in SRM pathogenesis. However, further clarity and unification on the mechanisms are required.

8.4. HMGCR Pathway Mediated Effects

Statin inhibition of HMGCR perturbs the mevalonate pathway (Figure 1). Whilst this perturbation has been linked to possible beneficial pleiotropic effects [12], importantly, the decreases in CoQ_{10}, protein prenylation, and cholesterol itself have all also been implicated in SRM.

8.4.1. Coenzyme Q_{10} Depletion

CoQ_{10} is an important cofactor in mitochondrial respiration [216]. Primary CoQ_{10} deficiency is a clinically and genetically heterogeneous condition, considered autosomal recessive, and has been associated with isolated myopathy, encephalopathy, nephrotic syndrome, cerebellar ataxia and severe infantile multisystemic disease [217]. In patients on statins, reduced circulating CoQ_{10} is routinely observed [216] and a modest decrease in muscle CoQ_{10} has been suggested in some [218] but not other studies [211,219]. *COQ2* encodes para-hydroxybenzoate-polyprenyl transferase, and defective *COQ2* has been associated with primary CoQ_{10} deficiency, which can improve with early CoQ_{10} supplementation [220]. *COQ2* variants, and in particular rs4693075 (1022C > G), have been investigated; some candidate gene studies [114,127], but not others [89], have reported an association with SRM. Importantly, a recent meta-analysis of RCTs found that CoQ_{10} supplementation likely does not reduce SRM, although larger trials are required to confirm this conclusion [221]. One possible explanation for this null result is that the Q_0 site of mitochondrial complex III is involved in the transfer of electrons from CoQ_{10} to cytochrome *c*, and Q_0 is also the off-target binding site for statin lactones (Section 8.3) [192]. Therefore, statins appear to both reduce circulating CoQ_{10} *and* compete for its pharmacodynamic (PD) target; thus CoQ_{10} supplementation alone may insufficiently counteract both statin actions.

8.4.2. Reduced Protein Prenylation

Farnesyl pyrophosphate (FPP) and geranylgeranyl pyrophosphate (GGPP) are both downstream metabolites of mevalonate, and facilitate post-translational prenylation of multiple proteins [222]. GGPP, rather than FPP, is consistently implicated in in vitro statin myotoxicity [213,223–225]. Experimental evidence has suggested that the statin-mediated decrease in GGPP reduces myotube ATP levels [213], blocks prenylation of small GTPases including Rab [213,224,226] and RhoA [225], induces atrogin-1 expression [227], and stimulates apoptosis [213,225]. The possible pathways that culminate in apoptosis include RhoA mis-localisation from the cell membrane to the cytoplasm (examined in fibroblasts) [225], inhibition of AKT (protein kinase B) phosphorylation and activation [228] likely via both statin-mediated ATP depletion through mitochondrial dysfunction and loss of Rab1 activity [229], and dose-dependent caspase-3 activation [225].

8.4.3. Cholesterol Depletion

The depletion of cholesterol itself has been posited as an aetiological factor in SRM pathogenesis. Slight skeletal muscle damage has been found by electron microscopy in skeletal muscle biopsies from asymptomatic statin-treated patients, with a characteristic pattern involving T-tubular system breakdown and sub-sarcolemmal rupture [230]; cholesterol extraction could reproduce these findings in vitro in skeletal muscle fibres [230]. Nevertheless, although statins inhibit de novo cholesterol production in C2C12 myotubes, total intracellular cholesterol pools remain unchanged [219]. Furthermore, the PCSK9 inhibitors, alirocumab and evolocumab, even more potently reduce LDL-C than statins, but do not currently appear to increase muscle-related adverse events [231,232]. This suggests that SRM is more statin-specific than cholesterol-specific.

8.5. Atrogin-1 Upregulation

The F-box protein, atrogin-1, is a tissue-specific ubiquitin protein E3 ligase that appears central to mediating the proteolysis associated with muscle atrophy observed in multiple diseases, including diabetes and renal failure [233]. Atrogin-1 expression is significantly higher in muscle biopsies from patients with SRM, and atrogin-1 knock down in zebrafish embryos prevented LVT-induced myotoxicity [234]. Moreover, it has been shown that SVT-mediated inhibition of AKT phosphorylation is associated with upregulation of atrogin-1 mRNA [229].

8.6. Calcium Signalling Disruption

RYR1 (chromosome 19) and RYR3 (chromosome 15) mediate the release of stored calcium ions from skeletal muscle sarcoplasmic reticulum, and thereby, play a role in triggering muscle contraction [235]. Deleterious *RYR1* variants are associated with anaesthesia-induced malignant hyperthermia, central core disease [236] and multi-minicore disease [237]. *CACNA1S* encodes the alpha-1 subunit of the L-type calcium channel (the dihydropyridine receptor) which associates with RYR1 in skeletal muscle, and *CACNA1S* mutations are associated with malignant hyperthermia and hypokalaemic periodic paralysis. Importantly, disease-causing mutations or variants in *RYR1* and *CACNA1S* have been found to be more frequent in statin myopathy patients than controls [135,136]. Furthermore, muscle biopsies from patients with SRM express significantly higher *RYR3* mRNA and have more severe structural damage, including intracellular T-tubular vacuolisation, than both statin-naïve and statin tolerant controls [238].

A recent study that examined statin-treated human and rat muscle tissue identified that statin treatment causes dissociation of the stabilising protein, FKBP12, from RYR1 in skeletal muscle, and this is associated with increased unwarranted calcium release sparks [197]. In vitro evidence further suggested that uptake of calcium by mitochondria stimulates reactive oxygen/reactive nitrogen species generation that, in turn, act on RYR1 to maintain and/or exacerbate this calcium release from the sarcoplasmic reticulum. Nevertheless, although the calcium sparks were associated with upregulation of pro-apoptotic signalling markers (caspase-3 and the proportion of TUNEL positive nuclei), statin treatment had no impact on muscle force production [197], and so other susceptibility factors are likely required for myotoxicity to manifest. In rats, running wheel exercise normalised FKBP12-RYR1 binding, which suggests a mechanism by which graduated exercise may improve statin tolerance. Statin treatment also had minimal effect on calcium sparks from statin-treated rat cardiac tissue [197].

Lastly, the intronic variant, rs2819742 (1559G > A), in *RYR2* (chromosome one) was suggestively associated with CVT severe myopathy by GWAS [115]. The minor A allele was associated with reduced myopathy risk (OR 0.48, 95% CI 0.36, 0.63, $p = 1.74 \times 10^{-7}$) [115]. Similarly, a small candidate gene study ($n = 19$) also identified the G allele of *RYR2* rs2819742 to be significantly more common in statin myalgia cases to statin-tolerant controls, in keeping with the GWAS finding [69]. However unlike RYR1/RYR3, RYR2 is expressed mainly in cardiac muscle tissue and deleterious *RYR2* mutations are associated with ventricular arrhythmias [239]. Therefore, the relevance of *RYR2* rs2819742 to SRM remains unclear.

8.7. Glycine Amidinotransferase (GATM)

A genome-wide expression quantitative expression loci (eQTL) analysis in lymphoblastoid cell lines derived from 480 clinical trial subjects identified rs9806699 as a cis-eQTL for *GATM*, which interacted with in vitro SVT exposure such that it was a significantly stronger eQTL under SVT-exposed versus control conditions [126]. GATM is involved in creatine synthesis, and phosphorylation of creatine by CK is a major mechanism for muscle energy storage. The *GATM* locus was associated with a reduced incidence of statin myopathy in two separate populations (combined SVT, ATV, PVT) with a meta-analysis OR for rs1719247 of 0.60 (95% CI 0.45–0.81, $p = 6.0 \times 10^{-4}$) [126]. Several subsequent SRM studies of SRM have not replicated this finding [110,111,240–242], although a recent candidate gene study of RVT myotoxicity in Han Chinese patients found a similar marginal protective effect of the *GATM* rs9806699 minor allele ($p = 0.024$) [109]. The lack of replication raises questions about the role of *GATM* in SRM; functional studies of *GATM* in human primary muscle cells may help resolve the discordant results.

8.8. Immunologically-Mediated Statin Myopathy

8.8.1. LILRB5

A GWAS of serum CK levels found strong signals with the muscle CK (*CKM*) gene and a missense variant, rs12975366 (D247G), within leukocyte immunoglobulin-like receptor subfamily B member 5 (*LILRB5*) [243]; these results were replicated in statin users and non-users [243]. Subsequently, D247 homozygosity has been associated with an increased risk of statin intolerance (a definition not reliant on CK), and replicated in two of three separate cohorts of patients with either myalgia on RVT, or statin myopathy (meta-analysis OR 1.34, 95% CI 1.16-1.54, $p = 7 \times 10^{-5}$) [139]. CK levels were included as a covariate, where appropriate. Subgroup analysis in the included RCT interestingly showed that, whilst D247 homozygosity was associated with myalgia with both placebo and RVT, those carrying 247G only had an increased myalgia risk if on RVT. Thus, whilst D247 homozygosity might confer an overall greater risk of myalgia, statin-induced myalgia appears associated with 247G. A randomized cross-over experimental medicine study to further investigate this drug-gene interaction is being undertaken [244]. Although the exact aetiology is unknown, the immune system is involved in the repair of skeletal muscles and the influx of Foxp3 + T regulatory cells are crucial to muscle regeneration [245]; interestingly, *LILRB5* D247 may associate with *FOXP3* expression [139].

8.8.2. HLA-DRB1*11:01

Interestingly, several research groups previously noted that symptoms and CK elevation in a few patients with SRM persist and/or progress after statin discontinuation, and furthermore, these patients benefit from immunosuppressive therapy [246–248]. These features are consistent with an autoimmune phenomenon. In 2011, it was reported that these patients, as well as a minority without prior statin exposure (less than 10% in myopathy patients ≥ 50 years old), are positive for anti-HMGCR autoantibodies [249]. Muscle biopsies often show necrotizing myopathy with minimal lymphocytic infiltration [137,250], and so anti-HMGCR positive myopathy is recognised as a distinct subtype of immune-mediated necrotizing myopathy [251]. Pharmacogenomic studies have provided further evidence of an autoimmune aetiology. Importantly, *HLA-DRB1*11:01* has been significantly associated with anti-HMGCR positive myopathy [137,138], and the ORs for the presence of *HLA-DRB1*11:01* in anti-HMGCR myopathy white or black patients, compared to controls, have been estimated to be ~25 and ~57, respectively [138]. *HLA-DRB1*11:01* has also been associated with the development of anti-Ro antibodies in neonatal lupus. Although the underlying aetiology of immune-mediated necrotizing myopathy remains incompletely resolved, a potential role for anti-HMGCR in its pathogenesis is suggested: muscle HMGCR expression is upregulated in anti-HMGCR positive myopathy patients [249], circulating anti-HMGCR levels correlate with CK concentration and disease activity [252], and anti-HMGCR can impair muscle regeneration and induce muscle atrophy [253].

8.9. Pain Perception

A family history of muscular symptoms with or without statin exposure increases the risk of SRM [58,69]. A candidate gene study in 195 statin-treated patients, of whom 51 experienced at least probable myalgia, found that rs2276307 and rs1935349 in the 5-hydroxytryptamine (5-HT, serotonin) receptor genes (*HTR*), *HTR3B* and *HTR7*, respectively, were significantly associated with myalgia score [140]. This suggests that variants that may produce individual differences in pain perception might play a role in statin-taking patients' reports of muscle pain [140]. No 5-HT-related candidate SNP was associated with serum CK level [140], suggesting that the associations are with pain perception rather than the extent of muscle breakdown. Nevertheless, these associations have not been replicated in SRM GWAS analyses [86,110,115], although these GWAS analyses used CK elevation (muscle breakdown) within their case definition [86,110,115]. Moreover, these associations were not identified in a small ($n = 19$) candidate gene study of statin myalgia [69]. Overall, an assessment in a larger cohort with statin myalgia cases will help finalise the relevance of these findings.

8.10. Muscle Transcriptomics

The multifaceted and complex pathogenesis of SRM has been underlined by a recent study that compared muscle transcriptomic profiles in 26 cases of strictly phenotyped statin myalgia undergoing statin re-challenge (75% re-developed muscle symptoms) to 10 statin-tolerant controls, with most taking SVT [69]. A robust separation in skeletal muscle differentially expressed genes was found that highlighted the roles of mitochondrial stress, cell senescence and apoptosis, localised activation of a pro-inflammatory immune response, and altered cell and calcium signalling mediated by protein prenylation and Ras-GTPase activation, in statin myalgia [69]. For example, the insulin/IGF/PI3K/AKT signalling network was the top perturbed canonical pathway. Within this network, calmodulin (*CALM*) was upregulated [69]. CALM is a calcium sensing protein that interacts with RYR1, and the calcium-calmodulin complex inhibits RYR1 [254]. Alternatively, inositol 1, 4, 5-triphosphate receptor 2 (*ITPR2*) can medicate calcium release from the sarcoplasmic reticulum [255], and was downregulated within this network [69]. These differential patterns of regulation likely influence calcium signalling and are conceivably an adaptive response to the increased RYR1-mediated calcium release sparks identified following statin-dependent FKBP12 dissociation from RYR1 (described in Section 8.6) [197]. The two most strongly upregulated genes were antisense RNA to the HECT domain E3 ubiquitin protein ligase 2 (*HECTD2-AS1*) and uncoupling protein 3 (*UCP3*). HECTD2 is pro-inflammatory, whilst UCP3 is a mitochondrial anion carrier protein posited to protect against oxidative stress [69]. Although atrogin-1 ubiquitin E3 ligase was not differentially expressed in this study, several genes of the ubiquitin ligase pathway (including HECTD2) did feature prominently in this study [69].

8.11. Vitamin D

The vitamin D family are a group of fat-soluble secosteroids that are instrumental in the regulation of calcium and phosphate levels, and bone mineralisation; the most important forms in humans are cholecalciferol (vitamin D_3) and ergocalciferol (vitamin D_2). The major natural source of vitamin D is via the conversion of 7-dehydrocholesterol (endogenously synthesised from cholesterol) to cholecalciferol by UV-B light, although ergocalciferol and cholecalciferol can also be obtained from plant and animal-derived dietary sources, respectively [256]. Vitamin D is inactive and so undergoes sequential hydroxylation, first to 25-hydroxycholecalciferol/25-hydroxyergocalciferol, which are the major circulating forms but also inactive, and then to 1, 25-dihydroxycholecalciferol (calcitriol)/1, 25-dihydroxyergocalciferol (collectively 1, 25(OH)2D) that constitute the biologically active vitamin D species [256]. 1,25(OH)2D acts through the vitamin D receptor, which is located in multiple tissues including bone, kidney, intestine, parathyroid glands and skeletal muscle, to mediate genomic and faster non-genomic actions [256,257].

There is controversy regarding the impact of statins on vitamin D level [258]. Nevertheless, 1, 25(OH)2D induces CYP3A4 [259,260] and consistent with this finding, the oral availability and systemic exposure of the CYP3A4 substrate, midazolam, trends higher in winter than summer [261]. Similarly, vitamin D supplementation reduces ATV exposure [262]. However, paradoxically, low vitamin D levels may blunt lipid-lowering response to ATV, perhaps because vitamin D derivatives can also inhibit HMGCR [256]. Vitamin D deficiency causes osteomalacia/rickets, as well as muscle weakness and myopathy. Importantly, a meta-analysis has confirmed that plasma vitamin D levels are significantly lower in statin-treated patients with myalgia, compared to those without [93]. Furthermore, several (non-randomized) clinical studies have reported that vitamin D supplementation effectively reduces incident SRM in patients previously statin intolerant undergoing re-challenge, particularly when previously low vitamin D levels are documented to become normalised [91,263–265]. Based on these findings, a double-blind adequately powered RCT is now required.

9. Management of SRM

As statins are widely prescribed, mild SRM is commonly encountered in clinical practice, although statin rhabdomyolysis remains rare. For a patient presenting with SRM, an initial CK level should be taken. During the consultation, the EAS recommend an evaluation of clinical risk factors for SRM (Table 2), other causes of muscular complaints (e.g., polymyalgia rheumatica), and to review the indication for statin therapy, particularly in those at low CVD risk [67]. The benefits and risks of continuing, temporarily suspending, and discontinuing statin treatment need to be weighed up. Additional patient counselling involves discussion about the nocebo effect and complimentary therapeutic lifestyle changes (e.g., smoking cessation, blood pressure control, adopting the Mediterranean diet) [67,266]. There is no gold-standard diagnostic method nor a validated questionnaire for SRM, although a myalgia clinical index score has been proposed by the NLA [267]. Nevertheless, the majority of patients that discontinue statin treatment after a statin-related event can subsequently tolerate some form of statin therapy if re-challenged [268]. In patients with SRM and an ongoing statin indication, temporary statin withdrawal is often appropriate, followed by one or more statin re-challenges (post washout), which can aid causality assessment. Re-challenges can use the same statin (at same dose), an alternate statin at usual dose, lower doses (with potential up-titration), and/or intermittent (non-daily) dosing using a high intensity statin with a long half-life (e.g., ATV, RVT) [67]. The aim should be to treat with the maximum tolerated dose required for the indication [7]. Patients should also be informed that any statin at any dose lowers CVD risk [7]. Nevertheless, whilst less intense approaches such as intermittent dosing are tolerated in at least 70% of patients, they lead to a variable and likely lower proportion of patients reaching LDL-C goals [269], which should also be discussed. In those that do not reach LDL-C goals, non-statin lipid lowering therapy can be considered in combination with the maximally tolerated statin dose or as monotherapy; available options include ezetimibe, a fibrate, or PCSK9 inhibitor. If considering fibrate therapy, fenofibrate is preferred, and gemfibrozil should be avoided because of its interaction with statins to increase rhabdomyolysis risk [67]. Alirocumab and evolocumab have demonstrated cardiovascular benefit in clinical outcomes trials [231,270]. Moreover, in statin-intolerant patients, these PCSK9 inhibitors are tolerated by > 80%, reduce LDL-C by 45–56%, and have fewer muscular adverse events than ATV re-challenge [232,271]. Nevertheless, the costs of PCSK9 inhibitors remain high. As a consequence, this often limits their use to select patients with severe dyslipidaemia [272], and is prohibitive for broader adoption in CVD prevention [273].

Recently, bempedoic acid has shown promise in patients unable to tolerate more than low-dose statin therapy. Bempedoic acid is a novel oral agent under development that inhibits ATP citrate lyase, and a phase 3 RCT showed it reduced LDL-C by 28.5% more than placebo, without a greater rate of muscle-related events. Of note, ATP citrate lyase is upstream of HMGCR, but bempedoic acid is a prodrug that requires very-long chain acyl-CoA synthetase-1 (ASCV1L) for bioactivation. ASCV1L is expressed predominantly in the liver and so it is plausible that the limited active bempedoic acid in muscle will reduce any potential for myotoxicity. It is also noteworthy that a large multicentre implementation initiative is pre-emptively genotyping patients starting one of 39 drugs for over 45 pharmacogenomic variants, and prospectively determining the incidence of ADRs compared to standard care [274]. For patients starting SVT (or ATV) with at least one *SLCO1B1* rs4149056 minor allele, the DPWG recommendations are provided to them and their healthcare team [274].

10. Conclusions

Despite the development of PCSK9 inhibitors, and ongoing development of novel promising therapeutics including bempedoic acid [275] and inclisiran [276], the undoubted efficacy, affordability, availability, and widespread experience with statins ensure they will likely remain the cornerstone of lipid lowering therapy for the foreseeable future. Thus, understanding and mitigating SRM remains clinically relevant. The majority of SRM is mild and ceases quickly after statin cessation. In patients in whom symptoms persist, a non-statin related diagnosis is most likely, although an unmasked metabolic myopathy, or immune-mediated anti-HMGCR positive myopathy, should also be considered. SRM can cause direct patient harm, and the links between muscular symptoms, suboptimal statin utilisation, and increased MACE are clear [61–63]. Several factors that increase systemic statin exposure are associated with SRM, including higher statin dose, advanced age, drug-drug interactions and, for SVT, *SLCO1B1* rs4149056. Increased systemic statin (lactone) exposure, in turn, predisposes to downstream deleterious effects on skeletal muscle. The most important appear to be mitochondrial dysfunction, calcium signalling disruption and reduced prenylation, whose sequelae include atrogin-1 mediated atrophy, apoptosis, and likely reduced immune-mediated muscle regeneration.

At present, our potential to predict SRM is limited. The parsimonious 'QStatin' model for statin moderate-severe myopathy [70] has been developed, which includes new statin use, ethnicity, co-morbidities (liver disease, hypothyroidism, diabetes mellitus) corticosteroids, age and BMI, although its area under the receiver operator curve of ~0.7 is modest [88]. The implementation of *SLCO1B1* rs4149056 testing [274] may help improve predictive power. Whilst the association between *HLA-DRB1*11:01* and anti-HMGCR positive myopathy is notably strong, *HLA-DRB1*11:01* will likely be insufficient to predict this condition alone given its rarity, but *HLA-DRB1*11:01* may have utility in excluding the diagnosis.

Overall, further research is critically needed to identify, validate and integrate novel risk factors for the different SRM phenotypes to improve predictive capability and harmonise understanding of SRM pathogenesis. We propose that the integration of strict clinical phenotyping to identify statin-induced myalgia through the N-of-1 trial paradigm [277], with systems pharmacology omics-based approaches, should be beneficial. Replication of the miR-499-5p and miR-145 signals is needed. The interactions between exercise and vitamin D status with statin use warrant further study. Increased research is also needed into the gut microbiome, as it has recently been shown to be significantly perturbed by statins [278,279] and might module statin response [280]. Much has been done; much work remains.

Supplementary Materials: The following are available online at http://www.mdpi.com/2077-0383/9/1/22/s1, Table S1: Clinical factors associated with statin exposure, Table S2: Genetic variants associated with statin exposure.

Author Contributions: R.M.T. drafted the manuscript; M.P. and R.M.T. reviewed the manuscript; both authors approved the final version. All authors have read and agreed to the published version of the manuscript.

Funding: R.M.T. was supported by the North West England Medical Research Council (MRC) Training Scheme in Clinical Pharmacology and Therapeutics (Grant number: G1000417), and by a Postdoctoral Research Fellowship from Health Education England Genomics Education Programme. The views expressed in this publication are those of the authors and not necessarily those of HEE GEP. M.P. is Emeritus NIHR Senior Investigator.

Conflicts of Interest: The authors declare no conflict of interest.

References

1. Postmus, I.; Verschuren, J.J.; de Craen, A.J.; Slagboom, P.E.; Westendorp, R.G.; Jukema, J.W.; Trompet, S. Pharmacogenetics of statins: Achievements, whole-genome analyses and future perspectives. *Pharmacogenomics* **2012**, *13*, 831–840. [CrossRef] [PubMed]
2. NHS Choices. Nice Publishes New Draft Guidelines on Statins Use. Available online: http://www.nhs.uk/news/2014/02February/Pages/NICE-publishes-new-draft-guidelines-on-statins-use.aspx (accessed on 19 October 2016).
3. Endo, A.; Kuroda, M.; Tsujita, Y. ML-236A, ML-236B, and ML-236C, new inhibitors of cholesterogenesis produced by penicillium citrinium. *J. Antibiot.* **1976**, *29*, 1346–1348. [CrossRef] [PubMed]

4. Endo, A. The origin of the statins. *Atherosclerosis. Suppl.* **2004**, *5*, 125–130. [CrossRef] [PubMed]
5. Liu, J.; Zhang, J.; Shi, Y.; Grimsgaard, S.; Alraek, T.; Fonnebo, V. Chinese red yeast rice (*Monascus purpureus*) for primary hyperlipidemia: A meta-analysis of randomized controlled trials. *Chin. Med.* **2006**, *1*, 4. [CrossRef]
6. Gunde-Cimerman, N.; Cimerman, A. Pleurotus fruiting bodies contain the inhibitor of 3-hydroxy-3-methylglutaryl-coenzyme a reductase—Lovastatin. *Exp. Mycol.* **1995**, *19*, 1–6. [CrossRef]
7. NICE. Cardiovascular Disease: Risk Assessment and Reduction, Including Lipid Modification (Clinical Guideline 181). Available online: https://www.nice.org.uk/guidance/cg181 (accessed on 23 October 2019).
8. National Statistics. Prescriptions Dispensed in the Community, England 2004-14. Available online: http://content.digital.nhs.uk/catalogue/PUB17644/pres-disp-com-eng-2004-14-rep.pdf (accessed on 19 July 2017).
9. Goldstein, J.L.; Brown, M.S. The LDL receptor. *Arterioscler. Thromb. Vasc. Biol.* **2009**, *29*, 431–438. [CrossRef]
10. Rosenson, R.S. Statins: Actions, Side Effects, and Administration. Available online: https://www.uptodate.com/contents/statins-actions-side-effects-and-administration (accessed on 15 March 2019).
11. Trialists, C.T. Efficacy and safety of more intensive lowering of LDL cholesterol: A meta-analysis of data from 170,000 participants in 26 randomised trials. *Lancet* **2010**, *376*, 1670–1681.
12. Kavalipati, N.; Shah, J.; Ramakrishan, A.; Vasnawala, H. Pleiotropic effects of statins. *Indian J. Endocrinol. Metab.* **2015**, *19*, 554–562.
13. Wu, L.M.; Wu, S.G.; Chen, F.; Wu, Q.; Wu, C.M.; Kang, C.M.; He, X.; Zhang, R.Y.; Lu, Z.F.; Li, X.H.; et al. Atorvastatin inhibits pyroptosis through the lncrna nexn-as1/nexn pathway in human vascular endothelial cells. *Atherosclerosis* **2019**, *293*, 26–34. [CrossRef]
14. Gorabi, A.M.; Kiaie, N.; Hajighasemi, S.; Banach, M.; Penson, P.E.; Jamialahmadi, T.; Sahebkar, A. Statin-induced nitric oxide signaling: Mechanisms and therapeutic implications. *J. Clin. Med.* **2019**, *8*, 2051. [CrossRef]
15. Cannon, C.P.; Braunwald, E.; McCabe, C.H.; Rader, D.J.; Rouleau, J.L.; Belder, R.; Joyal, S.V.; Hill, K.A.; Pfeffer, M.A.; Skene, A.M. Intensive versus moderate lipid lowering with statins after acute coronary syndromes. *N. Engl. J. Med.* **2004**, *350*, 1495–1504. [CrossRef] [PubMed]
16. Verdoodt, A.; Honore, P.M.; Jacobs, R.; De Waele, E.; Van Gorp, V.; De Regt, J.; Spapen, H.D. Do statins induce or protect from acute kidney injury and chronic kidney disease: An update review in 2018. *J. Transl. Int. Med.* **2018**, *6*, 21–25. [CrossRef] [PubMed]
17. Esmeijer, K.; Dekkers, O.M.; de Fijter, J.W.; Dekker, F.W.; Hoogeveen, E.K. Effect of different types of statins on kidney function decline and proteinuria: A network meta-analysis. *Sci Rep* **2019**, *9*, 16632. [CrossRef] [PubMed]
18. Kraker, K.; O'Driscoll, J.M.; Schutte, T.; Herse, F.; Patey, O.; Golic, M.; Geisberger, S.; Verlohren, S.; Birukov, A.; Heuser, A.; et al. Statins reverse postpartum cardiovascular dysfunction in a rat model of preeclampsia. *Hypertension* **2020**, *75*, 202–210. [CrossRef]
19. Schirris, T.J.; Ritschel, T.; Bilos, A.; Smeitink, J.A.; Russel, F.G. Statin lactonization by uridine 5′-diphospho-glucuronosyltransferases (UGTs). *Mol. Pharm.* **2015**, *12*, 4048–4055. [CrossRef]
20. Jacobsen, W.; Kuhn, B.; Soldner, A.; Kirchner, G.; Sewing, K.F.; Kollman, P.A.; Benet, L.Z.; Christians, U. Lactonization is the critical first step in the disposition of the 3-hydroxy-3-methylglutaryl-coa reductase inhibitor atorvastatin. *Drug Metab. Dispos. Biol. Fate Chem.* **2000**, *28*, 1369–1378.
21. Pfizer Inc. Lipitor- Atorvastatin Calcium Trihydrate Tablet, Film Coated. Highlights of Prescribing Information. Available online: http://labeling.pfizer.com/ShowLabeling.aspx?id=587 (accessed on 13 May 2019).
22. Catapano, A.L. Pitavastatin—Pharmacological profile from early phase studies. *Atheroscler. Suppl.* **2010**, *11*, 3–7. [CrossRef]
23. Black, A.E.; Sinz, M.W.; Hayes, R.N.; Woolf, T.F. Metabolism and excretion studies in mouse after single and multiple oral doses of the 3-hydroxy-3-methylglutaryl-coa reductase inhibitor atorvastatin. *Drug Metab. Dispos. Biol. Fate Chem.* **1998**, *26*, 755–763.
24. Knauer, M.J.; Urquhart, B.L.; Meyer zu Schwabedissen, H.E.; Schwarz, U.I.; Lemke, C.J.; Leake, B.F.; Kim, R.B.; Tirona, R.G. Human skeletal muscle drug transporters determine local exposure and toxicity of statins. *Circ. Res.* **2010**, *106*, 297–306. [CrossRef]
25. Generaux, G.T.; Bonomo, F.M.; Johnson, M.; Doan, K.M. Impact of *SLCO1B1* (OATP1B1) and *ABCG2* (BCRP) genetic polymorphisms and inhibition on LDL-C lowering and myopathy of statins. *Xenobiotica* **2011**, *41*, 639–651. [CrossRef]

26. Jemal, M.; Rao, S.; Salahudeen, I.; Chen, B.C.; Kates, R. Quantitation of cerivastatin and its seven acid and lactone biotransformation products in human serum by liquid chromatography-electrospray tandem mass spectrometry. *J. Chromatogr. B Biomed. Sci. Appl.* **1999**, *736*, 19–41. [CrossRef]
27. Muck, W. Clinical pharmacokinetics of cerivastatin. *Clin. Pharmacokinet.* **2000**, *39*, 99–116. [PubMed]
28. Muck, W.; Park, S.; Jager, W.; Voith, B.; Wandel, E.; Galle, P.R.; Schwarting, A. The pharmacokinetics of cerivastatin in patients on chronic hemodialysis. *Int. J. Clin. Pharmacol. Ther.* **2001**, *39*, 192–198. [CrossRef] [PubMed]
29. Novartis. Lescol (Fluvastatin Dosium)—Highlights of Prescribing Information. Available online: https://www.pharma.us.novartis.com/sites/www.pharma.us.novartis.com/files/Lescol.pdf (accessed on 7 July 2019).
30. Merck & Co. Mevacor (Lovastatin) Tablets Description. Available online: https://www.accessdata.fda.gov/drugsatfda_docs/label/2012/019643s085lbl.pdf (accessed on 19 December 2019).
31. Neuvonen, P.J.; Backman, J.T.; Niemi, M. Pharmacokinetic comparison of the potential over-the-counter statins simvastatin, lovastatin, fluvastatin and pravastatin. *Clin. Pharmacokinet.* **2008**, *47*, 463–474. [CrossRef] [PubMed]
32. Fujino, H.; Yamada, I.; Shimada, S.; Yoneda, M.; Kojima, J. Metabolic fate of pitavastatin, a new inhibitor of HMG-CoA reductase: Human UDP-Glucuronosyltransferase enzymes involved in lactonization. *Xenobiotica* **2003**, *33*, 27–41. [CrossRef] [PubMed]
33. Kowa Pharmaceuticals. Livalo (Pitavastatin) Tablet—Highlights of Prescribing Information. Available online: http://www.accessdata.fda.gov/drugsatfda_docs/label/2012/022363s008s009lbl.pdf (accessed on 7 July 2019).
34. Bristol-Myers Squibb Company. Pravachol (Pravastatin) Tablets—Highlights of Prescribing Information. Available online: http://packageinserts.bms.com/pi/pi_pravachol.pdf (accessed on 7 July 2019).
35. Hoffman, M.F.; Preissner, S.C.; Nickel, J.; Dunkel, M.; Preissner, R.; Preissner, S. The transformer database: Biotransformation of xenobiotics. *Nucleic Acids Res.* **2014**, *42*, 1113–1117. [CrossRef]
36. Van Haandel, L.; Gibson, K.T.; Leeder, J.S.; Wagner, J.B. Quantification of pravastatin acid, lactone and isomers in human plasma by UHPLC-MS/MS and its application to a pediatric pharmacokinetic study. *J. Chromatogr. B Anal. Technol. Biomed. Life Sci.* **2016**, *1012–1013*, 169–177. [CrossRef]
37. Riedmaier, S. Pharmacogenetic Determinants of Atorvastatin Metabolism and Response (Dissertation). Available online: https://publikationen.uni-tuebingen.de/xmlui/bitstream/handle/10900/49571/pdf/2011_Dissertation_Stephan_Riedmaier.pdf?sequence=1 (accessed on 7 July 2016).
38. Hirano, M.; Maeda, K.; Hayashi, H.; Kusuhara, H.; Sugiyama, Y. Bile salt export pump (BSEP/ABCB11) can transport a nonbile acid substrate, pravastatin. *J. Pharmacol. Exp. Ther.* **2005**, *314*, 876–882. [CrossRef]
39. McCormick, A.D.; McKillop, D.; Butters, C.J.; Miles, G.S.; Baba, T.; Touchi, A.; Yamaguchi, Y. Zd4522—An HMG-CoA reductase inhibitor free of metabolically mediated drug interactions: Metabolic studies in human in vitro systems (abstract 46). *J. Clin. Pharmacol.* **2000**, *40*, 1055.
40. Cooper, K.J.; Martin, P.D.; Dane, A.L.; Warwick, M.J.; Schneck, D.W.; Cantarini, M.V. The effect of fluconazole on the pharmacokinetics of rosuvastatin. *Eur. J. Clin. Pharmacol.* **2002**, *58*, 527–531.
41. Cooper, K.J.; Martin, P.D.; Dane, A.L.; Warwick, M.J.; Schneck, D.W.; Cantarini, M.V. Effect of itraconazole on the pharmacokinetics of rosuvastatin. *Clin. Pharmacol. Ther.* **2003**, *73*, 322–329. [CrossRef]
42. Finkelman, R.D.; Wang, T.D.; Wang, Y.; Azumaya, C.T.; Birmingham, B.K.; Wissmar, J.; Mosqueda-Garcia, R. Effect of *CYP2C19* polymorphism on the pharmacokinetics of rosuvastatin in healthy taiwanese subjects. *Clin. Pharmacol. Drug Dev.* **2015**, *4*, 33–40. [CrossRef] [PubMed]
43. AstraZeneca. Crestor (Rosuvastatin Calcium Tablets)—Highlights of Prescribing Information. Available online: http://www.accessdata.fda.gov/drugsatfda_docs/label/2010/021366s016lbl.pdf (accessed on 3 October 2019).
44. Jemnitz, K.; Veres, Z.; Tugyi, R.; Vereczkey, L. Biliary efflux transporters involved in the clearance of rosuvastatin in sandwich culture of primary rat hepatocytes. *Toxicol. In Vitro* **2010**, *24*, 605–610. [CrossRef] [PubMed]
45. Alakhali, K.; Hassan, Y.; Mohamed, N.; Mordi, M.N. Pharmacokinetic of simvastatin study in malaysian subjects. *ISOR J. Pharm.* **2013**, *3*, 46–51. [CrossRef]
46. Merck & Co. Zocor (Simvastatin) Tablets—Highlights of Prescribing Information. Available online: https://www.merck.com/product/usa/pi_circulars/z/zocor/zocor_pi.pdf (accessed on 17 October 2019).
47. Prueksaritanont, T.; Ma, B.; Yu, N. The human hepatic metabolism of simvastatin hydroxy acid is mediated primarily by *CYP3A*, and not CYP2D6. *Br. J. Clin. Pharmacol.* **2003**, *56*, 120–124. [CrossRef]

48. Kitzmiller, J.P.; Luzum, J.A.; Baldassarre, D.; Krauss, R.M.; Medina, M.W. CYP3A4*22 and CYP3A5*3 are associated with increased levels of plasma simvastatin concentrations in the cholesterol and pharmacogenetics study cohort. *Pharm. Genom.* **2014**, *24*, 486–491. [CrossRef]
49. DeGorter, M.K.; Tirona, R.G.; Schwarz, U.I.; Choi, Y.-H.; Dresser, G.K.; Suskin, N.; Myers, K.; Zou, G.; Iwuchukwu, O.; Wei, W.-Q.; et al. Clinical and pharmacogenetic predictors of circulating atorvastatin and rosuvastatin concentration in routine clinical care. *Circ. Cardiovasc. Genet.* **2013**, *6*, 400–408. [CrossRef]
50. Collins, R.; Reith, C.; Emberson, J.; Armitage, J.; Baigent, C.; Blackwell, L.; Blumenthal, R.; Danesh, J.; Smith, G.D.; DeMets, D.; et al. Interpretation of the evidence for the efficacy and safety of statin therapy. *Lancet* **2016**, *388*, 2532–2561. [CrossRef]
51. Golomb, B.A.; Evans, M.A. Statin adverse effects: A review of the literature and evidence for a mitochondrial mechanism. *Am. J. Cardiovasc. Drugs* **2008**, *8*, 373–418. [CrossRef]
52. The Electronic Medicines Compendium (eMC). Simvastatin 40 mg. Available online: https://www.medicines.org.uk/emc/product/7167/smpc (accessed on 17 July 2019).
53. Golomb, B.A.; Evans, M.A.; Dimsdale, J.E.; White, H.L. Effects of statins on energy and fatigue with exertion: Results from a randomized controlled trial. *Arch. Intern. Med.* **2012**, *172*, 1180–1182. [CrossRef]
54. Lee, D.S.; Markwardt, S.; Goeres, L.; Lee, C.G.; Eckstrom, E.; Williams, C.; Fu, R.; Orwoll, E.; Cawthon, P.M.; Stefanick, M.L.; et al. Statins and physical activity in older men: The osteoporotic fractures in men study. *JAMA Intern. Med.* **2014**, *174*, 1263–1270. [CrossRef]
55. Noyes, A.M.; Thompson, P.D. The effects of statins on exercise and physical activity. *J. Clin. Lipidol.* **2017**, *11*, 1134–1144. [CrossRef] [PubMed]
56. Gauthier, J.M.; Massicotte, A. Statins and their effect on cognition: Let's clear up the confusion. *Can. Pharm. J. Rev. des Pharm. du Can.* **2015**, *148*, 150–155. [CrossRef] [PubMed]
57. Samaras, K.; Makkar, S.R.; Crawford, J.D.; Kochan, N.A.; Slavin, M.J.; Wen, W.; Trollor, J.N.; Brodaty, H.; Sachdev, P.S. Effects of statins on memory, cognition, and brain volume in the elderly. *J. Am. Coll. Cardiol.* **2019**, *74*, 2554–2568. [CrossRef] [PubMed]
58. Bruckert, E.; Hayem, G.; Dejager, S.; Yau, C.; Begaud, B. Mild to moderate muscular symptoms with high-dosage statin therapy in hyperlipidemic patients—The primo study. *Cardiovasc. Drugs Ther.* **2005**, *19*, 403–414. [CrossRef] [PubMed]
59. Mendes, P.; Robles, P.G.; Mathur, S. Statin-induced rhabdomyolysis: A comprehensive review of case reports. *Physiother. Can.* **2014**, *66*, 124–132. [CrossRef] [PubMed]
60. Naderi, S.H.; Bestwick, J.P.; Wald, D.S. Adherence to drugs that prevent cardiovascular disease: Meta-analysis on 376,162 patients. *Am. J. Med.* **2012**, *125*, 882–887.e881. [CrossRef]
61. Wei, M.Y.; Ito, M.K.; Cohen, J.D.; Brinton, E.A.; Jacobson, T.A. Predictors of statin adherence, switching, and discontinuation in the usage survey: Understanding the use of statins in america and gaps in patient education. *J. Clin. Lipidol.* **2013**, *7*, 472–483. [CrossRef]
62. De Vera, M.A.; Bhole, V.; Burns, L.C.; Lacaille, D. Impact of statin adherence on cardiovascular disease and mortality outcomes: A systematic review. *Br. J. Clin. Pharmacol.* **2014**, *78*, 684–698. [CrossRef]
63. Turner, R.M.; Yin, P.; Hanson, A.; FitzGerald, R.; Morris, A.P.; Stables, R.H.; Jorgensen, A.L.; Pirmohamed, M. Investigating the prevalence, predictors, and prognosis of suboptimal statin use early after a non-st elevation acute coronary syndrome. *J. Clin. Lipidol.* **2017**, *11*, 204–214. [CrossRef]
64. Alfirevic, A.; Neely, D.; Armitage, J.; Chinoy, H.; Cooper, R.G.; Laaksonen, R.; Carr, D.F.; Bloch, K.M.; Fahy, J.; Hanson, A.; et al. Phenotype standardization for statin-induced myotoxicity. *Clin. Pharmacol. Ther.* **2014**, *96*, 470–476. [CrossRef] [PubMed]
65. Parker, B.A.; Capizzi, J.A.; Grimaldi, A.S.; Clarkson, P.M.; Cole, S.M.; Keadle, J.; Chipkin, S.; Pescatello, L.S.; Simpson, K.; White, C.M.; et al. Effect of statins on skeletal muscle function. *Circulation* **2013**, *127*, 96–103. [CrossRef] [PubMed]
66. Banach, M.; Rizzo, M.; Toth, P.P.; Farnier, M.; Davidson, M.H.; Al-Rasadi, K.; Aronow, W.S.; Athyros, V.; Djuric, D.M.; Ezhov, M.V.; et al. Statin intolerance—An attempt at a unified definition. Position paper from an international lipid expert panel. *Expert Opin. Drug Saf.* **2015**, *14*, 935–955. [CrossRef] [PubMed]
67. Stroes, E.S.; Thompson, P.D.; Corsini, A.; Vladutiu, G.D.; Raal, F.J.; Ray, K.K.; Roden, M.; Stein, E.; Tokgozoglu, L.; Nordestgaard, B.G.; et al. Statin-associated muscle symptoms: Impact on statin therapy-european atherosclerosis society consensus panel statement on assessment, aetiology and management. *Eur. Heart J.* **2015**, *36*, 1012–1022. [CrossRef]

68. Raju, S.B.; Varghese, K.; Madhu, K. Management of statin intolerance. *Indian J. Endocrinol. Metab.* **2013**, *17*, 977–982.
69. Elam, M.B.; Majumdar, G.; Mozhui, K.; Gerling, I.C.; Vera, S.R.; Fish-Trotter, H.; Williams, R.W.; Childress, R.D.; Raghow, R. Patients experiencing statin-induced myalgia exhibit a unique program of skeletal muscle gene expression following statin re-challenge. *PLoS ONE* **2017**, *12*, e0181308. [CrossRef]
70. Hippisley-Cox, J.; Coupland, C. Unintended effects of statins in men and women in england and wales: Population based cohort study using the qresearch database. *BMJ* **2010**, *340*, c2197. [CrossRef]
71. Kashani, A.; Phillips, C.O.; Foody, J.M.; Wang, Y.; Mangalmurti, S.; Ko, D.T.; Krumholz, H.M. Risks associated with statin therapy: A systematic overview of randomized clinical trials. *Circulation* **2006**, *114*, 2788–2797. [CrossRef]
72. Abd, T.T.; Jacobson, T.A. Statin-induced myopathy: A review and update. *Expert Opin. Drug Saf.* **2011**, *10*, 373–387. [CrossRef]
73. Davidson, M.H.; Robinson, J.G. Safety of aggressive lipid management. *J. Am. Coll. Cardiol.* **2007**, *49*, 1753–1762. [CrossRef]
74. Furberg, C.D.; Pitt, B. Withdrawal of cerivastatin from the world market. *Curr. Control. Trials Cardiovasc. Med.* **2001**, *2*, 205–207. [CrossRef] [PubMed]
75. Godlee, F. Adverse effects of statins. *BMJ* **2014**, *348*, g3306. [CrossRef] [PubMed]
76. Gupta, A.; Thompson, D.; Whitehouse, A.; Collier, T.; Dahlof, B.; Poulter, N.; Collins, R.; Sever, P. Adverse events associated with unblinded, but not with blinded, statin therapy in the anglo-scandinavian cardiac outcomes trial-lipid-lowering arm (ASCOT-LLA): A randomised double-blind placebo-controlled trial and its non-randomised non-blind extension phase. *Lancet* **2017**, *389*, 2473–2481.
77. Taylor, B.A.; Lorson, L.; White, C.M.; Thompson, P.D. A randomized trial of coenzyme Q10 in patients with confirmed statin myopathy. *Atherosclerosis* **2015**, *238*, 329–335. [CrossRef] [PubMed]
78. Nissen, S.E.; Stroes, E.; Dent-Acosta, R.E.; Rosenson, R.S.; Lehman, S.J.; Sattar, N.; Preiss, D.; Bruckert, E.; Ceska, R.; Lepor, N.; et al. Efficacy and tolerability of evolocumab vs ezetimibe in patients with muscle-related statin intolerance: The GAUSS-3 randomized clinical trial. *JAMA* **2016**, *315*, 1580–1590. [CrossRef]
79. Zhou, Q.; Ruan, Z.R.; Yuan, H.; Xu, D.H.; Zeng, S. ABCB1 gene polymorphisms, ABCB1 haplotypes and *ABCG2* c.421C > A are determinants of inter-subject variability in rosuvastatin pharmacokinetics. *Die Pharm.* **2013**, *68*, 129–134.
80. Birmingham, B.K.; Bujac, S.R.; Elsby, R.; Azumaya, C.T.; Wei, C.; Chen, Y.; Mosqueda-Garcia, R.; Ambrose, H.J. Impact of *ABCG2* and *SLCO1B1* polymorphisms on pharmacokinetics of rosuvastatin, atorvastatin and simvastatin acid in caucasian and asian subjects: A class effect? *Eur. J. Clin. Pharmacol.* **2015**, *71*, 341–355. [CrossRef]
81. Simonson, S.G.; Martin, P.D.; Mitchell, P.; Schneck, D.W.; Lasseter, K.C.; Warwick, M.J. Pharmacokinetics and pharmacodynamics of rosuvastatin in subjects with hepatic impairment. *Eur. J. Clin. Pharmacol.* **2003**, *58*, 669–675. [CrossRef]
82. Pasternak, R.C.; Smith, S.C.; Bairey-Merz, C.N.; Grundy, S.M.; Cleeman, J.I.; Lenfant, C. Acc/aha/nhlbi clinical advisory on the use and safety of statins. *Circulation* **2002**, *106*, 1024.
83. Simon, L.; Jolley, S.E.; Molina, P.E. Alcoholic myopathy: Pathophysiologic mechanisms and clinical implications. *Alcohol. Res.* **2017**, *38*, 207–217.
84. Appel-Dingemanse, S.; Smith, T.; Merz, M. Pharmacokinetics of fluvastatin in subjects with renal impairment and nephrotic syndrome. *J. Clin. Pharmacol.* **2002**, *42*, 312–318. [CrossRef] [PubMed]
85. Voora, D.; Shah, S.H.; Spasojevic, I.; Ali, S.; Reed, C.R.; Salisbury, B.A.; Ginsburg, G.S. The *SLCO1B1**5 genetic variant is associated with statin-induced side effects. *J. Am. Coll. Cardiol.* **2009**, *54*, 1609–1616. [CrossRef] [PubMed]
86. Link, E.; Parish, S.; Armitage, J.; Bowman, L.; Heath, S.; Matsuda, F.; Gut, I.; Lathrop, M.; Collins, R. *SLCO1B1* variants and statin-induced myopathy—A genomewide study. *N. Engl. J. Med.* **2008**, *359*, 789–799. [PubMed]
87. Schech, S.; Graham, D.; Staffa, J.; Andrade, S.E.; La Grenade, L.; Burgess, M.; Blough, D.; Stergachis, A.; Chan, K.A.; Platt, R.; et al. Risk factors for statin-associated rhabdomyolysis. *Pharmacoepidemiol. Drug Saf.* **2007**, *16*, 352–358. [CrossRef]
88. ClinRisk Ltd. Qstatin—2014 Update Information. Available online: http://qintervention.org/QStatin-2014-Update-Information.pdf (accessed on 24 July 2017).

89. Carr, D.F.; O'Meara, H.; Jorgensen, A.L.; Campbell, J.; Hobbs, M.; McCann, G.; van Staa, T.; Pirmohamed, M. SLCO1B1 genetic variant associated with statin-induced myopathy: A proof-of-concept study using the clinical practice research datalink. *Clin. Pharmacol. Ther.* **2013**, *94*, 695–701. [CrossRef]
90. Cziraky, M.J.; Willey, V.J.; McKenney, J.M.; Kamat, S.A.; Fisher, M.D.; Guyton, J.R.; Jacobson, T.A.; Davidson, M.H. Risk of hospitalized rhabdomyolysis associated with lipid-lowering drugs in a real-world clinical setting. *J. Clin. Lipidol.* **2013**, *7*, 102–108. [CrossRef]
91. Ahmed, W.; Khan, N.; Glueck, C.J.; Pandey, S.; Wang, P.; Goldenberg, N.; Uppal, M.; Khanal, S. Low serum 25 (OH) vitamin D levels (<32 ng/ml) are associated with reversible myositis-myalgia in statin-treated patients. *Transl. Res.* **2009**, *153*, 11–16.
92. Khayznikov, M.; Kumar, A.; Wang, P.; Glueck, C.J. Statin intolerance and vitamin d supplementation. *N. Am. J. Med. Sci.* **2015**, *7*, 339–340.
93. Michalska-Kasiczak, M.; Sahebkar, A.; Mikhailidis, D.P.; Rysz, J.; Muntner, P.; Toth, P.P.; Jones, S.R.; Rizzo, M.; Kees Hovingh, G.; Farnier, M.; et al. Analysis of vitamin d levels in patients with and without statin-associated myalgia—A systematic review and meta-analysis of 7 studies with 2420 patients. *Int. J. Cardiol.* **2015**, *178*, 111–116. [CrossRef]
94. Thompson, P.D.; Zmuda, J.M.; Domalik, L.J.; Zimet, R.J.; Staggers, J.; Guyton, J.R. Lovastatin increases exercise-induced skeletal muscle injury. *Metabolism* **1997**, *46*, 1206–1210. [CrossRef]
95. Meador, B.M.; Huey, K.A. Statin-associated myopathy and its exacerbation with exercise. *Muscle Nerve* **2010**, *42*, 469–479. [CrossRef] [PubMed]
96. Dreier, J.P.; Endres, M. Statin-associated rhabdomyolysis triggered by grapefruit consumption. *Neurology* **2004**, *62*, 670. [CrossRef] [PubMed]
97. Armitage, J. The safety of statins in clinical practice. *Lancet* **2007**, *370*, 1781–1790. [CrossRef]
98. Patel, A.M.; Shariff, S.; Bailey, D.G.; Juurlink, D.N.; Gandhi, S.; Mamdani, M.; Gomes, T.; Fleet, J.; Hwang, Y.J.; Garg, A.X. Statin toxicity from macrolide antibiotic coprescription: A population-based cohort study. *Ann. Intern. Med.* **2013**, *158*, 869–876. [CrossRef]
99. Neuvonen, P.J.; Niemi, M.; Backman, J.T. Drug interactions with lipid-lowering drugs: Mechanisms and clinical relevance. *Clin. Pharmacol. Ther.* **2006**, *80*, 565–581. [CrossRef]
100. Lees, R.S.; Lees, A.M. Rhabdomyolysis from the coadministration of lovastatin and the antifungal agent itraconazole. *N. Engl. J. Med.* **1995**, *333*, 664–665. [CrossRef]
101. Cheng, C.H.; Miller, C.; Lowe, C.; Pearson, V.E. Rhabdomyolysis due to probable interaction between simvastatin and ritonavir. *Am. J. Health Syst. Pharm. AJHP Off. J. Am. Soc. Health Syst. Pharm.* **2002**, *59*, 728–730. [CrossRef]
102. Chanson, N.; Bossi, P.; Schneider, L.; Bourry, E.; Izzedine, H. Rhabdomyolysis after ezetimibe/simvastatin therapy in an HIV-infected patient. *NDT Plus* **2008**, *1*, 157–161. [CrossRef]
103. Roten, L.; Schoenenberger, R.A.; Krahenbuhl, S.; Schlienger, R.G. Rhabdomyolysis in association with simvastatin and amiodarone. *Ann. Pharmacother.* **2004**, *38*, 978–981. [CrossRef]
104. Saliba, W.R.; Elias, M. Severe myopathy induced by the co-administration of simvastatin and itraconazole. *Eur. J. Intern. Med.* **2005**, *16*, 305. [CrossRef]
105. Mirosevic Skvrce, N.; Bozina, N.; Zibar, L.; Barisic, I.; Pejnovic, L.; Macolic Sarinic, V. CYP2C9 and ABCG2 polymorphisms as risk factors for developing adverse drug reactions in renal transplant patients taking fluvastatin: A case-control study. *Pharmacogenomics* **2013**, *14*, 1419–1431. [CrossRef] [PubMed]
106. Kitamura, S.; Maeda, K.; Wang, Y.; Sugiyama, Y. Involvement of multiple transporters in the hepatobiliary transport of rosuvastatin. *Drug Metab. Dispos.* **2008**, *36*, 2014–2023. [CrossRef] [PubMed]
107. Ho, R.H.; Tirona, R.G.; Leake, B.F.; Glaeser, H.; Lee, W.; Lemke, C.J.; Wang, Y.; Kim, R.B. Drug and bile acid transporters in rosuvastatin hepatic uptake: Function, expression, and pharmacogenetics. *Gastroenterology* **2006**, *130*, 1793–1806. [CrossRef] [PubMed]
108. Elsby, R.; Hilgendorf, C.; Fenner, K. Understanding the critical disposition pathways of statins to assess drug-drug interaction risk during drug development: It's not just about OATP1B1. *Clin. Pharmacol. Ther.* **2012**, *92*, 584–598. [CrossRef]
109. Bai, X.; Zhang, B.; Wang, P.; Wang, G.-L.; Li, J.-L.; Wen, D.-S.; Long, X.-Z.; Sun, H.-S.; Liu, Y.-B.; Huang, M.; et al. Effects of SLCO1B1 and gatm gene variants on rosuvastatin-induced myopathy are unrelated to high plasma exposure of rosuvastatin and its metabolites. *Acta Pharmacol. Sin.* **2019**, *40*, 492–499. [CrossRef]

110. Carr, D.F.; Francis, B.; Jorgensen, A.L.; Zhang, E.; Chinoy, H.; Heckbert, S.R.; Bis, J.C.; Brody, J.A.; Floyd, J.; Psaty, B.M.; et al. Genome-wide association study of statin-induced myopathy in patients recruited using the UK clinical practice research datalink. *Clin. Pharmacol. Ther.* **2019**, *106*, 1353–1361. [CrossRef]
111. Floyd, J.S.; Bloch, K.M.; Brody, J.A.; Maroteau, C.; Siddiqui, M.K.; Gregory, R.; Carr, D.F.; Molokhia, M.; Liu, X.; Bis, J.C.; et al. Pharmacogenomics of statin-related myopathy: Meta-analysis of rare variants from whole-exome sequencing. *PLoS ONE* **2019**, *14*, e0218115. [CrossRef]
112. Danik, J.S.; Chasman, D.I.; MacFadyen, J.G.; Nyberg, F.; Barratt, B.J.; Ridker, P.M. Lack of association between *SLCO1B1* polymorphisms and clinical myalgia following rosuvastatin therapy. *Am. Heart J.* **2013**, *165*, 1008–1014. [CrossRef]
113. De Keyser, C.E.; Peters, B.J.; Becker, M.L.; Visser, L.E.; Uitterlinden, A.G.; Klungel, O.H.; Verstuyft, C.; Hofman, A.; Maitland-van der Zee, A.H.; Stricker, B.H. The *SLCO1B1* c.521T > C polymorphism is associated with dose decrease or switching during statin therapy in the rotterdam study. *Pharm. Genom.* **2014**, *24*, 43–51. [CrossRef]
114. Puccetti, L.; Ciani, F.; Auteri, A. Genetic involvement in statins induced myopathy. Preliminary data from an observational case-control study. *Atherosclerosis* **2010**, *211*, 28–29. [CrossRef]
115. Marciante, K.D.; Durda, J.P.; Heckbert, S.R.; Lumley, T.; Rice, K.; McKnight, B.; Totah, R.A.; Tamraz, B.; Kroetz, D.L.; Fukushima, H.; et al. Cerivastatin, genetic variants, and the risk of rhabdomyolysis. *Pharm. Genom.* **2011**, *21*, 280–288. [CrossRef] [PubMed]
116. Xiang, Q.; Chen, S.Q.; Ma, L.Y.; Hu, K.; Zhang, Z.; Mu, G.Y.; Xie, Q.F.; Zhang, X.D.; Cui, Y.M. Association between SLCO1B1 T521C polymorphism and risk of statin-induced myopathy: A meta-analysis. *Pharm. J.* **2018**, *18*, 721–729. [CrossRef] [PubMed]
117. Ferrari, M.; Guasti, L.; Maresca, A.; Mirabile, M.; Contini, S.; Grandi, A.M.; Marino, F.; Cosentino, M. Association between statin-induced creatine kinase elevation and genetic polymorphisms in *SLCO1B1*, *ABCB1* and *ABCG2*. *Eur. J. Clin. Pharmacol.* **2014**, *70*, 539–547. [CrossRef] [PubMed]
118. Fiegenbaum, M.; da Silveira, F.R.; Van der Sand, C.R.; Van der Sand, L.C.; Ferreira, M.E.; Pires, R.C.; Hutz, M.H. The role of common variants of *ABCB1*, *CYP3A4*, and *CYP3A5* genes in lipid-lowering efficacy and safety of simvastatin treatment. *Clin. Pharmacol. Ther.* **2005**, *78*, 551–558. [CrossRef]
119. Hoenig, M.R.; Walker, P.J.; Gurnsey, C.; Beadle, K.; Johnson, L. The C3435T polymorphism in *ABCB1* influences atorvastatin efficacy and muscle symptoms in a high-risk vascular cohort. *J. Clin. Lipidol.* **2011**, *5*, 91–96. [CrossRef]
120. Mirosevic Skvrce, N.; Macolic Sarinic, V.; Simic, I.; Ganoci, L.; Muacevic Katanec, D.; Bozina, N. *ABCG2* gene polymorphisms as risk factors for atorvastatin adverse reactions: A case-control study. *Pharmacogenomics* **2015**, *16*, 803–815. [CrossRef]
121. Becker, M.L.; Visser, L.E.; van Schaik, R.H.; Hofman, A.; Uitterlinden, A.G.; Stricker, B.H. Influence of genetic variation in *CYP3A4* and *ABCB1* on dose decrease or switching during simvastatin and atorvastatin therapy. *Pharmacoepidemiol. Drug Saf.* **2010**, *19*, 75–81. [CrossRef]
122. Frudakis, T.N.; Thomas, M.J.; Ginjupalli, S.N.; Handelin, B.; Gabriel, R.; Gomez, H.J. CYP2D6*4 polymorphism is associated with statin-induced muscle effects. *Pharm. Genom.* **2007**, *17*, 695–707. [CrossRef]
123. Mulder, A.B.; van Lijf, H.J.; Bon, M.A.; van den Bergh, F.A.; Touw, D.J.; Neef, C.; Vermes, I. Association of polymorphism in the cytochrome *CYP2D6* and the efficacy and tolerability of simvastatin. *Clin. Pharmacol. Ther.* **2001**, *70*, 546–551. [CrossRef]
124. Wilke, R.A.; Moore, J.H.; Burmester, J.K. Relative impact of *CYP3A* genotype and concomitant medication on the severity of atorvastatin-induced muscle damage. *Pharm. Genom.* **2005**, *15*, 415–421. [CrossRef]
125. Zuccaro, P.; Mombelli, G.; Calabresi, L.; Baldassarre, D.; Palmi, I.; Sirtori, C.R. Tolerability of statins is not linked to CYP450 polymorphisms, but reduced *CYP2D6* metabolism improves cholesteraemic response to simvastatin and fluvastatin. *Pharmacol. Res.* **2007**, *55*, 310–317. [CrossRef] [PubMed]
126. Mangravite, L.M.; Engelhardt, B.E.; Medina, M.W.; Smith, J.D.; Brown, C.D.; Chasman, D.I.; Mecham, B.H.; Howie, B.; Shim, H.; Naidoo, D.; et al. A statin-dependent qtl for gatm expression is associated with statin-induced myopathy. *Nature* **2013**, *502*, 377–380. [CrossRef] [PubMed]
127. Oh, J.; Ban, M.R.; Miskie, B.A.; Pollex, R.L.; Hegele, R.A. Genetic determinants of statin intolerance. *Lipids Health Dis.* **2007**, *6*, 7. [CrossRef] [PubMed]

128. Ruano, G.; Windemuth, A.; Wu, A.H.; Kane, J.P.; Malloy, M.J.; Pullinger, C.R.; Kocherla, M.; Bogaard, K.; Gordon, B.R.; Holford, T.R.; et al. Mechanisms of statin-induced myalgia assessed by physiogenomic associations. *Atherosclerosis* **2011**, *218*, 451–456. [CrossRef] [PubMed]

129. Vladutiu, G.D.; Simmons, Z.; Isackson, P.J.; Tarnopolsky, M.; Peltier, W.L.; Barboi, A.C.; Sripathi, N.; Wortmann, R.L.; Phillips, P.S. Genetic risk factors associated with lipid-lowering drug-induced myopathies. *Muscle Nerve* **2006**, *34*, 153–162. [CrossRef]

130. Tsivgoulis, G.; Spengos, K.; Karandreas, N.; Panas, M.; Kladi, A.; Manta, P. Presymptomatic neuromuscular disorders disclosed following statin treatment. *Arch. Intern. Med.* **2006**, *166*, 1519–1524. [CrossRef]

131. Echaniz-Laguna, A.; Mohr, M.; Tranchant, C. Neuromuscular symptoms and elevated creatine kinase after statin withdrawal. *N. Engl. J. Med.* **2010**, *362*, 564–565. [CrossRef]

132. Knoblauch, H.; Schoewel, V.; Kress, W.; Rosada, A.; Spuler, S. Another side to statin-related side effects. *Ann. Intern. Med.* **2010**, *152*, 478–479. [CrossRef]

133. Voermans, N.C.; Lammens, M.; Wevers, R.A.; Hermus, A.R.; van Engelen, B.G. Statin-disclosed acid maltase deficiency. *J. Intern. Med.* **2005**, *258*, 196–197. [CrossRef]

134. Zeharia, A.; Shaag, A.; Houtkooper, R.H.; Hindi, T.; de Lonlay, P.; Erez, G.; Hubert, L.; Saada, A.; de Keyzer, Y.; Eshel, G.; et al. Mutations in lpin1 cause recurrent acute myoglobinuria in childhood. *Am. J. Hum. Genet.* **2008**, *83*, 489–494. [CrossRef]

135. Vladutiu, G.D.; Isackson, P.J.; Kaufman, K.; Harley, J.B.; Cobb, B.; Christopher-Stine, L.; Wortmann, R.L. Genetic risk for malignant hyperthermia in non-anesthesia-induced myopathies. *Mol. Genet. Metab.* **2011**, *104*, 167–173. [CrossRef] [PubMed]

136. Isackson, P.J.; Wang, J.; Zia, M.; Spurgeon, P.; Levesque, A.; Bard, J.; James, S.; Nowak, N.; Lee, T.K.; Vladutiu, G.D. Ryr1 and cacna1s genetic variants identified with statin-associated muscle symptoms. *Pharmacogenomics* **2018**, *19*, 1235–1249. [CrossRef] [PubMed]

137. Limaye, V.; Bundell, C.; Hollingsworth, P.; Rojana-Udomsart, A.; Mastaglia, F.; Blumbergs, P.; Lester, S. Clinical and genetic associations of autoantibodies to 3-hydroxy-3-methyl-glutaryl-coenzyme a reductase in patients with immune-mediated myositis and necrotizing myopathy. *Muscle Nerve* **2015**, *52*, 196–203. [CrossRef] [PubMed]

138. Mammen, A.L.; Gaudet, D.; Brisson, D.; Christopher-Stine, L.; Lloyd, T.E.; Leffell, M.S.; Zachary, A.A. Increased frequency of drb1*11:01 in anti-hydroxymethylglutaryl-coenzyme a reductase-associated autoimmune myopathy. *Arthritis Care Res.* **2012**, *64*, 1233–1237.

139. Siddiqui, M.K.; Maroteau, C.; Veluchamy, A.; Tornio, A.; Tavendale, R.; Carr, F.; Abelega, N.U.; Carr, D.; Bloch, K.; Hallberg, P.; et al. A common missense variant of *LILRB5* is associated with statin intolerance and myalgia. *Eur. Heart J.* **2017**, *38*, 3569–3575. [CrossRef]

140. Ruano, G.; Thompson, P.D.; Windemuth, A.; Seip, R.L.; Dande, A.; Sorokin, A.; Kocherla, M.; Smith, A.; Holford, T.R.; Wu, A.H. Physiogenomic association of statin-related myalgia to serotonin receptors. *Muscle Nerve* **2007**, *36*, 329–335. [CrossRef]

141. Isackson, P.J.; Ochs-Balcom, H.M.; Ma, C.; Harley, J.B.; Peltier, W.; Tarnopolsky, M.; Sripathi, N.; Wortmann, R.L.; Simmons, Z.; Wilson, J.D.; et al. Association of common variants in the human eyes shut ortholog (EYS) with statin-induced myopathy: Evidence for additional functions of EYS. *Muscle Nerve* **2011**, *44*, 531–538. [CrossRef]

142. Wienkers, L.C.; Heath, T.G. Predicting in vivo drug interactions from in vitro drug discovery data. *Nat. Rev. Drug Discov.* **2005**, *4*, 825–833. [CrossRef]

143. Gordon, A.S.; Tabor, H.K.; Johnson, A.D.; Snively, B.M.; Assimes, T.L.; Auer, P.L.; Ioannidis, J.P.; Peters, U.; Robinson, J.G.; Sucheston, L.E.; et al. Quantifying rare, deleterious variation in 12 human cytochrome P450 drug-metabolism genes in a large-scale exome dataset. *Hum. Mol. Genet.* **2014**, *23*, 1957–1963. [CrossRef]

144. Park, J.E.; Kim, K.B.; Bae, S.K.; Moon, B.S.; Liu, K.H.; Shin, J.G. Contribution of cytochrome P450 3A4 and 3A5 to the metabolism of atorvastatin. *Xenobiotica* **2008**, *38*, 1240–1251. [CrossRef]

145. Wang, D.; Guo, Y.; Wrighton, S.A.; Cooke, G.E.; Sadee, W. Intronic polymorphism in CYP3A4 affects hepatic expression and response to statin drugs. *Pharm. J.* **2011**, *11*, 274–286. [CrossRef] [PubMed]

146. Wang, D.; Sadee, W. CYP3A4 intronic snp rs35599367 (*CYP3A4*22*) alters RNA splicing. *Pharm. Genom.* **2016**, *26*, 40–43. [CrossRef] [PubMed]

147. Yates, A.; Akanni, W.; Amode, M.R.; Barrell, D.; Billis, K.; Carvalho-Silva, D.; Cummins, C.; Clapham, P.; Fitzgerald, S.; Gil, L.; et al. Ensembl 2016. *Nucleic Acids Res.* **2016**, *44*, D710–D716. [CrossRef] [PubMed]

148. Klein, K.; Thomas, M.; Winter, S.; Nussler, A.K.; Niemi, M.; Schwab, M.; Zanger, U.M. *PPARA*: A novel genetic determinant of CYP3A4 in vitro and in vivo. *Clin. Pharmacol. Ther.* **2012**, *91*, 1044–1052. [CrossRef]
149. Kozyra, M.; Ingelman-Sundberg, M.; Lauschke, V.M. Rare genetic variants in cellular transporters, metabolic enzymes, and nuclear receptors can be important determinants of interindividual differences in drug response. *Genet. Med.* **2017**, *19*, 20–29. [CrossRef]
150. Tsamandouras, N.; Dickinson, G.; Guo, Y.; Hall, S.; Rostami-Hodjegan, A.; Galetin, A.; Aarons, L. Identification of the effect of multiple polymorphisms on the pharmacokinetics of simvastatin and simvastatin acid using a population-modeling approach. *Clin. Pharmacol. Ther.* **2014**, *96*, 90–100. [CrossRef]
151. Elens, L.; van Gelder, T.; Hesselink, D.A.; Haufroid, V.; van Schaik, R.H. *CYP3A4*22*: Promising newly identified CYP3A4 variant allele for personalizing pharmacotherapy. *Pharmacogenomics* **2013**, *14*, 47–62. [CrossRef]
152. Shin, J.; Pauly, D.F.; Pacanowski, M.A.; Langaee, T.; Frye, R.F.; Johnson, J.A. Effect of cytochrome P450 3A5 genotype on atorvastatin pharmacokinetics and its interaction with clarithromycin. *Pharmacotherapy* **2011**, *31*, 942–950. [CrossRef]
153. Kim, K.A.; Park, P.W.; Lee, O.J.; Kang, D.K.; Park, J.Y. Effect of polymorphic *CYP3A5* genotype on the single-dose simvastatin pharmacokinetics in healthy subjects. *J. Clin. Pharmacol.* **2007**, *47*, 87–93. [CrossRef]
154. Yin, O.Q.; Chang, Q.; Tomlinson, B.; Chow, M.S. The effect of *CYP2D6* genotype on the pharmacokinetics of lovastatin in Chinese subjects. *Clin. Pharmacol. Ther.* **2004**, *75*, P18. [CrossRef]
155. Yin, O.Q.; Mak, V.W.; Hu, M.; Fok, B.S.; Chow, M.S.; Tomlinson, B. Impact of *CYP2D6* polymorphisms on the pharmacokinetics of lovastatin in Chinese subjects. *Eur. J. Clin. Pharmacol.* **2012**, *68*, 943–949. [CrossRef] [PubMed]
156. Choi, H.Y.; Bae, K.S.; Cho, S.H.; Ghim, J.L.; Choe, S.; Jung, J.A.; Jin, S.J.; Kim, H.S.; Lim, H.S. Impact of *CYP2D6*, *CYP3A5*, *CYP2C19*, *CYP2A6*, *SLCO1B1*, *ABCB1*, and *ABCG2* gene polymorphisms on the pharmacokinetics of simvastatin and simvastatin acid. *Pharm. Genom.* **2015**, *25*, 595–608. [CrossRef] [PubMed]
157. Prueksaritanont, T.; Gorham, L.M.; Ma, B.; Liu, L.; Yu, X.; Zhao, J.J.; Slaughter, D.E.; Arison, B.H.; Vyas, K.P. In vitro Metabolism of Simvastatin in Humans [sbt]Identification of metabolizing enzymes and effect of the drug on hepatic P450s. *Drug Metab. Dispos.* **1997**, *25*, 1191–1199. [PubMed]
158. Iyer, L.V.; Ho, M.N.; Furimsky, A.M.; Green, C.E.; Green, A.G.; Sharp, L.E.; Koch, S.; Li, Y.; Catz, P.; Furniss, M.; et al. In vitro metabolism and interaction studies with celecoxib and lovastatin. *Cancer Res.* **2004**, *64*, 488.
159. Kirchheiner, J.; Kudlicz, D.; Meisel, C.; Bauer, S.; Meineke, I.; Roots, I.; Brockmoller, J. Influence of *CYP2C9* polymorphisms on the pharmacokinetics and cholesterol-lowering activity of (−)-3s,5r-fluvastatin and (+)-3r,5s-fluvastatin in healthy volunteers. *Clin. Pharmacol. Ther.* **2003**, *74*, 186–194. [CrossRef]
160. Lee, C.R.; Goldstein, J.A.; Pieper, J.A. Cytochrome P450 2C9 polymorphisms: A comprehensive review of the in-vitro and human data. *Pharmacogenetics* **2002**, *12*, 251–263. [CrossRef]
161. Riedmaier, S.; Klein, K.; Hofmann, U.; Keskitalo, J.E.; Neuvonen, P.J.; Schwab, M.; Niemi, M.; Zanger, U.M. UDP-Glucuronosyltransferase (UGT) polymorphisms affect atorvastatin lactonization in vitro and in vivo. *Clin. Pharmacol. Ther.* **2010**, *87*, 65–73. [CrossRef]
162. Kearney, A.S.; Crawford, L.F.; Mehta, S.C.; Radebaugh, G.W. The interconversion kinetics, equilibrium, and solubilities of the lactone and hydroxyacid forms of the HMG-CoA reductase inhibitor, CI-981. *Pharm. Res.* **1993**, *10*, 1461–1465. [CrossRef]
163. Li, C.; Subramanian, R.; Yu, S.; Prueksaritanont, T. Acyl-coenzyme a formation of simvastatin in mouse liver preparations. *Drug Metab. Dispos.* **2006**, *34*, 102–110. [CrossRef]
164. Prueksaritanont, T.; Subramanian, R.; Fang, X.; Ma, B.; Qiu, Y.; Lin, J.H.; Pearson, P.G.; Baillie, T.A. Glucuronidation of statins in animals and humans: A novel mechanism of statin lactonization. *Drug Metab. Dispos.* **2002**, *30*, 505–512. [CrossRef]
165. Skottheim, I.B.; Gedde-Dahl, A.; Hejazifar, S.; Hoel, K.; Asberg, A. Statin induced myotoxicity: The lactone forms are more potent than the acid forms in human skeletal muscle cells in vitro. *Eur. J. Pharm. Sci.* **2008**, *33*, 317–325. [CrossRef] [PubMed]
166. Cho, S.K.; Oh, E.S.; Park, K.; Park, M.S.; Chung, J.Y. The *UGT1A3*2* polymorphism affects atorvastatin lactonization and lipid-lowering effect in healthy volunteers. *Pharm. Genom.* **2012**, *22*, 598–605. [CrossRef] [PubMed]

167. Stormo, C.; Bogsrud, M.P.; Hermann, M.; Asberg, A.; Piehler, A.P.; Retterstol, K.; Kringen, M.K. *UGT1A1*28* is associated with decreased systemic exposure of atorvastatin lactone. *Mol. Diagn. Ther.* **2013**, *17*, 233–237. [CrossRef] [PubMed]
168. Nies, A.T.; Niemi, M.; Burk, O.; Winter, S.; Zanger, U.M.; Stieger, B.; Schwab, M.; Schaeffeler, E. Genetics is a major determinant of expression of the human hepatic uptake transporter OATP1B1, but not of OATP1B3 and OATP2B1. *Genome Med.* **2013**, *5*, 1. [CrossRef] [PubMed]
169. Tornio, A.; Vakkilainen, J.; Neuvonen, M.; Backman, J.T.; Neuvonen, P.J.; Niemi, M. *SLCO1B1* polymorphism markedly affects the pharmacokinetics of lovastatin acid. *Pharm. Genom.* **2015**, *25*, 382–387. [CrossRef]
170. Pasanen, M.K.; Neuvonen, M.; Neuvonen, P.J.; Niemi, M. *SLCO1B1* polymorphism markedly affects the pharmacokinetics of simvastatin acid. *Pharm. Genom.* **2006**, *16*, 873–879. [CrossRef]
171. Ieiri, I.; Suwannakul, S.; Maeda, K.; Uchimaru, H.; Hashimoto, K.; Kimura, M.; Fujino, H.; Hirano, M.; Kusuhara, H.; Irie, S.; et al. *SLCO1B1* (OATP1B1, an uptake transporter) and *ABCG2* (BCRP, an efflux transporter) variant alleles and pharmacokinetics of pitavastatin in healthy volunteers. *Clin. Pharmacol. Ther.* **2007**, *82*, 541–547. [CrossRef]
172. Pasanen, M.K.; Fredrikson, H.; Neuvonen, P.J.; Niemi, M. Different effects of *SLCO1B1* polymorphism on the pharmacokinetics of atorvastatin and rosuvastatin. *Clin. Pharmacol. Ther.* **2007**, *82*, 726–733. [CrossRef]
173. Niemi, M.; Pasanen, M.K.; Neuvonen, P.J. *SLCO1B1* polymorphism and sex affect the pharmacokinetics of pravastatin but not fluvastatin. *Clin. Pharmacol. Ther.* **2006**, *80*, 356–366. [CrossRef]
174. Brunham, L.R.; Lansberg, P.J.; Zhang, L.; Miao, F.; Carter, C.; Hovingh, G.K.; Visscher, H.; Jukema, J.W.; Stalenhoef, A.F.; Ross, C.J.; et al. Differential effect of the rs4149056 variant in *SLCO1B1* on myopathy associated with simvastatin and atorvastatin. *Pharm. J.* **2012**, *12*, 233–237. [CrossRef]
175. Donnelly, L.A.; Doney, A.S.; Tavendale, R.; Lang, C.C.; Pearson, E.R.; Colhoun, H.M.; McCarthy, M.I.; Hattersley, A.T.; Morris, A.D.; Palmer, C.N. Common nonsynonymous substitutions in *SLCO1B1* predispose to statin intolerance in routinely treated individuals with type 2 diabetes: A Go-DARTS study. *Clin. Pharmacol. Ther.* **2011**, *89*, 210–216. [CrossRef] [PubMed]
176. Liu, J.-E.; Liu, X.-Y.; Chen, S.; Zhang, Y.; Cai, L.-Y.; Yang, M.; Lai, W.-H.; Ren, B.; Zhong, S.-L. *SLCO1B1* 521T > C polymorphism associated with rosuvastatin-induced myotoxicity in Chinese coronary artery disease patients: A nested case—Control study. *Eur. J. Clin. Pharmacol.* **2017**, *73*, 1409–1416. [CrossRef] [PubMed]
177. Santos, P.C.; Gagliardi, A.C.; Miname, M.H.; Chacra, A.P.; Santos, R.D.; Krieger, J.E.; Pereira, A.C. *SLCO1B1* haplotypes are not associated with atorvastatin-induced myalgia in brazilian patients with familial hypercholesterolemia. *Eur. J. Clin. Pharmacol.* **2012**, *68*, 273–279. [CrossRef] [PubMed]
178. Hubacek, J.A.; Dlouha, D.; Adamkova, V.; Zlatohlavek, L.; Viklicky, O.; Hruba, P.; Ceska, R.; Vrablik, M. *SLCO1B1* polymorphism is not associated with risk of statin-induced myalgia/myopathy in a czech population. *Med. Sci. Monit. Int. Med. J. Exp. Clin. Res.* **2015**, *21*, 1454–1459.
179. Food and Drug Administration. FDA Drug Safety Communication: New restrictions, contraindications, and dose limitations for Zocor (simvastatin) to reduce the risk of muscle injury. Available online: http://www.fda.gov/drugs/drug-safety-and-availability/fda-drug-safety-communication-new-restrictions-contraindications-and-dose-limitations-zocor (accessed on 19 December 2019).
180. Ramsey, L.B.; Johnson, S.G.; Caudle, K.E.; Haidar, C.E.; Voora, D.; Wilke, R.A.; Maxwell, W.D.; McLeod, H.L.; Krauss, R.M.; Roden, D.M.; et al. The clinical pharmacogenetics implementation consortium guideline for *SLCO1B1* and simvastatin-induced myopathy: 2014 update. *Clin. Pharmacol. Ther.* **2014**, *96*, 423–428. [CrossRef]
181. KNMP. Pharmacogenetic Recommendations. Available online: https://www.knmp.nl/patientenzorg/medicatiebewaking/farmacogenetica/pharmacogenetics-1/pharmacogenetics (accessed on 17 July 2019).
182. Krajcsi, P. Drug-transporter interaction testing in drug discovery and development. *World J. Pharmacol.* **2013**, *2*, 35–46. [CrossRef]
183. Ceckova-Novotna, M.; Pavek, P.; Staud, F. P-glycoprotein in the placenta: Expression, localization, regulation and function. *Reprod. Toxicol.* **2006**, *22*, 400–410. [CrossRef]
184. Mao, Q. BCRP/*ABCG2* in the placenta: Expression, function and regulation. *Pharm. Res.* **2008**, *25*, 1244–1255. [CrossRef]
185. Keskitalo, J.E.; Kurkinen, K.J.; Neuvoneni, P.J.; Niemi, M. *ABCB1* haplotypes differentially affect the pharmacokinetics of the acid and lactone forms of simvastatin and atorvastatin. *Clin. Pharmacol. Ther.* **2008**, *84*, 457–461. [CrossRef]

186. Amundsen, R.; Asberg, A.; Ohm, I.K.; Christensen, H. Cyclosporine A- and Tacrolimus-Mediated Inhibition of *CYP3A4* and *CYP3A5* In Vitro. *Drug Metab. Dispos.* **2012**, *40*, 655–661. [CrossRef]
187. Zhang, L. Transporter-Mediated Drug-Drug Interactions (DDIs). Available online: https://www.fda.gov/downloads/Drugs/DevelopmentApprovalProcess/DevelopmentResources/DrugInteractionsLabeling/UCM207267.pdf (accessed on 18 July 2017).
188. Merck Sharp & Dohme Corp. Prevymis (Letermovir) Highlights of Prescribing Information. Available online: https://www.accessdata.fda.gov/drugsatfda_docs/label/2017/209939Orig1s000,209940Orig1s000lbl.pdf (accessed on 7 November 2019).
189. Wiggins, B.S.; Lamprecht, D.G., Jr.; Page, R.L., II; Saseen, J.J. Recommendations for managing drug-drug interactions with statins and HIV medications. *Am. J. Cardiovasc. Drugs* **2017**, *17*, 375–389. [CrossRef] [PubMed]
190. Wiggins, B.S.; Saseen, J.J.; Page, R.L., II; Reed, B.N.; Sneed, K.; Kostis, J.B.; Lanfear, D.; Virani, S.; Morris, P.B. Recommendations for management of clinically significant drug-drug interactions with statins and select agents used in patients with cardiovascular disease: A scientific statement from the american heart association. *Circulation* **2016**, *134*, e468–e495. [CrossRef] [PubMed]
191. Sirvent, P.; Bordenave, S.; Vermaelen, M.; Roels, B.; Vassort, G.; Mercier, J.; Raynaud, E.; Lacampagne, A. Simvastatin induces impairment in skeletal muscle while heart is protected. *Biochem. Biophys. Res. Commun.* **2005**, *338*, 1426–1434. [CrossRef] [PubMed]
192. Schirris, T.J.; Renkema, G.H.; Ritschel, T.; Voermans, N.C.; Bilos, A.; van Engelen, B.G.; Brandt, U.; Koopman, W.J.; Beyrath, J.D.; Rodenburg, R.J.; et al. Statin-induced myopathy is associated with mitochondrial complex iii inhibition. *Cell Metab.* **2015**, *22*, 399–407. [CrossRef]
193. Parker, B.A.; Augeri, A.L.; Capizzi, J.A.; Ballard, K.D.; Troyanos, C.; Baggish, A.L.; D'Hemecourt, P.A.; Thompson, P.D. Effect of statins on creatine kinase levels before and after a marathon run. *Am. J. Cardiol.* **2012**, *109*, 282–287. [CrossRef]
194. Sinzinger, H.; O'Grady, J. Professional athletes suffering from familial hypercholesterolaemia rarely tolerate statin treatment because of muscular problems. *Br. J. Clin. Pharmacol.* **2004**, *57*, 525–528. [CrossRef]
195. Parker, B.A.; Thompson, P.D. Effect of statins on skeletal muscle: Exercise, myopathy, and muscle outcomes. *Exerc. Sport Sci. Rev.* **2012**, *40*, 188–194. [CrossRef]
196. Min, P.-K.; Park, J.; Isaacs, S.; Taylor, B.A.; Thompson, P.D.; Troyanos, C.; D'Hemecourt, P.; Dyer, S.; Chan, S.Y.; Baggish, A.L. Influence of statins on distinct circulating micrornas during prolonged aerobic exercise. *J. Appl. Physiol.* **2016**, *120*, 711–720. [CrossRef]
197. Lotteau, S.; Ivarsson, N.; Yang, Z.; Restagno, D.; Colyer, J.; Hopkins, P.; Weightman, A.; Himori, K.; Yamada, T.; Bruton, J.; et al. A mechanism for statin-induced susceptibility to myopathy. *JACC Basic Transl. Sci.* **2019**, *4*, 509–523. [CrossRef]
198. Bouitbir, J.; Daussin, F.; Charles, A.L.; Rasseneur, L.; Dufour, S.; Richard, R.; Piquard, F.; Geny, B.; Zoll, J. Mitochondria of trained skeletal muscle are protected from deleterious effects of statins. *Muscle Nerve* **2012**, *46*, 367–373. [CrossRef]
199. Rosenson, R.S.; Baker, S.K. Statin Muscle-Related Adverse Events. Available online: https://www.uptodate.com/contents/statin-muscle-related-adverse-events (accessed on 2 October 2019).
200. Brunham, L.R.; Baker, S.; Mammen, A.; Mancini, G.B.J.; Rosenson, R.S. Role of genetics in the prediction of statin-associated muscle symptoms and optimization of statin use and adherence. *Cardiovasc. Res.* **2018**, *114*, 1073–1081. [CrossRef] [PubMed]
201. Thomas, J.E.; Lee, N.; Thompson, P.D. Statins provoking melas syndrome. *Eur. Neurol.* **2007**, *57*, 232–235. [CrossRef] [PubMed]
202. Tay, S.K.H.; DiMauro, S.; Pang, A.Y.W.; Lai, P.-S.; Yap, H.-K. Myotoxicity of lipid-lowering agents in a teenager with melas mutation. *Pediatr. Neurol.* **2008**, *39*, 426–428. [CrossRef] [PubMed]
203. Cartwright, M.S.; Jeffery, D.R.; Nuss, G.R.; Donofrio, P.D. Statin-associated exacerbation of myasthenia gravis. *Neurology* **2004**, *63*, 2188. [CrossRef]
204. Al-Jubouri, M.A.; Briston, P.G.; Sinclair, D.; Chinn, R.H.; Young, R.M. Myxoedema revealed by simvastatin induced myopathy. *BMJ* **1994**, *308*, 588. [CrossRef]
205. Scalvini, T.; Marocolo, D.; Cerudelli, B.; Sleiman, I.; Balestrieri, G.P.; Giustina, G. Pravastatin-associated myopathy. Report of a case. *Recent. Progress. Med.* **1995**, *86*, 198–200.

206. Baker, S.K.; Tarnopolsky, M.A. Sporadic rippling muscle disease unmasked by simvastatin. *Muscle Nerve* **2006**, *34*, 478–481. [CrossRef]
207. Chariot, P.; Abadia, R.; Agnus, D.; Danan, C.; Charpentier, C.; Gherardi, R.K. Simvastatin-induced rhabdomyolysis followed by a melas syndrome. *Am. J. Med.* **1993**, *94*, 109–110. [CrossRef]
208. De Stefano, N.; Argov, Z.; Matthews, P.M.; Karpati, G.; Arnold, D.L. Impairment of muscle mitochondrial oxidative metabolism in mcardles's disease. *Muscle Nerve* **1996**, *19*, 764–769. [CrossRef]
209. Hur, J.; Liu, Z.; Tong, W.; Laaksonen, R.; Bai, J.P. Drug-induced rhabdomyolysis: From systems pharmacology analysis to biochemical flux. *Chem. Res. Toxicol.* **2014**, *27*, 421–432. [CrossRef]
210. Hermann, M.; Bogsrud, M.P.; Molden, E.; Asberg, A.; Mohebi, B.U.; Ose, L.; Retterstol, K. Exposure of atorvastatin is unchanged but lactone and acid metabolites are increased several-fold in patients with atorvastatin-induced myopathy. *Clin. Pharmacol. Ther.* **2006**, *79*, 532–539. [CrossRef] [PubMed]
211. Asping, M.; Stride, N.; Sogaard, D.; Dohlmann, T.L.; Helge, J.W.; Dela, F.; Larsen, S. The effects of 2 weeks of statin treatment on mitochondrial respiratory capacity in middle-aged males: The lifestat study. *Eur. J. Clin. Pharmacol.* **2017**, *73*, 679–687. [CrossRef] [PubMed]
212. Kwak, H.-B.; Thalacker-Mercer, A.; Anderson, E.J.; Lin, C.-T.; Kane, D.A.; Lee, N.-S.; Cortright, R.N.; Bamman, M.M.; Neufer, P.D. Simvastatin impairs adp-stimulated respiration and increases mitochondrial oxidative stress in primary human skeletal myotubes. *Free Radic. Biol. Med.* **2012**, *52*, 198–207. [CrossRef] [PubMed]
213. Wagner, B.K.; Gilbert, T.J.; Hanai, J.I.; Imamura, S.; Bodycombe, N.E.; Bon, R.S.; Waldmann, H.; Clemons, P.A.; Sukhatme, V.P.; Mootha, V.K. A small-molecule screening strategy to identify suppressors of statin myopathy. *ACS Chem. Biol.* **2011**, *6*, 900–904. [CrossRef]
214. Wagner, B.K.; Kitami, T.; Gilbert, T.J.; Peck, D.; Ramanathan, A.; Schreiber, S.L.; Golub, T.R.; Mootha, V.K. Large-scale chemical dissection of mitochondrial function. *Nat. Biotechnol.* **2008**, *26*, 343–351. [CrossRef]
215. Saito, S.; Nakanishi, T.; Shirasaki, Y.; Nakajima, M.; Tamai, I. Association of miR-145 with statin-induced skeletal muscle toxicity in human rhabdomyosarcoma RD cells. *J. Pharm. Sci.* **2017**, *106*, 2873–2880. [CrossRef]
216. Deichmann, R.; Lavie, C.; Andrews, S. Coenzyme Q10 and statin-induced mitochondrial dysfunction. *Ochsner J.* **2010**, *10*, 16–21.
217. Quinzii, C.M.; Hirano, M. Primary and secondary CoQ_{10} deficiencies in humans. *Biofactors* **2011**, *37*, 361–365. [CrossRef]
218. Lamperti, C.; Naini, A.B.; Lucchini, V.; Prelle, A.; Bresolin, N.; Moggio, M.; Sciacco, M.; Kaufmann, P.; DiMauro, S. Muscle coenzyme Q10 level in statin-related myopathy. *Arch. Neurol.* **2005**, *62*, 1709–1712. [CrossRef]
219. Mullen, P.J.; Luscher, B.; Scharnagl, H.; Krahenbuhl, S.; Brecht, K. Effect of simvastatin on cholesterol metabolism in C2C12 myotubes and HepG2 cells, and consequences for statin-induced myopathy. *Biochem. Pharmacol.* **2010**, *79*, 1200–1209. [CrossRef]
220. Montini, G.; Malaventura, C.; Salviati, L. Early coenzyme Q10 supplementation in primary coenzyme Q10 deficiency. *N. Engl. J. Med.* **2008**, *358*, 2849–2850. [CrossRef] [PubMed]
221. Banach, M.; Serban, C.; Sahebkar, A.; Ursoniu, S.; Rysz, J.; Muntner, P.; Toth, P.P.; Jones, S.R.; Rizzo, M.; Glasser, S.P.; et al. Effects of coenzyme Q10 on statin-induced myopathy: A meta-analysis of randomized controlled trials. *Mayo Clin. Proc.* **2015**, *90*, 24–34. [CrossRef] [PubMed]
222. Moßhammer, D.; Schaeffeler, E.; Schwab, M.; Mörike, K. Mechanisms and assessment of statin-related muscular adverse effects. *Br. J. Clin. Pharmacol.* **2014**, *78*, 454–466. [CrossRef] [PubMed]
223. Flint, O.P.; Masters, B.A.; Gregg, R.E.; Durham, S.K. HMG CoA reductase inhibitor-induced myotoxicity: Pravastatin and lovastatin inhibit the geranylgeranylation of low-molecular-weight proteins in neonatal rat muscle cell culture. *Toxicol. Appl. Pharmacol.* **1997**, *145*, 99–110. [CrossRef] [PubMed]
224. Sakamoto, K.; Honda, T.; Yokoya, S.; Waguri, S.; Kimura, J. Rab-small gtpases are involved in fluvastatin and pravastatin-induced vacuolation in rat skeletal myofibers. *FASEB J.* **2007**, *21*, 4087–4094. [CrossRef] [PubMed]
225. Itagaki, M.; Takaguri, A.; Kano, S.; Kaneta, S.; Ichihara, K.; Satoh, K. Possible mechanisms underlying statin-induced skeletal muscle toxicity in l6 fibroblasts and in rats. *J. Pharmacol. Sci.* **2009**, *109*, 94–101. [CrossRef]

226. Ronzier, E.; Parks, X.X.; Qudsi, H.; Lopes, C.M. Statin-specific inhibition of Rab-GTPase regulates cPKC-mediated IKs internalization. *Sci. Rep.* **2019**, *9*, 17747. [CrossRef]
227. Cao, P.; Hanai, J.-I.; Tanksale, P.; Imamura, S.; Sukhatme, V.P.; Lecker, S.H. Statin-induced muscle damage and atrogin-1 induction is the result of a geranylgeranylation defect. *FASEB J.* **2009**, *23*, 2844–2854. [CrossRef]
228. Mullen, P.J.; Zahno, A.; Lindinger, P.; Maseneni, S.; Felser, A.; Krähenbühl, S.; Brecht, K. Susceptibility to simvastatin-induced toxicity is partly determined by mitochondrial respiration and phosphorylation state of Akt. *Biochim. Biophys. Acta Mol. Cell Res.* **2011**, *1813*, 2079–2087. [CrossRef]
229. Bonifacio, A.; Sanvee, G.M.; Bouitbir, J.; Krähenbühl, S. The AKT/mTOR signaling pathway plays a key role in statin-induced myotoxicity. *Biochim. Biophys. Acta Mol. Cell Res.* **2015**, *1853*, 1841–1849. [CrossRef]
230. Draeger, A.; Monastyrskaya, K.; Mohaupt, M.; Hoppeler, H.; Savolainen, H.; Allemann, C.; Babiychuk, E.B. Statin therapy induces ultrastructural damage in skeletal muscle in patients without myalgia. *J. Pathol.* **2006**, *210*, 94–102. [CrossRef] [PubMed]
231. Sabatine, M.S.; Giugliano, R.P.; Keech, A.C.; Honarpour, N.; Wiviott, S.D.; Murphy, S.A.; Kuder, J.F.; Wang, H.; Liu, T.; Wasserman, S.M.; et al. Evolocumab and clinical outcomes in patients with cardiovascular disease. *N. Engl. J. Med.* **2017**, *376*, 1713–1722. [CrossRef] [PubMed]
232. Moriarty, P.M.; Thompson, P.D.; Cannon, C.P.; Guyton, J.R.; Bergeron, J.; Zieve, F.J.; Bruckert, E.; Jacobson, T.A.; Kopecky, S.L.; Baccara-Dinet, M.T.; et al. Efficacy and safety of alirocumab vs ezetimibe in statin-intolerant patients, with a statin rechallenge arm: The odyssey alternative randomized trial. *J. Clin. Lipidol.* **2015**, *9*, 758–769. [CrossRef] [PubMed]
233. Gomes, M.D.; Lecker, S.H.; Jagoe, R.T.; Navon, A.; Goldberg, A.L. Atrogin-1, a muscle-specific f-box protein highly expressed during muscle atrophy. *Proc. Natl. Acad. Sci. USA* **2001**, *98*, 14440–14445. [CrossRef]
234. Hanai, J.; Cao, P.; Tanksale, P.; Imamura, S.; Koshimizu, E.; Zhao, J.; Kishi, S.; Yamashita, M.; Phillips, P.S.; Sukhatme, V.P.; et al. The muscle-specific ubiquitin ligase atrogin-1/mafbx mediates statin-induced muscle toxicity. *J. Clin. Investig.* **2007**, *117*, 3940–3951. [CrossRef]
235. Protasi, F.; Takekura, H.; Wang, Y.; Chen, S.R.; Meissner, G.; Allen, P.D.; Franzini-Armstrong, C. Ryr1 and ryr3 have different roles in the assembly of calcium release units of skeletal muscle. *Biophys. J.* **2000**, *79*, 2494–2508. [CrossRef]
236. Robinson, R.; Carpenter, D.; Shaw, M.A.; Halsall, J.; Hopkins, P. Mutations in ryr1 in malignant hyperthermia and central core disease. *Hum. Mutat.* **2006**, *27*, 977–989. [CrossRef]
237. Jungbluth, H. Multi-minicore disease. *Orphanet J. Rare Dis.* **2007**, *2*, 31. [CrossRef]
238. Mohaupt, M.G.; Karas, R.H.; Babiychuk, E.B.; Sanchez-Freire, V.; Monastyrskaya, K.; Iyer, L.; Hoppeler, H.; Breil, F.; Draeger, A. Association between statin-associated myopathy and skeletal muscle damage. *CMAJ* **2009**, *181*, E11–E18. [CrossRef]
239. Laitinen, P.J.; Brown, K.M.; Piippo, K.; Swan, H.; Devaney, J.M.; Brahmbhatt, B.; Donarum, E.A.; Marino, M.; Tiso, N.; Viitasalo, M.; et al. Mutations of the cardiac ryanodine receptor (RYR2) gene in familial polymorphic ventricular tachycardia. *Circulation* **2001**, *103*, 485–490. [CrossRef]
240. Luzum, J.A.; Kitzmiller, J.P.; Isackson, P.J.; Ma, C.; Medina, M.W.; Dauki, A.M.; Mikulik, E.B.; Ochs-Balcom, H.M.; Vladutiu, G.D. Gatm polymorphism associated with the risk for statin-induced myopathy does not replicate in case-control analysis of 715 dyslipidemic individuals. *Cell Metab.* **2015**, *21*, 622–627. [CrossRef] [PubMed]
241. Carr, D.F.; Alfirevic, A.; Johnson, R.; Chinoy, H.; van Staa, T.; Pirmohamed, M. Gatm gene variants and statin myopathy risk. *Nature* **2014**, *513*, E1. [CrossRef] [PubMed]
242. Floyd, J.S.; Bis, J.C.; Brody, J.A.; Heckbert, S.R.; Rice, K.; Psaty, B.M. Gatm locus does not replicate in rhabdomyolysis study. *Nature* **2014**, *513*, E1–E3. [CrossRef] [PubMed]
243. Dube, M.P.; Zetler, R.; Barhdadi, A.; Brown, A.; Mongrain, I.; Normand, V.; Laplante, N.; Asselin, G.; Feroz Zada, Y.; Provost, S.; et al. *CKM* and *LILRB5* are associated with serum levels of creatine kinase. *Circ. Cardiovasc. Genet.* **2014**, *7*, 880–886. [CrossRef] [PubMed]
244. ClinicalTrials.gov. Statin Immune Study (Immunostat) nct02984293. Available online: https://clinicaltrials.gov/ct2/show/NCT02984293 (accessed on 24 July 2019).
245. Kuswanto, W.; Burzyn, D.; Panduro, M.; Wang, K.K.; Jang, Y.C.; Wagers, A.J.; Benoist, C.; Mathis, D. Poor repair of skeletal muscle in aging mice reflects a defect in local, interleukin-33-dependent accumulation of regulatory t cells. *Immunity* **2016**, *44*, 355–367. [CrossRef] [PubMed]

246. Needham, M.; Fabian, V.; Knezevic, W.; Panegyres, P.; Zilko, P.; Mastaglia, F.L. Progressive myopathy with up-regulation of MHC-I associated with statin therapy. *Neuromuscul. Disord.* **2007**, *17*, 194–200. [CrossRef] [PubMed]
247. Grable-Esposito, P.; Katzberg, H.D.; Greenberg, S.A.; Srinivasan, J.; Katz, J.; Amato, A.A. Immune-mediated necrotizing myopathy associated with statins. *Muscle Nerve* **2010**, *41*, 185–190. [CrossRef]
248. Christopher-Stine, L.; Casciola-Rosen, L.A.; Hong, G.; Chung, T.; Corse, A.M.; Mammen, A.L. A novel autoantibody recognizing 200-kd and 100-kd proteins is associated with an immune-mediated necrotizing myopathy. *Arthritis Rheum.* **2010**, *62*, 2757–2766. [CrossRef]
249. Mammen, A.L.; Chung, T.; Christopher-Stine, L.; Rosen, P.; Rosen, A.; Casciola-Rosen, L.A. Autoantibodies against 3-hydroxy-3-methylglutaryl-coenzyme a reductase (HMGCR) in patients with statin-associated autoimmune myopathy. *Arthritis Rheum.* **2011**, *63*, 713–721. [CrossRef]
250. Mammen, A.L. Statin-associated autoimmune myopathy. *N. Engl. J. Med.* **2016**, *374*, 664–669. [CrossRef]
251. Pinal-Fernandez, I.; Casal-Dominguez, M.; Mammen, A.L. Immune-mediated necrotizing myopathy. *Curr. Rheumatol. Rep.* **2018**, *20*, 21. [CrossRef] [PubMed]
252. Werner, J.L.; Christopher-Stine, L.; Ghazarian, S.R.; Pak, K.S.; Kus, J.E.; Daya, N.R.; Lloyd, T.E.; Mammen, A.L. Antibody levels correlate with creatine kinase levels and strength in anti-3-hydroxy-3-methylglutaryl-coenzyme a reductase-associated autoimmune myopathy. *Arthritis Rheum.* **2012**, *64*, 4087–4093. [CrossRef] [PubMed]
253. Arouche-Delaperche, L.; Allenbach, Y.; Amelin, D.; Preusse, C.; Mouly, V.; Mauhin, W.; Tchoupou, G.D.; Drouot, L.; Boyer, O.; Stenzel, W.; et al. Pathogenic role of anti-signal recognition protein and anti-3-hydroxy-3-methylglutaryl-coa reductase antibodies in necrotizing myopathies: Myofiber atrophy and impairment of muscle regeneration in necrotizing autoimmune myopathies. *Ann. Neurol.* **2017**, *81*, 538–548. [CrossRef] [PubMed]
254. Huang, X.; Fruen, B.; Farrington, D.T.; Wagenknecht, T.; Liu, Z. Calmodulin-binding locations on the skeletal and cardiac ryanodine receptors. *J. Biol. Chem.* **2012**, *287*, 30328–30335. [CrossRef]
255. Wiel, C.; Lallet-Daher, H.; Gitenay, D.; Gras, B.; Le Calvé, B.; Augert, A.; Ferrand, M.; Prevarskaya, N.; Simonnet, H.; Vindrieux, D.; et al. Endoplasmic reticulum calcium release through itpr2 channels leads to mitochondrial calcium accumulation and senescence. *Nat. Commun.* **2014**, *5*, 3792. [CrossRef]
256. Gupta, A.; Thompson, P.D. The relationship of vitamin d deficiency to statin myopathy. *Atherosclerosis* **2011**, *215*, 23–29. [CrossRef]
257. Bikle, D.D. Vitamin d metabolism, mechanism of action, and clinical applications. *Chem. Biol.* **2014**, *21*, 319–329. [CrossRef]
258. Mazidi, M.; Rezaie, P.; Vatanparast, H.; Kengne, A.P. Effect of statins on serum vitamin d concentrations: A systematic review and meta-analysis. *Eur. J. Clin. Investig.* **2017**, *47*, 93–101. [CrossRef]
259. Thummel, K.E.; Brimer, C.; Yasuda, K.; Thottassery, J.; Senn, T.; Lin, Y.; Ishizuka, H.; Kharasch, E.; Schuetz, J.; Schuetz, E. Transcriptional control of intestinal cytochrome P-4503A by 1α,25-Dihydroxy vitamin D_3. *Mol. Pharmacol.* **2001**, *60*, 1399–1406. [CrossRef]
260. Wang, Z.; Schuetz, E.G.; Xu, Y.; Thummel, K.E. Interplay between vitamin d and the drug metabolizing enzyme CYP3A4. *J. Steroid Biochem. Mol. Biol.* **2013**, *136*, 54–58. [CrossRef]
261. Thirumaran, R.K.; Lamba, J.K.; Kim, R.B.; Urquhart, B.L.; Gregor, J.C.; Chande, N.; Fan, Y.; Qi, A.; Cheng, C.; Thummel, K.E.; et al. Intestinal CYP3A4 and midazolam disposition in vivo associate with vdr polymorphisms and show seasonal variation. *Biochem. Pharmacol.* **2012**, *84*, 104–112. [CrossRef] [PubMed]
262. Schwartz, J.B. Effects of vitamin d supplementation in atorvastatin-treated patients: A new drug interaction with an unexpected consequence. *Clin. Pharmacol. Ther.* **2009**, *85*, 198–203. [CrossRef] [PubMed]
263. Glueck, C.J.; Lee, K.; Prince, M.; Milgrom, A.; Makadia, F.; Wang, P. Low serum vitamin d, statin associated muscle symptoms, vitamin d supplementation. *Atherosclerosis* **2017**, *256*, 125–127. [CrossRef] [PubMed]
264. Jetty, V.; Glueck, C.J.; Wang, P.; Shah, P.; Prince, M.; Lee, K.; Goldenberg, M.; Kumar, A. Safety of 50,000-100,000 units of vitamin d3/week in vitamin D-Deficient, hypercholesterolemic patients with reversible statin intolerance. *N. Am. J. Med. Sci.* **2016**, *8*, 156–162. [PubMed]
265. Kang, J.H.; Nguyen, Q.N.; Mutka, J.; Le, Q.A. Rechallenging statin therapy in veterans with statin-induced myopathy post vitamin d replenishment. *J. Pharm. Pract.* **2017**, *30*, 521–527. [CrossRef]
266. Alonso, R.; Cuevas, A.; Cafferata, A. Diagnosis and management of statin intolerance. *J. Atheroscler. Thromb.* **2019**, *26*, 207–215. [CrossRef] [PubMed]

267. Rosenson, R.S.; Baker, S.K.; Jacobson, T.A.; Kopecky, S.L.; Parker, B.A. The National Lipid Association's Muscle Safety Expert Panel. An assessment by the statin muscle safety task force: 2014 update. *J. Clin. Lipidol.* **2014**, *8*, S58–S71. [CrossRef]
268. Zhang, H.; Plutzky, J.; Skentzos, S.; Morrison, F.; Mar, P.; Shubina, M.; Turchin, A. Discontinuation of statins in routine care settings: A cohort study. *Ann. Intern. Med.* **2013**, *158*, 526–534. [CrossRef]
269. Keating, A.J.; Campbell, K.B.; Guyton, J.R. Intermittent nondaily dosing strategies in patients with previous statin-induced myopathy. *Ann. Pharmacother.* **2013**, *47*, 398–404. [CrossRef]
270. Schwartz, G.G.; Steg, P.G.; Szarek, M.; Bhatt, D.L.; Bittner, V.A.; Diaz, R.; Edelberg, J.M.; Goodman, S.G.; Hanotin, C.; Harrington, R.A.; et al. Alirocumab and cardiovascular outcomes after acute coronary syndrome. *N. Engl. J. Med.* **2018**, *379*, 2097–2107. [CrossRef]
271. Stroes, E.; Colquhoun, D.; Sullivan, D.; Civeira, F.; Rosenson, R.S.; Watts, G.F.; Bruckert, E.; Cho, L.; Dent, R.; Knusel, B.; et al. Anti-PCSK9 antibody effectively lowers cholesterol in patients with statin intolerance: The GAUSS-2 randomized, placebo-controlled phase 3 clinical trial of evolocumab. *J. Am. Coll. Cardiol.* **2014**, *63*, 2541–2548. [CrossRef] [PubMed]
272. Oren, O.; Kludtke, E.L.; Kopecky, S.L. Characteristics and outcomes of patients treated with proprotein convertase subtilisin/kexin type 9 inhibitors (the mayo clinic experience). *Am. J. Cardiol.* **2019**, *124*, 1669–1673. [CrossRef] [PubMed]
273. Patel, R.S.; Scopelliti, E.M.; Olugbile, O. The role of PCSK9 inhibitors in the treatment of hypercholesterolemia. *Ann. Pharmacother.* **2018**, *52*, 1000–1018. [CrossRef] [PubMed]
274. Van der Wouden, C.H.; Cambon-Thomsen, A.; Cecchin, E.; Cheung, K.C.; Davila-Fajardo, C.L.; Deneer, V.H.; Dolzan, V.; Ingelman-Sundberg, M.; Jonsson, S.; Karlsson, M.O.; et al. Implementing pharmacogenomics in europe: Design and implementation strategy of the ubiquitous pharmacogenomics consortium. *Clin. Pharmacol. Ther.* **2017**, *101*, 341–358. [CrossRef]
275. Ray, K.K.; Bays, H.E.; Catapano, A.L.; Lalwani, N.D.; Bloedon, L.T.; Sterling, L.R.; Robinson, P.L.; Ballantyne, C.M. Safety and efficacy of bempedoic acid to reduce LDL cholesterol. *N. Engl. J. Med.* **2019**, *380*, 1022–1032. [CrossRef]
276. Ray, K.K.; Stoekenbroek, R.M.; Kallend, D.; Leiter, L.A.; Landmesser, U.; Wright, R.S.; Wijngaard, P.; Kastelein, J.J.P. Effect of an siRNA therapeutic targeting PCSK9 on atherogenic lipoproteins. *Circulation* **2018**, *138*, 1304–1316. [CrossRef]
277. Herrett, E.; Williamson, E.; Beaumont, D.; Prowse, D.; Youssouf, N.; Brack, K.; Armitage, J.; Goldacre, B.; MacDonald, T.; Staa, T.V.; et al. Study protocol for statin web-based investigation of side effects (statinwise): A series of randomised controlled N-of-1 trials comparing atorvastatin and placebo in UK primary care. *BMJ Open* **2017**, *7*, e016604. [CrossRef]
278. Maier, L.; Pruteanu, M.; Kuhn, M.; Zeller, G.; Telzerow, A.; Anderson, E.E.; Brochado, A.R.; Fernandez, K.C.; Dose, H.; Mori, H.; et al. Extensive impact of non-antibiotic drugs on human gut bacteria. *Nature* **2018**, *555*, 623. [CrossRef]
279. Khan, T.J.; Ahmed, Y.M.; Zamzami, M.A.; Mohamed, S.A.; Khan, I.; Baothman, O.A.S.; Mehanna, M.G.; Yasir, M. Effect of atorvastatin on the gut microbiota of high fat diet-induced hypercholesterolemic rats. *Sci. Rep.* **2018**, *8*, 662. [CrossRef]
280. Morelli, M.B.; Wang, X.; Santulli, G. Functional role of gut microbiota and PCSK9 in the pathogenesis of diabetes mellitus and cardiovascular disease. *Atherosclerosis* **2019**, *289*, 176–178. [CrossRef]

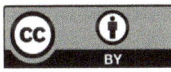

© 2019 by the authors. Licensee MDPI, Basel, Switzerland. This article is an open access article distributed under the terms and conditions of the Creative Commons Attribution (CC BY) license (http://creativecommons.org/licenses/by/4.0/).

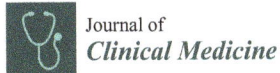

Article

Effects of Fructose or Glucose on Circulating ApoCIII and Triglyceride and Cholesterol Content of Lipoprotein Subfractions in Humans

Bettina Hieronimus [1], Steven C. Griffen [2], Nancy L. Keim [3,4], Andrew A. Bremer [5], Lars Berglund [2], Katsuyuki Nakajima [6,7,8,9], Peter J. Havel [1,4] and Kimber L. Stanhope [1,*]

1. Department of Molecular Biosciences, School of Veterinary Medicine, University of California, Davis, CA 95616, USA
2. Department of Internal Medicine, School of Medicine, University of California, Davis, Sacramento, CA 95817, USA
3. United States Department of Agriculture, Western Human Nutrition Research Center, Davis, CA 95616, USA
4. Department of Nutrition, University of California, Davis, CA 95616, USA
5. Department of Pediatrics, School of Medicine, University of California, Davis, Sacramento, CA 95817, USA
6. Department of Clinical Laboratory Medicine, Gunma University Graduate School of Medicine, Maebashi, Gunma 371-8510, Japan
7. Hidaka Hospital, Takasaki, Gunma 370-0001, Japan
8. General Internal Medicine, Kanazawa Medical University, Kanazawa 920-0265, Japan
9. Laboratory of Clinical Nutrition and Medicine, Kagawa Nutrition University, Tokyo 350-0288, Japan
* Correspondence: klstanhope@ucdavis.edu; Tel.: +1-530-752-3720

Received: 25 May 2019; Accepted: 24 June 2019; Published: 26 June 2019

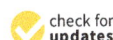

Abstract: ApoCIII and triglyceride (TG)-rich lipoproteins (TRL), particularly, large TG-rich lipoproteins particles, have been described as important mediators of cardiovascular disease (CVD) risk. The effects of sustained consumption of dietary fructose compared with those of sustained glucose consumption on circulating apoCIII and large TRL particles have not been reported. We measured apoCIII concentrations and the TG and cholesterol content of lipoprotein subfractions separated by size in fasting and postprandial plasma collected from men and women (age: 54 ± 8 years) before and after they consumed glucose- or fructose-sweetened beverages for 10 weeks. The subjects consuming fructose exhibited higher fasting and postprandial plasma apoCIII concentrations than the subjects consuming glucose ($p < 0.05$ for both). They also had higher concentrations of postprandial TG in all TRL subfractions ($p < 0.05$, effect of sugar), with the highest increases occurring in the largest TRL particles ($p < 0.0001$ for fructose linear trend). Compared to glucose consumption, fructose consumption increased postprandial TG in low-density lipoprotein (LDL) particles ($p < 0.05$, effect of sugar), especially in the smaller particles ($p < 0.0001$ for fructose linear trend). The increases of both postprandial apoCIII and TG in large TRL subfractions were associated with fructose-induced increases of fasting cholesterol in the smaller LDL particles. In conclusion, 10 weeks of fructose consumption increased the circulating apoCIII and postprandial concentrations of large TRL particles compared with glucose consumption.

Keywords: sugar; atherosclerosis risk factors; lipoprotein fractions; TG-rich lipoproteins; clinical studies; LDL; lipid and lipoprotein metabolism; nutrition/carbohydrates

1. Introduction

The incidence and prevalence of undesirable health outcomes including obesity, type-2 diabetes, cardiovascular disease (CVD), and metabolic syndrome are increasing in developing and developed countries alike, with CVD being the number one cause of death globally [1]. Dietary habits affect cardiometabolic risk [2], but we lack a full understanding of how dietary patterns influence the development of undesirable lipid profiles that lead to metabolic diseases. Understanding the mechanisms that link specific dietary components and patterns to atherogenic dyslipidemia will promote the implementation of dietary policies to reduce CVD risk.

We earlier reported the results from a 10-week intervention trial with women and men (age: 54 ± 8 years; body mass index (BMI): 29.1 ± 2.9 kg/m^2 (mean ± SD)) who consumed 25% of their energy requirement from fructose- or glucose-sweetened beverages [3]. Despite comparable weight gain in both groups, fructose consumption promoted lipid dysregulation, while glucose consumption did not [3]. Compared with glucose, the consumption of fructose increased the circulating concentrations of postprandial triglycerides (TG), remnant-like particle lipoprotein (RLP)-TG, and RLP-cholesterol (chol), as well as those of fasting total chol, low-density lipoprotein (LDL)-chol, apolipoprotein B (apoB), small dense LDL-chol (sdLDL-chol), and oxidized LDL [3]. Subjects consuming fructose also exhibited increased postprandial hepatic de novo lipogenesis (DNL) and decreased insulin sensitivity compared with subjects consuming glucose [3].

We and others have suggested that these results are mediated by the preferential and unregulated metabolism of fructose in the liver [4–7]. Hepatic fructose overload leads to upregulated DNL [3,8–10], reduced fat oxidation [8,9,11], and increased liver fat content [8,9,12], which are associated with increased synthesis and secretion of TG-rich VLDL$_1$ (very low density lipoprotein) [13]. At high concentrations, VLDL$_1$ becomes the favored substrate of cholesteryl ester transfer protein (CETP) [14] that catalyzes lipid transfer between lipoproteins. This leads to TG enrichment of LDL. TG-enriched LDL particles are the preferential substrate for the lipolytic action of hepatic lipase, which leads to smaller, denser particles [15]. However, whether sustained fructose consumption causes an increase in large TRL or TG enrichment of LDL particles has not been determined. Furthermore, apoCIII has been implicated as a major mediator of the metabolic processes that increase CVD risk [16,17] by causing reduced lipoprotein flux through clearance pathways and increased flux through the lipolysis pathways that lead to sdLDL [17]. In support of this, it was recently reported that the increase in LDL particle size caused by a weight loss intervention and the decrease in LDL particle size caused by a high-carbohydrate (32.5% of energy as complex, 32.5% as simple) dietary intervention, were both inversely correlated to the changes in apoCIII concentrations [18]. While it has been shown that consumption of both fructose [8,19] and fructose-containing sugar [20] leads to increased plasma apoCIII concentrations, it is not known if this effect is general for all carbohydrates or specific to fructose. Therefore, our objective was to determine the effects of sustained consumption of fructose-sweetened compared with glucose-sweetened beverages on fasting and postprandial circulating apoCIII and the TG-enrichment of large lipoproteins and LDL. We analyzed apoCIII concentrations and the TG and chol content of 20 lipoprotein fractions separated by size in fasting and postprandial plasma collected before and after intervention from subjects who consumed glucose- or fructose-sweetened beverages for 10 weeks [3].

2. Experimental Section

As previously reported [3], this was a matched, parallel-arm, dietary intervention study that consisted of three phases: (1) a two-week inpatient baseline period during which the subjects consumed an energy-balanced diet; (2) an eight-week outpatient intervention period during which the subjects consumed 25% of daily energy requirement as either glucose- (n = 15) or fructose-sweetened (n = 17) beverages, divided into three servings, along with their usual ad libitum diet; and (3) a two-week inpatient intervention period during which the subjects consumed 25% of their daily energy requirement as the assigned sugar-sweetened beverage along with an energy-balanced diet (Figure 1). Daily energy requirement was calculated by the Mifflin equation ([21]), with an adjustment of 1.3 for the days of the 24 h blood collections and an adjustment of 1.5 for the other days. Subjects resided in the University of California, Davis, (UCD), Clinical and Translational Science Center's Clinical Research

Center (CCRC) during the two-week baseline and two-week intervention inpatient periods of the study (Figure 1). Energy-balanced breakfast accounted for 25% of the subjects' energy requirement, lunch for 35%, and dinner for 40%. The baseline diet consisted of 55% of energy as mainly complex carbohydrate, 30% fat, and 15% protein. Intervention meals mimicked the respective baseline meals in all but the carbohydrate composition, which consisted of 30% complex carbohydrate and 25% glucose- or fructose-sweetened beverages. During the eight-week outpatient intervention period, the subjects were instructed to drink three servings of the assigned beverages, one with each meal, and to refrain from drinking other sugar-containing beverages including fruit juices. We have previously reported that during the eight-week outpatient period, both groups gained comparable amounts of body weight (approximately 1.4 kg) [3].

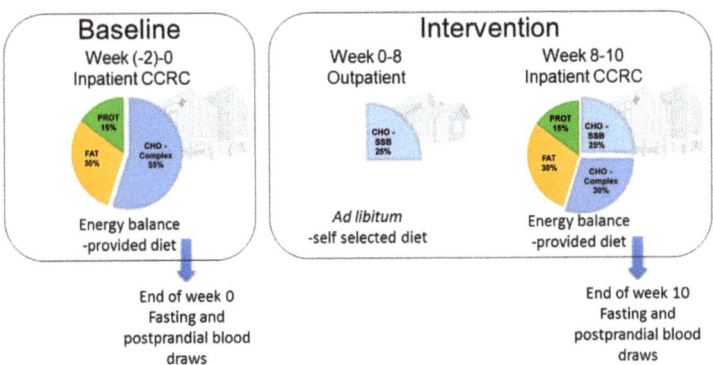

Figure 1. Study design and dietary protocol. CCRC: Clinical and Translational Science Center's Clinical Research Center.

Subjects: Participants were recruited through newspaper advertisements and underwent a telephone and an in-person interview with medical history, a complete blood count, and a serum biochemistry panel to assess eligibility. Inclusion criteria included age 40–72 years and BMI 25–35 kg/m^2, with a self-report of stable body weight during the prior six months. Women were post-menopausal on the basis of a self-report of no menstruation for at least one year. Exclusion criteria included: evidence of diabetes, renal or hepatic disease, fasting serum TG concentrations >400 mg/dL, hypertension (>140/90 mg Hg), and surgery for weight loss. Also excluded were individuals who smoked, reported exercise of more than 3.5 h/week at a level more vigorous than walking, or having used thyroid, lipid-lowering, glucose-lowering, anti-hypertensive, anti-depressant, or weight loss medications. Diet-related exclusion criteria included habitual consumption of more than one sugar-sweetened beverage/day or more than two alcoholic beverages/day. All experimental procedures were in accordance with the Helsinki Declaration and approved by the UCD Institutional Review Board. All subjects provided informed written consent to participate in the study. Thirty-nine subjects enrolled in the study, and experimental groups were matched for gender, BMI, and fasting TG and insulin concentrations. Seven subjects (three in the glucose group, four in the fructose group) failed to complete the study due to inability/unwillingness to comply with the protocol or due to personal or work-related conflicts. The baseline anthropometric and metabolic parameters of the subjects were previously reported [3] and were equal between the experimental groups. The mean age, BMI, and baseline fasting plasma TG concentration of all subjects was 53.7 ± 1.4 years, 30.8 ± 1.0 kg/m^2, and 145.2 ± 12.3 mg/dL, respectively.

After 10 days of energy-balanced feeding, 24 h serial blood collections were conducted during baseline (0 week) and the 10th week of intervention (10 week). Meals were served at 9:00 a.m., 1:00 p.m. and 6:00 p.m. The plasma from the three fasting samples (8:00 a.m., 8:30 a.m., 9:00 a.m.) was pooled, as was the plasma from three postprandial blood samples (10:00 p.m., 11:00 p.m., 11:30 p.m.).

We chose 10:00–11:30 p.m. as the postprandial time-points because it was during this period that fructose had the most marked effects on TG concentrations compared with glucose during our previous study [22]. The 0-week and 10-week fasting and postprandial plasma samples from 31 of the 32 subjects (insufficient plasma obtained from one subject in the fructose group) were classified and quantified for chol and TG concentrations in 20 subfractions by high-performance liquid chromatography at Skylight Biotech (LipoSEARCH; Skylight Bio-tech Inc., Akita, Japan) to examine the lipoprotein profiles by subclass [23–25]. The subfractions were termed TRLp1-7, LDLp1-6, and HDLp1-7, respectively, and were classified by particle diameter (Table 1). The results pertaining to the HDLp1-7 subfractions are not reported in this paper. Apolipoprotein CIII (apoCIII) was measured in the same pooled samples used to determine fasting (8:00, 8:30, 9:00 a.m.) and postprandial (10:00, 11:00, 11:30 p.m.) lipoproteins. The concentrations were assessed with a Polychem Chemistry Analyzer (PolyMedCo Inc., Cortlandt Manor, NY, USA) with reagents from MedTest DX.

The effects of 2-, 8- and 10-week glucose and fructose consumption on the plasma concentrations of fasting and postprandial TG and apoB100, and fasting total, LDL, high-density lipoprotein (HDL), and sdLDL-chol were previously reported [3].

Statistical Analysis: Differences in the percent changes (delta Δ) in the TRL, LDL fractions (Table 2), and apoCIII (Figure 2) were analyzed with a generalized linear two-factor (sugar and gender) method. The percent changes of chol and TG in TRL (chylomicron, VLDL) and LDL subfractions at 10 weeks compared to baseline (Figures 3 and 4) were analyzed by three-factor (sugar, subfraction size, gender), mixed procedures (PROC MIXED) repeated measures (subfraction size) ANOVA (SAS 9.4). Significant within-group changes from baseline for the individual subfractions were identified by least-squares means (LS means) of the percent changes significantly different from zero. Trend contrasts were used to identify linear relationships between particle size and glucose or fructose consumption. The symbols designating a significant effect of ANOVA factors are consistent for Figures 2–4: a = sugar, b = particle size, c = gender, d = sugar × size, f = fructose-induced linear trend, g = glucose-induced linear trend. Pearson's correlation coefficients were calculated for the changes of total postprandial TG, total and subfraction TRL TG, fasting and postprandial apoCIII, and total fasting LDL and LDLp3-6 chol (SAS 9.4). The data are presented as mean ± SEM.

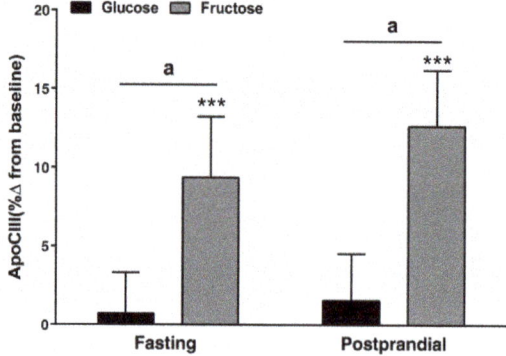

Figure 2. Percent (%) changes (10 weeks vs. 0 weeks) of apoCIII in the serum of subjects consuming glucose- ($n = 15$) or fructose-sweetened beverages ($n = 16$) for 10 weeks. ^{a} $p < 0.05$ effect of sugar, least squares (LS) means different from zero; *** $p < 0.001$, LS means different from zero—change from baseline. Data shown as mean ± SEM.

Table 1. Baseline values of fasting and postprandial cholesterol (chol) and triglycerides (TG) in TG-rich lipoproteins (TRL) and low-density lipoprotein (LDL) subfractions.

	Diameter (nm)	Cholesterol (mg/dL)				TG (mg/dL)			
		Fasting		Postprandial		Fasting		Postprandial	
		Glucose	Fructose	Glucose	Fructose	Glucose	Fructose	Glucose	Fructose
TRLp1	>90	2.7 ± 0.6	3.2 ± 0.8	3.4 ± 0.7	3.6 ± 0.9	10.0 ± 2.6	14.1 ± 3.4	19.0 ± 4.1	22.1 ± 5.0
TRLp2	75	1.4 ± 0.2	1.5 ± 0.3	1.6 ± 0.2	1.6 ± 0.3	6.6 ± 1.3	6.9 ± 1.3	10.1 ± 1.7	10.3 ± 2.1
TRLp3	64	3.8 ± 0.5	3.7 ± 0.5	4.1 ± 0.5	3.7 ± 0.6	14.9 ± 2.6	14.1 ± 2.3	18.4 ± 2.7	17.9 ± 2.9
TRLp4	53.6	7.4 ± 0.7	6.8 ± 0.7	7.1 ± 0.7	6.4 ± 0.8	27.1 ± 4.0	23.9 ± 3.4	29.7 ± 4.0	28.0 ± 4.0
TRLp5	44.5	16.5 ± 1.0	14.6 ± 1.0	14.4 ± 1.2	12.6 ± 1.1	33.9 ± 4.4	28.9 ± 3.5	35.0 ± 4.3	32.7 ± 3.9
TRLp6	36.8	12.9 ± 1.1	11.5 ± 1.2	10.6 ± 1.4	9.5 ± 1.3	17.7 ± 2.0	15.1 ± 1.7	18.5 ± 2.0	17.6 ± 1.9
TRLp7	31.3	6.0 ± 0.4	5.5 ± 0.6	6.4 ± 0.5	6.0 ± 0.5	5.0 ± 0.5	4.3 ± 0.5	5.6 ± 0.5	5.5 ± 0.5
LDLp1	28.6	19.4 ± 1.1	18.2 ± 1.2	20.7 ± 1.6	19.1 ± 1.2	7.6 ± 0.6	6.9 ± 0.7	8.7 ± 0.7	8.5 ± 0.7
LDLp2	25.5	39.0 ± 1.3	36.3 ± 2.1	36.6 ± 1.6	35.7 ± 2.1	8.4 ± 0.6	8.0 ± 0.8	9.4 ± 0.7	9.6 ± 1.0
LDLp3	23.0	21.7 ± 1.3	20.2 ± 1.9	19.0 ± 1.6	18.6 ± 1.7	5.5 ± 0.5	5.1 ± 0.6	5.9 ± 0.6	6.0 ± 0.8
LDLp4	20.7	6.3 ± 0.5	5.8 ± 0.6	5.6 ± 0.7	5.2 ± 0.5	2.1 ± 0.2	1.9 ± 0.2	2.2 ± 0.3	2.2 ± 0.3
LDLp5	18.6	2.5 ± 0.2	2.4 ± 0.2	2.3 ± 0.2	2.2 ± 0.2	1.1 ± 0.1	1.1 ± 0.1	1.4 ± 0.2	1.3 ± 0.2
LDLp6	16.7	1.4 ± 0.1	1.3 ± 0.1	1.3 ± 0.1	1.2 ± 0.1	0.7 ± 0.1	0.7 ± 0.1	1.0 ± 0.1	0.9 ± 0.1

Mean ± SEM.

Table 2. Total fasting (FST) and postprandial (PP) TG and cholesterol concentrations in TRL and LDL fractions before and after consumption of glucose- and fructose-sweetened beverages for 10 weeks.

	Glucose			Fructose		
	0 weeks	10 weeks	% change	0 weeks	10 weeks	% change
Lipoprotein TG (mg/dL)						
TRL TG–FST	116.4 ± 17.3	122.8 ± 16.6	14.3 ± 6.0 *	107.3 ± 14.5	111.9 ± 15.4	7.2 ± 6.8
TRL TG–PP	138.3 ± 19.4	149.8 ± 18.9	11.4 ± 6.1	134.2 ± 18.8	180.9 ± 22.4	42.9 ± 8.3 [aa,****]
LDL TG–FST	24.7 ± 2.3	26.1 ± 2.2	6.3 ± 6.3	23.7 ± 2.5	26.8 ± 2.9	13.9 ± 5.3 ****
LDL TG–PP	27.3 ± 2.7	30.6 ± 2.2	8.8 ± 4.4 *	28.5 ± 2.9	33.2 ± 3.1	18.6 ± 3.1 ****
Lipoprotein Chol (mg/dL)						
TRL Chol–FST	51.3 ± 43.7	46.3 ± 5.3	−4.1 ± 3.0	46.7 ± 4.0	47.9 ± 4.7	2.6 ± 3.8
TRL Chol–PP	48.1 ± 4.3	46.4 ± 6.1	−2.7 ± 3.6	43.4 ± 4.5	49.8 ± 4.7	16.3 ± 5.1 [aa,***]
LDL Chol–FST	90.4 ± 3.3	96.1 ± 3.9	7.0 ± 3.7	84.3.0 ± 5.3	101 ± 7	19.3 ± 2.9 [a,****]
LDL Chol–PP	86.0 ± 3.9	90.3 ± 3.4	7.1 ± 2.6 **	82.1 ± 5.0	94.3 ± 6.1	14.7 ± 1.9 [a,****]

[a] $p < 0.05$, [aa] $p < 0.01$, effect of sugar. * $p < 0.05$, ** $p < 0.01$, *** $p < 0.001$, **** $p < 0.0001$, LS mean of % change different than zero. Mean ± SEM.

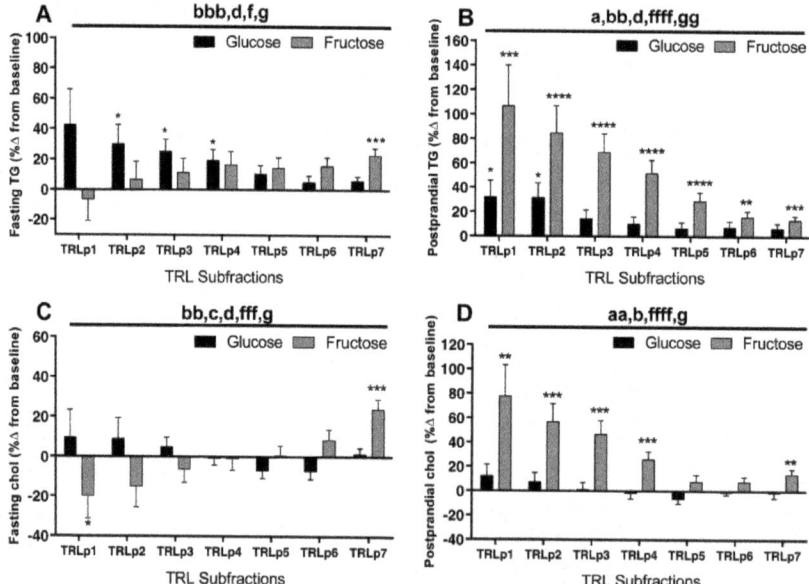

Figure 3. Percent (%) changes (10 weeks vs. 0 weeks) of fasting (**A**) and postprandial (**B**) TG and fasting (**C**) and postprandial (**D**) chol in TRL subfractions (chylomicrons (CM) and very low density lipoprotein (VLDL)) in subjects consuming glucose- ($n = 15$) or fructose-sweetened beverages ($n = 16$) for 10 weeks. [a] $p < 0.05$, [aa] $p < 0.01$, effect of sugar; [b] $p < 0.05$, [bb] $p < 0.01$, [bbb] $p < 0.001$, effect of particle size, [c] $p < 0.05$, effect of gender, [d] $p < 0.05$, effect of sugar × size; [f] $p < 0.05$, [fff] $p < 0.00$, [ffff] $p < 0.0001$ for fructose-induced lineal trend, [g] $p < 0.05$, [gg] $p < 0.01$ for glucose-induced lineal trend. * $p < 0.05$, ** $p < 0.01$, *** $p < 0.001$, **** $p < 0.0001$, LS means different from zero—within-group change from baseline. Data shown as mean ± SEM. Note the differences in scales.

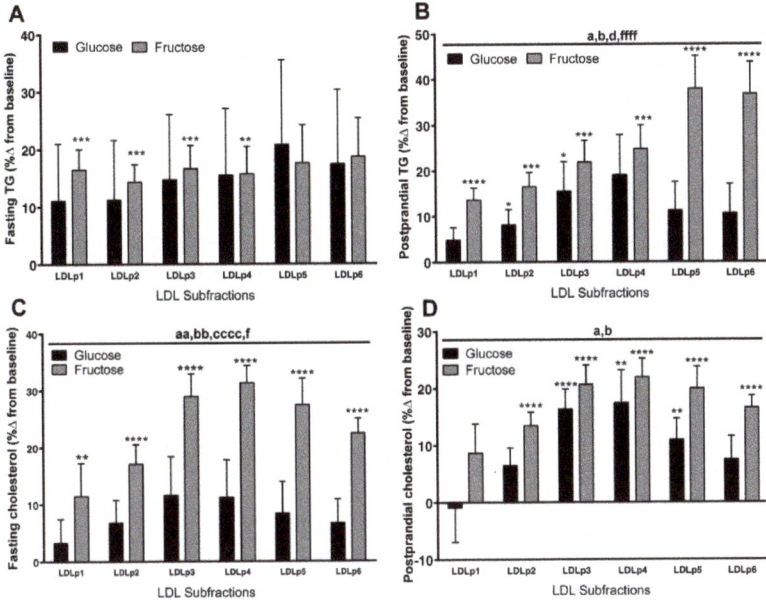

Figure 4. Percent (%) changes (10 weeks vs. 0 weeks) of fasting (**A**) and postprandial (**B**) TG and fasting (**C**) and postprandial (**D**) chol in LDL subfractions in subjects consuming glucose-sweetened beverages ($n = 15$) or fructose-sweetened beverages ($n = 16$) for 10 weeks. [a] $p < 0.05$, [aa] $p < 0.01$, effect of sugar; [b] $p < 0.05$, [bb] $p < 0.01$, effect of particle size; [cccc] $p < 0.0001$, effect of gender, [d] $p < 0.05$, effect of sugar × size, [f] $p < 0.05$; [ffff] $p < 0.0001$ for fructose-induced lineal trend, [g] $p < 0.05$ for glucose-induced lineal trend. * $p < 0.05$, ** $p < 0.01$, *** $p < 0.001$, **** $p < 0.0001$, LS means different from zero—within group change from baseline. Data shown as mean ± SEM. Note the differences in scales.

3. Results

Figure 2 shows the percent changes of plasma apoCIII concentrations after glucose or fructose intervention. Fasting and postprandial apoCIII levels increased in subjects consuming fructose compared with subjects consuming glucose ($p < 0.05$ for both fasting and postprandial, effect of sugar).

The baseline fasting and postprandial contents of chol and TG were not significantly different between the groups in any of the TRL or LDL subfractions (Table 1). The baseline and intervention values and percent changes in the overall TRL and LDL fractions are shown in Table 2. The subjects consuming fructose had increased postprandial levels of chol and TG in both overall particle fractions. In addition, chol and TG were increased in fasting LDL fractions after fructose consumption. In the glucose group, fasting TRL TG and postprandial LDL TG and chol levels increased after the intervention compared to baseline. The fructose-induced increases were significantly higher than those induced by glucose for postprandial TG in TRL, postprandial chol in TRL and LDL, and fasting chol in LDL.

The percent changes of TG and chol (week 10 compared to baseline) in the TRL subfractions are shown in Figure 3. The two sugars induced opposite linear trends for the changes of fasting TG within the TRL subfractions (Figure 3A: $p < 0.05$, sugar × size; $p < 0.05$, both fructose and glucose linear trend). The subjects consuming glucose had increased TG content in the larger TRL particles (TRLp2–4), while those consuming fructose had increased TG content only in the smallest particles (TRLp7). The same opposing linear trends occurred for fasting chol in TRL (Figure 3C: $p < 0.001$, fructose linear trend; $p < 0.05$, glucose linear trend). In the postprandial state, the subjects consuming fructose had increased TG content in all TRL subfractions, with the highest changes in the largest TRL subfractions. This increase exhibited a highly significant linear trend (Figure 3B; $p < 0.0001$, fructose linear trend) in the opposite direction of the fasting trend. The effects of glucose consumption on postprandial TG content in the TRL subfractions were significantly lower, ($p < 0.05$, effect of sugar; $p < 0.05$ effect of sugar × size), with only TRLp1 and 2 showing a significant increase. The postprandial changes in TRL chol content (Figure 3D) paralleled the changes in TRL TG. The increases induced by fructose showed the same linear trend ($p < 0.0001$ for linear trend) and were higher than those induced by glucose ($p < 0.01$, effect of sugar).

The percent change at 10 weeks compared with baseline of fasting and postprandial chol and TG in the six LDL subfractions are shown in Figure 4. The fructose-induced increases of fasting TG content in LDL were comparable among the subfractions and were not significantly higher than those induced by glucose (Figure 4A). In contrast to the fasting state (Figure 4A), the fructose-induced increases in postprandial LDL TG were higher than those induced by glucose ($p < 0.05$, effect of sugar, effect of sugar × size) and displayed a highly significant linear trend with higher increases in the smaller particles (Figure 4B; $p < 0.0001$). Compared with glucose, fructose consumption significantly increased fasting chol content in the LDL subfractions, especially in the smaller subfractions (small dense (sd)LDL) (Figure 4C; $p < 0.01$, effect of sugar). The changes were higher in men than in women (Figure 4C; $p < 0.0001$, effect of gender). In the postprandial state, both sugars increased LDL TG and chol content, but the increases were higher and more significant in subjects consuming fructose than in subjects consuming glucose (Figure 4B-TG: $p < 0.05$, effect of sugar; $p < 0.05$, effect of sugar × size; Figure 4D-chol: $p < 0.05$, effect of sugar).

In order to compare the relationships of postprandial TG-rich particles and apoCIII to fasting sdLDL-chol, we performed regression analysis. Table 3 lists the regression coefficients and p-values for the relationships between the changes of fasting and postprandial apoCIII, total TG, total TLR TG, and TG in each TRL subfraction and the changes of total fasting LDL chol and fasting chol in the small LDL particles (LDLp3–6). In subjects consuming fructose, postprandial apoCIII correlated with total fasting LDL-chol ($p < 0.03$), while the individual TRL subfractions and total TG did not. There were significant associations (all $p < 0.05$) between the increase in fasting LDLp3–6 chol (sdLDL-chol) and the increase in postprandial apoCIII and postprandial TG in TRLp2 and TRLp3 in subjects consuming fructose, but not in subjects consuming glucose. In multivariate regression that included both postprandial apoCIII and TRLp2 or TRLp3, the significance of both were attenuated (apoCIII and TRLp2 $p = 0.16$ and $p = 0.13$; apoCIII and TRLp3 $p = 0.20$ and $p = 0.20$). There were significant positive correlations between postprandial apoCIII and total TRL TG ($p < 0.0001$) and between postprandial apoCIII and TRLp2 or TRLp3 TG ($p < 0.05$ for both).

Table 3. The relationship of percent change of postprandial total, TRL subfraction TG, and fasting and postprandial apoCIII to the absolute increase of total fasting LDL and LDLp3–6 cholesterol.

	Total FST LDL Cholesterol				FST LDLp3-6 Cholesterol			
	Glucose r	P Value	Fructose r	P Value	Glucose r	P Value	Fructose r	P Value
Total TG–PP	0.03	0.91	0.21	0.44	−0.13	0.65	0.21	0.43
Total TRL TG–PP	0.04	0.88	0.01	0.97	−0.14	0.64	0.28	0.29
TRLp1 TG–PP	−0.07	0.82	−0.08	0.77	−0.21	0.47	0.40	0.12
TRLp2 TG–PP	0.02	0.94	−0.04	0.88	−0.23	0.42	0.53	**0.04**
TRLp3 TG–PP	0.10	0.72	0.01	0.96	0.03	0.91	0.51	**0.05**
TRLp4 TG–PP	0.06	0.83	0.07	0.78	−0.04	0.88	0.39	0.14
TRLp5 TG–PP	0.08	0.78	0.06	0.84	−0.09	0.75	0.33	0.21
TRLp6 TG–PP	0.04	0.88	−0.17	0.53	−0.14	0.63	0.16	0.54
TRLp7 TG–PP	−0.07	0.82	−0.27	0.30	−0.22	0.44	−0.06	0.82
ApoCIII FST	−0.27	0.36	0.44	0.09	−0.37	0.20	0.44	0.09
ApoCIII PP	−0.32	0.26	0.53	**0.03**	−0.48	0.08	0.51	**0.04**

r: Pearson's correlation coefficient; FST: fasting state; PP: postprandial state. Bold: indicates significance ($p < 0.05$).

4. Discussion

In the present study, we explored differences between circulating apoCIII and the TG and chol composition of lipoprotein fractions in subjects consuming glucose- or fructose-sweetened beverages for 10 weeks. The changes in apoCIII and in the patterns of TG and chol within the different lipoprotein fractions varied markedly between the two groups, despite their consuming standardized inpatient diets for 10 days prior to both baseline and 10-week intervention blood collections. The intervention diets differed solely in the composition of the beverages, specifically, in the type of added sugar, i.e., glucose or fructose.

ApoCIII is associated with increased CVD risk through various mechanisms, and several studies suggest it to be a robust and reliable predictor of CVD risk [26,27]. Our data show fasting and postprandial apoCIII levels increased after fructose consumption compared with the levels after glucose consumption. To the best of our knowledge, this is the first study to report increased responses of circulating apoCIII to fructose consumption compared with glucose consumption. The results suggest that the previously reported increases of plasma apoCIII concentrations in human subjects consuming fructose [8] or fructose-containing sugar [20] are specific to fructose rather than to carbohydrate in general. A possible explanation for these results may involve insulin, which is a negative transcriptional regulator of apoCIII expression [28]. We have previously reported that the two sugars had highly significant and opposite effects on circulating insulin, with glucose consumption increasing, and fructose consumption decreasing 24 h area under the curve (AUC) and post-meal insulin responses [29]. Cell culture experiments showed apoCIII expression is induced by glucose via hepatocyte nuclear factor 4 alpha (HNF-4α) and carbohydrate-responsive element-binding protein (ChREBP) [30] and is reduced by insulin via Forkhead Box O1 (FOXO1) [28]. This regulation takes place in the liver but not in the intestine, which are the two main sites of apoCIII expression [31]. Thus, it is possible that the failure of glucose consumption to increase circulating apoCIII is due to insulin's negative feedback on hepatic apoCIII transcription. Fructose also activates ChREBP [32,33]. This activation, in the absence of negative feedback by insulin on apoCIII transcription [34], may explain the increased levels of circulating apoCIII after fructose consumption compared with glucose consumption.

It has been recently reported that apoCIII is the strongest predictor of hypertriglyceridemia in a large cohort of rhesus primates and that inhibition of apoCIII by RNA interference lowered fructose-induced hypertriglyceridemia [35]. ApoCIII may affect the lipid metabolism by promoting hepatic DNL and VLDL$_1$ production [27,34,36–40] and by interfering with hepatic clearance of TRL through masking apoB/apoE receptors [16,17,41,42]. Both processes lead to increased and sustained TRL levels in the circulation, which are associated with CVD development and progression [43,44]. Therefore, to investigate the effects of fructose on the fasting and postprandial levels of TRL and other indicators of CVD risk, we measured TG and chol in lipoprotein particles separated by size. The subjects consuming glucose had increased fasting TG in large TRL particles, while those consuming fructose had increased fasting TG in small TRL particles. Thus, if our study only investigated the changes that occurred in the fasting state, these results could lead to the suggestion that consumption of glucose is associated with CVD risk to a larger extent than consumption of fructose. However, the postprandial changes induced by the two sugars in the TG content of the TRL subfractions differed dramatically from the changes in the fasting state with regard to the direction of the linear trend, the magnitude of the increases, and the differential effects of the beverages. Overall, they clearly demonstrate that, compared with glucose consumption, the consumption of fructose increased postprandial TG content in all TRL subfractions, with the increases being most marked in the largest particles. Given that people spend up to 18 h per day in a nonfasted state [45], these results from samples collected postprandially are likely to be more relevant to CVD risk than the fasting results. Furthermore, epidemiology studies provide evidence that non-fasting TG is a more reliable index of CVD risk than fasting TG [46,47]. Compared with glucose, fructose also increased postprandial chol content in the TRL subfractions, with the increases being most marked in the largest particles. This too may promote CVD risk. A prospective study on 90,000 individuals showed a dose-dependent effect of non-fasted remnant cholesterol on later ischemic heart disease and myocardial infarction [48].

The prominently increased postprandial TRL TG and chol in the subjects consuming fructose may result from impaired TRL clearance or increased TRL synthesis—or a combination of both. As stated above, apoCIII could be involved in TRL clearance and/or increased TRL synthesis. Other possible mechanisms not involving apoCIII include a direct effect of fructose overload on the upregulation of hepatic DNL. We have previously reported that postprandial hepatic DNL was significantly increased in the subjects consuming fructose compared to those consuming glucose [3]. Also, it has been suggested, although the available evidence to date is limited, that disruption of enterocyte lipid metabolism may make a meaningful contribution to the hypertriglyceridemia often associated with fructose consumption [49,50]. Fructose feeding has been shown to increase chylomicron synthesis in enterocytes via upregulated DNL and reduced apoB48 degradation in a hamster model of insulin resistance [49]. Impaired TRL clearance could be mediated by decreased lipoprotein lipase (LPL) activity [3], which catalyzes the lipolysis of TG from TRL in the circulation. ApoCII is an important cofactor for LPL activation [51,52] and could be involved in the in differential effects of the two beverages on TRL clearance; however, the effects of fructose compared with those of glucose on apoCII have yet to be investigated.

We previously reported that sdLDL cholesterol was increased in the subjects consuming fructose compared with those consuming glucose [3], and the current data confirm this. The high levels of apoCIII may be involved in generating sdLDL by inhibiting lipoprotein clearance pathways and promoting the lipolytic conversion of TRL, IDL, and LDL to smaller, denser LDL particles [17]. However, the traditional view on the generation of sdLDL involves cholesteryl ester transfer protein (CETP) -mediated TG transfer from TRL to LDL [15,53,54]. Supportive of this, our results showed an increase in the TG content of all LDL subfractions during the postprandial period after fructose consumption compared to glucose consumption. TG-enriched LDL has reduced affinity for the LDL receptor and a longer residence time in the circulation compared to LDL with normal TG content [55]. It is therefore exposed to hepatic lipase, which lyses TG. Accordingly, the LDL particles from subjects consuming fructose were less enriched with TG in the fasting state than in the postprandial state ($p < 0.001$ for all individual LDL subfractions, paired t tests). At the same time, these fasting particles had increased cholesterol content compared to the LDL particles from subjects consuming glucose, especially in the smaller particles (LDLp3-6).

Regression analyses showed associations between the changes in fasting sdLDL-chol and postprandial apoCIII and large particle TRLs (TRLp2 and TRLp3) only in subjects consuming fructose. The results are in agreement with the hypothesis that increased and sustained concentrations of large TRL particles lead to lipoprotein changes that result in the formation of sdLDL-chol [15,56,57] and the possibility that apoCIII has a major role in mediating these metabolic processes [17]. A recent intervention trial showed apoCIII was positively associated with sdLDL formation after a high-carbohydrate diet that contained equal amounts of complex and simple carbohydrate [18]. Here, we expand on these results showing that the elevation of apoCIII and its association with sdLDL formation occurred after fructose, but not glucose, consumption. The results showing that apoCIII also correlated with the changes in total LDL-chol may suggest that apoCIII impairs clearance of all LDL particles. In contrast, neither TRLp2 nor TRLp3 correlated with total LDL-chol. Possibly, the effects of TRLp2 and TRLp3 were more specific to LDLp3–6 because they mediated higher TG-enrichment in LDLp3-6 than in LDLp1 ($p = 0.003$–0.04) or p2 ($p = 0.003$–0.06, all comparisons, paired t tests)). However, the attenuated effects of both apoCIII and TRLp2 or TRLp3, when included in the same multi-regression analysis, suggests that their effects on the increase in fasting chol in LDLp3–6 are mediated by dependent pathways.

Elevated levels of sdLDL have been described as independent predictors of cardiovascular events in patients with non-coronary atherosclerosis [58–60] and also of cardio- and cerebro-vascular events in patients with metabolic syndrome [59]. Increased sdLDL, along with elevated levels of TRL,

LDL cholesterol, oxidized LDL, and apoB and low levels of HDL-chol constitute the 'atherogenic dyslipidemia complex', a feature of type 2 diabetes and the metabolic syndrome [61]. The subjects consuming fructose-sweetened beverages for 10 weeks exhibited adverse changes in all components of the 'atherogenic dyslipidemia complex', excepting lowered HDL-chol concentrations. As previously reported, plasma HDL concentrations were unchanged at 10 weeks in the subjects consuming fructose- or glucose-sweetened beverages [3].

A limitation to our study is the selective inclusion of older and overweight subjects, which may limit our findings to this group. However, as this demographic is increasing and already at a high risk for CVD, our reported findings are valuable even if younger and healthier subjects react differently to sugar consumption. The modest sample size limited the exploration of gender effects, which should be studied further with increased subject numbers. Finally, this study does not investigate the effects of sugar-sweetened beverage consumption as they are commonly consumed in this country, with regard to both the amount of sugar consumed and the types of sugars consumed. Self-reported intake data suggest that only 13% of the US population consumes >25% of energy from added sugars (41), and the majority of the added sugar is not pure fructose or glucose, but rather high fructose corn syrup (HFCS) (55% fructose, 45% glucose) and sucrose (50% fructose, 50% glucose). However, the study of fructose and glucose separately allowed us to demonstrate that fructose increases circulating apoCIII compared to glucose, thus, it is the likely mediator of the increases in apoCIII induced by a high-carbohydrate diet [18] or HFCS-sweetened beverages [20].

Furthermore, mechanistic insights gleaned from investigations of fructose compared to glucose are relevant to explaining the observed increases in postprandial TG, fasting and/or postprandial apoCIII, LDL-chol, sdLDL, and apoB observed in subjects consuming HFCS or sucrose-sweetened beverages [12,20,62,63].

5. Conclusions

The results from this study demonstrate that consumption of fructose increases fasting and postprandial plasma concentrations of apoCIII compared with the consumption of glucose and support the involvement of apoCIII in the development of sdLDL and CVD risk [17]. The results also show that fructose markedly increases large TRL particles and the TG-enrichment of LDL in the late postprandial period, which may also affect the development of sdLDL and CVD risk [3,15,56,57]. As the adverse effects of fructose compared with glucose occurred after 10 days of controlled dietary conditions, the results do not support the often-repeated belief that "a calorie is a calorie" independent of its source. While more research is required to determine the levels of fructose-containing sugar that can be consumed without increased risk, it is prudent to advise patients at risk for CVD to refrain from drinking beverages sweetened with fructose-containing sugars.

Author Contributions: Conceptualization, P.J.H. and K.L.S.; Data curation, B.H.; Formal analysis, K.L.S.; Funding acquisition, N.L.K., L.B., P.J.H., and K.L.S.; Investigation, S.C.G., N.L.K., A.A.B., L.B., K.N., and K.L.S.; Methodology, S.C.G., A.A.B., K.A., P.J.H., and K.L.S.; Project administration, K.L.S.; Supervision, K.L.S.; Visualization, B.H.; Writing, original draft, B.H. and K.L.S.; Writing, review & editing, B.H., S.C.G., N.L.K., A.A.B., L.B., K.A., P.J.H., and K.L.S.

Funding: This research was supported with funding from NIH grant R01 HL-075675. The project also received support from Grant Number UL1 RR024146 from the National Center for Research Resources (NCRR), a component of the National Institutes of Health (NIH), and NIH Roadmap for Medical Research. BH is supported by a research fellowship from the German Research Foundation HI 2113/1-1. PJH's laboratory also received support during the project period from NIH grants HL-091333, HL-107256, DK-095960 and the American Diabetes Association. The content is solely the responsibility of the authors and does not necessarily represent the official views of the National Institutes of Health.

Conflicts of Interest: KN has consulted for Denka Seiken Co., Tokyo, Japan, and Otsuka Pharmaceutical Co., Ltd., Tokyo, Japan. The remaining authors declare no conflict of interest.

References

1. World Heal Organ (WHO). *Global Status Report on Noncommunicable Diseases 2014*; World Heal Organ: Geneva, Switzerland, 2014; p. 176.
2. Mozaffarian, D.; Benjamin, E.J.; Go, A.S.; Arnett, D.K.; Blaha, M.J.; Cushman, M.; Das, S.R.; De Ferranti, S.; Després, J.P.; Fullerton, H.J.; et al. Executive summary: Heart disease and stroke statistics-2016 update: A Report from the American Heart Association. *Circulation* **2016**, *133*, 447–454. [CrossRef] [PubMed]
3. Stanhope, K.L.; Schwarz, J.M.; Keim, N.L.; Griffen, S.C.; Bremer, A.A.; Graham, J.L.; Hatcher, B.; Cox, C.L.; Dyachenko, A.; Zhang, W.; et al. Consuming fructose-sweetened, not glucose-sweetened, beverages increases visceral adiposity and lipids and decreases insulin sensitivity in overweight/obese humans. *J. Clin. Investig.* **2009**, *119*, 1322–1334. [CrossRef] [PubMed]
4. Stanhope, K.L.; Havel, P.J. Fructose consumption: Potential mechanisms for its effects to increase visceral adiposity and induce dyslipidemia and insulin resistance. *Curr. Opin. Lipidol.* **2008**, *19*, 16–24. [CrossRef] [PubMed]
5. Stanhope, K.L. Sugar consumption, metabolic disease and obesity: The state of the controversy. *Crit. Rev. Clin. Lab. Sci.* **2016**, *53*, 52–67. [CrossRef] [PubMed]
6. Softic, S.; Cohen, D.E.; Kahn, C.R. Role of Dietary Fructose and Hepatic De Novo Lipogenesis in Fatty Liver Disease. *Dig. Dis. Sci.* **2016**, *61*, 1282–1293. [CrossRef] [PubMed]
7. Mirtschink, P.; Jang, C.; Arany, Z.; Krek, W. Fructose metabolism, cardiometabolic risk, and the epidemic of coronary artery disease. *Eur. Heart J.* **2018**, *39*, 2497–2505. [CrossRef] [PubMed]
8. Taskinen, M.-R.; Söderlund, S.; Bogl, L.H.; Hakkarainen, A.; Matikainen, N.; Pietiläinen, K.H.; Räsänen, S.; Lundbom, N.; Björnson, E.; Eliasson, B.; et al. Adverse effects of fructose on cardiometabolic risk factors and hepatic lipid metabolism in subjects with abdominal obesity. *J. Intern. Med.* **2017**, *140*, 874–888. [CrossRef] [PubMed]
9. Schwarz, J.M.; Noworolski, S.M.; Wen, M.J.; Dyachenko, A.; Prior, J.L.; Weinberg, M.E.; Herraiz, L.A.; Tai, V.W.; Bergeron, N.; Bersot, T.P.; et al. Effect of a high-fructose weight-maintaining diet on lipogenesis and liver fat. *J. Clin. Endocrinol. Metab.* **2015**, *100*, 2434–2442. [CrossRef] [PubMed]
10. Faeh, D.; Minehira, K.; Schwarz, J.M.; Periasami, R.; Seongsu, P.; Tappy, L. Effect of fructose overfeeding and fish oil administration on hepatic de novo lipogenesis and insulin sensitivity in healthy men. *Diabetes* **2005**, *54*, 1907–1913. [CrossRef] [PubMed]
11. Cox, C.L.; Stanhope, K.L.; Schwarz, J.M.; Graham, J.L.; Hatcher, B.; Griffen, S.C.; Bremer, A.A.; Berglund, L.; McGahan, J.P.; Havel, P.J.; et al. Consumption of fructose-sweetened beverages for 10 weeks reduces net fat oxidation and energy expenditure in overweight/obese men and women. *Eur. J. Clin. Nutr.* **2012**, *66*, 201–208. [CrossRef]
12. Maersk, M.; Belza, A.; Stodkilde-Jorgensen, H.; Ringgaard, S.; Chabanova, E.; Thomsen, H.; Pedersen, S.B.; Astrup, A.; Richelsen, B. Sucrose-sweetened beverages increase fat storage in the liver, muscle, and visceral fat depot: A 6-mo randomized intervention study. *Am. J. Clin. Nutr.* **2012**, *95*, 283–289. [CrossRef] [PubMed]
13. Adiels, M.; Taskinen, M.-R.; Packard, C.; Caslake, M.J.; Soro-Paavonen, A.; Westerbacka, J.; Vehkavaara, S.; Hakkinen, A.; Olofsson, S.-O.; Yki-Jarvinen, H.; et al. Overproduction of large VLDL particles is driven by increased liver fat content in man. *Diabetologia* **2006**, *49*, 755–765. [CrossRef] [PubMed]
14. Chapman, M.J.; Le Goff, W.; Guerin, M.; Kontush, A. Cholesteryl ester transfer protein: At the heart of the action of lipid-modulating therapy with statins, fibrates, niacin, and cholesteryl ester transfer protein inhibitors. *Eur. Heart J.* **2010**, *31*, 149–164. [CrossRef] [PubMed]
15. Packard, C.J. Triacylglycerol-rich lipoproteins and the generation of small, dense low-density lipoprotein. *Biochem. Soc. Trans.* **2003**, *31*, 1066–1069. [CrossRef] [PubMed]
16. Zheng, C.; Khoo, C.; Furtado, J.; Sacks, F.M. Apolipoprotein C-III and the metabolic basis for hypertriglyceridemia and the dense low-density lipoprotein phenotype. *Circulation* **2010**, *121*, 1722–1734. [CrossRef] [PubMed]
17. Sacks, F.M. The crucial roles of apolipoproteins E and C-III in apoB lipoprotein metabolism in normolipidemia and hypertriglyceridemia. *Curr. Opin. Lipidol.* **2015**, *26*, 56–63. [CrossRef] [PubMed]
18. Mendoza, S.; Trenchevska, O.; King, S.M.; Nelson, R.W.; Nedelkov, D.; Krauss, R.M.; Yassine, H.N. Changes in low-density lipoprotein size phenotypes associate with changes in apolipoprotein C-III glycoforms after dietary interventions. *J. Clin. Lipidol.* **2017**, *11*, 224–233.e2. [CrossRef]

19. Bremer, A.A.; Stanhope, K.L.; Graham, J.L.; Cummings, B.P.; Wang, W.; Saville, B.R.; Havel, P.J. Fructose-fed rhesus monkeys: A nonhuman primate model of insulin resistance, metabolic syndrome, and type 2 diabetes. *Clin. Transl. Sci.* **2011**, *4*, 243–252. [CrossRef] [PubMed]
20. Stanhope, K.L.; Medici, V.; Bremer, A.A.; Lee, V.; Lam, H.D.; Nunez, M.V.; Chen, G.X.; Keim, N.L.; Havel, P.J. A dose-response study of consuming high-fructose corn syrup-sweetened beverages on lipid/lipoprotein risk factors for cardiovascular disease in young adults. *Am. J. Clin. Nutr.* **2015**, *101*, 1144–1154. [CrossRef]
21. Gonzalez-granda, A.; Damms-machado, A.; Basrai, M.; Bischoff, S.C. Changes in Plasma Acylcarnitine and Lysophosphatidylcholine Levels Following a High-Fructose Diet: A Targeted Metabolomics Study in Healthy Women. *Nutrients* **2018**, *10*, 1254. [CrossRef]
22. Teff, K.L.; Elliott, S.S.; Tschöp, M.; Kieffer, T.J.; Rader, D.; Heiman, M.; Townsend, R.R.; Keim, N.L.; D'Alessio, D.; Havel, P.J. Dietary fructose reduces circulating insulin and leptin, attenuates postprandial suppression of ghrelin, and increases triglycerides in women. *J. Clin. Endocrinol. Metab.* **2004**, *89*, 2963–2972. [CrossRef] [PubMed]
23. Okazaki, M.; Usui, S.; Ishigami, M.; Sakai, N.; Nakamura, T.; Matsuzawa, Y.; Yamashita, S. Identification of unique lipoprotein subclasses for visceral obesity by component analysis of cholesterol profile in high-performance liquid chromatography. *Arterioscler. Thromb. Vasc. Biol.* **2005**, *25*, 578–584. [CrossRef] [PubMed]
24. Toshima, G.; Iwama, Y.; Kimura, F.; Matsumoto, Y.; Miura, M. LipoSEARCH®; Analytical GP-HPLC method for lipoprotein profiling and its applications. *J. Biol. Macromol.* **2013**, *13*, 21–32.
25. Araki, E.; Yamashita, S.; Arai, H.; Yokote, K.; Satoh, J.; Inoguchi, T.; Nakamura, J.; Maegawa, H.; Yoshioka, N.; Yukio, T.; et al. Effects of Pemafibrate, a Novel Selective PPARα Modulator, on Lipid and Glucose Metabolism in Patients With Type 2 Diabetes and Hypertriglyceridemia: A Randomized, Double-Blind, Placebo-Controlled, Phase 3 Trial. *Diabetes Care* **2018**, *41*, 538–546. [CrossRef] [PubMed]
26. Lee, S.J.; Campos, H.; Moye, L.A.; Sacks, F.M. LDL containing apolipoprotein CIII is an independent risk factor for coronary events in diabetic patients. *Arterioscler. Thromb. Vasc. Biol.* **2003**, *23*, 853–858. [CrossRef] [PubMed]
27. Ooi, E.M.M.; Barrett, P.H.R.; Chan, D.C.; Watts, G.F. Apolipoprotein C-III: Understanding an emerging cardiovascular risk factor. *Clin. Sci.* **2008**, *114*, 611–624. [CrossRef] [PubMed]
28. Altomonte, J.; Cong, L.; Harbaran, S.; Richter, A.; Xu, J.; Meseck, M.; Dong, H.H. Foxo1 mediates insulin action on apoC-III and triglyceride metabolism. *J. Clin. Investig.* **2004**, *114*, 1493–1503. [CrossRef] [PubMed]
29. Stanhope, K.L.; Griffen, S.C.; Bremer, A.A.; Vink, R.G.; Schaefer, E.J.; Nakajima, K.; Schwarz, J.M.; Beysen, C.; Berglund, L.; Keim, N.L.; et al. Metabolic responses to prolonged consumption of glucose- and fructose-sweetened beverages are not associated with postprandial or 24-h glucose and insulin excursions. *Am. J. Clin. Nutr.* **2011**, *94*, 112–119. [CrossRef]
30. Caron, S.; Verrijken, A.; Mertens, I.; Samanez, C.H.; Mautino, G.; Haas, J.T.; Duran-Sandoval, D.; Prawitt, J.; Francque, S.; Vallez, E.; et al. Transcriptional activation of apolipoprotein CIII expression by glucose may contribute to diabetic dyslipidemia. *Arterioscler. Thromb. Vasc. Biol.* **2011**, *31*, 513–519. [CrossRef]
31. West, G.; Rodia, C.; Li, D.; Johnson, Z.; Dong, H.; Kohan, A.B. Key differences between apoC-III regulation and expression in intestine and liver. *Biochem. Biophys. Res. Commun.* **2017**, *491*, 747–753. [CrossRef]
32. Kim, M.; Lai, M.; Herman, M.A.; Kim, M.; Krawczyk, S.A.; Doridot, L.; Fowler, A.J.; Wang, J.X.; Trauger, S.A.; Noh, H.; et al. ChREBP regulates fructose-induced glucose production independently of insulin signaling. *J. Clin. Investig.* **2016**, *126*, 4372–4386. [CrossRef] [PubMed]
33. Koo, H.Y.; Wallig, M.A.; Chung, B.H.; Nara, T.Y.; Cho, B.H.S.; Nakamura, M.T. Dietary fructose induces a wide range of genes with distinct shift in carbohydrate and lipid metabolism in fed and fasted rat liver. *Biochim. Biophys. Acta Mol. Basis Dis.* **2008**, *1782*, 341–348. [CrossRef] [PubMed]
34. Ramms, B.; Gordts, P.L.S.M. Apolipoprotein C-III in triglyceride-rich lipoprotein metabolism. *Curr. Opin. Lipidol.* **2018**, *29*, 171–179. [CrossRef] [PubMed]
35. Butler, A.A.; Price, C.A.; Graham, J.L.; Stanhope, K.L.; King, S.; Hung, Y.-H.; Sethupathy, P.; Wong, S.; Hamilton, J.; Krauss, R.M.; et al. Fructose-induced hypertriglyceridemia in rhesus macaques is attenuated with fish oil or apoC3 RNA interference. *J. Lipid Res.* **2019**, *60*, jlr.M089508. [CrossRef] [PubMed]
36. Batal, R.; Tremblay, M.; Barrett, P.H.R.; Jacques, H.; Fredenrich, A.; Mamer, O.; Davignon, J.; Cohn, J.S. Plasma kinetics of apoC-III and apoE in normolipidemic and hypertriglyceridemic subjects. *J. Lipid Res.* **2000**, *41*, 706–718. [PubMed]

37. Yao, Z. Human apolipoprotein C-III—A new intrahepatic protein factor promoting assembly and secretion of very low density lipoproteins. *Cardiovasc. Hematol. Disord. Drug Targets* **2012**, *12*, 133–140. [CrossRef] [PubMed]
38. Sundaram, M.; Yao, Z. Recent progress in understanding protein and lipid factors affecting hepatic VLDL assembly and secretion. *Nutr. Metab.* **2010**, *7*, 1–17. [CrossRef]
39. Sundaram, M.; Curtis, K.R.; Amir Alipour, M.; LeBlond, N.D.; Margison, K.D.; Yaworski, R.A.; Parks, R.J.; McIntyre, A.D.; Hegele, R.A.; Fullerton, M.D.; et al. The apolipoprotein C-III (Gln38Lys) variant associated with human hypertriglyceridemia is a gain-of-function mutation. *J. Lipid Res.* **2017**, *58*, 2188–2196. [CrossRef]
40. Matikainen, N.; Adiels, M.; Söderlund, S.; Stennabb, S.; Ahola, T.; Hakkarainen, A.; Borén, J.; Taskinen, M.R. Hepatic lipogenesis and a marker of hepatic lipid oxidation, predict postprandial responses of triglyceride-rich lipoproteins. *Obesity* **2014**, *22*, 1854–1859. [CrossRef]
41. Gordts, P.L.S.M.; Nock, R.; Son, N.-H.; Ramms, B.; Lew, I.; Gonzales, J.C.; Thacker, B.E.; Basu, D.; Lee, R.G.; Mullick, A.E.; et al. ApoC-III Modulates Clearance of Triglyceride-Rich Lipoproteins in Mice Through Low Density Lipoprotein Family Receptors. *J. Clin. Investig.* **2016**, *126*, 2855–2866. [CrossRef]
42. Talayero, B.; Wang, L.; Furtado, J.; Carey, V.J.; Bray, G.A.; Sacks, F.M. Obesity favors apolipoprotein E- and C-III-containing high density lipoprotein subfractions associated with risk of heart disease. *J. Lipid Res.* **2014**, *55*, 2167–2177. [CrossRef] [PubMed]
43. Hodis, H.N. Triglyceride-rich lipoprotein remnant particles and risk of atherosclerosis. *Circulation* **1999**, *99*, 2852–2854. [CrossRef] [PubMed]
44. Sacks, F.M.; Alaupovic, P.; Moye, L.A.; Cole, T.G.; Sussex, B.; Stampfer, M.J.; Pfeffer, M.A.; Braunwald, E. VLDL, apolipoproteins B, CIII, and E, and risk of recurrent coronary events in the Cholesterol and Recurrent Events (CARE) trial. *Circulation* **2000**, *102*, 1886–1892. [CrossRef] [PubMed]
45. Sharrett, A.R.; Heiss, G.; Chambless, L.E.; Boerwinkle, E.; Coady, S.A.; Folsom, A.R.; Patsch, W. Metabolic and lifestyle determinants of postprandial lipemia differ from those of fasting triglycerides the Atherosclerosis Risk in Communities (ARIC) study. *Arterioscler. Thromb. Vasc. Biol.* **2001**, *21*, 275–281. [CrossRef] [PubMed]
46. Bansal, S.; Buring, J.E.; Rifai, N.; Mora, S.; Sacks, F.M.; Ridker, P.M. Fasting compared with nonfasting triglyceride and risk of cardiovascular events in women. *JAMA* **2007**, *298*, 309–316. [CrossRef] [PubMed]
47. Nordestgaard, B.G.; Benn, M.; Schnohr, P.; Tybjærg-hansen, A. Nonfasting Triglycerides and Risk of Myocardial Infarction, Ischemic Heart. *JAMA* **2007**, *298*, 299–308. [CrossRef] [PubMed]
48. Varbo, A.; Freiberg, J.J.; Nordestgaard, B.G. Extreme nonfasting remnant cholesterol vs extreme LDL cholesterol as contributors to cardiovascular disease and all-cause mortality in 90000 individuals from the general population. *Clin. Chem.* **2015**, *61*, 533–543. [CrossRef]
49. Haidari, M.; Leung, N.; Mahbub, F.; Uffelman, K.D.; Kohen-Avramoglu, R.; Lewis, G.F.; Adeli, K. Fasting and postprandial overproduction of intestinally derived lipoproteins in an animal model of insulin resistance: Evidence that chronic fructose feeding in the hamster is accompanied by enhanced intestinal de novo lipogenesis and ApoB48-containing li. *J. Biol. Chem.* **2002**, *277*, 31646–31655. [CrossRef]
50. Steenson, S.; Umpleby, A.M.; Lovegrove, J.A.; Jackson, K.G.; Fielding, B.A. Role of the enterocyte in fructose-induced hypertriglyceridaemia. *Nutrients* **2017**, *9*, 349. [CrossRef]
51. Nestel, P.J.; Fidge, N.H. Apoprotein C Metabolism in Man. *Adv. Lipid Res.* **1982**, *19*, 55–83.
52. Wolska, A.; Dunbar, R.L.; Freeman, L.A.; Ueda, M.; Amar, M.J.; Sviridov, D.O.; Remaley, A.T. Apolipoprotein C-II: New findings related to genetics, biochemistry, and role in triglyceride metabolism. *Atherosclerosis* **2017**, *267*, 49–60. [CrossRef] [PubMed]
53. Taskinen, M.R. Diabetic dyslipidaemia: From basic research to clinical practice. *Diabetologia* **2003**, *46*, 733–749. [CrossRef] [PubMed]
54. Eisenberg, S. Preferential enrichment of large-sized very low density lipoprotein populations with transferred cholesteryl esters. *J. Lipid Res.* **1985**, *26*, 487–494. [PubMed]
55. Krauss, R.M. Dietary and genetic probes of atherogenic dyslipidemia. *Arterioscler. Thromb. Vasc. Biol.* **2005**, *25*, 2265–2272. [CrossRef] [PubMed]
56. Adiels, M.; Olofsson, S.O.; Taskinen, M.R.; Borén, J. Overproduction of very low-density lipoproteins is the hallmark of the dyslipidemia in the metabolic syndrome. *Arterioscler. Thromb. Vasc. Biol.* **2008**, *28*, 1225–1236. [CrossRef] [PubMed]
57. Berneis, K.K.; Krauss, R.M. Metabolic origins and clinical significance of LDL heterogeneity. *J. Lipid Res.* **2002**, *43*, 1363–1379. [CrossRef] [PubMed]

58. Berneis, K.; Rizzo, M.; Spinas, G.A.; Di Lorenzo, G.; Di Fede, G.; Pepe, I.; Pernice, V.; Rini, G.B. The predictive role of atherogenic dyslipidemia in subjects with non-coronary atherosclerosis. *Clin. Chim. Acta* **2009**, *406*, 36–40. [CrossRef]
59. Rizzo, M.; Pernice, V.; Frasheri, A.; Di Lorenzo, G.; Rini, G.B.; Spinas, G.A.; Berneis, K. Small, dense low-density lipoproteins (LDL) are predictors of cardio- and cerebro-vascular events in subjects with the metabolic syndrome. *Clin. Endocrinol.* **2009**, *70*, 870–875. [CrossRef]
60. Ivanova, E.A.; Myasoedova, V.A.; Melnichenko, A.A.; Grechko, A.V.; Orekhov, A.N. Small Dense Low-Density Lipoprotein as Biomarker for Atherosclerotic Diseases. *Oxid. Med. Cell. Longev.* **2017**, *2017*, 1273042. [CrossRef]
61. Xiao, C.; Dash, S.; Morgantini, C.; Hegele, R.A.; Lewis, G.F. Pharmacological targeting of the atherogenic dyslipidemia complex: The next frontier in CVD prevention beyond lowering LDL cholesterol. *Diabetes* **2016**, *65*, 1767–1778. [CrossRef]
62. Aeberli, I.; Hochuli, M.; Gerber, P. Moderate Amounts of Fructose Consumption Impair Insulin Sensitivity in Healthy Young Men A randomized controlled trial. *Diabetes Care* **2013**, *36*, 150–156. [CrossRef] [PubMed]
63. Aeberli, I.; Gerber, P.A.; Hochuli, M.; Kohler, S.; Haile, S.R.; Gouni-Berthold, I.; Berthold, H.K.; Spinas, G.A.; Berneis, K. Low to moderate sugar-sweetened beverage consumption impairs glucose and lipid metabolism and promotes inflammation in healthy young men: A randomized controlled trial. *Am. J. Clin. Nutr.* **2011**, *94*, 479–485. [CrossRef] [PubMed]

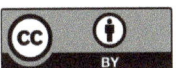 © 2019 by the authors. Licensee MDPI, Basel, Switzerland. This article is an open access article distributed under the terms and conditions of the Creative Commons Attribution (CC BY) license (http://creativecommons.org/licenses/by/4.0/).

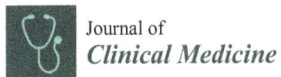

Article

The Polymorphisms of the Peroxisome-Proliferator Activated Receptors' Alfa Gene Modify the Aerobic Training Induced Changes of Cholesterol and Glucose

Agnieszka Maciejewska-Skrendo [1], Maciej Buryta [1], Wojciech Czarny [2], Pawel Król [2], Michal Spieszny [3], Petr Stastny [4,*], Miroslav Petr [4], Krzysztof Safranow [5] and Marek Sawczuk [6]

1. Department of Molecular Biology, Faculty of Physical Education, Gdansk University of Physical Education and Sport, 80-336 Gdansk, Poland
2. Department of Anatomy and Anthropology, Faculty of Physical Education, University of Rzeszow, 35-310 Rzeszow, Poland
3. Institute of Sports, Faculty of Physical Education, University of Physical Education and Sport, 31-571 Kraków, Poland
4. Department of Sport Games, Faulty of Physical Education and Sport, Charles University, 162-52 Prague, Czech Republic
5. Department of Biochemistry and Medical Chemistry, Pomeranian Medical University, 70-204 Szczecin, Poland
6. Unit of Physical Medicine, Faculty of Tourism and Recreation, Gdansk University of Physical Education and Sport, 80-336 Gdansk, Poland
* Correspondence: stastny@ftvs.cuni.cz; Tel.: +420-777198764

Received: 4 June 2019; Accepted: 15 July 2019; Published: 17 July 2019

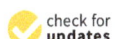

Abstract: Background: PPARα is a transcriptional factor that controls the expression of genes involved in fatty acid metabolism, including fatty acid transport, uptake by the cells, intracellular binding, and activation, as well as catabolism (particularly mitochondrial fatty acid oxidation) or storage. *PPARA* gene polymorphisms may be crucial for maintaining lipid homeostasis and in this way, being responsible for developing specific training-induced physiological reactions. Therefore, we have decided to check if post-training changes of body mass measurements as well as chosen biochemical parameters are modulation by the *PPARA* genotypes. Methods: We have examined the genotype and alleles' frequencies (described in *PPARA* rs1800206 and rs4253778 polymorphic sites) in 168 female participants engaged in a 12-week training program. Body composition and biochemical parameters were measured before and after the completion of a whole training program. Results: Statistical analyses revealed that *PPARA* intron 7 rs4253778 CC genotype modulate training response by increasing low-density lipoproteins (LDL) and glucose concentration, while *PPARA* Leu162Val rs1800206 CG genotype polymorphism interacts in a decrease in high-density lipoproteins (HDL) concentration. Conclusions: Carriers of *PPARA* intron 7 rs4253778 CC genotype and Leu162Val rs1800206 CG genotype might have potential negative training-induced cholesterol and glucose changes after aerobic exercise.

Keywords: human performance; aerobic training; genetic predisposition; lipid metabolism; glucose tolerance; VO$_2$max; mitochondria activity; cholesterol levels

1. Introduction

PPARα is a transcriptional factor that controls the expression of genes involved in fatty acid metabolism, including fatty acid transport, uptake by the cells, intracellular binding, and activation, as well as catabolism (particularly mitochondrial fatty acid oxidation) or storage [1]. PPARα is expressed at moderate levels, mainly in the liver and skeletal muscles, but also in the heart, kidney, brown fat, and large intestine [2–4]. PPARα-dependent transcriptional activity results from a direct interaction of the nuclear receptor with its ligands [5]. The primary natural PPARα ligands are unsaturated fatty acids that directly bind to the PPARα via ligand binding domain (LBD) and enable its heterodimerization with the retinoid X receptor (RXR)-α. Such PPAR:RXR complex binds via PPARα DNA binding domain (DBD) to the PPRE (peroxisome proliferator response element) sequence in the promoter region of target genes [6]. In comparison with the unsaturated fatty acids, saturated fatty acids are poor PPAR ligands [7]. Moreover, synthetic compounds, such as hypolipidemic agents, prostaglandin 12 analogs, leukotriene B4 analogs, leukotriene D4 antagonist, carnitine palmitoyl transferase I (CPT1) inhibitors, fatty acyl-CoA dehydrogenase inhibitors, can activate PPAR [8–10]. It is worth noting that an alternative activation pathway of PPAR:RXR may also occur through ligand binding to RXR [11,12]. In addition to ligand-dependent activation, PPARα may also be regulated by insulin-induced trans-activation that occurs through the phosphorylation of two mitogen-activated protein (MAP) kinase sites at positions 12 and 21 located in the activation function (AF)-1-like domain within PPARα receptor [13].

The *PPARA* gene has been mapped on the human chromosome 22 (locus 22q12-q13.1) and comprises a total of eight exons encoding PPARα protein [14]. Within the entire gene, several polymorphic sites have been identified, with the most studied variant, a missense mutation C/G (rs1800206), resulting in Leu162Val amino acids substitution. This polymorphic site is located in the exon 5 of the *PPARA* gene that encodes the second zinc finger of the DNA binding domain in the PPARα protein. Despite the fact that Leu to Val is a conservative change, this amino acids substitution has functional consequences on protein activity, because the 162 position is next to a cysteine which coordinates the zinc atom and, at the same time, Leu162Val is located upstream of a region determining the specificity and polarity of PPARα binding to different PPREs [15]. In vitro experiments revealed that PPARα isoform with Val in the 162 position has increased PPRE-dependent transcriptional activity compared with the PPARα isoform with Leu in the same position when treated with the PPARα ligand [16]. Interestingly, observed differences were ligand concentration-dependence: At higher concentrations of the ligand, the 162Val variant's transactivation activity was five-fold greater as compared with Leu162 variant [17]. In addition, in vivo observations confirmed that Leu162Val polymorphism exerts an effect on plasma lipoprotein–lipid profile. Carriers of the minor G allele (for Val in the 162 position) compared with homozygotes of the C allele (for Leu162) had significantly higher concentrations of plasma total and low-density lipoproteins (LDL)-apolipoprotein B as well as and LDL cholesterol [18]. In Type II diabetic patients, G allele carriers had higher levels of total cholesterol, high-density lipoproteins (HDL) cholesterol, and apoAI [16]. Moreover, G allele carriers were characterized by a better response to lipid-lowering drugs, showing a greater lowering effect with regard to total cholesterol and non-HDL-cholesterol than C allele homozygotes treated with the same drug [19]. Furthermore, other studies revealed that Leu162Val polymorphism influences the conversion from impaired glucose tolerance to type 2 diabetes [20] as well as being associated with progression of coronary atherosclerosis and the risk of coronary artery disease [21].

The second polymorphic site that has been studied in many contexts is a C/G substitution in *PPARA* intron 7 (rs4253778). It was described for the first time in 2002 in the publications focused on genetic modulators influencing the progression of coronary atherosclerosis and the risk of coronary artery disease [21] as well as left ventricular growth [22]. It has been revealed that *PPARA* rs4253778 polymorphism influences human left ventricular growth observed in response to exercise and hypertension: The C allele carriers had significantly higher left ventricular mass. Moreover, the observed effect was additive: CC homozygotes had a 3-fold greater, and GC heterozygotes had a 2-fold greater increase in left ventricular mass than G allele homozygotes [22]. Taking into account that one of the molecular adaptations described in the hypertrophied heart is reduced PPARα activity [23] and, at the same time, an increase in glucose utilization and a decrease in fatty acid oxidation (FAO) is observed [24,25], it has been hypothesized that the *PPARA* intron 7 C allele affects PPARα function and is connected with downregulation of the expression of mitochondrial FAO enzymes, leading to reduced FAO and impaired cellular lipid homeostasis [22]. Study with diabetic patients has confirmed that C allele carriers are characterized by reduced the lipid-lowering response to fenofibrate treatment in comparison with GG homozygotes [26]. Next, studies with athletes representing different sports disciplines revealed that GG homozygotes were more prevalent in the groups of endurance-type athletes engaged in prolonged aerobic exertion [27,28], while the C allele was frequently observed in power-oriented athletes who were involved in shorter and very intense anaerobic exertion [29]. These results were partly explained by muscle biopsies showing the association between *PPARA* rs4253778 polymorphism and fiber type composition, particularly the correlation between G allele and increased proportion of type I (oxidative) fibers as well as the association of the C allele with the propensity to skeletal muscle hypertrophy, and a facilitation of glucose utilization in response to anaerobic exercise [29].

All the aforementioned facts suggest that *PPARA* polymorphisms may be crucial for maintaining lipid homeostasis and in this way, be responsible for developing specific training-induced physiological reactions. Therefore, we have decided to check if post-training changes of body composition measurements, as well as chosen biochemical parameters (LDL, HDL, glucose), are modulated by the *PPARA* genotypes. To test this hypothesis, we have examined the genotype and alleles' frequencies (described in *PPARA* rs1800206 and rs4253778 polymorphic sites) in female participants engaged in a 12-week training program.

2. Experimental Section

2.1. Ethics Statement

The procedures followed in the study were conducted ethically according to the principles of the World Medical Association Declaration of Helsinki and ethical standards in sport and exercise science research. The study was approved by the Ethics Committee of the Regional Medical Chamber in Szczecin (Approval number 09/KB/IV/2011). All participants were given a consent form and a written information sheet concerning the study, providing all pertinent information (purpose, procedures, risks, and benefits of participation). The experimental procedures were conducted in accordance with the set of guiding principles for reporting the results of genetic association studies defined by the Strengthening the Reporting of Genetic Association studies (STREGA) Statement [30].

2.2. Participants

Out of 201 recruited Polish Caucasian women (range 19–24 years) we have obtained 182 full sets of pre-training and post-training body composition and biochemical data in those who completed a 12-week training program. From these 182 participants, the genetic material was isolated and 168 samples (age 21.6 ± 1.3 years, body mass 60.6 ± 7.6 kg, 21.6 ± 2.4) were successfully genotyped for PPARA rs1800206 and rs4253778. None of the included individuals had engaged in regular physical activity in the previous 6 months. The level of physical activity over the last 6 months has been estimated in every participant according to Global Physical Activity Questionnaire (GPAQ) as well as the individual recording of the subject's own activity, such as direct observation and activity diaries [31]. They had no history of any metabolic or cardiovascular diseases. Participants were nonsmokers and refrained from taking any medications or supplements known to affect metabolism. Before the training phase, all participants were included in a dietary program and had received an individual dietary plan. For every participant, the Basal Metabolic Rate (BMR) as well as the Physical Activity Level (PAL, calculated as the ratio of Total Energy Expenditure (TEE) to BMR), was defined. Every participant was asked to keep a balanced diet customized for the individual's PAL coefficient and body mass according to nutrition standards described for the Polish population [32] during the study and for 2 months before the study. The participants were asked to keep a food diary every day. Weekly consultations were held in which the quality and quantity of meals were analyzed and, if necessary, minor adjustments were made. The nutrition and general lifestyle conditions for all participants during the training phase were considered as similar. During the last weekly session before the 12-week training program, the participants underwent the graded exercise VO$_2$max test and body composition screen.

2.3. Training Intervention

Maximum heart rate (HRmax) was calculated directly in every subject by a continuous graded exercise test on an electronically braked cycle ergometer (Oxycon Pro, Erich JAEGER GmbH, Hoechberg, Germany) which was performed to determine their aerobic capacity (VO2max). The heart rate (HR) at each step of the training program was measured in every subject using HR personal monitoring devices (Polar T31 straps and CE0537 Watches, Lake Success, NY, USA) with customized setup. The training stage was preceded by a week-long familiarization stage, when the examined women exercised 3 times a week for 30 min, at an intensity of about 50% of their HRR (HR Reserve) calculated according to the Karvonen formula. After the week-long familiarization stage, proper training has started. Each training unit consisted of a warm-up routine (10 min), the main aerobic routine (43 min), and stretching and breathing exercise (7 min). The main aerobic routine was a combination of two alternating styles—low and high impact as described by Zarebska et al. [33–35]. Low impact style comprised movements with at least one foot on the floor at all times, whereas high impact styles included running, hopping, and jumping with a variety of flight phases [36]. Music of variable rhythm intensity (tempo) was incorporated into both styles. A 12-week program of low–high impact aerobics was divided as follows: (1) 3 weeks (9 training units), 60 min each, at about 50–60% of HRR, music tempo 135–140 BPM (beats per min), (2) 3 weeks (9 training units), 60 min each, at 55–65% of HRR, music tempo 135–140 BPM, (3) 3 weeks (9 training units), 60 min with the intensity of 60–70% of HRR, music tempo 140–152 BPM, and (4) 3 weeks (9 training units), 60 min with an intensity of 65–75% of HRR, music tempo 140–152 BPM. All 36 training units were administered and supervised by the same instructor.

2.4. Body Composition Measurements

Body mass and body composition were assessed by the bioimpedance method (body's inherent resistance to an electrical current) with the use of the electronic scale "Tanita TBF 300M" (Horton Health Initiatives, Orland Park, IL, USA) as described by Zarebska et al. [33]. The device was plugged in and calibrated with the consideration of the weight of the clothes (0.2 kg). Afterward, data regarding age, body height, and sex of the subject were inserted. Then, the subjects stood on the scale with their bare feet on the marked places without leaning any body part. The device analyses body composition based on the differences in the ability to conduct electrical current by body tissues (different resistance) due to different water content. Body mass and body composition measurements were taken with the use of the electronic scale "Tanita" are as follows: total body mass (kg), fat free mass (FFM, kg), fat mass (kg), body mass index (BMI = body mass (kg)/(body height (m))^2, in kg.m^{-2}), tissue impedance (Ohm), total body water (TBW, kg), and basal metabolic rate (BMR, kJ).

2.5. Biochemical Analyses

Fasting blood samples were obtained in the morning from the elbow vein before the start of the aerobic fitness training program and repeated at the 12th week of this training program (after the 36th training unit). Compete blood samples (taken before and after 12-week training period) were obtained for 182 participants. The analyses were performed immediately after the blood collection, as described by Leońska-Duniec et al. [37]. Blood samples from each participant were collected in 2 tubes. For biochemical analyses, a 4.9 mL·S-Monovette tube with ethylenediaminetetraacetic acid (K 3 EDTA; 1.6 mg EDTA/mL blood) and separating gel (SARSTEDT AG and Co., Nümbrecht, Germany) were used. Blood samples for biochemical analyses were centrifuged 300× g for 15 min at room temperature to receive blood plasma. All biochemical analyses were conducted using Random Access Automatic Biochemical Analyzer for Clinical Chemistry and Turbidimetry A15 (BIO-SYSTEMS S.A., Barcelona,

Spain). Blood plasma was used to determine lipid profile: triglycerides (TGL), total cholesterol, high-density lipoproteins (HDL) and low-density lipoproteins (LDL) concentrations. Plasma TGL and total cholesterol concentrations were determined using a diagnostic colorimetric enzymatic method according to the manufacturer's protocol (BioMaxima S.A., Lublin, Poland). The manufacturer's declared intra-assay coefficients of variation (CV) of the method were <2.5% and <1.5% for the TGL and total cholesterol determinations, respectively. HDL plasma concentration was determined using the human anti-β-lipoprotein antibody and colorimetric enzymatic method according to the manufacturer's protocol (BioMaxima S.A.). The manufacturer's declared intra-assay CV of the method was <1.5%. Plasma concentrations of LDL were determined using a direct method according to the manufacturer's protocol (PZ Cormay S.A., Lomianki, Poland). The manufacturer's declared intra-assay CV of the method was 4.97%. All analysis procedures were verified with the use of a multi-parametric control serum (BIOLABO S.A.S, Maizy, France), as well as control serum of normal level (BioNormL) and high level (BioPathL) lipid profiles (BioMaxima S.A.).

2.6. Genetic Analyses

The buccal cells donated by the subjects were collected in Resuspension Solution (GenElute Mammalian Genomic DNA Miniprep Kit, Sigma-Aldrich Chemie Gmbh, Munich, Germany) with the use of sterile foam-tipped applicators (Puritan, Holbrook, NY 11741, USA). DNA was extracted from the buccal cells using a GenElute Mammalian Genomic DNA Miniprep Kit (Sigma-Aldrich Chemie Gmbh, Munich, Germany) according to the manufacturer's protocol. DNA isolates were evaluated for quantity, quality, and integrity of DNA using the spectrophotometer BioPhotometer Plus (Eppendorf, Wesseling-Berzdorf, Germany). Only 168 isolates passed the evaluation and were used for subsequent genotyping.

To discriminate *PPARA* I7 rs4253778 (G > C) as well as Leu162Val rs1800206 (C > G) alleles, TaqMan Pre-Designed SNP Genotyping Assays were used (Applied Biosystems, Waltham, MA, USA) (assay IDs: C___2985251_10 and C___8817670_20, respectively) including primers and fluorescently labeled (FAM and VIC) MGBTM TaqMan probes to detect alleles. All samples were genotyped in duplicate on a StepOne Real-Time Polymerase Chain Reaction (RT-PCR) instrument (Applied Biosystems, Waltham, MA, USA) as previously described [37]. PCR products were then subjected to Endpoint-genotyping analysis using an allelic discrimination assay at StepOne Software v2.3 (Applied Biosystems, Carlsbad, CA, USA) to measure the relative amount of allele-specific fluorescence (FAM or VIC), which leads directly to the determination of individual genotypes. Genotypes were assigned using all of the data from the study simultaneously.

2.7. Statistical Analyses

Allele frequencies were determined by gene counting. An χ^2 test was used to test the Hardy–Weinberg equilibrium. To examine the hypothesis that the *PPARA* I7 rs4253778 polymorphism modulate training response, we conducted a repeated measure 2 × 3 ANOVA for genes and 2 × 2 ANOVA for alleles comparison with one between-subject factor (*PPARA* I7 rs4253778 genotype: GG vs. GC vs. CC, GG vs. GC + CC, GG + GC vs. CC) and one within-subject factor (time: before training versus after training) for twelve dependent variables. To examine the hypothesis that *PPARA* Leu162Val rs1800206 modulate training response, we conducted a repeated measure of 2 × 2 ANOVA. Kolmogorov–Smirnov test was used to check for data normality, Mauchly's test for data sphericity, and a post hoc Tukey test was applied when interaction was significant and was used to perform pair-wise comparisons. The effect size (partial eta squared–η^2) of each test was calculated for all analyses and was classified according to Larson-Hall [38], where η^2: 0.01, 0.06, 0.14 were estimated for small, moderate, and large effect, respectively. All statistics were performed in STATISTICA software (version 13; StatSoft, Tulsa, OK, USA) with the level of statistical significance set at $p < 0.05$.

3. Results

PPARA I7 rs4253778, as well as Leu162Val rs1800206 genotypes, conformed to Hardy–Weinberg equilibrium ($p = 0.887$ and $p = 0.572$, respectively) and phenotype outcomes were normally distributed, with no disruption of sphericity (Supplementary File S1). The genotyping error was assessed as 1%, while the call rate (the proportion of samples in which the genotyping provided unambiguous reading) exceeded 95%.

The ANOVA showed genotype × training interactions in *PPARA* I7 rs4253778 for LDL ($F_{1, 165} = 5.12$, $p = 0.025$, $\eta^2 = 0.03$) (Table 1), where post hoc test showed that LDL increased in *PPARA* I7 rs4253778 CC homozygotes after training intervention (79.17 ± 14.16 vs. 95.48 ± 15.35 mg/dL), which did not appear in other genotypes (Figure 1). ANOVA in *PPARA* I7 rs4253778 allele × training interactions showed differences in LDL ($F_{1, 166} = 4.59$, $p = .034$, $\eta^2 = 0.03$), where post hoc analyses showed that CC homozygotes and not G allele carriers increased the LDL concentration after training intervention (Table 1).

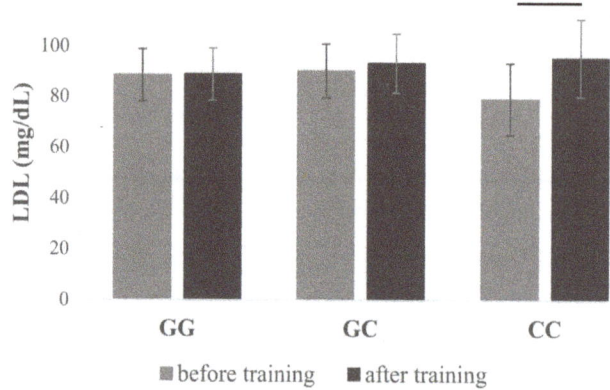

Figure 1. Changes in plasma low-density lipoproteins (LDL) concentrations measured before and after the completion of the 12-week training program in carriers of different *PPARA* I7 rs4253778 genotypes. The values are mean ± SD.

Other *PPARA* I7 rs4253778 genotype × training interactions were found in glucose plasma concentrations ($F_{2, 165} = 3.99$, $p = 0.02$, $\eta^2 = 0.05$) (Table 1), where post hoc showed that carriers of GG and GC genotypes decreased glucose concentration over the period of training (78.83 ± 10.20 vs. 76.44 ± 10.21 and 77.62 ± 8.92 vs. 73.34 ± 9.28, respectively, mg/dL), while for CC homozygotes were characterized by the opposite effect of training and demonstrated a significant increase of glucose concentration (70.50 ± 7.76 vs. 78.17 ± 12.58 mg/dL) (Figure 2) (Table 1). Furthermore, ANOVA in PPARA I7 rs4253778 allele × training interactions showed differences in glucose concentration ($F_{1, 166} = 6.68$, $p = 0.011$, $\eta^2 = 0.06$), where post hoc showed that G allele carriers decreased glucose concentration and CC homozygotes increased glucose concentration (Table 1).

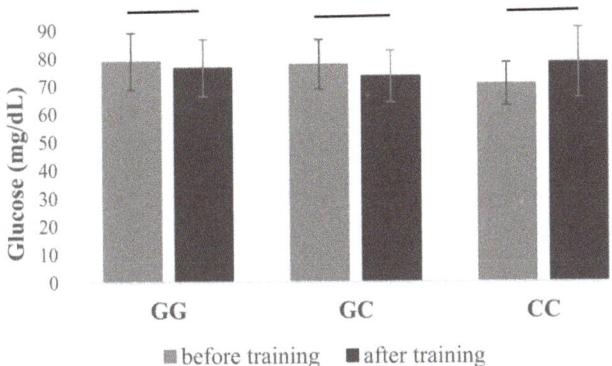

Figure 2. Changes in plasma glucose concentrations measured before and after the completion of the 12-week training program in carriers of different *PPARA* I7 rs4253778 genotypes. The values are mean ± SD.

HDL plasma concentration resulted in statistical differences in *PPARA* Leu162Val rs1800206 genotype ($F_{1, 166}$ = 22.68, $p < 0.001$, $\eta^2 = 0.12$) and training interactions ($F_{1, 166}$ = 6.30, $p = 0.013$, $\eta^2 = 0.04$) (Table 2), where post hoc showed that HDL decreased in both *PPARA* Leu162Val rs1800206 genotypes (CC and CG) in the course of training (65.12 ± 13.51 vs. 61.78 ± 13.48 and 64.82 ± 11.83 vs. 54.03 ± 12.08, respectively) (Figure 3) and this training decrease was bigger in CG genotype (only G allele carriers) when compared to CC homozygotes (Table 2). There were no other effects of training or *PPARA* Leu162Val rs1800206 genotypes observed in dependent variables.

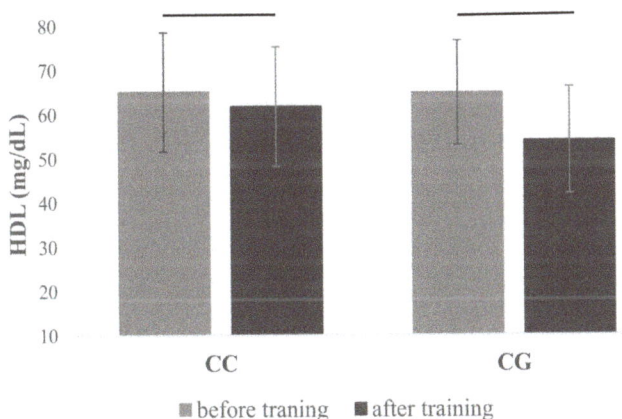

Figure 3. Changes in plasma high-density lipoproteins (HDL) concentrations measured before and after the completion of the 12-week training program in carriers of different *PPARA* Leu162Val rs1800206 genotypes. The values are mean ± SD.

Table 1. The *PPARA I7* rs4253778 genotypes and response to training.

Variable	GG (n = 109)			GC (n = 53)			CC (n = 6)			p Values for Genotypes		p Values for Allele × Training Interaction	
	Before Training	After Training		Before Training	After Training		Before Training	After Training		Genotype	Training	GG vs. GC+CC	GG+GC vs. CC
Body mass (kg)	59.82 ± 7.45	59.12 ± 7.31		62.35 ± 7.93	61.51 ± 7.86		58.93 ± 6.92	58.27 ± 7.35		0.130	0.859	0.220	0.544
BMI (kg/m^2)	21.36 ± 2.36	21.14 ± 2.30		22.06 ± 2.51	21.82 ± 2.48		21.47 ± 2.85	21.25 ± 2.87		0.226	0.984	0.964	0.510
BMR (kJ)	6027.11 ± 322.75	5988.31 ± 301.69		6117.87 ± 333.88	6087.24 ± 337.16		6035.00 ± 309.97	5970.17 ± 322.14		0.194	0.855	0.889	0.602
Tissue impedance (Ohm)	556.21 ± 64.49	542.09 ± 62.98		536.09 ± 62.33	524.34 ± 62.26		557.17 ± 50.41	543.50 ± 42.88		0.257	0.382	0.643	0.578
FM (kg)	14.42 ± 4.98	13.54 ± 4.97		15.67 ± 5.21	14.59 ± 5.35		14.32 ± 5.15	13.10 ± 5.53		0.565	0.647	0.955	0.979
FFM (kg)	45.38 ± 3.10	45.79 ± 3.06		46.45 ± 3.34	46.91 ± 3.58		44.62 ± 2.57	45.17 ± 2.38		0.084	0.936	0.874	0.491
TBW (kg)	33.32 ± 2.46	33.56 ± 2.28		33.84 ± 2.88	34.32 ± 2.69		32.67 ± 1.88	33.37 ± 1.51		0.229	0.481	0.813	0.429
Total cholesterol (mg/dL)	169.11 ± 22.86	167.16 ± 24.21		172.30 ± 29.33	170.53 ± 33.83		165.00 ± 10.18	172.67 ± 10.65		0.671	0.549	0.983	0.076
TGL (mg/dL)	81.90 ± 35.08	85.27 ± 36.75		76.15 ± 24.53	81.55 ± 32.75		85.50 ± 38.52	73.50 ± 15.54		0.825	0.475	0.679	0.414
HDL (mg/dL)	64.09 ± 12.29	61.21 ± 12.65		66.75 ± 15.18	60.86 ± 15.46		68.80 ± 14.95	62.28 ± 12.26		0.059	0.211	0.085	0.481
LDL (mg/dL)	88.54 ± 20.31	88.91 ± 20.34		90.26 ± 25.69	93.32 ± 29.70		79.17 ± 14.16	95.48 ± 15.35		0.648	**0.025**	0.171	**0.033**
Glucose (mg/dL)	78.83 ± 10.20	76.44 ± 10.21		77.62 ± 8.92	73.34 ± 9.28		70.50 ± 7.76	78.17 ± 12.58		0.298	**0.020**	0.101	**0.011**

The values are mean ± SD; p values (analyzed by two-way mixed ANOVA test) for main effects (genotype and training) genotype × training interaction; bold p values-statistically significant differences (p < 0.05); BMI–body mass index; BMR–basal metabolic rate; FM–fat mass; FFM–fat free mass; TBW–total body water; TGL–triglycerides; HDL–high-density lipoproteins; LDL–low-density lipoproteins.

Table 2. The *PPARA* Leu162Val rs18000206 genotypes and response to training.

Variable	CC (n = 154)		CG (n = 14)		p Values for Main Effects	
	Before Training	After Training	Before Training	After Training	Genotype	Training
Body mass (kg)	60.57 ± 7.69	59.90 ± 7.58	60.77 ± 7.37	59.21 ± 7.13	0.063	0.052
BMI (kg/m^2)	21.55 ± 2.46	21.34 ± 2.39	22.03 ± 2.16	21.58 ± 2.39	0.0.64	0.099
BMR (kJ)	6055.80 ± 328.86	6021.35 ± 317.31	6058.43 ± 304.72	5991.64 ± 304.76	0.064	0.303
Tissue impedance (Ohm)	548.23 ± 62.99	535.32 ± 62.33	568.21 ± 71.46	549.93 ± 64.19	0.233	0.582
FM (kg)	14.73 ± 5.09	13.85 ± 5.10	15.63 ± 4.89	13.98 ± 5.34	0.098	0.163
FFM (kg)	45.77 ± 3.19	46.20 ± 3.25	44.79 ± 3.20	45.24 ± 3.15	0.716	0.090
TBW (kg)	33.52 ± 2.60	33.86 ± 2.41	32.81 ± 2.36	33.13 ± 2.32	0.096	0.950
Total cholesterol (mg/dL)	170.99 ± 24.67	169.36 ± 27.58	158.78 ± 23.55	158.07 ± 21.24	0.690	0.876
TGL (mg/dL)	80.86 ± 32.29	85.12 ± 35.55	73.14 ± 31.21	67.71 ± 22.64	0.900	0.294
HDL (mg/dL)	65.12 ± 13.51	61.78 ± 13.48	64.82 ± 11.83	54.03 ± 12.08	**0.001**	**0.013**
LDL (mg/dL)	89.60 ± 21.69	90.55 ± 23.39	79.43 ± 23.59	90.43 ± 26.16	0.259	0.587
Glucose (mg/dL)	78.41 ± 9.74	75.32 ± 10.02	75.36 ± 10.59	77.71 ± 10.67	0.795	0.053

The values are mean ± SD; *p* values (analyzed by two-way mixed ANOVA test) for genotype × training interaction; BMI–body mass index; BMR–basal metabolic rate; FM–fat mass; FFM–fat free mass; TBW–total body water; TGL–triglycerides; HDL–high-density lipoproteins; LDL–low-density lipoproteins.

Our statistical analyses revealed that *PPARA* intron 7 rs4253778 polymorphism modulate training response in reference to plasma LDL and glucose concentration, while *PPARA* Leu162Val rs1800206 polymorphism interacts with HDL concentration. Taken together, our results supply additional information about the potential role played by genetic variants described in the *PPARA* gene in training-induced biochemical changes.

4. Discussion

This study aimed to check if post-training changes of body mass measurements, as well as chosen biochemical parameters observed in physically active women, are modulated by specific genotypes. The verified hypothesis assumed that in the presence of specific genotypes and alleles in the *PPARA* gene would influence the post-training response observed in biochemical parameter changes in the course of the 12-week training program. Taking onto account *PPARA* intron 7 (rs4253778) genotype × training interactions, there were two statistically significant effects: for LDL and glucose plasma concentrations. For all genotypes, a slight increase in LDL level was observed. However, the rise of LDL concentration reached the highest point in intron 7 CC homozygotes when compared to G allele carriers. Moreover, the CC homozygotes were characterized by an unexpected increase in glucose plasma concentration, while in GC and GG participants, the reverse trend of decreasing glucose concentration was noted. It is commonly expected that LDL, as well as glucose plasma levels, would decrease after regular physical activity [39]. However, more detailed analyses revealed that beneficial changes of the lipid profile are achieved only when the intensity of training is moderate (the exercises are performed below the anaerobic threshold), while the training above the anaerobic threshold intensity may not lead to such healthy effects; what is more it may even reverse these beneficial trends in the context of plasma lipid concentrations [40]. A meta-analysis of studies on the impact of aerobic training on plasma HDL concentration revealed that the minimum duration of aerobic exercises necessary for achieving the beneficial effect of HDL level elevation is about 120 minutes per week, which is an equivalent of 900 kcal energy expenditure [41]. In the exercise protocol used in our study, we had about 180 min exercises per week, and the intensity of the exercises was gradually increased from 50% to 60% to 65% to 75% heart rate reserve. Each training unit consisted of a warm-up, the main aerobic routine, and the ending phase, including stretching and a breathing exercise [33–35]. The structure of the main routine that was a combination of two alternating styles of low and high intensity may resemble interval training, in which the high-intensity workouts are similar to anaerobic exercises, while low-intensity sets correspond to a restitution phase. The summary volume of aerobic exercises probably was not enough to achieve the expected beneficial changes in the lipid profile and glucose level, especially in *PPARA* intron 7 CC homozygotes.

The functional role of *PPARA* intron 7 polymorphism was suggested for the first time in the prospective study of healthy middle-aged men in the United Kingdom [21] as well as in the study of male British Army recruits undergoing a 10-week physical training program [22]. It has been demonstrated that intron 7 C allele is associated with progression of atherosclerosis [21] and is positively correlated with left ventricular growth in response to exercise [22]. Based on the results of the studies showing that hypertrophied heart is characterized by reduced PPARα activity [23] and, in the same time, downregulation of the expression of mitochondrial FAO enzymes [25] with accompanying increases in expression of genes encoding glycolytic enzymes [24], it has been speculated that intron 7 C allele is responsible for lowering the expression of the *PPARA* gene and in this way, is indirectly connected with downregulation of the expression of key metabolic enzymes, leading to impairment of cellular lipid and glucose homeostasis. Another issue is, of course, the question of how the polymorphism located in the non-coding region influences the gene's expression. One possible answer could be that *PPARA* intron 7 alleles are not direct casual variants, but are rather in linkage disequilibrium with an unidentified polymorphism (within the *PPARA* gene or in its regulatory region) that alters encoded protein levels and, as a consequence, may change the expression of PPARα target genes [27,29,42,43]. There is also a hypothesis that, considering this SNP location, the *PPARA* intron 7 polymorphism may change and disrupt a microRNA site [44].

Considering that the proper expression of the *PPARA* gene, necessary for maintaining the appropriate level of PPARα protein, is crucial for regulation of carbohydrate/lipid metabolism, and that the intron 7 C allele may affect this expression process, it is may be expected that the lipid profile and glucose levels would be altered in C allele carriers. Indeed, our results seem to confirm this assumption because we have observed that LDL and glucose levels in CC homozygotes were different from the normal range, with the surprising effect of a post-training increase of plasma glucose concentration as well as the highest rise of LDL levels observed in CC participants. These results suggest that *PPARA* intron 7 CC genotype may be in the group of disadvantageous factors responsible for developing unexpected post-training effects. Probably the CC homozygotes should undergo a different training program with increased volume of aerobic exercises to achieve the expected beneficial results.

When *PPARA* Leu162Val (rs1800206) genotype × training interactions were taken into account, only one statistically significant effect was observed: for post-training changes of HDL levels. In the case of both recorded measurements in these SNP genotypes (CC and CG) we have observed a slight decrease of HDL levels. However, this lowering effect was more pronounced in G allele carriers, in which at least half of the PPARα protein amount comprised the Val amino acid in the 162 position. It is worth noting that rs1800206 GG homozygotes are very rare in the human population, in our study, there were no such individuals in the whole study group.

The C→G substitution, described as *PPARA* rs1800206 polymorphism, is placed within the coding region of the gene, what makes it functional "by definition", causing an amino acid change in the 162 position (Leu162Val) that is located within DNA binding domain (DBD) of the PPARα protein [18]. DBD is directly involved in the interaction between the PPARα transcription factor and PPRE sequences in the promoter region of target genes [6]. Detailed in vitro analyses revealed that PPARα constructs with Val amino acid in the 162 position is activated by the endogenous ligands to a lesser extent when compared with "wild type" PPARα with Leu amino acid residue in the same localization [45]. The PPARα Leu form, that is produced in CC homozygotes, is considered as an active form of this transcriptional factor, displaying a higher transcriptional activity [45] and being able to stimulate the expression of the genes encoding β-oxidation enzymes more efficiently, which cause the shift of the metabolic balance toward catabolic pathways [46,47].

In vivo studies have shown that Leu162Val polymorphism is associated with total plasma cholesterol [16,48,49], LDL [18,49], HDL [16], as well as apolipoprotein B (apoB) [18,48,49], apolipoprotein A-I (apoA-I) [16], and apolipoprotein C-III (apoC-III) [49] concentrations. Moreover, Leu162Val is involved in diabetes and arteriosclerosis progression [16,20,21]. To be more specific, the studies of diabetic patients and non-diabetic subjects revealed that the rs1800206 G allele (also designed as the 162Val allele) carriers were characterized by higher levels of plasma total cholesterol, LDL, and apoB levels in comparison with CC homozygotes [18]. The large population-based study confirmed that the presence of the rs1800206 G allele is correlated with higher levels of total cholesterol, LDL, apoB, and apoC [49]. Moreover, the study of men with metabolic syndrome showed that the frequency of the rs1800206 G allele was higher in subjects having simultaneously abdominal obesity, hypertriglyceridemia, and low HDL levels. The same study demonstrated that carriers of the G allele were characterized by higher plasma apoB and triglyceride (TG) levels and the presence of G allele was associated with components of metabolic syndrome [50]. In another relative large-scale study of middle-aged whites, the G allele was also correlated with an increase in fasting levels of serum lipids [51]. In a controlled dietary intervention trial, in which saturated fat was replaced with either monounsaturated fat or carbohydrate in isoenergetic diets, the effects of *PPARA* Leu162Val genotypes in the determination of plasma lipid concentrations were assessed. The results of this study revealed that Leu162Val variants influence plasma LDL cholesterol concentration, especially being a determinant of small dense LDL (sdLDL) [52]. It has been confirmed in several independent studies showing that rs1800206 CC homozygotes are characterized by a larger LDL particle with reduced density and by an increased general proportion of large LDL particles in the total cholesterol pool [53,54]. Such larger and more buoyant LDL particles are less prone to oxidation processes which create protecting conditions in case of atherosclerosis progression, while small dense LDLs are considered as risk factors of atherosclerosis and coronary artery disease [55,56]. Studies in patients demonstrated that fibrate ligands of PPARα can reduce production of sdLDL, so in carriers of the less active PPARα Val form (that is produced in rs1800206 G allele carriers), activation by dietary ligands could result in a shift to a higher proportion of sdLDL [47,57].

All the aforementioned studies led us to the suggestion that the *PPARA* rs1800206 G allele (producing PPARα protein with Val amino acid in the 162 position) may be associated with developing in its carriers the adverse effects in the context of lipid metabolism. Our results, at least in part, confirm this hypothesis, because the unfavorable post-training effects expressed by an increase of the HDL level was pointed out most firmly in GC heterozygotes, while in CC homozygotes these disadvantageous changes were significantly restricted.

We are aware that our study has some limitations. The first issue of almost every genetic association study has a proper number of participants in the study group. In our case, this could also be a problem, and we see the need for replicating our results in another, preferably larger, population. Especially, *PPARA* I7 rs4253778 CC genotype was rare ($n = 6$) and might cause statistical bias. On the other hand, this rs4253778 CC genotype has been rare in previous studies on the Caucasian population, where it was shown to influence physical condition level [58,59]. The second question is whether the analyzed *PPARA* polymorphisms are true causative factors or perhaps only in linkage disequilibrium with variants directly engaged in developing a specific trait. This problem has been brought up in many studies, and in most cases, the conclusion is that the variation within the *PPARA* gene does not influence any physiological traits alone. Thus, it should be underlined that *PPARA* diversity probably accounts for only a small portion of phenotypic variability, due to the polygenic character of the traits connected with body mass and biochemical parameters measured in our experiment, implying that multiple gene-environment interactions may contribute to the observed differential effects.

5. Conclusions

The results obtained in the current study support our initial hypothesis and suggest that *PPARA* intron 7 rs4253778, as well as Leu162Val rs1800206 variants, play a role in differentiating the beneficial effects of physical activity between the specific genotype carriers. We have demonstrated that harboring a specific *PPARA* intron 7 rs4253778 as well as Leu162Val rs1800206 genotypes may be associated with different post-training changes of measured biochemical parameters. We have observed the surprising effect of a post-training increase of plasma glucose concentration as well as the highest rise of LDL levels in rs4253778 CC participants, which led us to the suggestion that rs4253778 C allele may affect the lipid profile and glucose levels. On the other hand, we have also indicated that some individuals may benefit from being an rs1800206 CC homozygote because in such participants the unfavorable training effects were significantly restricted.

The information obtained in this study can be used as an additional source of precise information about a person undertaking physical effort, determining at the molecular level its inherent metabolic characteristics. Potentially, such information may help design individualized forms of training and more effective optimization and control of the obtained post-training or other treatment effects. Due to the importance of the polymorphic forms analyzed in *PPARA* gene in the etiology of many human diseases, they can be used as a molecular tool of pro-health prophylaxis, helpful in estimating the risk of disorders, such as obesity.

Supplementary Materials: The following are available online at http://www.mdpi.com/2077-0383/8/7/1043/s1, Table S1: *PPARA* I7 rs4253778 and Leu162Val rs1800206 genotypes and phenotype outcomes.

Author Contributions: A.M.-S., P.S., M.B., M.P., and M.S. conceived and designed the experiments; A.M.-S., W.C., P.K., M.S., M.B. and K.S. performed the experiments; A.M.-S., P.S., M.B., M.P., W.C., P.K., M.S. and M.S., K.S. analyzed the data; A.M.-S. and M.S. contributed reagents/materials/analysis tools; A.M.-S., P.S., M.B., M.P., and M.S. wrote the paper.

Funding: This research was funded by Charles University in Prague (funding number: UNCE\HUM\032) and the Polish Ministry of Science and Higher Education (Grant UM0-2012/07/B/NZ7/ 01155).

Acknowledgments: This experiment was supported by Grant UM0-2012/07/B/NZ7/ 01155 founded by the Polish Ministry of Science and Higher Education (http://www.nauka.gov.pl/). This article was written during a scientific training session in the Faculty of Physical Education and Sport of Charles University in Prague (Czech Republic), and the study was supported by a research grant from Charles University UNCE\HUM\032. The funders had no role in study design, data collection, and analysis, decision to publish, or preparation of the paper. The experiments comply with the current laws of the country in which they were performed. The authors would like to thank all participants who decided to spend time to take part in their study and make the research possible.

Conflicts of Interest: The authors declare no conflict of interest.

References

1. Desvergne, B.; Wahli, W. Peroxisome proliferator-activated receptors: Nuclear control of metabolism. *Endocr. Rev.* **1999**, *20*, 649–688. [PubMed]
2. Auboeuf, D.; Rieusset, J.; Fajas, L.; Vallier, P.; Frering, V.; Riou, J.P.; Staels, B.; Auwerx, J.; Laville, M.; Vidal, H. Tissue distribution and quantification of the expression of mRNAs of peroxisome proliferator–activated receptors and liver X receptor-α in humans: No alteration in adipose tissue of obese and NIDDM patients. *Diabetes* **1997**, *46*, 1319–1327.
3. Mukherjee, R.; Jow, L.; Croston, G.E.; Paterniti, J.R. Identification, characterization, and tissue distribution of human peroxisome proliferator-activated receptor (PPAR) isoforms PPARγ2 versus PPARγ1 and activation with retinoid X receptor agonists and antagonists. *J. Biol. Chem.* **1997**, *272*, 8071–8076. [CrossRef] [PubMed]
4. Palmer, C.N.; Hsu, M.-H.; Griffin, K.J.; Raucy, J.L.; Johnson, E.F. Peroxisome proliferator activated receptor-α expression in human liver. *Mol. Pharm.* **1998**, *53*, 14–22. [CrossRef]
5. Willson, T.M.; Wahli, W. Peroxisome proliferator-activated receptor agonists. *Curr. Opin. Chem. Biol.* **1997**, *1*, 235–241. [CrossRef]
6. Dowell, P.; Peterson, V.J.; Zabriskie, T.M.; Leid, M. Ligand-induced peroxisome proliferator-activated receptor α conformational change. *J. Biol. Chem.* **1997**, *272*, 2013–2020. [CrossRef] [PubMed]
7. Kliewer, S.A.; Sundseth, S.S.; Jones, S.A.; Brown, P.J.; Wisely, G.B.; Koble, C.S.; Devchand, P.; Wahli, W.; Willson, T.M.; Lenhard, J.M.; et al. Fatty acids and eicosanoids regulate gene expression through direct interactions with peroxisome proliferator-activated receptors α and γ. *Proc. Natl. Acad. Sci. USA* **1997**, *94*, 4318–4323. [CrossRef] [PubMed]

8. Brown, P.J.; Smith-Oliver, T.A.; Charifson, P.S.; Tomkinson, N.C.; Fivush, A.M.; Sternbach, D.D.; Wade, L.E.; Orband-Miller, L.; Parks, D.J.; Blanchard, S.G.; et al. Identification of peroxisome proliferator-activated receptor ligands from a biased chemical library. *Chem. Biol.* **1997**, *4*, 909–918. [CrossRef]
9. Henke, B.R.; Blanchard, S.G.; Brackeen, M.F.; Brown, K.K.; Cobb, J.E.; Collins, J.L.; Harrington, W.W., Jr.; Hashim, M.A.; Hull-Ryde, E.A.; Kaldor, I.; et al. N-(2-benzoylphenyl)-L-tyrosine PPARγ agonists. 1. Discovery of a novel series of potent antihyperglycemic and antihyperlipidemic agents. *J. Med. Chem.* **1998**, *41*, 5020–5036. [CrossRef]
10. Lehmann, J.M.; Moore, L.B.; Smith-Oliver, T.A.; Wilkison, W.O.; Willson, T.M.; Kliewer, S.A. An antidiabetic thiazolidinedione is a high affinity ligand for peroxisome proliferator-activated receptor γ (PPARγ). *J. Biol. Chem.* **1995**, *270*, 12953–12956. [CrossRef]
11. Gearing, K.; Göttlicher, M.; Teboul, M.; Widmark, E.; Gustafsson, J.-A. Interaction of the peroxisome-proliferator-activated receptor and retinoid X receptor. *Proc. Natl. Acad. Sci. USA* **1993**, *90*, 1440–1444. [CrossRef]
12. Keller, H.R.; Dreyer, C.; Medin, J.; Mahfoudi, A.; Ozato, K.; Wahli, W. Fatty acids and retinoids control lipid metabolism through activation of peroxisome proliferator-activated receptor-retinoid X receptor heterodimers. *Proc. Natl. Acad. Sci. USA* **1993**, *90*, 2160–2164. [CrossRef] [PubMed]
13. Juge-Aubry, C.E.; Hammar, E.; Siegrist-Kaiser, C.; Pernin, A.; Takeshita, A.; Chin, W.W.; Burger, A.G.; Meier, C.A. Regulation of the transcriptional activity of the peroxisome proliferator-activated receptor α by phosphorylation of a ligand-independent trans-activating domain. *J. Biol. Chem.* **1999**, *274*, 10505–10510. [CrossRef] [PubMed]
14. Sher, T.; Yi, H.F.; McBride, O.W.; Gonzalez, F.J. cDNA cloning, chromosomal mapping, and functional characterization of the human peroxisome proliferator activated receptor. *Biochemistry* **1993**, *32*, 5598–5604. [CrossRef] [PubMed]
15. Hsu, M.-H.; Palmer, C.N.; Song, W.; Griffin, K.J.; Johnson, E.F. A carboxyl-terminal extension of the zinc finger domain contributes to the specificity and polarity of peroxisome proliferator-activated receptor DNA binding. *J. Biol. Chem.* **1998**, *273*, 27988–27997. [CrossRef]
16. Flavell, D.; Torra, I.P.; Jamshidi, Y.; Evans, D.; Diamond, J.; Elkeles, R.; Bujac, S.R.; Miller, G.; Talmud, P.J.; Staels, B.; et al. Variation in the PPARα gene is associated with altered function in vitro and plasma lipid concentrations in Type II diabetic subjects. *Diabetologia* **2000**, *43*, 673–680. [CrossRef] [PubMed]
17. Sapone, A.; Peters, J.M.; Sakai, S.; Tomita, S.; Papiha, S.S.; Dai, R.; Friedman, F.K.; Gonzalez, F.J. The human peroxisome proliferator-activated receptor α gene: identification and functional characterization of two natural allelic variants. *Pharm. Genom* **2000**, *10*, 321–333. [CrossRef]
18. Vohl, M.-C.; Lepage, P.; Gaudet, D.; Brewer, C.G.; Bétard, C.; Perron, P.; Houde, G.; Cellier, C.; Faith, J.M.; Després, J.P.; et al. Molecular scanning of the human PPARα gene: Association of the L162V mutation with hyperapobetalipoproteinemia. *J. Lipid Res.* **2000**, *41*, 945–952.
19. Elkeles, R.S.; Diamond, J.R.; Poulter, C.; Dhanjil, S.; Nicolaides, A.N.; Mahmood, S.; Richmond, W.; Mather, H.; Sharp, P.; Feher, M.D.; et al. Cardiovascular outcomes in type 2 diabetes: A double blind placebo controlled study of bezafibrate: The St. Mary's, Ealing, Northwick Park Diabetes Cardiovascular Disease Prevention (SENDCAP) Study. *Diabetes Care* **1998**, *21*, 641–648. [CrossRef]
20. Andrulionytė, L.; Kuulasmaa, T.; Chiasson, J.-L.; Laakso, M. Single Nucleotide Polymorphisms of the Peroxisome Proliferator–Activated Receptor-α Gene (PPARA) Influence the Conversion From Impaired Glucose Tolerance to Type 2 Diabetes: The STOP-NIDDM Trial. *Diabetes* **2007**, *56*, 1181–1186. [CrossRef]
21. Flavell, D.M.; Jamshidi, Y.; Hawe, E.; Pineda Torra, I.S.; Taskinen, M.-R.; Frick, M.H.; Nieminen, M.S.; Kesäniemi, Y.A.; Pasternack, A.; Staels, B.; et al. Peroxisome proliferator-activated receptor α gene variants influence progression of coronary atherosclerosis and risk of coronary artery disease. *Circulation* **2002**, *105*, 1440–1445. [CrossRef]
22. Jamshidi, Y.; Montgomery, H.E.; Hense, H.-W.; Myerson, S.G.; Torra, I.P.; Staels, B.; World, M.J.; Doering, A.; Erdmann, J.; Hengstenberg, C.; et al. Peroxisome proliferator–activated receptor α gene regulates left ventricular growth in response to exercise and hypertension. *Circulation* **2002**, *105*, 950–955. [CrossRef] [PubMed]
23. Barger, P.M.; Brandt, J.M.; Leone, T.C.; Weinheimer, C.J.; Kelly, D.P. Deactivation of peroxisome proliferator–activated receptor-α during cardiac hypertrophic growth. *J. Clin. Investig.* **2000**, *105*, 1723–1730. [CrossRef] [PubMed]

24. Allard, M.; Schonekess, B.; Henning, S.; English, D.; Lopaschuk, G.D. Contribution of oxidative metabolism and glycolysis to ATP production in hypertrophied hearts. *Am. J. Physiol. Heart Circ. Physiol.* **1994**, *267*, H742–H750. [CrossRef] [PubMed]
25. Sack, M.N.; Rader, T.A.; Park, S.; Bastin, J.; McCune, S.A.; Kelly, D.P. Fatty acid oxidation enzyme gene expression is downregulated in the failing heart. *Circulation* **1996**, *94*, 2837–2842. [CrossRef] [PubMed]
26. Foucher, C.; Rattier, S.; Flavell, D.M.; Talmud, P.J.; Humphries, S.E.; Kastelein, J.J.; Ayyobi, A.; Pimstone, S.; Frohlich, J.; Ansquer, J.C.; et al. Response to micronized fenofibrate treatment is associated with the peroxisome–proliferator-activated receptors alpha G/C intron7 polymorphism in subjects with type 2 diabetes. *Pharmacogenetics* **2004**, *14*, 823–829. [CrossRef]
27. Maciejewska, A.; Sawczuk, M.; Cieszczyk, P. Variation in the PPARalpha gene in Polish rowers. *J. Sci. Med. Sport* **2011**, *14*, 58–64. [CrossRef] [PubMed]
28. Eynon, N.; Meckel, Y.; Sagiv, M.; Yamin, C.; Amir, R.; Sagiv, M.; Goldhammer, E.; Duarte, J.A.; Oliveira, J. Do PPARGC1A and PPARalpha polymorphisms influence sprint or endurance phenotypes? *Scand. J. Med. Sci. Sports* **2010**, *20*, e145–e150. [CrossRef]
29. Ahmetov, I.I.; Mozhayskaya, I.A.; Flavell, D.M.; Astratenkova, I.V.; Komkova, A.I.; Lyubaeva, E.V.; Tarakin, P.P.; Shenkman, B.S.; Vdovina, A.B.; Netreba, A.I.; et al. PPARalpha gene variation and physical performance in Russian athletes. *Eur. J. Appl. Physiol.* **2006**, *97*, 103–108. [CrossRef]
30. Little, J.; Higgins, J.P.; Ioannidis, J.P.; Moher, D.; Gagnon, F.; Von Elm, E.; Khoury, M.J.; Cohen, B.; Davey-Smith, G.; Grimshaw, J.; et al. STrengthening the REporting of Genetic Association studies (STREGA)—An extension of the STROBE statement. *Genet. Epidemiol.* **2009**, *33*, 581–598. [CrossRef]
31. Hills, A.P.; Mokhtar, N.; Byrne, N.M. Assessment of physical activity and energy expenditure: An overview of objective measures. *Front. Nutr.* **2014**, *16*, 5. [CrossRef]
32. Jarosz, M. *Normy żywienia dla Populacji Polski*; Instytut Żywności I Żywienia: Warszawa, Poland, 2017.
33. Zarebska, A.; Jastrzebski, Z.; Cieszczyk, P.; Leonska-Duniec, A.; Kotarska, K.; Kaczmarczyk, M.; Sawczuk, M.; Maciejewska-Karlowska, A. The Pro12Ala polymorphism of the peroxisome proliferator-activated receptor gamma gene modifies the association of physical activity and body mass changes in Polish women. *PPAR Res.* **2014**, *2014*, 1–7. [CrossRef] [PubMed]
34. Zarebska, A.; Jastrzebski, Z.; Kaczmarczyk, M.; Ficek, K.; Maciejewska-Karlowska, A.; Sawczuk, M.; Leońska-Duniec, A.; Krol, P.; Cieszczyk, P.; Zmijewski, P.; et al. The GSTP1 c. 313A> G polymorphism modulates the cardiorespiratory response to aerobic training. *Biol. Sport* **2014**, *31*, 261–266. [CrossRef] [PubMed]
35. Zarębska, A.; Jastrzębski, Z.; Moska, W.; Leońska-Duniec, A.; Kaczmarczyk, M.; Sawczuk, M.; Maciejewska-Skrendo, A.; Zmijewski, P.; Ficek, K.; Trybek, G.; et al. The AGT gene M235T polymorphism and response of power-related variables to aerobic training. *J. Sports Sci. Med.* **2016**, *15*, 616–624.
36. De Angelis, M.; Vinciguerra, G.; Gasbarri, A.; Pacitti, C. Oxygen uptake, heart rate and blood lactate concentration during a normal training session of an aerobic dance class. *Eur. J. Appl. Physiol. Occup. Physiol.* **1998**, *78*, 121–127. [CrossRef] [PubMed]
37. Leońska-Duniec, A.; Jastrzębski, Z.; Zarębska, A.; Maciejewska, A.; Ficek, K.; Cięszczyk, P. Assessing effect of interaction between the FTO A/T polymorphism (rs9939609) and physical activity on obesity-related traits. *J. Sport Health Sci.* **2018**, *7*, 459–464. [CrossRef] [PubMed]
38. Larson-Hall, J. A Guide to Doing Statistics in Second Language Research Using SPSS. *Ibérica* **2010**, *20*, 167–204.
39. Fikenzer, K.; Fikenzer, S.; Laufs, U.; Werner, C. Effects of endurance training on serum lipids. *Vasc. Pharm.* **2018**, *101*, 9–20. [CrossRef]
40. Aellen, R.; Hollmann, W.; Boutellier, U. Effects of aerobic and anaerobic training on plasma lipoproteins. *Int. J. Sports Med.* **1993**, *14*, 396–400. [CrossRef]
41. Kodama, S.; Tanaka, S.; Saito, K.; Shu, M.; Sone, Y.; Onitake, F.; Suzuki, E.; Shimano, H.; Yamamoto, S.; Kondo, K.; et al. Effect of aerobic exercise training on serum levels of high-density lipoprotein cholesterol: A meta-analysis. *Arch. Intern. Med.* **2007**, *167*, 999–1008. [CrossRef]
42. Chen, E.S.; Mazzotti, D.R.; Furuya, T.K.; Cendoroglo, M.S.; Ramos, L.R.; Araujo, L.Q.; Burbano, R.R.; Smith Mde, A. Association of PPARα gene polymorphisms and lipid serum levels in a Brazilian elderly population. *Exp. Mol. Pathol.* **2010**, *88*, 197–201. [CrossRef]

43. Doney, A.S.; Fischer, B.; Lee, S.P.; Morris, A.D.; Leese, G.; Palmer, C.N. Association of common variation in the PPARA gene with incident myocardial infarction in individuals with type 2 diabetes: A Go-DARTS study. *Nucl. Recept.* **2005**, *3*, 4. [CrossRef]
44. Cresci, S.; Jones, P.G.; Sucharov, C.C.; Marsh, S.; Lanfear, D.E.; Garsa, A.; Courtois, M.; Weinheimer, C.J.; Wu, J.; Province, M.A.; et al. Interaction between PPARA genotype and β-blocker treatment influences clinical outcomes following acute coronary syndromes. *Pharmacogenomics* **2008**, *9*, 1403–1417. [CrossRef] [PubMed]
45. Rudkowska, I.; Verreault, M.; Barbier, O.; Vohl, M.-C. Differences in Transcriptional Activation by the Two Allelic (L162V Polymorphic) Variants of PPAR after Omega-3 Fatty Acids Treatment. *Ppar. Res.* **2009**, *2009*, 369602. [CrossRef] [PubMed]
46. Berneis, K.; Rizzo, M. LDL size: Does it matter? *Swiss. Med. Wkly.* **2004**, *134*, 720–724. [PubMed]
47. Caslake, M.; Packard, C.; Gaw, A.; Murray, E.; Griffin, B.; Vallance, B.; Shepherd, J. Fenofibrate and LDL metabolic heterogeneity in hypercholesterolemia. *Arter. Thromb* **1993**, *13*, 702–711. [CrossRef]
48. Lacquemant, C.; Lepretre, F.; Torra, I.P.; Manraj, M.; Charpentier, G.; Ruiz, J.; Staels, B.; Froguel, P. Mutation screening of the PPARalpha, gene in type 2 diabetes associated with coronary heart disease. *Diabetes Metab.* **2000**, *26*, 393–402. [PubMed]
49. Tai, E.; Demissie, S.; Cupples, L.; Corella, D.; Wilson, P.; Schaefer, E.; Ordovas, J.M. Association between the PPARA L162V polymorphism and plasma lipid levels: the Framingham Offspring Study. *Arter. Thromb. Vasc. Biol.* **2002**, *22*, 805–810. [CrossRef]
50. Robitaille, J.; Brouillette, C.; Houde, A.; Lemieux, S.; Pérusse, L.; Tchernof, A.; Gaudet, D.; Vohl, M.-C. Association between the PPARα-L162V polymorphism and components of the metabolic syndrome. *J. Hum. Gen.* **2004**, *49*, 482.
51. Sparsø, T.; Hussain, M.S.; Andersen, G.; Hainerova, I.; Borch-Johnsen, K.; Jørgensen, T.; Hansen, T.; Pedersen, O. Relationships between the functional PPARα Leu162Val polymorphism and obesity, type 2 diabetes, dyslipidaemia, and related quantitative traits in studies of 5799 middle-aged white people. *Mol. Genet. Metab.* **2007**, *90*, 205–209. [CrossRef]
52. AlSaleh, A.; Frost, G.S.; Griffin, B.A.; Lovegrove, J.A.; Jebb, S.A.; Sanders, T.A.; O'Dell, S.D.; RISCK Study Investigators. PPARγ2 gene Pro12Ala and PPARα gene Leu162Val single nucleotide polymorphisms interact with dietary intake of fat in determination of plasma lipid concentrations. *J. Nutr. Nutr.* **2011**, *4*, 354–366. [CrossRef]
53. Bouchard-Mercier, A.; Godin, G.; Lamarche, B.; Pérusse, L.; Vohl, M.-C. Effects of peroxisome proliferator-activated receptors, dietary fat intakes and gene–diet interactions on peak particle diameters of low-density lipoproteins. *J. Nutr. Nutr.* **2011**, *4*, 36–48. [CrossRef] [PubMed]
54. Egert, S.; Kratz, M.; Kannenberg, F.; Fobker, M.; Wahrburg, U. Effects of high-fat and low-fat diets rich in monounsaturated fatty acids on serum lipids, LDL size and indices of lipid peroxidation in healthy non-obese men and women when consumed under controlled conditions. *Eur. J. Nutr.* **2011**, *50*, 71–79. [CrossRef] [PubMed]
55. Lamarche, B.; Lemieux, I.; Despres, J. The small, dense LDL phenotype and the risk of coronary heart disease: Epidemiology, patho-physiology and therapeutic aspects. *Diabetes Metab.* **1999**, *25*, 199–212.
56. Berneis, K.K.; Krauss, R.M. Metabolic origins and clinical significance of LDL heterogeneity. *J. Lipid Res.* **2002**, *43*, 1363–1379. [CrossRef] [PubMed]
57. Jakob, T.; Nordmann, A.J.; Schandelmaier, S.; Ferreira-González, I.; Briel, M. Fibrates for primary prevention of cardiovascular disease events. *Cochrane Database Syst. Rev.* **2016**, *11*, CD009753. [CrossRef] [PubMed]
58. Stastny, P.; Lehnert, M.; De Ste Croix, M.; Petr, M.; Svoboda, Z.; Maixnerova, E.; Varekova, R.; Botek, M.; Petrek, M.; Kocourkova, L.; et al. Effect of COL5A1, GDF5, and PPARA Genes on a Movement Screen and Neuromuscular Performance in Adolescent Team Sport Athletes. *J. Strength Cond. Res.* **2019**. [CrossRef] [PubMed]
59. Petr, M.; Stastny, P.; Pecha, O.; Šteffl, M.; Šeda, O.; Kohlíková, E. PPARA intron polymorphism associated with power performance in 30-s anaerobic Wingate Test. *PLoS ONE* **2014**, *9*, e107351. [CrossRef]

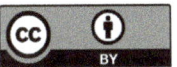

© 2019 by the authors. Licensee MDPI, Basel, Switzerland. This article is an open access article distributed under the terms and conditions of the Creative Commons Attribution (CC BY) license (http://creativecommons.org/licenses/by/4.0/).

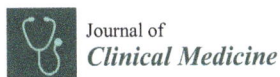

Review

A Mechanistic and Pathophysiological Approach for Stroke Associated with Drugs of Abuse

Aristides Tsatsakis [1,†], **Anca Oana Docea** [2,*,†], **Daniela Calina** [3,*,†], **Konstantinos Tsarouhas** [4,†], **Laura-Maria Zamfira** [3], **Radu Mitrut** [5,6], **Javad Sharifi-Rad** [7], **Leda Kovatsi** [8], **Vasileios Siokas** [9], **Efthimios Dardiotis** [9], **Nikolaos Drakoulis** [10], **George Lazopoulos** [11], **Christina Tsitsimpikou** [12], **Panayiotis Mitsias** [13,14] and **Monica Neagu** [15,16,*]

1. Center of Toxicology Science & Research, Medical School, University of Crete, 71003 Heraklion, Crete, Greece
2. Department of Toxicology, University of Medicine and Pharmacy of Craiova, 200349 Craiova, Romania
3. Department of Clinical Pharmacy, University of Medicine and Pharmacy of Craiova, 200349 Craiova, Romania
4. Department of Cardiology, University Hospital of Larissa, 41221 Larissa, Greece
5. Department of Pathology, University of Medicine and Pharmacy of Craiova, 200349 Craiova, Romania
6. Department of Cardiology, University and Emergency Hospital, 050098 Bucharest, Romania
7. Zabol Medicinal Plants Research Center, Zabol University of Medical Sciences, Zabol 61615-585, Iran
8. Laboratory of Forensic Medicine and Toxicology, School of Medicine, Aristotle University of Thessaloniki, 54248 Thessaloniki, Greece
9. Department of Neurology, Stroke Unit, University of Thessaly, University Hospital of Larissa, 41221 Larissa, Greece
10. Research Group of Clinical Pharmacology and Pharmacogenomics, Faculty of Pharmacy, School of Health Sciences, National and Kapodistrian University of Athens, 15771 Athens, Greece
11. Department of Cardiothoracic Surgery, University General Hospital of Heraklion, University of Crete, Medical School, 71003 Heraklion, Crete, Greece
12. Department of Hazardous Substances, Mixtures and Articles, General Chemical State Laboratory of Greece, 10431 Athens, Greece
13. Department of Neurology, School of Medicine, University of Crete, 71003 Heraklion, Greece
14. Comprehensive Stroke Center and Department of Neurology, Henry Ford Hospital, Detroit, MI 48202, USA
15. Department of Immunology, Victor Babes National Institute of Pathology, 050096 Bucharest, Romania
16. Department of Pathology, Colentina Clinical Hospital, 021183 Bucharest, Romania
* Correspondence: ancadocea@gmail.com (A.O.D.); calinadaniela@gmail.com (D.C.); neagu.monica@gmail.com (M.N.)
† These authors contributed to this paper equally.

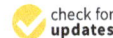

Received: 31 July 2019; Accepted: 21 August 2019; Published: 23 August 2019

Abstract: Drugs of abuse are associated with stroke, especially in young individuals. The major classes of drugs linked to stroke are cocaine, amphetamines, heroin, morphine, cannabis, and new synthetic cannabinoids, along with androgenic anabolic steroids (AASs). Both ischemic and hemorrhagic stroke have been reported due to drug abuse. Several common mechanisms have been identified, such as arrhythmias and cardioembolism, hypoxia, vascular toxicity, vascular spasm and effects on the thrombotic mechanism, as causes for ischemic stroke. For hemorrhagic stroke, acute hypertension, aneurysm formation/rupture and angiitis-like changes have been implicated. In AAS abuse, the effect of blood pressure is rather substance specific, whereas increased erythropoiesis usually leads to thromboembolism. Transient vasospasm, caused by synthetic cannabinoids, could lead to ischemic stroke. Opiates often cause infective endocarditis, resulting in ischemic stroke and hypereosinophilia accompanied by pyogenic arthritis, provoking hemorrhagic stroke. Genetic variants are linked to increased risk for stroke in cocaine abuse. The fact that case reports on cannabis-induced stroke usually refer to the young population is very alarming.

Keywords: stroke; amphetamines; cocaine; cannabis; morphine; heroin; synthetic cannabinoids; anabolic androgenic steroids

1. Introduction

1.1. Stroke Definitions

According to the World Health Organization, a stroke is defined as 'a clinical syndrome consisting of rapidly developing clinical signs of focal (or global in case of coma) disturbance of cerebral function lasting more than 24 h or leading to death with no apparent cause other than a vascular origin'. On the other hand, a transient ischemic attack (TIA) presents the signs and symptoms of a stroke, but without tissue damage and the symptoms usually resolve within 24 h [1,2]. A stroke can be defined as a rupture or blockage of an artery of the brain, which results in bleeding into the brain parenchyma or in decreased blood supply and ischemic damage to specific brain areas respectively [3].

1.2. Epidemiology of Illicit Drugs of Abuse Use and Stroke

The use of psychoactive substances has been known for thousands of years: From the ingestion of plant derivatives, such as the mushroom *Psilocybe hispanica* used in religious rituals performed 6000 years ago, to the abuse of synthetic drugs, such as heroin that was first synthesized in 1874 by C. R. Alder Wright, an English chemist working at St. Mary's Hospital Medical School in London. Nowadays, substance abuse constitutes a major social and medical problem. According to the World Drug Report 2017, issued by the United Nations Office on Drugs and Crime, the number of estimated drug users worldwide has increased by 23% in 11 years, reaching 255 million individuals in 2015. At the same time, drug users with various health disorders, such as lung or heart disease, mental health diseases, infectious diseases, stroke and cancer, reached 29.5 million in 2015, with an increase of 13.5% compared to 2006. The number of deaths attributed to drug abuse has also significantly increased. Out of the total registered deaths due to drug abuse, 67.5% are attributed to amphetamine use, 49.7% to cocaine, 29.6% to opioids and the remaining 23% to other drugs [4].

Stroke is the second leading cause of death in the world, responsible for 5.7 million deaths every year, which is expected to reach approximately 7.8 million by 2030 [5–8]. Moreover, stroke is the leading cause of major disability. A timely diagnosis by computed tomography (CT) and, depending on the circumstances, by CT angiography and CT perfusion is necessary to assure effective management [3,7].

1.3. Classic Concept of Stroke Pathophysiology

A stroke occurs when blood circulation of the brain is disturbed. There are two types of strokes: Ischemic stroke/transient ischemic attack (TIA) and hemorrhagic stroke. Brain tissue destruction is caused by different mechanisms with multifactorial character in the two types of strokes.

Ischemic stroke represents the loss of brain function caused by a decreased blood flow and consequently reduced oxygen supply to the affected brain tissue [9].

The knowledge of the latest physiopathological mechanisms in ischemic stroke is important for the development of new pharmacotherapies. Recent experimental studies in mice with transient middle cerebral artery occlusion (tMCAO) have shown the involvement of the Von Willebrandt factor (vWF) which interacts with and binds to the GPI platelet glycoprotein and the collagen receptor GP VI [10]. This vWF–GPIb axis combined with activated coagulation factor XII triggers the thrombo-inflammatory cascade in acute ischemic stroke [10,11]. In this thrombo-inflammatory process, platelets interact with T cells, which aggravate ischemia-reperfusion injury after recanalization [10,11]. However, targeting stroke-related neuroinflammation with anti-inflammatory drugs may be used with caution in order to detect any potential adverse effects to be avoided [11].

Numerous other pathophysiological studies performed on patients with ischemic stroke demonstrated hemostatic abnormalities such as low serum levels of coagulation factor VII, FVII-activated antithrombin complex, tissue factor and increased serum levels of tissue factor-bearing microparticles (MPs-TF) [12,13].

In hemorrhagic stroke the neuronal injury is supplemented by the compressive effect exerted by the hematoma, the systemic inflammatory response, the neuronal toxicity of the hemoglobin and the effect thrombolysis inside the intracerebral thrombus [14,15].

A key role in controlling stroke mortality lies in controlling the so-called modifiable stroke risk factors [3]. There are several risk factors for stroke including age, gender, hypertension, diabetes mellitus, dyslipidemia, atheromatosis, thrombophilia, atrial fibrillation, sick sinus syndrome, patent foramen ovale or family history of cardiovascular events, hyperhomocysteinemia as well as lifestyle habits, such as low physical activity, obesity, tobacco smoking, poor diet, and alcohol consumption [3,5,6,8,16–18]. Controlling blood pressure and blood glucose levels, using statins for elevated blood lipid levels and reducing the use of oral contraceptives, along with lifestyle changes, can drastically reduce the risk for stroke [5].

Drugs of abuse are also associated with stroke, especially in younger individuals. It has been shown that drug users, between 15 and 44 years old, were 6.5 times more likely to have a stroke compared with non-users [19]. The major classes of drugs linked to stroke are cocaine, amphetamines, heroin, morphine, cannabis, and the new synthetic cannabinoids, along with androgenic anabolic steroids, which are widely used both by professional and recreational athletes but also by the general public.

This article aims to review epidemiological evidence related to drug abuse-associated stroke and elucidate the possible underlying mechanisms of stroke induced by different classes of drugs of abuse.

2. Stroke Linked to Illicit Drugs of Abuse

In general, drugs of abuse can provoke stroke either by causing direct damage to cerebral vessels or indirectly, by affecting other organs, such as the liver (affecting blood coagulation pathways) or the heart, thus negatively affecting cerebral circulation [20,21]. There are substance-specific mechanisms involved. For example, stimulants such as amphetamines, cocaine and their derivatives are associated with both types of stroke, acute ischemic (cerebral infarcts) and hemorrhagic (intracerebral hemorrhages, subarachnoid hemorrhages), where the involved mechanisms differ [21,22].

The increase in blood pressure, caused by stimulants, could lead to a cerebral vessel rupture or aneurysm rupture and a subsequent hemorrhagic stroke. On the other hand, acute ischemic stroke can be attributed to stimulant-induced cerebral vasoconstriction, which reduces blood flow, promotes platelet aggregation and accelerates atherosclerosis and cardiac disturbances [21].

The pathophysiology of stroke, related to drugs of abuse, will be discussed hereafter separately for each class identified.

2.1. Amphetamines and Amphetamine Derivatives

Amphetamines are weak bases, chemically similar to natural neurotransmitters, adrenaline, and dopamine. They are synthetic sympathomimetics, which are used as mental stimulants. Their use has increased significantly, mainly because of the euphoria they induce [23]. Amphetamine derivatives include 3,4-methylenedioxymeth-amphetamine (MDMA), N-ethyl-3,4-methylenedioxyamphetamine (MDEA), 3,4-methylenedioxy-amphetamine (MDA) and methylenedioxymethylpropyl-amphetamine (MDMPA).

2.1.1. Mechanisms of Actions of Amphetamines and Amphetamine Derivatives

All amphetamines are rapidly absorbed when taken orally and even faster when they are smoked, chewed or injected [24]. Tolerance develops to standard and designer amphetamines, leading to the need to increase the dose by the consumer. Classical amphetamines, dextroamphetamine, methamphetamine and methylphenidate produce their primary effects through the release of catecholamines, especially dopamine, in the brain [24,25].

These effects are particularly strong in the brain areas associated with pleasure, especially in the cerebral cortex and limbic system. The effect of this pathway is probably responsible for the amphetamine addiction [24]. Catecholamines are similar to natural body compounds and act as neurotransmitters in the central nervous system [25]. Dopamine, an intermediate derived from epinephrine and norepinephrine biosynthesis is one of these compounds [26]. "Designer amphetamines", especially Ecstasy, cause the release of catecholamines, dopamine and norepinephrine, in addition to serotonin, a neurotransmitter that produces hallucinogens effects [27].

The main effects of amphetamines are euphoria, increased productivity and motor movements and decreased appetite. In chronic users, amphetamines create tolerance, addiction, and craving [28].

2.1.2. Influence of Amphetamines and Amphetamine Derivatives on Stroke

Amphetamines, which were initially used to increase intellectual performance and weight loss, are associated with both types of stroke [29–31].

There is also limited evidence that links a delayed ischemic stroke with amphetamine use, such as the case of a 19-year-old woman who developed right occipital infarction 3 months after methamphetamine use [32]. The mechanism involved in triggering delayed ischemic stroke remains unknown but it seems to be associated with chronic vasculitis [32,33].

Intracranial hemorrhage, following amphetamine abuse, is associated with a transient increase in blood pressure [34]. High blood pressure and vasoconstriction may also occur after consuming the so-called "diet pills" containing the amphetamine-like substance [31,35].

An in vivo study on mice revealed that even a single, acute exposure to methamphetamine can induce a biphasic effect in cerebral blood flow: An initial transient increase, followed by a prolonged decrease, 30 min after exposure, that induces vasoconstriction of pial arterioles [36]. Moreover, stroke may be attributed to the direct toxic effect of amphetamines on cerebral vessels, causing necrotizing vasculitis [37]. Many studies report intracranial hemorrhage following the use of amphetamines [38,39]. Figure 1 summarizes the main pathophysiological mechanisms of stroke associated with amphetamines and amphetamine derivative abuse.

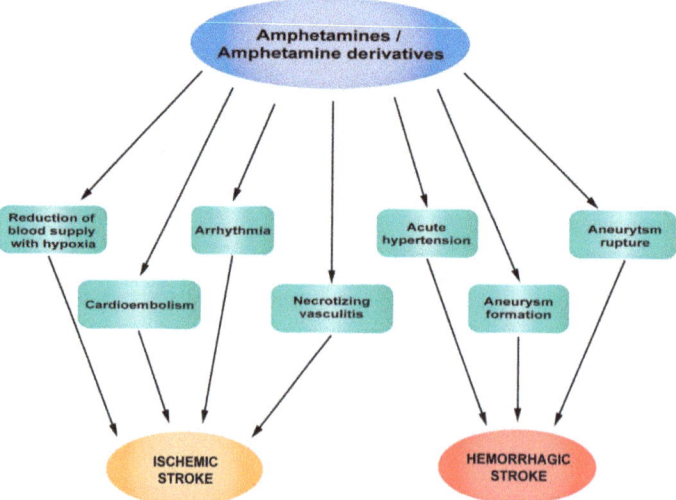

Figure 1. Pathophysiological mechanisms of stroke associated with amphetamines and amphetamine derivative abuse.

2.1.3. Clinical Studies, Case Reports and Epidemiology of Stroke Related to Amphetamines and Amphetamine Derivatives abuse

Amphetamines were first used during World War II by soldiers in order to suppress fatigue. In the 1950s, the legal prescription of amphetamines in the US increased. Worldwide, there are over 35 million people who abuse amphetamines, compared to 15 million cocaine users [28]. The route of administration can be intravenous, oral, intranasal and by inhalation (smoking) [40]. The half-life is between 10 and 30 h and they are metabolized through the liver. Studies have shown that adolescents who use amphetamines have a 5-fold higher risk of stroke than those who do not use these drugs [24,41].

Apart from thrombosis and cerebrovascular pathology, several other side effects of amphetamines and amphetamine derivatives have been reported, including cardiomyopathy and arrhythmias, liver failure, renal failure, suicide, confusion, memory loss, psychosis and premature mortality [40]. The risk of stroke is four times higher in amphetamine users than in nonusers and the hemorrhagic stroke may occur twice as often, as in the case of cocaine users [29]. Although it is less frequent compared to amphetamine-associated hemorrhagic stroke, amphetamine-associated ischemic stroke is also described in the literature (Table 1). De Silva reported the case of a 30-year-old woman who developed acute left middle cerebral artery infarction after acute intake of amphetamine [33]. Christensen et al. reported the case of a 33-year-old Caucasian male addicted to amphetamines who died due to bilateral cerebral infarction [42]. In the past, it was believed that amphetamine derivatives were a safer option compared with other stimulants, because it was thought that intracranial hemorrhages occurred only in combination with other stimulant drugs [39]. However, it was later shown that a clear association exists between intracerebral hemorrhage in young people, without comorbidities, and amphetamine, methamphetamine or their derivative intake [43–45]. The most interesting and recent studies that report amphetamine-associated hemorrhagic stroke and amphetamine-associated ischemic stroke are summarized in Table 1.

Table 1. Characteristic case reports that associate amphetamines and amphetamine derivatives abuse with stroke.

Subject/Age	Substance Exposure	Symptoms	Diagnostic Approach	Diagnosis	Intervention	Evolution	Reference
Female, 23, no previous medical history	Took 4-fluoroamphetamine 4 h before, concomitant use of cannabis 7 h before	Collapsed at a dance event, no neurological deficits, sleepy and headache, decreased consciousness 1.5 h later, weakness of the right arm and leg	Plain computed tomography scan (computed tomography (CT) scan); CT angiography	Intracerebral hemorrhage in the left hemisphere; dilated non-responsive right pupil (false localizing sign)	Acute neurosurgical intervention: Hematoma evacuation, removal of the bone flap due to persistent intraoperative brain swelling	Right-sided hemiparalysis and severe aphasia. Replacement of the autologous bone graft after 4 months without complications. Able to talk in her native language and walk with supportive measures	[44]
Female, 23, no medical history	Took 110 mg 4-fluoroamphetamine the night before, concomitant use of four units of alcohol	Severe headache, nausea, followed by vomiting 5 h after the intake, dizziness, photophobia	CT scan	Small subarachnoid hemorrhage at the right frontal side	Discharged after 24 h	Headache for weeks that gradually declined cognitive problems. Inability to work for several months	[44]
Female, 29, progressive headache and diplopia for 2 weeks, no medical history	Intravenous methamphetamine use	A 2-day history of left-sided hemiparesis and dysarthria	Cranial nerve examination, CT brain imaging without contrast medium, magnetic resonance imaging (MRI), angiogram	A 25 × 25 × 20-mm hyperdense lesion within the right cerebellopontine angle Initially thought to represent an extra-axial mass (meningioma), confirmed to be a large brainstem hemorrhage, extended from the inferior midbrain to the pontomedullary junction	Transferred to rehabilitation	Deterioration of left hemiparesis, dysarthria and dysphagia after 1 month. No underlying vascular abnormality observed	[45]
Male, Caucasian, 53, history of head and neck squamous cell carcinoma post-surgery and radiation (13 years before), hypothyroidism, hyperlipidemia, gastrointestinal reflux disease	Treatment for Attention Deficit Hyperactivity Disorder (ADHD) with mixed amphetamine salts, starting 5 mg/day to 15 mg/day over 4 months	Posterior headache with left-face numbness, diplopia 2.5 months after last dosing scheme	Head CT without contrast agent; MRI; transthoracic echocardiogram	Right posterior paramedian midbrain hematoma with cerebral aqueduct effacement and mild ventriculomegaly. No hypertension, arteriovenous malformation, cavernous malformation, or aneurysms	-	-	[46]
Male, 31	Amphetamine abuse	-	Transcranial color-coded Doppler sonography; angiography	Intracerebral hemorrhage, diffuse cerebral vasospasm	Surgical removal of intracerebral hemorrhage, pharmaceutical treatment	-	[47]

Table 1. *Cont.*

Subject/Age	Substance Exposure	Symptoms	Diagnostic Approach	Diagnosis	Intervention	Evolution	Reference
Male, African-American, 20	Took 3,4-methylenedioxymeth-amphetamine (MDMA), concomitant use of marijuana and beer	Non-verbal, vomiting and aphasic upon presentation, no sign of trauma, 18 h after ingestion developed right-sided weakness, left-sided facial droop and bilateral hyperreflexia in the lower extremities	MRI; carotid ultrasound; magnetic resonance angiogram of the brain	Left middle cerebral artery complete infarction, no significant stenosis, mild to moderate stenosis observed on the distal left internal carotid artery	Transferred to rehabilitation	-	[48]
Female, 36, history of migraine	Methamphetamine use, concomitant use of oral contraceptives	Sudden onset of speech difficulty and right-sided weakness	Head CT; MRI of the brain; MR angiography	Small infarct in the left frontal lobe, focal narrowing in the left internal carotid artery	Pharmaceutical treatment: IV heparin, discharged on warfarin 5 days after stroke; after 8 months, warfarin was replaced with aspirin 81 mg/day	Recovered after 4 months with only mild expressive aphasia	[49]
Female, 29	History of methamphetamine use for 10 years	Sudden right-sided weakness and speech difficulty 4 days after last use of methamphetamine	Head CT, MRI, MR angiography	Large left middle cerebral artery (MCA) infarct with hemorrhagic transformation	Discharged after 4 days on aspirin treatment, on day 5th showed worsening deficit, hospitalized; stent-assisted transformation applied	Recovered only with moderate expression aphasia and mild right-hand weakness within 4 months	[49]
Male, 31	Methamphetamine ingestion approximately 0.25 and 0.5 g Urine screen positive also for tetrahydrocannabinol (THC)	Severe headache, nausea, vomiting, left-side of the body felt numb, slurred speech, died the next day	Autopsy	Cerebral edema, subarachnoid hemorrhage over the cerebral convexities bilaterally, intracerebral hemorrhage lateral to the basal ganglia extending to involve the lateral aspect of the putamen, external capsule claustrum, insula, and superior longitudinal fasciculus of the right cerebral hemisphere (3.5 cm by 4.5 cm) No evidence of inflammation or vasculitis		Death	[38]

191

Table 1. *Cont.*

Subject/Age	Substance Exposure	Symptoms	Diagnostic Approach	Diagnosis	Intervention	Evolution	Reference
Male, Caucasian, 33, amphetamine addict	Amphetamine and methamphetamine ingestion. Low concentrations of methadone and codeine in the blood	Bilateral cerebral infarction associated with multi-organ failure	CT scan, autopsy	Extensive infarction of both cerebral hemispheres; symmetrical necrosis of the white matter of both cerebral hemispheres in the autopsy		Died 19 days after hospital admission	[42]
Female, 30, no significant medical history, non-smoker, very light alcohol consumer	Ecstasy ingestion one night before the presentation	Right-sided weakness, global aphasia, right neglect, and right hemiparesis	Brain CT scan; ultrasound of the extracranial carotid arteries; transcranial color-coded Doppler (TCCD); MRI	Left parietal hypodensity consistent with left middle cerebral artery (MCA) infarction; irregularity of the left MCA	Aspirin 100 mg/day	TCCD studies showed normal velocities in the MCA 3 months after onset	[33]
Female, 19, duodenal ulcer at 16, no other medical history, no family history of stroke	Methamphetamine intravenously four times over 2 months, wash-out for 3 months, concomitant use of cigarettes and alcohol	Severe right-sided headache, blurred vision on the left side and numbness of the left arm and leg upon admission, severe headache every time associated with use	Brain CT, MRI and magnetic resonance angiography	Right occipital infarction, segmental narrowing of the right posterior cerebral artery with characteristics of vasculitis	Discharged one week after admission	The right occipital infarction faded with mild atrophy, left superior quadrant hemianopia remained and had persistent headaches 4 months later	[32]

2.2. Cocaine

Cocaine, also known as benzoylmethylecgonine, is extracted from the leaves of the *Erythroxylum coca* shrub, which usually grows in Peru, Bolivia, and Ecuador [50]. In the past, the leaves of this plant were chewed or sucked in order to decrease hunger or obtain euphoric effect. Its use increased after the 1970s. After 2007, cocaine has become one of the most abused drugs, regularly used by five million Americans [50]. Cocaine has two chemical forms: Cocaine hydrochloride and alkaloidal cocaine [50]. Cocaine hydrochloride is water soluble and is readily absorbed after nasal administration [50]. Alkaloidal cocaine is lipid soluble and is a free base. It is synthesized by mixing cocaine hydrochloride with water and ammonia. Another form is produced by mixing cocaine hydrochloride with sodium bicarbonate, known as 'crack cocaine' in street language.

2.2.1. The Mechanism of Action of Cocaine

The main mechanism of action of cocaine is the blockage of noradrenaline reuptake [51]. The side effect is increased norepinephrine release. These effects act synergistically to increase the level of norepinephrine in the nerve endings. Cocaine also causes moderate release and blocking the reuptake of serotonin and dopamine [51]. It is a local anesthetic with effects caused by the blocking of the sodium channels, which determines the inhibition of nerve conduction by decreasing the amplitude of the action potential of the membranes but increasing its duration. Cocaine also blocks the potassium channels and, in some cells, it also blocks the sodium–calcium pump [52]. The drug is soluble in lipids and, therefore, crosses the blood–brain barrier. Cocaine stimulates the central nervous system, especially the limbic system where it potentiates dopaminergic transmission in the basal ventral nuclei, producing the sensation of pleasure, which has led to its widespread use [52]. Cocaine substitutes dopamine, the neurotransmitter involved in mood management [53]. Cocaine use is associated with myocardial infarction, vasoconstriction, chronic uncontrolled hypertension, nervous system stimulation and stroke [53]. Cocaine is associated with vascular toxicity. Various mechanisms are involved, such as hypertension, disturbance of platelet aggregation and homeostasis, effects on cerebral blood flow, and thromboembolism [54].

2.2.2. Influence of Cocaine on Stroke

The risk of stroke is twice as high in cocaine users, compared to age-matched non-users [29,54].

Ischemic stroke related to cocaine is associated with large vessel atherosclerosis, advanced atherosclerosis of intracranial vessels, increased platelet activation and arrhythmias, especially bradyarrhythmias, which can be explained by the ability of cocaine to depress sinus node automaticity and to block the atrioventricular node conduction [53,55].

Although it is well documented that cocaine can cause cerebral ischemia, researchers could not explain the exact mechanism. Cerebral vasospasm is attributed to the sympathomimetic effect of cocaine and the increase in circulating endothelin-1 [56]. Endothelin-1 is a vasoconstrictor protein produced by vascular endothelial cells. When elevated, it leads to nitric oxide decrease and vasoconstriction. In addition, cocaine effects on vasoconstriction are also related to elevated calcium in the vessels [57]. Other causes of stroke, related to acute cocaine use, cervicocephalic or intracranial arterial dissection are additional causes of stroke related to acute cocaine use [53]. A study by You et al. revealed that cocaine can cause a stroke by reducing blood flow to the brain. The researchers visualized exactly what happens in the brain when it is exposed to cocaine. Using quantitative laser-based visualization, it was possible to see exactly how cocaine affects small blood vessels in the brains of mice. Following 30 days of exposure to cocaine (by injection), or even after several injections performed at different time points with short intervals between them, a drastic reduction in blood circulation could be demonstrated. It was shown that in some vessels, cocaine induced micro-ischemia, a state in which blood flow to the brain is not adequate and cerebral hypoxia and ischemic stroke occur. These findings could help physicians to improve neurosurgical techniques and develop more effective methods for treating cocaine users [58].

In a large cohort study on cocaine-related stroke, during a period of 10 years, atherosclerosis of large vessels was found to be the common mechanism of stroke [59]. Cocaine use creates an elevated immune system inflammatory state. Various basal anti-inflammatory markers, like interleukin-10 (IL 10) have been found to be decreased, while pro-inflammatory cytokines (tumor necrosis factor alpha, Interleukin 1β) are increased, thus contributing to vascular disease [60,61].

Acute cocaine use induces acute hypertension, which is implicated in the occurrence of hemorrhagic stroke in users. The implication of cocaine in aneurysm formation and rupture is supported by the high incidence of aneurysmal subarachnoid hemorrhage (SAH) in cocaine users. Only less than half of them have a family history of hypertension [59].

Figure 2 summarizes the main pathophysiological mechanisms of stroke associated with cocaine abuse.

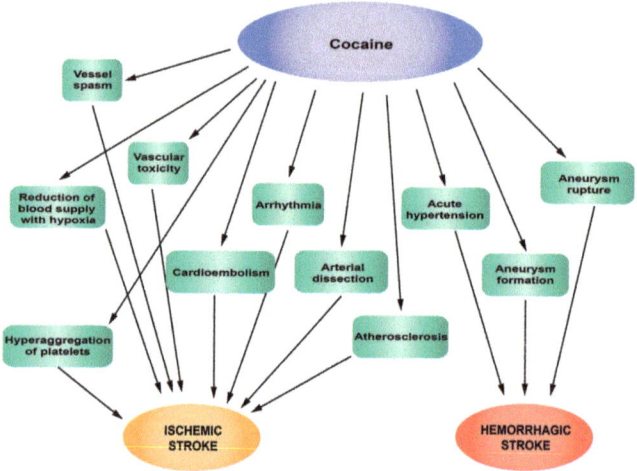

Figure 2. Pathophysiological mechanisms of stroke associated with cocaine abuse.

2.2.3. Clinical Studies, Case Reports and Epidemiology of Stroke Related to Cocaine Abuse

In order to evaluate the net effect of cocaine abuse on stroke risk, co-triggers, predictors, and co-morbidities of stroke (and other vascular diseases) should be taken into account [62]. Factors such as infections with human immunodeficiency virus type 1 (HIV-1) and hepatitis C virus (HCV) are of great importance [63,64]. So far, studies have supported the fact that cocaine use is prevalent in individuals infected with HIV and/or HCV, and vice versa [63–65]. Moreover, a few clinical studies suggested that cocaine abuse may increase HIV-1 viral load, and thus increase acquired immune deficiency syndrome (AIDS)-related mortality, even among patients under antiretroviral therapy (ART) [65]. In a study by Lucas et al. (2015), HIV and HCV infection were associated with carotid plaque progression. Furthermore, cocaine use was associated with higher odds of carotid plaque at baseline, suggesting that it is a risk factor for stroke [62].

Genetic variants are linked to increased risk for stroke in cocaine users. However, their precise impact on stroke risk remains unknown, as the association of the identified variants is considered relatively weak [66]. One of these genetic factors is the histone deacetylase 9 (*HDAC9*) gene, which has been associated with large vessel stroke [66,67]. *HDAC9* belongs to the family of epigenetic molecules, known as the histone deacetylases (HDACs), which are involved in the regulation of maladaptive behavioral changes induced by cocaine use [68,69]. There is evidence that overexpression of *HDAC4* (another member of this family) in the nucleus accumbens of the brain can modulate cocaine reward [69]. Moreover, the single nucleotide polymorphism (SNP) rs3791398 on *HDAC4* is associated with carotid intima–media thickness [70]. Based on the above, it is possible that carriers of particular variants on HDACs are more prone to cocaine abuse and have an inherent susceptibility for stroke.

Among 584,115 patients with stroke, identified from the data of the National Inpatient Sample of the Healthcare Cost and Utilization Project, in-hospital outcomes, mortality and comorbidities between patients with stroke following cocaine use and patients with stroke without cocaine use were compared. The results showed that in the users group, cardiovascular incidences were higher than in the non-users group, including valvular disorders (13.2% versus 9.7%, $p < 0.001$), venous thromboembolism (3.5% versus 2.6%, $p < 0.03$), vasculitis (0.9% versus 0.4%, $p < 0.003$), and sudden cardiac death (0.4% versus 0.2%, $p < 0.02$). In the users group, the incidence of epilepsy and major depression was also higher. In the non-users group, the incidence of certain risk factors for stroke (atherosclerosis, elevated cholesterol, hypertension, cardiac circulatory anomalies, diabetes, family history of stroke, paralysis, transient ischemic attack, coagulopathy, deficiency anemia, and disorders of fluid and electrolytes) was higher. Users also presented higher in-hospital mortality, while venous thromboembolism or vasospasm seemed to be connected to cocaine administration. The chronic use of cocaine seems to make users more vulnerable to stroke, but further research is necessary in order to assess cocaine-induced stroke [71].

The frequency and the route of administration seem to play an important role, when assessing the link between cocaine use and the risk of stroke. Following the acute use of cocaine, a 6.4-fold higher incidence of stroke within 24 h for users is reported, compared to those who had never used cocaine. Furthermore, acute cocaine use has also proven more detrimental compared to chronic use. In addition, smoking cocaine presents the highest risk for stroke. In 26 patients, suffering from stroke following acute cocaine use, the prominent route of administration was smoking ("crack"), while in all cases, typical risk factors for stroke, such as hypertension, myocardial infarction, hyperlipidemia, diabetes mellitus, and tobacco use, co-existed. Some patients were multidrug users (heroin and marijuana) [72]. It is rather likely that stroke can occur following cocaine use, even without other risk factors [73].

Neurovascular implications are rather common among cocaine abusers. Among 96 active or former cocaine users, 45 cases of ischemic stroke/TIA were reported, while intracerebral hemorrhage (ICH) and SAH occurred with a similar prevalence of approximately 25%. ICH and SAH were associated with active cocaine use, while ischemic stroke/TIA was more likely to occur in former cocaine users. Regarding the different forms of cocaine, crack is implicated equally in both types of strokes, while cocaine is implicated more in hemorrhagic stroke [59]. In a paper published by Martin-Schild et al., the authors compared the location, demographics, and outcome of patients with ICH. Out of 3241 patients with stroke, 132 (4.1%) were cocaine users, according to the urine drug screen, and 45 had ICH. Six of the 45 cocaine users with ICH were also using other illicit drugs (such as marijuana and amphetamines). The control group consisted of 105 non-users with ICH. The study showed that cocaine users with ICH had a male predominance and were less likely to be Hispanic (11% vs. 28%; $p = 0.022$) and more likely to be African-American (69% vs. 44%). Cocaine users had a higher median diastolic blood pressure (121 (100–126) vs. 110 (107–141)); $p = 0.024$). Furthermore, cocaine users had more severe ICH, compared to the control group. In addition, cocaine use seems to correlate with the emergence of intraventricular hemorrhage (IVH). This study also showed that cocaine users are more likely to die during their hospitalization, compared to the control group [74]. One study investigated the outcome of strokes related to cocaine abuse, compared with strokes that are not related to cocaine. They concluded that younger age and cardiac arrhythmias are associated with cocaine-related strokes. Regarding other traditional cerebrovascular risk factors, no differences were found between cocaine and non-cocaine related strokes [55].

There are several case reports on hemorrhagic or ischemic stroke after cocaine use and the most recent and interesting are presented in Table 2.

Table 2. Characteristic case reports studies that associate cocaine abuse and stroke.

Subject/Age	Substance Exposure	Symptoms	Diagnostic Approach	Diagnosis	Intervention	Evolution	Reference
Male, African American, 65, diabetes, heart diseases, hepatitis C	Smoking crack cocaine before symptom onset, admitted to intermittent cocaine abuse	Left arm pain described as feeling like "jumping out of the window"	Head CT scan; carotid ultrasound; CT angiography of head and neck	Acute 2.2-cm intraparenchymal hemorrhage that presented in the posterior right parietal lobe vasogenic edema	Send to the rehabilitation unit	Left arm pain resolved after 24 h	[75]
Female, African-American, 66, multi-substance abuser, hepatitis C, heart diseases	Urine samples positive for cocaine	Somnolent a day prior to admission, confused in the day of admission, short-term memory loss, unable to perform usual daily activities	Brain CT; CT angiogram of the head and neck; MRI of the brain associated with MR venogram	Infarction in bilateral posterior inferior cerebellar artery and hippocamp showing multifocal punctate infarcts in the basal ganglia and bilateral posterior cerebral artery secondary to severe vasoconstriction	Neurosurgery consult for possible external ventricular drain placement and posterior fossa decompression	Mental status improved during hospitalization; discharged to a rehabilitation center after 7 days with persistent problems of memory and inability to recognize faces	[76]
Male, 22, hypertension and cocaine abuser	Positive for cocaine and tetrahydrocannabinol	Right hemiplegia associated with motor and sensitive aphasia	CT scan	The ischemic region in the left medial cerebral artery region with increased cerebral edema and cerebral midline displacement of 9 mm on the subfalcine region	Not suitable for surgery due to complications	Died in the hospital	[77]
Female, 39, smoker, no other risk factors for stroke	Urine screening positive for cocaine	Global aphasia, left-side total gaze paresis, 7th cranial nerve right-side partial paresis and right hemiplegia	Non-contrast brain CT	Left ischemic stroke—hyperdensity in the left middle cerebral artery (MCA); occlusion in the left and right MCA and an irregular profile of the left internal carotid artery (ICA)	Endovascular treatment, intra-arterial administration of 40 mg of recombinant tissue plasminogen activator (rtPA) associated with a self-expandable and retrievable stent	After 3 months from the event, ischemia at the left basal ganglia	[78]
Male, 31, no medical history	Positive urine screening for cocaine and negative for other drugs	Found unresponsive 6 h after excessive alcohol and intranasal cocaine abuse	MRI; intra- and extracranial CT angiography	Globus pallidus and the vascular watershed zones presents acute bilateral ischemia	—	Consciousness improved progressively; clinical improvements, but mental slowing, executive dysfunction, hypophonia, and verbal fluency deficit persisted	[79]
Female, 31, no medical history, occasional alcohol consumer and smoker	First time snorted cocaine hydrochloride associated with 500 mL of vodka	Acute onset of right hemiplegia and left hemiparesis evolving into quadriplegia	MRI	Thickened pons with focus localized in his central part on the left side (20 mm) (ischemic change)	After 17 days of hospitalization, transferred to rehabilitation	The movements of the left side of the body improved slowly and the rehabilitation continues in ambulatory	[80]

2.3. Cannabis

Cannabis is extracted from the plant *Cannabis sativa* and its varieties, *Cannabis Americana* and *Cannabis Indica*, and has two principal preparations, marijuana and hashish, which can be smoked, ingested or inhaled. Delta 9-tetrahydrocannabinol (THC) is the psychoactive cannabinoid in cannabis. Based on the THC content, potency varies in the preparations of cannabis and it is usually higher in hashish than in marijuana [81]. Cannabis substitutes anandamide, a neurotransmitter involved in mechanisms of appetite regulation, memory, reproduction and cell proliferation (the basis of tumor development).

2.3.1. The Mechanism of Action of Cannabis

The mechanism of action of THC has also been controversial. At first, it was thought that, due to the lipophilic nature, it causes the disruption of the membranes of the cell components. In the 1990s, researchers discovered cannabinoid receptors located in the brain and in the cells of the body, responsible for many of the effects of THC [82]. The molecular mechanism was initially considered nonspecific, of an anesthetic type, for which the lack of stereospecificity of the activity of delta-9-THC and also its lipophilicity was advocated [82]. The first evidence for the specific action of cannabinoids was brought by Howlett, who showed that delta-9-THC inhibits adenylate-cyclase activity in N18TG2 neuroblastoma cells cultured in vitro, and the use of a radiolabeled analogue allowed the detection of cannabinoid sites, specific in the brain [82,83].

There are two types of cannabinoid receptors (CB): CB_1 in the central nervous system and CB_2 in the immune system cells [82,84]. High densities of cannabinoid receptors are found in the frontal cortex, basal ganglia, cerebellum, and hippocampus. They are absent in the brain nuclei. The stimulation of these receptors causes the release of neurotransmitters [82]. The main effects of cannabis are relaxation, euphoria and increased self-confidence. Its side effects include cardiovascular complications, peripheral events (such as kidney infarction or peripheral arteritis) and neurological complications [82,84].

2.3.2. The Influence of Cannabis on Stroke

Cannabis causes transient cerebral ischemic attacks (TIAs) and ischemic strokes.

The possible mechanisms through which cannabis can induce stroke include cerebral vasoconstriction, hypotension, vasospasm, impaired cerebral vasomotor function and fluctuations in blood pressure [81,85]. It is possible that all the above could be attributed to the potential of cannabis to induce sympathetic stimulation and decrease parasympathetic activity [8,86]. There is currently increasing scientific interest towards the determination of the dose and duration of cannabis abuse that would lead to a stroke. In a study conducted on the National Inpatient Sample database from USA, a significant increase in symptomatic cerebral vasospasm was observed in marijuana users [87]. In a case of basal ganglia hemorrhage, reported after an increased intake of cannabis, the proposed mechanism for the pathogenesis of intracerebral hemorrhage was the capacity of cannabis to impair autoregulation and to induce transient arterial hypertension [88,89].

Regarding the mechanism by which cannabis induces thrombotic events, one should consider the fact that platelets synthesize endogenous cannabinoids, mainly the Δ 9-tetrahydrocannabinol (THC) metabolite [90]. Via CB1 and CB2 receptors, the platelet membranes are targets for exogenous cannabinoids, resulting in aggregation, which is nonreversible, at high cannabinoid levels [90,91]. Moreover, cannabinoids lead to the increased reactivation of factor VII and elevated ADP-induced aggregation in platelet-rich plasma [91]. An additional procoagulatory effect appears to be the elevated expression of glycoprotein IIb-IIIa and P selectin on the surfaces of the platelets by THC, dependent though by concentration [90]. The stimulation of the sympathetic system and the inhibition of the parasympathetic system, and the inflammatory processes at the level of at the arterial wall, have been described as other possible THC mechanisms of action, resulting to thrombus formation and endothelial erosion at both cerebral and coronary arteries [92–94]. Finally, cannabinoids can also lead to the activation, adhesion and aggregation of platelets, as a result of the decreased availability of nitric oxide, due to oxidative stress (which is induced by cannabinoids [90,91]. Figure 3 summarizes the main pathophysiological mechanisms of stroke associated with cannabis abuse.

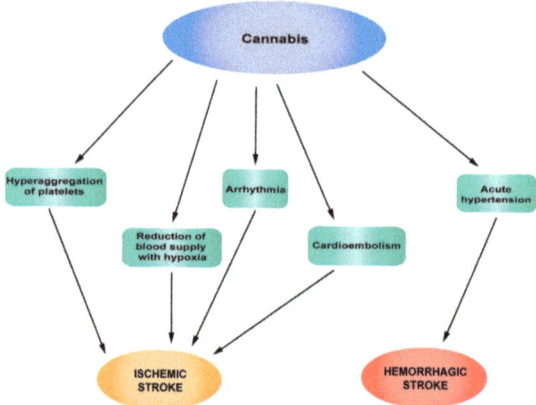

Figure 3. Main pathophysiological mechanisms of stroke associated with cannabis abuse.

2.3.3. Clinical Studies, Case Reports and Epidemiology of Stroke Related to Cannabis

The most widely used psychoactive substance in the world is cannabis, with almost 180 million annual consumers [8]. Most users believe that cannabis is a safe recreational drug. Furthermore, because of its therapeutic applications, 15 states of the US have approved it for medical use [81]. In Europe, countries such as Cyprus, Finland, Germany, Greece, Italy, Israel, Norway, Netherlands, Croatia, Czech Republic, Denmark, Georgia, Luxembourg, Malta, Poland, Portugal, San Marino, Switzerland, United Kingdom have already legalized the use of cannabis for medical purposes and other countries are in the process of legalizing it [95].

Following the chronic use of cannabis, psychological and physical dependence are encountered and the withdrawal syndrome includes sleep difficulties and anxiety [81].

In recent years, there have been several case reports, case series and studies that show a link between cerebrovascular events and cannabis use [96–98]. It seems that cannabis users are more likely to present with neurological conditions, such as multifocal intracranial arterial stenosis, reversible cerebral vasoconstriction syndrome and chronic use of cannabis can lead to increased cerebrovascular resistance. There seems to be a link between cannabis use and stroke/TIA (odds ratio, 2.30; 95% confidence intervals, 1.08–5.08) [96].

In 48 patients (under 45 years of age) admitted to hospital for ischemic stroke, cardiovascular investigations, blood tests and urine screens for cannabinoids were performed, in order to study stroke in young adults. Urine tests were positive for cannabis in 13 patients. Out of these 13 patients, 21% had a distinctive form of multifocal intracranial stenosis (MIS) and suffered from a severe headache. In seven patients, ischemic stroke was located in the vertebrobasilar territory; in nine patients, MIS was in the posterior cerebral arteries; and in seven patients, it was located in the superior cerebellar arteries. The link between MIS and cannabis was statistically significant (odds ratio, 113 (9–5047); $p < 0.001$) [99].

Studies showed that cannabis can be related to stroke, especially in smokers. Interestingly, in a large cohort of 49,321 Swedish men, born between 1949 and 1951, who had been in the military service between 1969 and 1970, alcohol consumption, cannabis use or tobacco smoking and their association with stroke were studied. Among men who have had a stroke before 60 years of age, the risk factors were often common and included a family history of cardiovascular disease, obesity, high alcohol consumption, and tobacco smoking. Cannabis use was associated with elevated blood pressure and was more prevalent in stroke at a younger age (< 45 years), but cannabis use alone was not reported as a risk factor for stroke in individuals younger than 45 years old [8]. Rumalla et al., conducted a study on patients between 15 and 54 years old, with a primary diagnosis of acute ischemic stroke (AIS). Data were obtained from the Nationwide Inpatient Sample, the largest inpatient database in the US. The purpose of this study was to evaluate the correlation between marijuana use and hospitalization for AIS. The researchers identified an increased incidence of AIS in the marijuana cohort, especially in young patients, who were African American males. Multivariable analysis was applied to investigate the risk factor for the occurrence of AIS involving marijuana use alone or in combination with other risk factors. The analysis showed that marijuana use represented a significant risk factor for AIS hospitalization [87].

Cannabis use has been mainly associated with ischemic stroke. Nevertheless, more recent studies show an association between cannabis use and hemorrhagic stroke. Several recent case reports on cannabis-associated stroke are presented in Table 3. A very interesting case is that reported by Atchaneeyasakul et al., It refers to a 27-year-old man who presented right basal ganglia intracerebral hemorrhage (ICH) following the ingestion of cannabis. No vascular abnormality was observed on digital subtraction angiography (DSA) of the cerebral vasculature, CT angiography of the head, and magnetic resonance imaging (MRI) of the brain. The toxicological tests were positive for cannabinoids, with a serum level of 9-carboxy tetrahydrocannabinol of 222 ng/mL. The patient was not diagnosed with secondary hypertension. The fact that no other risk factor for the basal ganglia hemorrhage was identified in this case supports the role of cannabis in the risk of stroke with robustness [88].

Table 3. Characteristic case reports that associate cannabis abuse with stroke.

Subject/Age	Substance Exposure	Symptoms	Diagnostic Approach	Diagnosis	Intervention	Evolution	Reference
Female, 51, asthma	Long-term cannabis user, positive urine screening for cannabis, a large amount of cannabis was consumed prior to the onset of symptoms	Left-side upper and lower extremities weakness	Head CT scan	Acute right cerebral infarct; after 30 min from arrival, developed in the left pons new hemorrhage associated with decompression on the lateral and left ventricles	Pharmaceutical treatment: Labetalol, recombinant tissue plasminogen activator	Died	[100]
Male, 27, without any known medical history	Single raw cannabis consumption (confirmed by a blood test) just before symptom onset	Sudden progressive left-sided weakness, degradation in mentation, nausea, and vomiting	Brain CT without contrast media; CT angiography; MRI of the brain	Right basal ganglia ICH measuring 32 × 24 mm with extension into the ventricles with mild hydrocephalus, no vasculature abnormality	Intubation and placement of an external ventricular drain, treatment on recombinant tissue plasminogen activator	Improvement of motor function, left hemiparesis	[88]
Female, 14, no remarkable medical history	Toxicological screening positive for cannabis 2-year history of daily cannabis use	Generalized tonic–clonic seizures	Head CT, electroencephalography (EEG); MRI	Multiple ischemic infarcts located in basal ganglia, left frontal lobe, and genu of corpus callosum, which had both chronic and acute features	After stabilization, transferred to rehabilitation	Complained of chronic headache, learning disabilities	[101]
Male, 25	Cannabis ingestion one night before Concomitant ingestion of alcohol	Drowsy, talking irrelevantly and the state degraded	Non-contrast CT of the brain; Coronary CT angiogram	Acute infarct in the right frontoparietal region	After hospitalization was discharged in a stable condition	Left-sided weakness improved	[102]
Male	Marijuana History of smoking marijuana from the age of 1	Presented with weakness of leg, arm and face associated with slurred speech 90 min after smoking marijuana Recurrence of the symptoms twice	Brain CT scan, CT angiogram and MRI	Right lentiform nucleus presents subtle hypodensity; no evidence of vasospasm, thrombus or dissection	Heparin treatment after a recurrent episode of focal neurological deficits	After 2 months, he presented residual weakness in the left arm and leg, left facial droop and spastic tone	[103]
Male, 33, smoker	Urine toxicologic screening positive for cannabis Heavy user of cannabis for 15 years	Transient left hemiparesis and dysarthria, no altered consciousness, chest pain one day before	Brain MRI and CT angiography	The presence of multi focal acute infarctions in the bilateral watershed zones between middle and anterior cerebral artery territories and the right middle cerebral artery territory. Cardioembolic stroke produced by acute myocardial infarction (likely related to cannabis use)	-	No recurrence in the following 6 months of cardiac or neurologic symptoms	[104]
Male, Caucasian French, 24, no medical history	Urine toxicology positive for cannabis; heavy cannabis use one night before admission Regular cannabis smoker for four years	Non-reactive state, with seizures	Cerebral CT scan, EEG, MRI, Doppler examination, magnetic resonance angiography, and angiography	Infarcts in the insular mantle and the lenticular and caudate nuclear structures exclude all other causes of stroke in young people	Treated in the hospital until recovery and transferred to the psychiatric department to be treated for behavioral disorders	In the following 1 and a half years, he returned on seven occasions for generalized tonic–clonic seizures	[98]
Male, 36, with no history of migraine or other known vascular risk factors	Urine toxicological screening positive for cannabis Heavy hashish consumption and alcohol before the symptoms Sporadically hashish user	An acute episode of isolated aphasia, followed by convulsive seizures	Cranial MRI and MR angiography	Had 2 acute ischemic infarcts, one on the left parietal lobe, and another area of silent ischemia in the right parietal lobe	Treatment with ticlopidine	After 1 year, a new episode of aphasia and right hemiparesis immediately after hashish smoking and a new episode after 1 and a half years again after hashish use Between the two episodes, he denied consumption	[93]

2.4. Synthetic Cannabinoids

Synthetic cannabinoids are a new class of psychoactive chemicals, similar in pharmacological action with THC, the active component of *Cannabis sativa* [105]. Synthetic cannabinoids are not derived from cannabis. They are synthetized in the laboratory and they manifest a full agonist activity on cannabinoid receptors, in contrast to THC which is only a partial agonist [105]. They are metabolized to active metabolites that give them a higher potency compared to THC [106]. Although they are labeled "not for human consumption", they are available in the market as herbal mixtures sprayed with synthetic cannabinoids, in street language known as "spice", "K2", "herbal incense". They are used for recreational purposes and they are called "legal drugs" [106]. Their use has increased in the last years, along with concerns regarding their safety. The market of synthetic cannabinoids is growing very fast and a new compound is synthetized as soon as the previous one is classified as illegal by legislation.

2.4.1. The Mechanism of Action of the Synthetic Cannabinoids

Synthetic cannabinoids act as CB1 and CB2 cannabinoid receptor agonists, similar to tetrahydrocannabinol (THC) but they have a different chemical structure [107]. They cause agitation, anxiety, paranoia, hypertension, rarely myocardial infarction or renal failure [107].

2.4.2. The Influence of Synthetic Cannabinoids on Stroke

Synthetic cannabinoids have been associated with ischemic stroke through various case reports. Unfortunately, epidemiological studies are hard to conduct because these substances are not detected in routine toxicological screen tests [106]. Their increased potency on cannabinoid receptors, their active metabolites, and their cross-reactivity with other receptors induce a strong prothrombotic state, which, in combination with other minor risk factors for stroke, can lead to ischemic stroke [108]. Two case reports that associate AIS with synthetic cannabinoids, support the embolic etiology of stroke which is in agreement with previous reports on severe adverse cardiac events following spice use [109]. In some cases of AIS attributed to synthetic cannabinoid use, past use of cannabis was also reported. In these cases, one could question whether acute synthetic cannabinoid overdose is the actual cause of stroke, or whether chronic cannabis use is also implicated. This theory could be supported by the similarity in the structure of THC and synthetic cannabinoids, which could lead to the same mechanism of cardiovascular injury [106]. Further studies are needed to elucidate the exact mechanism.

The reported cases of hemorrhagic strokes following acute use of synthetic cannabinoids can be explained by the transient vasospasm observed immediately after use [110]. The capacity of synthetic cannabinoids to alter neurotransmitter release from nerve terminals can lead to activation of smooth muscle cells which are associated with disruption of endothelial cell function and can, therefore, lead to ischemia or hemorrhage [111].

Figure 4 summarizes the main pathophysiological mechanisms of strokes associated with synthetic cannabinoid abuse.

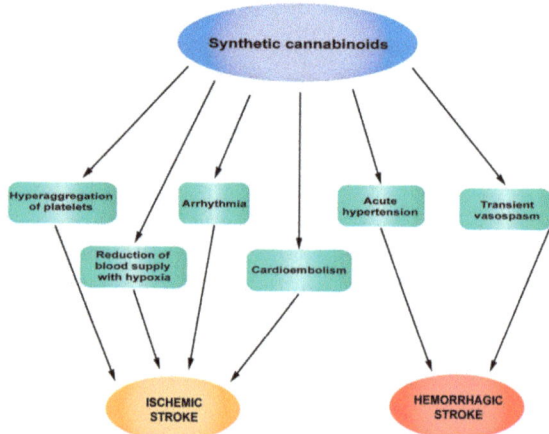

Figure 4. Main pathophysiological mechanisms of strokes associated with synthetic cannabinoid abuse.

2.4.3. Clinical Studies, Case Reports and Epidemiology of Stroke Related to Synthetic Cannabinoid Abuse

To date, only a few studies have investigated the toxic effects of synthetic cannabinoids. Case reports correlate their use with severe adverse and toxic effects, different from those observed after marijuana use. Even deaths have been reported [112].

The association of synthetic cannabinoid consumption and ischemic stroke/TIA was first reported by Bernson-Leung et al.. The group has published two cases of ischemic stroke in young people, pathologies that occurred within hours after a first-time exposure to synthetic cannabinoids. One patient was a 22-year-old woman who developed right middle cerebral artery AIS a few hours after smoking "K2" and the other patient was a 26-year-old woman who developed middle cerebral artery territory infarction after smoking "Peak Extreme". In both cases, the tests for serum vascular risk factors and hypercoagulability were negative. Both cases presented other minor risk factors for stroke: The 22-year-old woman was taking oral contraceptives and the 26-year-old woman had migraine with aura, took oral contraceptives, was an active smoker and had a family history of superficial thrombophlebitis. Even so, both were young and healthy and, most importantly, AIS occurred within a few hours after the first use of synthetic cannabinoids [113]. Another study reported two cases of middle cerebral artery location of AIS in a 26-year-old man and a 19-year-old woman immediately after smoking "spice". Both had positive urine tests for cannabinoids and they confirmed the use of synthetic cannabinoids in the past but not in the days that preceded stroke. The synthetic cannabinoid JWH-018 was found in their urine [109]. Faroqui et al. described a case of a 36-year-old African American man, without a medical history with risk factors for stroke, who showed extensive left cervical and intracranial internal carotid artery occlusion AIS after smoking "K2". He also reported smoking marijuana in the past, but not recently [114].

Only recently, there have been reports linking synthetic cannabinoids to hemorrhagic stroke. Rose et al. reported two cases of SAH after smoking "spice": A 31-year-old man, for whom the consumption of XLR-11((1-(5-fluoropentyl)-1H-indol-3-yl) (2,2,3,3-tetramethylcyclo-propyl) methanone) was confirmed, and a 25-year-old woman [110]. A summary of the main studies is presented in Table 4.

It is interesting to note that case reports on cannabis-associated stroke increased after the appearance of synthetic cannabinoids on the market. Based on the fact that synthetic cannabinoids are usually used together with cannabis and that they cannot be detected in urine through standard screening tests, further studies are needed to elucidate if cannabis is the real cause of these strokes, or whether a synergistic effect is caused by the concurrent use of cannabis and synthetic cannabinoids.

Table 4. Characteristic case reports that associate synthetic cannabinoid use with stroke.

Subject/Age	Substance Exposure	Symptoms	Diagnostic Approach	Diagnosis	Intervention	Evolution	Reference
Male, African American, 36, no history of stroke or coagulopathy or blood disorders	Reported taking K2 on the night before symptom onset; concomitant use of marijuana in the past	Had a 1-day history of aphasia and weakness in the right side of the body	Non-contrast CT of the head; computed tomography angiography (CTA); MRI; MR angiography	A thrombotic event that lead to an acute ischemic infarct with left MCA distribution characterized by hypodensity in the left basal ganglia and a left hyperdense MCA; a large filling defect observed from the origin of the left ICA into the intracranial portions of the ICA	Aspirin, clopidogrel and enoxaparin	After 10 days, the patient was discharged for short-term rehabilitation after gradual improvement	[114]
Female, 22, in treatment with atomoxetine and estrogen-containing oral contraceptive	Smoked K2; concomitant use of THC, benzodiazepine and salicylates as they were positive at urine toxicological test	While smoking, K2 presented dyspnea, palpitations and angor animi. Few hours later after smoking K2, developed dysarthria and difficulty standing	Head CT, MRI, and CT angiogram	Right middle cerebral artery AIS; proximal right M1 occlusion with distal reconstruction	Aspirin	In follow-up, presented limited ambulation and no use of her spastic left arm	[113]
Female, 26, estrogen-containing oral contraceptive, suffering from migraine with aura	Smoked 'Peak Extreme'	The next morning after smoking drugs, presented with felt-sided numbness, left facial weakness and dysfluency	CT angiogram, MRI, and head CT	Near occlusion of the right M1 segment with extensive infarction in the middle cerebral artery territory	Warfarin	Improved speech and comprehension	[113]
Male, 33, no medical history	Smoked two "joints" of synthetic cannabinoid product 10 min prior to the onset of symptoms; urine positive also for opiates; synthetic cannabinoid XLR-11-1-(5-fluoropentyl)-1H-indol-3-yl) (2,2,3,3-tetramethylcyclopropyl) methanone was confirmed in the product used	Right-sided weakness and aphasia	Non-contrast head CT, and electrocardiography	Acute infarction located in the left insular cortex	Aspirin	The neurological problems were completely resolved in 3 days in the hospital; no return to follow-up	[115]
Male, 26, no family history of any stroke risk factors, non-smoker, non-alcohol consumer	Smoked spice "a few hours prior" to his symptom onset; concomitant use of marijuana in the past but not recent	Weakness of right side of face and arm, dysarthria, expressive aphasia that occur suddenly	Non-contrast head CT; CT perfusion; CT angiography; MRI	Hyperdense left middle cerebral artery (MCA); a large area of penumbra without core infarction; left MCA clot	Received IV tissue plasminogen activator (t-PA)	Improved clinically and did not return to follow-up	[109]
Female, 19, smoker, anxiety disorder and panic attacks	Smoked spice; urine drug screening positive for cannabinoids and confirmed for JWH-018	A few minutes after smoking spice, the patient lost consciousness and started vomiting; mental status was persistently altered for several hours; presented with "shaking movements" of the legs and arms according to witnesses	CT angiogram and MRI	Infarctions in the left MCA with large distribution associated with punctate infarcts localized in the right cerebral hemisphere	-	She stabilized neurologically, but right hemiparesis and expressive aphasia remained at a follow-up office visit	[109]

Table 4. *Cont.*

Subject/Age	Substance Exposure	Symptoms	Diagnostic Approach	Diagnosis	Intervention	Evolution	Reference
Male, 31	Smoked spice; toxicological tests confirmed XLR-11	Generalized seizure	Head CT and digital subtraction angiography (DSA)	Hemorrhage in the bifrontal subarachnoid associated with left frontal and right parieto-occipital intraparenchymal hemorrhage	Intra-arterial verapamil	After 10 days from the event the paralysis of left leg, left homonymous hemianopsia and mentation improved	[110]
Female, 25, preeclampsia	Smoked synthetic marijuana; concomitant use of marijuana	Seizure after smoking synthetic and nonsynthetic marijuana; left leg monoplegia	CT, MRI, and DSA	SAH in the bilateral Sylvian fissures and interpeduncular and prepontine cisterns; restricted diffusion localized in the right frontal lobe, left cerebellum, left temporal lobe and bilateral parietal and occipital lobes, which is consistent with the diagnosis of multifocal AIS	Intra-arterial verapamil	Follow-up DSA showed worsening vertebrobasilar vasospasm	[110]

2.5. Opiates/Heroin

The most well-known substances belonging to the class of narcotic analgesics are morphine and heroin. Morphine is a natural substance extracted from some poppy species grown in South-East and South-West Asia, Mexico and Colombia [116]. Heroin (diacetylmorphine) is a semi-synthetic opioid drug, obtained by a chemical reaction between morphine and acetic anhydride [117]. Originally conceived as a substitute for morphine, heroin has been used in the past for the amelioration of withdrawal symptoms in alcohol-addicted individuals. Unfortunately, the synthetic drug is extremely addictive, causing both physical and psychological dependence [117].

2.5.1. The Mechanism of Action of Opiates/Heroin

Narcotic analgesics have a direct action on the vasomotor center and augment parasympathetic activity, reduce sympathetic activity and induce histamine release from mast cells [118]. These effects cause bradycardia, stimulating cardiac automatism, triggering atrial ectopic, atrial fibrillation, idioventricular rhythm or malignant ventricular arrhythmias. A complication of intravenous use is deep venous thrombosis, originating in the deep or superficial femoral vein, with the consequent risk of massive pulmonary embolism and stroke [9,119].

Morphine is rapidly absorbed and metabolized in the liver, and the main active metabolite is 6-glucuronide-morphine. It has a 2-fold increased potency compared to morphine. At the cerebral level, this metabolite has a 100-fold increased potency compared to morphine [116]. The metabolite 6-glucuronide-morphine is responsible for the analgesic action. Morphine has a plasma half-life of 2–3 h with rapid hepatic metabolism. Urinary excretion of metabolites can be detected in urine for up to 48 h (for occasional users) and for up to a few days (for chronic users) [120]. Due to the fact that heroin is more lipid soluble than morphine, it has an increased mode of action [121].

2.5.2. The Influence of Opiates/Heroin on Stroke

A proposed mechanism for heroin-associated ischemic stroke is cardioembolism.

This can occur secondary to infectious endocarditis (which is common in intravenous users), or due to other adulterants found in drugs [122]. The cardiogenic embolic effect of infectious endocarditis is further reinforced by the direct toxic effect of heroin on cerebral arteries [123]. Furthermore, post-anoxic encephalopathy and global hypoperfusion of the brain, due to heroin-induced hypotension, bradycardia, cardiopulmonary arrest, and hypoxia, can also be a possible mechanism [122,124]. Recent reports indicate that heroin-induced hypereosinophilia could be the cause of heroin-induced cerebral infarction. Heroin is known to induce hypereosinophilia in chronic users. Bolz et al. describe the case of a 29-year-old man who admitted sniffing heroin for seven years. He was diagnosed with heroin-induced hypereosinophilia and presented with multiple cerebral infarctions, without having any other cardiovascular risk factors [125]. The mechanism involved in cerebral ischemia could be associated with focal damage of the endothelium of the endocardium and of both small and larger arteries, determined by eosinophilic-associated proteins. This can be associated with increased blood clotting and local hypercoagulation, determined by components of eosinophilic granule [126]. In a study conducted in 2009, Hamzei Moqaddam et al. report that opioid dependence may be considered as an independent risk factor for stroke. The suggested underlying mechanism was that opioid dependence may increase plasma fibrinogen levels, which are known to represent a risk factor for the development of atherosclerosis in the coronary arteries, as well as in peripheral and cerebral vessels, and may, therefore, lead to heart infarctions or stroke [127].

Hemorrhagic stroke induced by heroin has also been reported. The possible pathogenic mechanisms could be: a) the hemorrhagic transformation of ischemic infarction or a hemorrhage determined by pyogenic arteritis and b) the rupture of a mycotic aneurysm [124,128].

Figure 5 summarizes the main pathophysiological mechanisms of strokes associated with opiate/heroin abuse.

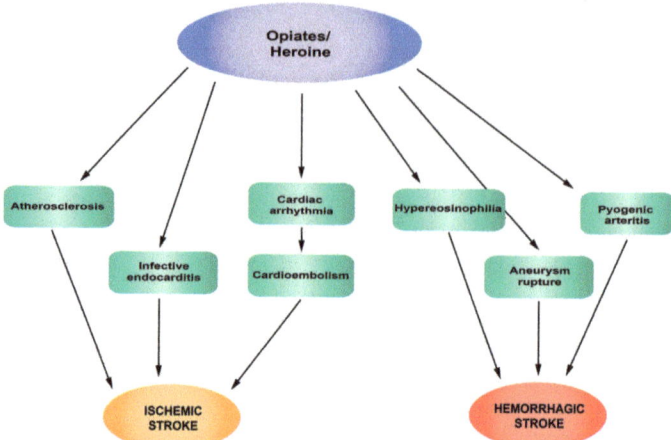

Figure 5. Pathophysiological mechanisms of stroke associated with opiate/heroin abuse.

2.5.3. Clinical Studies, Case Reports and Epidemiology of Stroke Related to Opiates/Heroin Abuse

Heroin-associated stroke has rarely been reported, but intranasal administration can lead to ischemic lesions of globus pallidus [129]. The ischemic pathology of heroin-associated stroke is more common than hemorrhagic forms [130]. Kumar et al. described a case of a 28-year-old woman who admitted using heroin and presented with intraparenchymal hemorrhage in the left frontal lobe without cardioembolic, vasculitic or other etiologies for stroke [128]. In the literature, there are only a couple of other cases of hemorrhagic stroke in young people who use heroin: A 42-year-old man who presented with massive left intracerebral hemorrhage and a 45-year-old man who presented with right basal ganglia hemorrhage [131]. Chronic morphine treatment may be associated with an increased incidence of stroke in patients with malignancies. A higher correlation is encountered in prostate cancer patients, as shown in a 2013 study in Taiwan [132].

Opiate-addicted individuals have a higher risk of stroke than the general population [133]. In Table 5, the most recent case reports that associate narcotic analgesic use and stroke are presented.

Table 5. Case reports that associate narcotic analgesic use with stroke.

Subject/Age	Substance Exposure	Symptoms	Diagnostic Approach	Diagnosis	Intervention	Evolution	Reference
Female, 28	Admitted to using heroin	Altered mental status	Head CT	A large 5.1 × 5-cm intraparenchymal hemorrhage in the left frontal lobe, vasogenic edema, and a 5-mm midline shift	Surgical intervention was unnecessary. After discharge, was transferred to rehabilitation	Improvement in cognitive function was mild; the patient continue to be confused and presented significant memory loss	[128]
Male, 29, without cardiovascular risk factors	Sniffed heroin with regularity in the last seven years	Left-sided hemikypesthesia and gait disturbance	MRI and MR angiography	Multiple cerebral and cerebellar areas of diffusion restriction in different territories; heroin-induced eosinophilia	Steroid pulse treatment (methylprednisolone 250 mg IV) in the first three days followed by another 21 days of oral prednisolone (60 mg)—for eosinophilia and antiplatelet therapy with aspirin	A slight improvement in his sensorium and gait but only incomplete recovery	[125]
Male, 33	Heroin inhalation	Amnesia 48 h after first heroin inhalation	MRI	Cortical laminar necrosis of the left hippocampus without vascular abnormality	-	Impaired performance on the verbal and visual level	[134]
Male, 33	Used heroin for 13 years. Concomitant use of methamphetamine. For 6 months, started methadone treatment to quit heroin	Found unconsciousness	Brain CT and MRI	Acute ischemic strokes localized in bilateral fronto-parieto-temporal white matter and in bilateral corona radiate. Damage was noted in the bilateral globus pallidus and left cerebral peduncle; rhabdomyolysis	Active treatment in the intensive care unit	-	[135]

2.6. Androgenic Anabolic Steroids

Anabolic androgenic steroids (AASs) are either endogenous (e.g., testosterone) or synthetic, exogenous substances (e.g., nandrolone and stanozolol), acting through specific androgen receptors. AASs are used for the treatment of several disorders, such as hypogonadism, cachexia of various etiologies, hypercalcemia, hypercalciuria, and along with other chronic diseases also in oncology as a supportive treatment [136].

2.6.1. The Mechanism of Action of AASs

The mechanism is complex and is associated with several parameters. More specifically, changes in the lipid profile have also been observed, both at chronic therapeutic doses and during short term treatment, with the reduction in high-density lipoprotein (HDL) cholesterol being the most profound change. Interestingly, molecular biology tests revealed that a concomitant increase in total cholesterol was accompanied by increased mRNA and protein expression of HMG-CoA reductase, a key enzyme in the formation of cholesterol by the liver [137]. The decrease in HDL cholesterol may reach 20% and, similarly, the increase in low-density lipoprotein (LDL) cholesterol may reach 20%, possibly as a result of the lipoproteins' lipolytic degradation and their subtraction by receptors due to the modification of apolipoprotein A-I and B synthesis [138]. Apolipoprotein B has been connected to atherosclerosis, via the interaction between the arterial wall and LDL cholesterol [139]. Abnormalities in lipoprotein expand the hazard of coronary artery disease by 3–6 fold and it may occur within 9 weeks of AAS use. In addition to its atherogenic effects, the excess of LDL-C may be oxidized at the arterial endothelium leading to impaired endothelium-dependent arterial relaxation via inhibition of nitric oxide production. This could predispose to the development of coronary vasospasm [140]. Fortunately, the effects of lipids appear to be reversible [141].

The effects of anabolic steroids on blood pressure remain conflicting. A few studies have reported elevated blood pressure levels in anabolic steroid users [142], which might be maintained even 5 to 12 months after discontinuation [143]. The mechanism involved could be the ability of AASs to increase the activity of the sympathetic nervous system activity, to baroreflex control and to endothelial dysfunction as well [144]. The mode of action seems to be substance specific. For example, nandrolone has no effects on blood pressure, while the cardiac hypertrophy caused by nandrolone administration was not associated with the systemic renin–angiotensin system but with its effects at a local level. Unfortunately, data so far are not sufficient to settle on whether the prolonged AAS use can lead to irreversible elevated levels of blood pressure [145].

2.6.2. The Influence of AASs on Stroke

Atherothrombosis or embolization could lead to thromboembolic ischemic strokes. Peripheral vascular disease can occur through the same mechanisms. The main action of AASs is anabolism. It is involved in growth-promoting effects on cardiac tissue, following AAS administration and causes hypertrophic cardiomyopathy. Probably as a counteracting effect, apoptotic cell death has also been observed—a process that is mediated by membrane receptor second messenger cascades that increase intracellular Ca^{2+} influx and mobilization, leading to the release of apoptogenic factors [146–148]. In vitro studies performed in isolated human myocytes have shown that AASs bind to androgen receptors. Therefore, it is possible that hypertrophy may be induced directly, via tissue upregulation of the renin–angiotensin system [149]. Supporting evidence lies in the fact that the AT1 receptor antagonist prevented similar effects induced by nandrolone administration [150]. Moreover, nandrolone treatment, in combination with swimming training, increased left ventricular angiotensin-converting enzyme (LV-ACE) activity and CYP11B2 expression, implying an elevation in both angiotensin II and aldosterone and the promotion of cardiac dysfunction [151].

Sex hormone-related mechanisms also seem to be involved in the pathogenesis of various cardiovascular disorders, with ischemic stroke included, particularly for men. However, these findings are not specifically informative about endogenous testosterone or testosterone supplementation [152]. Testosterone supplementation for therapeutic purposes has not been conclusively linked with a high thrombotic risk. In a cohort of 3422 male US military service members, aged 40–64 years, treated with testosterone for low testosterone levels, there was no difference in event-free survival with regard to thromboembolism, compared to an appropriately matched control group [153]. On the other hand, elevated testosterone was independently associated with an increased risk for both ischemic stroke (odds ratio 3.9) and cerebral venous thrombosis (odds ratio 5.5) [154]. Nevertheless, the Guidelines of the Endocrine Society suggest that testosterone therapy should be avoided in patients with, among other clinical conditions, elevated hematocrit, myocardial infarction or stroke within the last 6 months or thrombophilia. Furthermore, measuring serum testosterone concentrations and hematocrit is highly recommended [155].

The effect of AASs on the hemostatic system may lead to a prothrombotic profile, depending on the dose and the duration of AAS administration. Low doses decrease platelet threshold activation to collagen. In addition, androgens reduce plasminogen activator inhibitor-1 (PAI-1) levels and increase fibrinolytic activity via high tissue plasminogen activator (t-PA) levels. Both the release of t-PA from endothelial cells into the circulation and the amount of t-PA inhibitor (PAI-1) that is present in the circulation regulate fibrinolytic activity [156,157]. Possible vascular thrombosis due to increased fibrinolytic activity as a result of decreased PAI-1 levels can consequently be speculated [158]. Higher doses have been associated with the elevated aggregation of platelets and possibly affect the activity of vascular cyclooxygenase enzyme, which may lead to a procoagulant state [159]. Several AASs appear to be involved in procoagulatory pathways, by increasing plasma levels of factor VIII and IX [160]. They also increase the aggregation of platelets and the formation of thrombus formation via increased platelet production of thromboxane A2, and via decreased production of prostacyclin and increased fibrinogen levels [139]. At the same time, as animal experiments have shown, extracellular matrix, nitric oxide production and the arachidonic metabolism of endothelial cells and platelets are also influenced [161]. Moreover, both exogenous and endogenous AASs can provoke polycythemia and consequent ischemic cardiovascular events through the reduction of hepcidin and the stimulation of erythropoiesis, by recalibrating the erythropoietin set point [162,163]. Testosterone has also been shown to stabilize telomeres in bone marrow progenitors, which may play a role in increased red cell production [164].

Figure 6 summarizes the main pathophysiological mechanisms of stroke associated with anabolic androgenic steroid abuse.

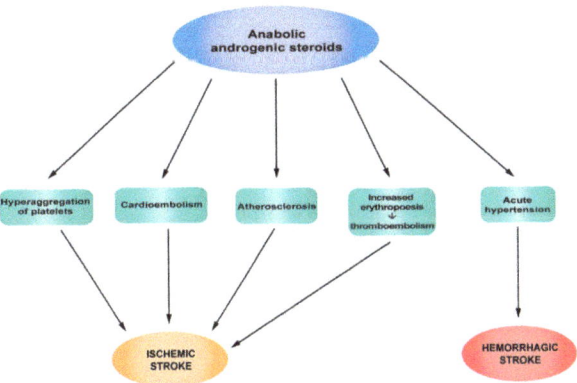

Figure 6. Pathophysiological mechanisms of strokes associated with anabolic androgenic steroid abuse.

2.6.3. Clinical Studies, Case Reports and Epidemiology of Stroke Related to AAS Abuse

Since the early 1930s, AASs have been extensively used by amateur or professional athletes and the general public for the improvement of physical conditions and athletic performance [165–168]. When used for ergogenic or recreational purposes, the doses are usually 5–15 times higher than the recommended therapeutic ones [145,167,169]. At such high levels, AASs can cause a number of serious side effects, including liver dysfunction, renal disorders, cardiotoxicity and potentially stroke [136].

Indeed, athletes abusing AASs for years have a high probability to develop atherothrombotic phenomena (cardiovascular and cerebrovascular disorders, such as cerebral ischemia, i.e., transitory ischemic attacks resulting in stroke, peripheral artery occlusive disease and venous thromboembolism) [143]. These phenomena can be attributed to arterial hypertension, lipid metabolism disorders, increased vascular tone and increased platelet counts and hematocrit [139,145,170]. The reversibility of such myocardial and vascular effects after discontinuation is still controversial [171]. Several case reports describe stroke in AAS abusers, and the most interesting ones are summarized in Table 6.

Table 6. Case reports that associate androgenic anabolic steroid (AAS) abuse with stroke.

Subject/Age	Substance Exposure	Symptoms	Diagnostic Approach	Diagnosis	Reference
Male, 27, with an American father and a mother who was half Japanese, no known stroke risk factors, regularly training, AAS user	Methasterone, prostanozol for the past 6 months	Sudden right hemiparalysis, homonymous hemianopia, dysarthria, tinnitus, and double vision in the middle of muscle training	MRI with and without gadolinium enhancement, MR angiography, three-dimensional CT angiography, carotid ultrasonography, transcranial Doppler and transesophageal echocardiography, and duplex ultrasonography	Cardiogenic embolism and atrial septal aneurysm and large patent foramen ovule, suspected deep vein thrombosis	[170]
Male, 37, no history of alcohol or any other substance abuse, negative medical and family histories	Methandienone, methenolone acetate for the past 2 years	Acute right-sided hemiparesis (grade 3) with right-sided facial weakness, associated with a confused state followed a first-ever experience of generalized tonic–clonic seizure	Brain CT and MRI, ECG, chest X-ray, abdominal ultrasound, and echocardiography	Chronic infarction in the left frontal lobe and subacute left temporoparietal infarction Dilated cardiomyopathy and multiple thrombi in the left ventricle Hepatomegaly, mild ascites and bilateral pleural effusion in addition to a grade I nephropathy	[140]
Male, 16, healthy bodybuilder (weight 87 kg and height 181 cm), unremarkable past medical record	Concomitant use of cannabis (up to 1.5 g/day) and methandrostenolone (40 mg/day) for the past 5 months	Sudden dizziness and right hemiparesis	Cerebral CT, MRI, conventional and magnetic resonance angiography, transesophageal echocardiography, cervical Doppler duplex ultrasound, transcranial Doppler, and ECG	Acute ischemic stroke	[156]
Male, 39, bodybuilder, 3 months earlier sudden loss of vision in the left eye, weakness and numbness in the left upper and lower limbs, lasting less than 1 h, refused admission to hospital	Intramuscular injections of nandrolone twice weekly for the past three years	Dizziness and expressive aphasia for the last 6 h	Brain CT and MRI, ECG, chest X-ray, echocardiography, and magnetic resonance angiography	Dilated cardiomyopathy with LV thrombus formation; embolic stroke and peripheral vascular disease as a complication of the former	[141]
Male, 31, kickboxer	Nandrolone, testosterone clenbuterol since the age of 16; cocaine, ecstasy and alcohol abuser for three years	Patient disoriented in space, mild dysarthria without aphasic elements, oculocephalic preference to right, left homonymous hemianopsia, paresis (3/5), hemicorporal anesthesia on the left side and somatoagnosia	Cranial CT, cerebral arteriography, transesophageal and transthoracic echocardiography, and magnetic resonance angiography	Acute ischemic stroke: Cerebral infarction due to occlusion of the artery cerebral media of unknown etiology	[172]
Male	Injectable (nandrolone decanoate) and oral (methandrostenolone/danabol) three months prior to the incidence Previous intravenous (heroin), and inhaled (marijuana) drug use	Visual disturbances and left-sided weakness commencing 24 h prior to presentation Homonymous hemianopia, mild left-sided weakness in his upper limbs and ataxia in his left upper limb, and high hemoglobin (200 g/L)	Brain magnetic resonance, magnetic resonance angiography, transthoracic echocardiogram, and 24-h Holter monitoring, extensive hematological screening, and thrombophilia screening	Cerebral infarction: Extensive region of acute infarction in the right posterior cerebral artery territory and ongoing occlusion in his right posterior cerebral artery Polycythemia	[173]

Table 7 summarizes the association between the different classes of drugs of abuse with different types of stroke.

Table 7. The incidence of ischemic stroke and hemorrhagic stroke in different classes of drugs of abuse.

Drugs of Abuse			Ischemic Stroke	Hemorrhagic Stroke
Amphetamines			+	+++
Amphetamine derivatives			+	+++ Risk in young people without comorbidities
Cocaine	Cocaine		In those with a history of use	In active users
	Hydrochloride		+	+++
	Crack		++	++
Cannabis			++	+ In recent case reports
Synthetic cannabinoids			++	+In recent case reports
Opiates/Heroin			++	+In recent case reports
Anabolic androgenic steroids			++	

+ mild evidence. ++ medium evidence. +++ high evidence.

3. Management

Stroke can occur either in minutes/hours following illicit drug use or later as a consequence of complications, such as vasculitis or endocarditis, resulting in septic emboli [45,174].

Acute stroke is a medical emergency. Patients should be transported by ambulance to a medical facility that is organized and equipped to manage acute stroke as soon as possible after symptom onset and capable of offering emergency treatments such as intravenous thrombolysis and endovascular thrombectomy—organized acute stroke unit management. These treatments are typically offered in departments of neurology with organized stroke centers [40].

The outcome of ICH depends on the hematoma location and volume, the promptness of treatment, and the management of associated diseases. The mortality of ICH remains very high. For those who survive, recovery is difficult and long lasting, with a negative impact on quality of life. Risk factors, such as high blood pressure, smoking, obesity and drug use, play an important role. Prevention plays a central role and can be favorably influenced by changing lifestyle and taking therapeutic measures, especially for hypertension control.

4. Conclusions

Drug abuse represents a major social and public health problem, with huge financial implications. Epidemiological studies and case reports have shown that drug abuse is a risk factor for both hemorrhagic and ischemic stroke. Stimulants, such as amphetamines, amphetamine derivatives, and cocaine have been associated with both types of stroke—more so of the hemorrhagic type. "Crack" cocaine can cause both acute ischemic stroke and hemorrhagic strokes, while cocaine hydrochloride is more likely to cause hemorrhagic strokes. Stroke can emerge after cocaine use, even in the absence of other traditional stroke risk factors. The association between cannabis, synthetic cannabinoids, or opioid/heroin use and stroke has not been entirely proven by epidemiological studies that offer contradictory findings. New case reports describe the correlation between cannabinoids and synthetic cannabinoids and hemorrhagic stroke. Anabolic androgenic steroids are associated with cardiotoxicity and atherothrombotic phenomena which can lead to ischemic stroke. Given the epidemic of illicit drug use, we recommend that every hospitalized stroke patient, and especially those who are young for stroke, is subjected to toxicological screening.

Author Contributions: All the authors contributed equally to conceiving and designing the manuscript. A.O.D., D.C., L.-M.Z. and C.T. searched the literature for inclusion in the study that was then checked and reviewed by A.T., K.T., R.M., L.K., J.S.R., P.D.M. and N.D. D.C., A.O.D., G.L., C.T. and M.N. drafted and wrote the manuscript. A.T., P.D.M., L.K., V.S., E.D. critically revised the manuscript. A.O.D., D.C., J.S.-R. and L.M.D. designed the figures. A.O.D., C.T. and R.M. designed the tables. All the authors have read and approved the final version of the manuscript.

Acknowledgments: This paper and APC was supported by Grants PN-III-P1-1.2-PCCDI-2017-0341/2018, PN 19.29.01.01 and by the Ministry of Research and Innovation in Romania under Program 1: The Improvement of the National System of Research and Development, Subprogram 1.2: Institutional Excellence—Projects of Excellence Funding in RDI, Contract No. 7PFE/16.10.2018.

Conflicts of Interest: The authors declare no conflict of interest.

References

1. Easton, J.D.; Saver, J.L.; Albers, G.W.; Alberts, M.J.; Chaturvedi, S.; Feldmann, E.; Hatsukami, T.S.; Higashida, R.T.; Johnston, S.C.; Kidwell, C.S.; et al. Definition and evaluation of transient ischemic attack: A scientific statement for healthcare professionals from the American Heart Association/American Stroke Association Stroke Council; Council on Cardiovascular Surgery and Anesthesia; Council on Cardiovascular Radiology and Intervention; Council on Cardiovascular Nursing; and the Interdisciplinary Council on Peripheral Vascular Disease. The American Academy of Neurology affirms the value of this statement as an educational tool for neurologists. *Stroke* **2009**, *40*, 2276–2293. [CrossRef] [PubMed]
2. National Collaborating Centre for Chronic Conditions. National Collaborating Centre for Chronic Conditions. National Institute for Health and Clinical Excellence: Guidance. In *Stroke: National Clinical Guideline for Diagnosis and Initial Management of Acute Stroke and Transient Ischaemic Attack (TIA)*; Royal College of Physicians (UK) Royal College of Physicians of London: London, UK, 2008.
3. Johnson, W.; Onuma, O.; Owolabi, M.; Sachdev, S. Stroke: A global response is needed. *Bull. World Health Organ.* **2016**, *94*. [CrossRef] [PubMed]
4. United Nations Oddice on Drugs and Crime. World Drug Report 2017. Available online: https://www.unodc.org/wdr2017/field/WDR_2017_presentation_lauch_version.pdf (accessed on 26 February 2019).
5. Smajlovic, D. Strokes in young adults: Epidemiology and prevention. *Vasc. Health Risk Manag.* **2015**, *11*, 157–164. [CrossRef] [PubMed]
6. Mendis, S. Stroke disability and rehabilitation of stroke: World Health Organization perspective. *Int. J. Stroke* **2013**, *8*, 3–4. [CrossRef] [PubMed]
7. Jivan, K.; Ranchod, K.; Modi, G. Management of ischaemic stroke in the acute setting: Review of the current status. *Cardiovasc. J. Afr.* **2013**, *24*, 86–92. [CrossRef] [PubMed]
8. Falkstedt, D.; Wolff, V.; Allebeck, P.; Hemmingsson, T.; Danielsson, A.K. Cannabis, Tobacco, Alcohol Use, and the Risk of Early Stroke: A Population-Based Cohort Study of 45,000 Swedish Men. *Stroke* **2017**, *48*, 265–270. [CrossRef] [PubMed]
9. Sloan, M.A. Illicit drug use/abuse and stroke. *Handb. Clin. Neurol.* **2009**, *93*, 823–840. [CrossRef] [PubMed]
10. Nieswandt, B.; Kleinschnitz, C.; Stoll, G. Ischaemic stroke: A thrombo-inflammatory disease? *J. Physiol.* **2011**, *589*, 4115–4123. [CrossRef]
11. Stoll, G.; Nieswandt, B. Thrombo-inflammation in acute ischaemic stroke—Implications for treatment. *Nat. Rev. Neurol.* **2019**, *15*, 473–481. [CrossRef]
12. Slomka, A.; Switonska, M.; Sinkiewicz, W.; Zekanowska, E. Assessing Circulating Factor VIIa-Antithrombin Complexes in Acute Ischemic Stroke: A Pilot Study. *Clin. Appl. Thromb. Hemost.* **2017**, *23*, 351–359. [CrossRef]
13. Switonska, M.; Slomka, A.; Sinkiewicz, W.; Zekanowska, E. Tissue-factor-bearing microparticles (MPs-TF) in patients with acute ischaemic stroke: The influence of stroke treatment on MPs-TF generation. *Eur. J. Neurol.* **2015**, *22*, e328–e399. [CrossRef] [PubMed]
14. Brouwers, H.B.; Greenberg, S.M. Hematoma expansion following acute intracerebral hemorrhage. *Cerebrovasc. Dis.* **2013**, *35*, 195–201. [CrossRef] [PubMed]
15. Sonni, S.; Lioutas, V.A.; Selim, M.H. New avenues for treatment of intracranial hemorrhage. *Curr. Treat. Options Cardiovasc. Med.* **2014**, *16*, 277. [CrossRef] [PubMed]

16. Dardiotis, E.; Aloizou, A.M.; Markoula, S.; Siokas, V.; Tsarouhas, K.; Tzanakakis, G.; Libra, M.; Kyritsis, A.P.; Brotis, A.G.; Aschner, M.; et al. Cancer-associated stroke: Pathophysiology, detection and management (Review). *Int. J. Oncol.* **2019**, *54*, 779–796. [CrossRef]
17. Teodoro, M.; Briguglio, G.; Fenga, C.; Costa, C. Genetic polymorphisms as determinants of pesticide toxicity: Recent advances. *Toxicol. Rep.* **2019**. [CrossRef] [PubMed]
18. Kaye, S.; Darke, S.; Duflou, J.; McKetin, R. Methamphetamine-related fatalities in Australia: Demographics, circumstances, toxicology and major organ pathology. *Addiction* **2008**, *103*, 1353–1360. [CrossRef]
19. Kaku, D.A.; Lowenstein, D.H. Emergence of recreational drug abuse as a major risk factor for stroke in young adults. *Ann. Intern. Med.* **1990**, *113*, 821–827. [CrossRef]
20. Ho, E.L.; Josephson, S.A.; Lee, H.S.; Smith, W.S. Cerebrovascular complications of methamphetamine abuse. *Neurocrit. Care* **2009**, *10*, 295–305. [CrossRef]
21. Buttner, A. Review: The neuropathology of drug abuse. *Neuropathol. Appl. Neurobiol.* **2011**, *37*, 118–134. [CrossRef]
22. Sloan, M.A.; Kittner, S.J.; Rigamonti, D.; Price, T.R. Occurrence of stroke associated with use/abuse of drugs. *Neurology* **1991**, *41*, 1358–1364. [CrossRef]
23. Parrott, A.C.; Milani, R.M.; Gouzoulis-Mayfrank, E.; Daumann, J. Cannabis and Ecstasy/MDMA (3,4-methylenedioxymethamphetamine): An analysis of their neuropsychobiological interactions in recreational users. *J. Neural Transm. (Vienna, Austria: 1996)* **2007**, *114*, 959–968. [CrossRef] [PubMed]
24. Heal, D.J.; Smith, S.L.; Gosden, J.; Nutt, D.J. Amphetamine, past and present—A pharmacological and clinical perspective. *J. Psychopharmacol. (Oxford, UK)* **2013**, *27*, 479–496. [CrossRef] [PubMed]
25. Walker-Batson, D.; Mehta, J.; Smith, P.; Johnson, M. Amphetamine and other pharmacological agents in human and animal studies of recovery from stroke. *Prog. Neuropsychopharmacol. Biol. Psychiatry* **2016**, *64*, 225–230. [CrossRef] [PubMed]
26. Calipari, E.S.; Ferris, M.J. Amphetamine mechanisms and actions at the dopamine terminal revisited. *J. Neurosci.* **2013**, *33*, 8923–8925. [CrossRef] [PubMed]
27. Christophersen, A.S. Amphetamine designer drugs—An overview and epidemiology. *Toxicol. Lett.* **2000**, *112–113*, 127–131. [CrossRef]
28. Albertson, T.E.; Derlet, R.W.; Van Hoozen, B.E. Methamphetamine and the expanding complications of amphetamines. *West. J. Med.* **1999**, *170*, 214–219. [PubMed]
29. Westover, A.N.; McBride, S.; Haley, R.W. Stroke in young adults who abuse amphetamines or cocaine: A population-based study of hospitalized patients. *Arch. Gen. Psychiatry* **2007**, *64*, 495–502. [CrossRef]
30. Phillips, M.C.; Leyden, J.M.; Chong, W.K.; Kleinig, T.; Czapran, P.; Lee, A.; Koblar, S.A.; Jannes, J. Ischaemic stroke among young people aged 15 to 50 years in Adelaide, South Australia. *Med. J. Aust.* **2011**, *195*, 610–614. [CrossRef]
31. Indave, B.I.; Sordo, L.; Bravo, M.J.; Sarasa-Renedo, A.; Fernandez-Balbuena, S.; De la Fuente, L.; Sonego, M. Risk of stroke in prescription and other amphetamine-type stimulants use: A systematic review. *Drug Alcohol Rev.* **2018**, *37*, 56–69. [CrossRef]
32. Ohta, K.; Mori, M.; Yoritaka, A.; Okamoto, K.; Kishida, S. Delayed ischemic stroke associated with methamphetamine use. *J. Emerg. Med.* **2005**, *28*, 165–167. [CrossRef]
33. De Silva, D.A.; Wong, M.C.; Lee, M.P.; Chen, C.L.; Chang, H.M. Amphetamine-associated ischemic stroke: Clinical presentation and proposed pathogenesis. *J. Stroke Cerebrovasc. Dis.* **2007**, *16*, 185–186. [CrossRef] [PubMed]
34. Weiss, S.R.; Raskind, R.; Morganstern, N.L.; Pytlyk, P.J.; Baiz, T.C. Intracerebral and subarachnoid hemorrhage following use of methamphetamine ("speed"). *Int. J. Surg.* **1970**, *53*, 123–127.
35. Yakoot, M. Phenylpropanolamine and the hemorrhagic stroke: A new search for the culprit. *J. Pharmacol. Pharmacother.* **2012**, *3*, 4–6. [CrossRef] [PubMed]
36. Polesskaya, O.; Silva, J.; Sanfilippo, C.; Desrosiers, T.; Sun, A.; Shen, J.; Feng, C.; Polesskiy, A.; Deane, R.; Zlokovic, B.; et al. Methamphetamine causes sustained depression in cerebral blood flow. *Brain Res.* **2011**, *1373*, 91–100. [CrossRef] [PubMed]
37. Berlit, P. Diagnosis and treatment of cerebral vasculitis. *Ther. Adv. Neurol. Disord.* **2010**, *3*, 29–42. [CrossRef] [PubMed]

38. McGee, S.M.; McGee, D.N.; McGee, M.B. Spontaneous intracerebral hemorrhage related to methamphetamine abuse: Autopsy findings and clinical correlation. *Am. J. Forensic Med. Pathol.* **2004**, *25*, 334–337. [CrossRef] [PubMed]
39. Pilgrim, J.L.; Gerostamoulos, D.; Drummer, O.H.; Bollmann, M. Involvement of amphetamines in sudden and unexpected death. *J. Forensic Sci.* **2009**, *54*, 478–485. [CrossRef] [PubMed]
40. Lappin, J.M.; Darke, S.; Farrell, M. Stroke and methamphetamine use in young adults: A review. *J. Neurol. Neurosurg. Psychiatry* **2017**, *88*, 1079–1091. [CrossRef]
41. Huang, M.C.; Yang, S.Y.; Lin, S.K.; Chen, K.Y.; Chen, Y.Y.; Kuo, C.J.; Hung, Y.N. Risk of Cardiovascular Diseases and Stroke Events in Methamphetamine Users: A 10-Year Follow-Up Study. *J. Clin. Psychiatry* **2016**, *77*, 1396–1403. [CrossRef]
42. Christensen, M.R.; Lesnikova, I.; Madsen, L.B.; Rosendal, I.; Banner, J. Drug-induced bilateral ischemic infarction in an amphetamine addict. *Forensic Sci. Med. Pathol.* **2013**, *9*, 458–461. [CrossRef]
43. Kahn, D.E.; Ferraro, N.; Benveniste, R.J. 3 cases of primary intracranial hemorrhage associated with "Molly", a purified form of 3,4-methylenedioxymethamphetamine (MDMA). *J. Neurol. Sci.* **2012**, *323*, 257–260. [CrossRef] [PubMed]
44. Wijers, C.H.W.; Visser, M.C.; van Litsenburg, R.T.H.; Niesink, R.J.M.; Willemse, R.B.; Croes, E.A. Haemorrhagic stroke related to the use of 4-fluoroamphetamine. *J. Neurol.* **2018**, *265*, 1607–1611. [CrossRef] [PubMed]
45. Chiu, Z.K.; Bennett, I.E.; Chan, P.; Rosenfeld, J.V. Methamphetamine-related brainstem haemorrhage. *J. Clin. Neurosci.* **2016**, *32*, 137–139. [CrossRef] [PubMed]
46. Kapetanovic, S.; Kim, M.A. Hemorrhagic stroke in a patient recently started on mixed amphetamine salts. *Am. J. Psychiatry* **2010**, *167*, 1277–1278. [CrossRef] [PubMed]
47. Lyson, T.; Kochanowicz, J.; Rutkowski, R.; Turek, G.; Lewko, J. Cerebral vasospasm in patient with hemorrhagic stroke after amphetamine intake—Case report. *Pol. Merkur. Lek. Organ Pol. Tow. Lek.* **2008**, *24*, 265–267.
48. Muntan, C.D.; Tuckler, V. Cerebrovascular accident following MDMA ingestion. *J. Med. Toxicol.* **2006**, *2*, 16–18. [CrossRef] [PubMed]
49. McIntosh, A.; Hungs, M.; Kostanian, V.; Yu, W. Carotid artery dissection and middle cerebral artery stroke following methamphetamine use. *Neurology* **2006**, *67*, 2259–2260. [CrossRef]
50. Treadwell, S.D.; Robinson, T.G. Cocaine use and stroke. *Postgrad. Med. J.* **2007**, *83*, 389–394. [CrossRef]
51. Kishi, T.; Matsuda, Y.; Iwata, N.; Correll, C.U. Antipsychotics for cocaine or psychostimulant dependence: Systematic review and meta-analysis of randomized, placebo-controlled trials. *J. Clin. Psychiatry* **2013**, *74*, e1169–e1180. [CrossRef]
52. Riezzo, I.; Fiore, C.; De Carlo, D.; Pascale, N.; Neri, M.; Turillazzi, E.; Fineschi, V. Side effects of cocaine abuse: Multiorgan toxicity and pathological consequences. *Curr. Med. Chem.* **2012**, *19*, 5624–5646. [CrossRef]
53. Bachi, K.; Mani, V.; Jeyachandran, D.; Fayad, Z.A.; Goldstein, R.Z.; Alia-Klein, N. Vascular disease in cocaine addiction. *Atherosclerosis* **2017**, *262*, 154–162. [CrossRef] [PubMed]
54. Sordo, L.; Indave, B.I.; Barrio, G.; Degenhardt, L.; de la Fuente, L.; Bravo, M.J. Cocaine use and risk of stroke: A systematic review. *Drug Alcohol Depend.* **2014**, *142*, 1–13. [CrossRef] [PubMed]
55. Bhattacharya, P.; Taraman, S.; Shankar, L.; Chaturvedi, S.; Madhavan, R. Clinical Profiles, Complications, and Disability in Cocaine-Related Ischemic Stroke. *J. Stroke Cerebrovasc. Dis.* **2011**, *20*, 443–449. [CrossRef] [PubMed]
56. Pradhan, L.; Mondal, D.; Chandra, S.; Ali, M.; Agrawal, K.C. Molecular analysis of cocaine-induced endothelial dysfunction: Role of endothelin-1 and nitric oxide. *Cardiovasc. Toxicol.* **2008**, *8*, 161–171. [CrossRef] [PubMed]
57. He, G.Q.; Zhang, A.; Altura, B.T.; Altura, B.M. Cocaine-induced cerebrovasospasm and its possible mechanism of action. *J. Pharmacol. Exp. Ther.* **1994**, *268*, 1532–1539. [PubMed]
58. You, J.; Du, C.; Volkow, N.D.; Pan, Y. Optical coherence Doppler tomography for quantitative cerebral blood flow imaging. *Biomed. Opt. Express* **2014**, *5*, 3217–3230. [CrossRef] [PubMed]
59. Toossi, S.; Hess, C.P.; Hills, N.K.; Josephson, S.A. Neurovascular Complications of Cocaine Use at a Tertiary Stroke Center. *J. Stroke Cerebrovasc. Dis.* **2010**, *19*, 273–278. [CrossRef]
60. Narvaez, J.C.; Magalhaes, P.V.; Fries, G.R.; Colpo, G.D.; Czepielewski, L.S.; Vianna, P.; Chies, J.A.; Rosa, A.R.; Von Diemen, L.; Vieta, E.; et al. Peripheral toxicity in crack cocaine use disorders. *Neurosci. Lett.* **2013**, *544*, 80–84. [CrossRef]

61. Fox, H.C.; D'Sa, C.; Kimmerling, A.; Siedlarz, K.M.; Tuit, K.L.; Stowe, R.; Sinha, R. Immune system inflammation in cocaine dependent individuals: Implications for medications development. *Hum. Psychopharmacol.* **2012**, *27*, 156–166. [CrossRef]
62. Lucas, G.M.; Atta, M.G.; Fine, D.M.; McFall, A.M.; Estrella, M.M.; Zook, K.; Stein, J.H. HIV, Cocaine Use, and Hepatitis C Virus: A Triad of Nontraditional Risk Factors for Subclinical Cardiovascular Disease. *Arterioscler. Thromb. Vasc. Biol.* **2016**, *36*, 2100–2107. [CrossRef]
63. Harsch, H.H.; Pankiewicz, J.; Bloom, A.S.; Rainey, C.; Cho, J.K.; Sperry, L.; Stein, E.A. Hepatitis C virus infection in cocaine users—A silent epidemic. *Community Ment. Health J.* **2000**, *36*, 225–233. [CrossRef] [PubMed]
64. Kalichman, S.C.; Washington, C.; Kegler, C.; Grebler, T.; Kalichman, M.O.; Cherry, C.; Eaton, L. Continued Substance Use Among People Living With HIV-Hepatitis-C Co-Infection and Receiving Antiretroviral Therapy. *Subst. Use Misuse* **2015**, *50*, 1536–1543. [CrossRef] [PubMed]
65. Dash, S.; Balasubramaniam, M.; Villalta, F.; Dash, C.; Pandhare, J. Impact of cocaine abuse on HIV pathogenesis. *Front. Microbiol.* **2015**, *6*, 1111. [CrossRef] [PubMed]
66. Boehme, A.K.; Esenwa, C.; Elkind, M.S. Stroke Risk Factors, Genetics, and Prevention. *Circ. Res.* **2017**, *120*, 472–495. [CrossRef] [PubMed]
67. Gretarsdottir, S.; Thorleifsson, G.; Manolescu, A.; Styrkarsdottir, U.; Helgadottir, A.; Gschwendtner, A.; Kostulas, K.; Kuhlenbaumer, G.; Bevan, S.; Jonsdottir, T.; et al. Risk variants for atrial fibrillation on chromosome 4q25 associate with ischemic stroke. *Ann. Neurol.* **2008**, *64*, 402–409. [CrossRef] [PubMed]
68. Kouzarides, T. Histone acetylases and deacetylases in cell proliferation. *Curr. Opin. Genet. Dev.* **1999**, *9*, 40–48. [CrossRef]
69. Penrod, R.D.; Carreira, M.B.; Taniguchi, M.; Kumar, J.; Maddox, S.A.; Cowan, C.W. Novel role and regulation of HDAC4 in cocaine-related behaviors. *Addict. Biol.* **2018**, *23*, 653–664. [CrossRef] [PubMed]
70. Lanktree, M.B.; Hegele, R.A.; Yusuf, S.; Anand, S.S. Multi-ethnic genetic association study of carotid intima-media thickness using a targeted cardiovascular SNP microarray. *Stroke* **2009**, *40*, 3173–3179. [CrossRef]
71. Desai, R.; Patel, U.; Rupareliya, C.; Singh, S.; Shah, M.; Patel, R.S.; Patel, S.; Mahuwala, Z. Impact of Cocaine Use on Acute Ischemic Stroke Patients: Insights from Nationwide Inpatient Sample in the United States. *Cureus* **2017**, *9*, e1536. [CrossRef]
72. Cheng, Y.C.; Ryan, K.A.; Qadwai, S.A.; Shah, J.; Sparks, M.J.; Wozniak, M.A.; Stern, B.J.; Phipps, M.S.; Cronin, C.A.; Magder, L.S.; et al. Cocaine Use and Risk of Ischemic Stroke in Young Adults. *Stroke* **2016**, *47*, 918–922. [CrossRef]
73. Daras, M.; Tuchman, A.J.; Marks, S. Central nervous system infarction related to cocaine abuse. *Stroke* **1991**, *22*, 1320–1325. [CrossRef] [PubMed]
74. Martin-Schild, S.; Albright, K.C.; Hallevi, H.; Barreto, A.D.; Philip, M.; Misra, V.; Grotta, J.C.; Savitz, S.I. Intracerebral hemorrhage in cocaine users. *Stroke* **2010**, *41*, 680–684. [CrossRef] [PubMed]
75. Lucerna, A.; Espinosa, J.; Zaman, T.; Hertz, R.; Stranges, D. Limb Pain as Unusual Presentation of a Parietal Intraparenchymal Bleeding Associated with Crack Cocaine Use: A Case Report. *Case Rep. Neurol. Med.* **2018**, *2018*, 9598675. [CrossRef] [PubMed]
76. Mullaguri, N.; Battineni, A.; Narayan, A.; Guddeti, R. Cocaine Induced Bilateral Posterior Inferior Cerebellar Artery and Hippocampal Infarction. *Cureus* **2018**, *10*, e2576. [CrossRef] [PubMed]
77. Rico-Mesa, J.S.; Rico-Mesa, M.A.; Berrouet, M.C. Ischemic stroke related to acute consumption of cocaine. *CES Medicina* **2017**, *31*, 207–214. [CrossRef]
78. Vidale, S.; Peroni, R.; Di Palma, F.; Sampietro, A.; Gozzi, G.; Arnaboldi, M. Intra-arterial thrombolysis in a young patient with cocaine-associated stroke. *Neurol. Sci.* **2014**, *35*, 1465–1466. [CrossRef] [PubMed]
79. Renard, D.; Brunel, H.; Gaillard, N. Bilateral haemorrhagic infarction of the globus pallidus after cocaine and alcohol intoxication. *Acta Neurol. Belg.* **2009**, *109*, 159–161. [PubMed]
80. Sein Anand, J.; Chodorowski, Z.; Wisniewski, M.; Golska, A. A cocaine-associated quadriplegia and motor aphasia after first use of cocaine. *Przegl. Lek.* **2007**, *64*, 316–317. [PubMed]
81. Wolff, V.; Armspach, J.P.; Lauer, V.; Rouyer, O.; Bataillard, M.; Marescaux, C.; Geny, B. Cannabis-related stroke: Myth or reality? *Stroke* **2013**, *44*, 558–563. [CrossRef]
82. Zou, S.; Kumar, U. Cannabinoid Receptors and the Endocannabinoid System: Signaling and Function in the Central Nervous System. *Int. J. Mol. Sci.* **2018**, *19*, 833. [CrossRef]

83. Howlett, A.C.; Fleming, R.M. Cannabinoid inhibition of adenylate cyclase. Pharmacology of the response in neuroblastoma cell membranes. *Mol. Pharmacol.* **1984**, *26*, 532–538. [PubMed]
84. Pertwee, R.G. The pharmacology of cannabinoid receptors and their ligands: An overview. *Int. J. Obes.* **2006**, *30*, S13–S18. [CrossRef] [PubMed]
85. Wolff, V.; Armspach, J.P.; Lauer, V.; Rouyer, O.; Ducros, A.; Marescaux, C.; Geny, B. Ischaemic strokes with reversible vasoconstriction and without thunderclap headache: A variant of the reversible cerebral vasoconstriction syndrome? *Cerebrovasc. Dis.* **2015**, *39*, 31–38. [CrossRef] [PubMed]
86. Hemachandra, D.; McKetin, R.; Cherbuin, N.; Anstey, K.J. Heavy cannabis users at elevated risk of stroke: Evidence from a general population survey. *Aust. N. Z. J. Public Health* **2016**, *40*, 226–230. [CrossRef] [PubMed]
87. Rumalla, K.; Reddy, A.Y.; Mittal, M.K. Recreational marijuana use and acute ischemic stroke: A population-based analysis of hospitalized patients in the United States. *J. Neurol. Sci.* **2016**, *364*, 191–196. [CrossRef] [PubMed]
88. Atchaneeyasakul, K.; Torres, L.F.; Malik, A.M. Large Amount of Cannabis Ingestion Resulting in Spontaneous Intracerebral Hemorrhage: A Case Report. *J. Stroke Cerebrovasc. Dis.* **2017**, *26*, e138–e139. [CrossRef] [PubMed]
89. Ince, B.; Benbir, G.; Yuksel, O.; Koseoglu, L.; Uluduz, D. Both hemorrhagic and ischemic stroke following high doses of cannabis consumption. *Presse Med.* **2015**, *44*, 106–107. [CrossRef] [PubMed]
90. Deusch, E.; Kress, H.G.; Kraft, B.; Kozek-Langenecker, S.A. The procoagulatory effects of delta-9-tetrahydrocannabinol in human platelets. *Anesth. Analg.* **2004**, *99*, 1127–1130. [CrossRef]
91. Levy, R.; Schurr, A.; Nathan, I.; Dvilansky, A.; Livn, A. Impairment of ADP-Induced Platelet Aggregation by Hashish Components. *Thromb. Haemost.* **1976**, *36*, 634–640. [CrossRef]
92. Thanvi, B.R.; Treadwell, S.D. Cannabis and stroke: Is there a link? *Postgrad. Med. J.* **2009**, *85*, 80–83. [CrossRef]
93. Mateo, I.; Pinedo, A.; Gomez-Beldarrain, M.; Basterretxea, J.M.; Garcia-Monco, J.C. Recurrent stroke associated with cannabis use. *J. Neurol. Neurosurg. Psychiatry* **2005**, *76*, 435–437. [CrossRef] [PubMed]
94. Bailly, C.; Merceron, O.; Hammoudi, N.; Dorent, R.; Michel, P.L. Cannabis induced acute coronary syndrome in a young female. *Int. J. Cardiol.* **2010**, *143*, e4–e6. [CrossRef] [PubMed]
95. EMCDDA. *Medical Use of Cannabis and Cannabinoids: Questions and Answers for Policymaking*; Publications Office of the European Union: Luxembourg, Luxembourg, 2018.
96. Barber, P.A.; Pridmore, H.M.; Krishnamurthy, V.; Roberts, S.; Spriggs, D.A.; Carter, K.N.; Anderson, N.E. Cannabis, ischemic stroke, and transient ischemic attack: A case-control study. *Stroke* **2013**, *44*, 2327–2329. [CrossRef] [PubMed]
97. Jamil, M.; Zafar, A.; Adeel Faizi, S.; Zawar, I. Stroke from Vasospasm due to Marijuana Use: Can Cannabis Synergistically with Other Medications Trigger Cerebral Vasospasm? *Case Rep. Neurol. Med.* **2016**, *2016*, 5313795. [CrossRef] [PubMed]
98. Trojak, B.; Leclerq, S.; Meille, V.; Khoumri, C.; Chauvet-Gelinier, J.C.; Giroud, M.; Bonin, B.; Gisselmann, A. Stroke with neuropsychiatric sequelae after cannabis use in a man: A case report. *J. Med. Case Rep.* **2011**, *5*, 264. [CrossRef]
99. Wolff, V.; Lauer, V.; Rouyer, O.; Sellal, F.; Meyer, N.; Raul, J.S.; Sabourdy, C.; Boujan, F.; Jahn, C.; Beaujeux, R.; et al. Cannabis use, ischemic stroke, and multifocal intracranial vasoconstriction: A prospective study in 48 consecutive young patients. *Stroke* **2011**, *42*, 1778–1780. [CrossRef]
100. Shere, A.; Goyal, H. Cannabis can augment thrombolytic properties of rtPA: Intracranial hemorrhage in a heavy cannabis user. *Am. J. Emerg. Med.* **2017**, *35*, 1988-e1. [CrossRef]
101. Volpon, L.C.; Sousa, C.; Moreira, S.K.K.; Teixeira, S.R.; Carlotti, A. Multiple Cerebral Infarcts in a Young Patient Associated With Marijuana Use. *J. Addict. Med.* **2017**, *11*, 405–407. [CrossRef]
102. Tirkey, N.K.; Gupta, S. Acute Antero-Inferior Wall Ischaemia with Acute Ischaemic Stroke Caused by Oral Ingestion of Cannabis in a Young Male. *J. Assoc. Physicians India* **2016**, *64*, 93–94.
103. Baharnoori, M.; Kassardjian, C.D.; Saposnik, G. Cannabis use associated with capsular warning syndrome and ischemic stroke. *Can. J. Neurol. Sci.* **2014**, *41*, 272–273. [CrossRef]
104. Renard, D.; Taieb, G.; Gras-Combe, G.; Labauge, P. Cannabis-related myocardial infarction and cardioembolic stroke. *J. Stroke Cerebrovasc. Dis.* **2012**, *21*, 82–83. [CrossRef] [PubMed]
105. Castaneto, M.S.; Gorelick, D.A.; Desrosiers, N.A.; Hartman, R.L.; Pirard, S.; Huestis, M.A. Synthetic cannabinoids: Epidemiology, pharmacodynamics, and clinical implications. *Drug Alcohol Depend.* **2014**, *144*, 12–41. [CrossRef] [PubMed]

106. Seely, K.A.; Lapoint, J.; Moran, J.H.; Fattore, L. Spice drugs are more than harmless herbal blends: A review of the pharmacology and toxicology of synthetic cannabinoids. *Prog. Neuropsychopharmacol. Biol. Psychiatry* **2012**, *39*, 234–243. [CrossRef] [PubMed]
107. Tai, S.; Fantegrossi, W.E. Synthetic Cannabinoids: Pharmacology, Behavioral Effects, and Abuse Potential. *Curr. Addict. Rep.* **2014**, *1*, 129–136. [CrossRef] [PubMed]
108. Brents, L.K.; Reichard, E.E.; Zimmerman, S.M.; Moran, J.H.; Fantegrossi, W.E.; Prather, P.L. Phase I hydroxylated metabolites of the K2 synthetic cannabinoid JWH-018 retain in vitro and in vivo cannabinoid 1 receptor affinity and activity. *PLoS ONE* **2011**, *6*, e21917. [CrossRef] [PubMed]
109. Freeman, M.J.; Rose, D.Z.; Myers, M.A.; Gooch, C.L.; Bozeman, A.C.; Burgin, W.S. Ischemic stroke after use of the synthetic marijuana "spice". *Neurology* **2013**, *81*, 2090–2093. [CrossRef] [PubMed]
110. Rose, D.Z.; Guerrero, W.R.; Mokin, M.V.; Gooch, C.L.; Bozeman, A.C.; Pearson, J.M.; Burgin, W.S. Hemorrhagic stroke following use of the synthetic marijuana "spice". *Neurology* **2015**, *85*, 1177–1179. [CrossRef] [PubMed]
111. Hillard, C.J. Endocannabinoids and vascular function. *J. Pharmacol. Exp. Ther.* **2000**, *294*, 27–32. [PubMed]
112. Brents, L.K.; Prather, P.L. The K2/Spice phenomenon: Emergence, identification, legislation and metabolic characterization of synthetic cannabinoids in herbal incense products. *Drug Metab. Rev.* **2014**, *46*, 72–85. [CrossRef] [PubMed]
113. Bernson-Leung, M.E.; Leung, L.Y.; Kumar, S. Synthetic cannabis and acute ischemic stroke. *J. Stroke Cerebrovasc. Dis.* **2014**, *23*, 1239–1241. [CrossRef] [PubMed]
114. Faroqui, R.; Mena, P.; Wolfe, A.R.; Bibawy, J.; Visvikis, G.A.; Mantello, M.T. Acute carotid thrombosis and ischemic stroke following overdose of the synthetic cannabinoid K2 in a previously healthy young adult male. *Radiol. Case Rep.* **2018**, *13*, 747–752. [CrossRef] [PubMed]
115. Takematsu, M.; Hoffman, R.S.; Nelson, L.S.; Schechter, J.M.; Moran, J.H.; Wiener, S.W. A case of acute cerebral ischemia following inhalation of a synthetic cannabinoid. *Clin. Toxicol.* **2014**, *52*, 973–975. [CrossRef] [PubMed]
116. Lachenmeier, D.W.; Sproll, C.; Musshoff, F. Poppy seed foods and opiate drug testing—Where are we today? *Ther. Drug Monit.* **2010**, *32*, 11–18. [CrossRef] [PubMed]
117. Mars, S.G.; Bourgois, P.; Karandinos, G.; Montero, F.; Ciccarone, D. The Textures of Heroin: User Perspectives on "Black Tar" and Powder Heroin in Two U.S. Cities. *J. Psychoact. Drugs* **2016**, *48*, 270–278. [CrossRef] [PubMed]
118. Freye, E.; Levy, J. *Opioids in Medicine—A Comprehensive Review on the Mode of Action and the Use of Analgesics in Different Clinical Pain States*; Springer Science + Business Media BV: Dordrecht, The Netherlands, 2008.
119. Dinis-Oliveira, R.J.; Carvalho, F.; Moreira, R.; Duarte, J.A.; Proenca, J.B.; Santos, A.; Magalhaes, T. Clinical and forensic signs related to opioids abuse. *Curr. Drug Abus. Rev.* **2012**, *5*, 273–290. [CrossRef]
120. Yeh, S.Y. Urinary excretion of morphine and its metabolites in morphine-dependent subjects. *J. Pharmacol. Exp. Ther.* **1975**, *192*, 201–210. [PubMed]
121. Meyer, M.R.; Schutz, A.; Maurer, H.H. Contribution of human esterases to the metabolism of selected drugs of abuse. *Toxicol. Lett.* **2015**, *232*, 159–166. [CrossRef] [PubMed]
122. Fonseca, A.C.; Ferro, J.M. Drug abuse and stroke. *Curr. Neurol. Neurosci. Rep.* **2013**, *13*, 325. [CrossRef]
123. Niehaus, L.; Roricht, S.; Meyer, B.U.; Sander, B. Nuclear magnetic resonance tomography detection of heroin-associated CNS lesions. *Aktuelle Radiol.* **1997**, *7*, 309–311.
124. Enevoldson, T.P. Recreational drugs and their neurological consequences. *J. Neurol. Neurosurg. Psychiatry* **2004**, *75*, iii9–iii15. [CrossRef]
125. Bolz, J.; Meves, S.H.; Kara, K.; Reinacher-Schick, A.; Gold, R.; Krogias, C. Multiple cerebral infarctions in a young patient with heroin-induced hypereosinophilic syndrome. *J. Neurol. Sci.* **2015**, *356*, 193–195. [CrossRef] [PubMed]
126. Prick, J.J.; Gabreels-Festen, A.A.; Korten, J.J.; van der Wiel, T.W. Neurological manifestations of the hypereosinophilic syndrome (HES). *Clin. Neurol. Neurosurg.* **1988**, *90*, 269–273. [CrossRef]
127. Hamzei Moqaddam, A.; Ahmadi Musavi, S.M.R.; Khademizadeh, K. Relationship of opium dependency and stroke. *Addict. Health* **2009**, *1*, 6–10. [PubMed]
128. Kumar, N.; Bhalla, M.C.; Frey, J.A.; Southern, A. Intraparenchymal hemorrhage after heroin use. *Am. J. Emerg. Med.* **2015**, *33*, 1109-e3. [CrossRef] [PubMed]
129. Alquist, C.R.; McGoey, R.; Bastian, F.; Newman, W., 3rd. Bilateral globus pallidus lesions. *J. La. State Med. Soc.* **2012**, *164*, 145–146. [PubMed]

130. Vila, N.; Chamorro, A. Ballistic movements due to ischemic infarcts after intravenous heroin overdose: Report of two cases. *Clin. Neurol. Neurosurg.* **1997**, *99*, 259–262. [CrossRef]
131. Brust, J.C.; Richter, R.W. Stroke associated with addiction to heroin. *J. Neurol. Neurosurg. Psychiatry* **1976**, *39*, 194–199. [CrossRef]
132. Lee, C.W.; Muo, C.H.; Liang, J.A.; Sung, F.C.; Kao, C.H. Association of intensive morphine treatment and increased stroke incidence in prostate cancer patients: A population-based nested case-control study. *Jpn. J. Clin. Oncol.* **2013**, *43*, 776–781. [CrossRef]
133. Hamzei-Moghaddam, A.; Shafa, M.A.; Khanjani, N.; Farahat, R. Frequency of Opium Addiction in Patients with Ischemic Stroke and Comparing their Cerebrovascular Doppler Ultrasound Changes to Non-Addicts. *Addict. Health* **2013**, *5*, 95–101.
134. Benoilid, A.; Collongues, N.; de Seze, J.; Blanc, F. Heroin inhalation-induced unilateral complete hippocampal stroke. *Neurocase* **2013**, *19*, 313–315. [CrossRef]
135. Hsu, W.Y.; Chiu, N.Y.; Liao, Y.C. Rhabdomyolysis and brain ischemic stroke in a heroin-dependent male under methadone maintenance therapy. *Acta Psychiatr. Scand.* **2009**, *120*, 76–79. [CrossRef] [PubMed]
136. Brenu, E.W.; McNaughton, L.; Marshall-Gradisnik, S.M. Is there a potential immune dysfunction with anabolic androgenic steroid use: A review. *Mini Rev. Med. Chem.* **2011**, *11*, 438–445. [CrossRef] [PubMed]
137. Kenna, G.A.; Lewis, D.C. Risk factors for alcohol and other drug use by healthcare professionals. *Subst. Abus. Treat. Prev. Policy* **2008**, *3*, 3. [CrossRef] [PubMed]
138. Hartgens, F.; Rietjens, G.; Keizer, H.A.; Kuipers, H.; Wolffenbuttel, B.H. Effects of androgenic-anabolic steroids on apolipoproteins and lipoprotein (a). *Br. J. Sports Med.* **2004**, *38*, 253–259. [CrossRef] [PubMed]
139. Santamarina, R.D.; Besocke, A.G.; Romano, L.M.; Ioli, P.L.; Gonorazky, S.E. Ischemic stroke related to anabolic abuse. *Clin. Neuropharmacol.* **2008**, *31*, 80–85. [CrossRef] [PubMed]
140. Shamloul, R.M.; Aborayah, A.F.; Hashad, A.; Abd-Allah, F. Anabolic steroids abuse-induced cardiomyopathy and ischaemic stroke in a young male patient. *BMJ Case Rep.* **2014**, *2014*. [CrossRef] [PubMed]
141. Youssef, M.Y.; Alqallaf, A.; Abdella, N. Anabolic androgenic steroid-induced cardiomyopathy, stroke and peripheral vascular disease. *BMJ Case Rep.* **2011**, *2011*. [CrossRef] [PubMed]
142. Pearson, A.C.; Schiff, M.; Mrosek, D.; Labovitz, A.J.; Williams, G.A. Left ventricular diastolic function in weight lifters. *Am. J. Cardiol.* **1986**, *58*, 1254–1259. [CrossRef]
143. Lippi, G.; Banfi, G. Doping and thrombosis in sports. *Semin. Thromb. Hemost.* **2011**, *37*, 918–928. [CrossRef]
144. Beutel, A.; Bergamaschi, C.T.; Campos, R.R. Effects of chronic anabolic steroid treatment on tonic and reflex cardiovascular control in male rats. *J. Steroid Biochem. Mol. Biol.* **2005**, *93*, 43–48. [CrossRef]
145. Santos, M.A.; Oliveira, C.V.; Silva, A.S. Adverse cardiovascular effects from the use of anabolic-androgenic steroids as ergogenic resources. *Subst. Use Misuse* **2014**, *49*, 1132–1137. [CrossRef] [PubMed]
146. Achar, S.; Rostamian, A.; Narayan, S.M. Cardiac and metabolic effects of anabolic-androgenic steroid abuse on lipids, blood pressure, left ventricular dimensions, and rhythm. *Am. J. Cardiol.* **2010**, *106*, 893–901. [CrossRef] [PubMed]
147. D'Ascenzo, S.; Millimaggi, D.; Di Massimo, C.; Saccani-Jotti, G.; Botre, F.; Carta, G.; Tozzi-Ciancarelli, M.G.; Pavan, A.; Dolo, V. Detrimental effects of anabolic steroids on human endothelial cells. *Toxicol. Lett.* **2007**, *169*, 129–136. [CrossRef] [PubMed]
148. Hartgens, F.; Kuipers, H. Effects of androgenic-anabolic steroids in athletes. *Sports Med.* **2004**, *34*, 513–554. [CrossRef] [PubMed]
149. Liu, P.Y.; Death, A.K.; Handelsman, D.J. Androgens and cardiovascular disease. *Endocr. Rev.* **2003**, *24*, 313–340. [CrossRef] [PubMed]
150. Rocha, F.L.; Carmo, E.C.; Roque, F.R.; Hashimoto, N.Y.; Rossoni, L.V.; Frimm, C.; Aneas, I.; Negrao, C.E.; Krieger, J.E.; Oliveira, E.M. Anabolic steroids induce cardiac renin-angiotensin system and impair the beneficial effects of aerobic training in rats. *Am. J. Physiol. Heart Circ. Physiol.* **2007**, *293*, H3575–H3583. [CrossRef] [PubMed]
151. Do Carmo, E.C.; Fernandes, T.; Koike, D.; Da Silva, N.D., Jr.; Mattos, K.C.; Rosa, K.T.; Barretti, D.; Melo, S.F.; Wichi, R.B.; Irigoyen, M.C.; et al. Anabolic steroid associated to physical training induces deleterious cardiac effects. *Med. Sci. Sports Exerc.* **2011**, *43*, 1836–1848. [CrossRef] [PubMed]
152. Schooling, C.M.; Luo, S.; Au Yeung, S.L.; Thompson, D.J.; Karthikeyan, S.; Bolton, T.R.; Mason, A.M.; Ingelsson, E.; Burgess, S. Genetic predictors of testosterone and their associations with cardiovascular disease and risk factors: A Mendelian randomization investigation. *Int. J. Cardiol.* **2018**, *267*, 171–176. [CrossRef] [PubMed]

153. Cole, A.P.; Hanske, J. Impact of testosterone replacement therapy on thromboembolism, heart disease and obstructive sleep apnoea in men. *BJU Int.* **2018**, *121*, 811–818. [CrossRef] [PubMed]
154. Normann, S.; de Veber, G.; Fobker, M.; Langer, C.; Kenet, G.; Bernard, T.J.; Fiedler, B.; Sträter, R.; Goldenberg, N.A.; Nowak-Göttl, U. Role of endogenous testosterone concentration in pediatric stroke. *Ann. Neurol.* **2009**, *66*, 754–758. [CrossRef] [PubMed]
155. Bhasin, S.; Brito, J.P.; Cunningham, G.R.; Hayes, F.J.; Hodis, H.N.; Matsumoto, A.M.; Snyder, P.J.; Swerdloff, R.S.; Wu, F.C.; Yialamas, M.A. Testosterone Therapy in Men With Hypogonadism: An Endocrine Society Clinical Practice Guideline. *J. Clin. Endocrinol. Metab.* **2018**, *103*, 1715–1744. [CrossRef] [PubMed]
156. El Scheich, T.; Weber, A.A.; Klee, D.; Schweiger, D.; Mayatepek, E.; Karenfort, M. Adolescent ischemic stroke associated with anabolic steroid and cannabis abuse. *J. Pediatr. Endocrinol. Metab.* **2013**, *26*, 161–165. [CrossRef] [PubMed]
157. Juhan-Vague, I.; Pyke, S.D.; Alessi, M.C.; Jespersen, J.; Haverkate, F.; Thompson, S.G. Fibrinolytic factors and the risk of myocardial infarction or sudden death in patients with angina pectoris. ECAT Study Group. European Concerted Action on Thrombosis and Disabilities. *Circulation* **1996**, *94*, 2057–2063. [CrossRef] [PubMed]
158. Siokas, V.; Dardiotis, E.; Sokolakis, T.; Kotoula, M.; Tachmitzi, S.V.; Chatzoulis, D.Z.; Almpanidou, P.; Stefanidis, I.; Hadjigeorgiou, G.M.; Tsironi, E.E. Plasminogen Activator Inhibitor Type-1 Tag Single-Nucleotide Polymorphisms in Patients with Diabetes Mellitus Type 2 and Diabetic Retinopathy. *Curr. Eye Res.* **2017**, *42*, 1048–1053. [CrossRef] [PubMed]
159. Winkler, U.H. Effects of androgens on haemostasis. *Maturitas* **1996**, *24*, 147–155. [CrossRef]
160. Nieminen, M.S.; Ramo, M.P.; Viitasalo, M.; Heikkila, P.; Karjalainen, J.; Mantysaari, M.; Heikkila, J. Serious cardiovascular side effects of large doses of anabolic steroids in weight lifters. *Eur. Heart J.* **1996**, *17*, 1576–1583. [CrossRef] [PubMed]
161. Kalin, M.F.; Zumoff, B. Sex hormones and coronary disease: A review of the clinical studies. *Steroids* **1990**, *55*, 330–352. [CrossRef]
162. Bachman, E.; Feng, R.; Travison, T.; Li, M.; Olbina, G.; Ostland, V.; Ulloor, J.; Zhang, A.; Basaria, S.; Ganz, T.; et al. Testosterone suppresses hepcidin in men: A potential mechanism for testosterone-induced erythrocytosis. *J. Clin. Endocrinol. Metab.* **2010**, *95*, 4743–4747. [CrossRef]
163. Bachman, E.; Travison, T.G.; Basaria, S.; Davda, M.N.; Guo, W.; Li, M.; Connor Westfall, J.; Bae, H.; Gordeuk, V.; Bhasin, S. Testosterone induces erythrocytosis via increased erythropoietin and suppressed hepcidin: Evidence for a new erythropoietin/hemoglobin set point. *J. Gerontol. A Biol. Sci. Med. Sci.* **2014**, *69*, 725–735. [CrossRef]
164. Young, N.S. Telomere biology and telomere diseases: Implications for practice and research. *Hematol. Am. Soc. Hematol. Educ. Program* **2010**, *2010*, 30–35. [CrossRef]
165. Tsarouhas, K.; Kioukia-Fougia, N.; Papalexis, P.; Tsatsakis, A.; Kouretas, D.; Bacopoulou, F.; Tsitsimpikou, C. Use of nutritional supplements contaminated with banned doping substances by recreational adolescent athletes in Athens, Greece. *Food Chem. Toxicol. Int. J. Publ. Br. Ind. Biol. Res. Assoc.* **2018**, *115*, 447–450. [CrossRef] [PubMed]
166. Tsitsimpikou, C.; Chrisostomou, N.; Papalexis, P.; Tsarouhas, K.; Tsatsakis, A.; Jamurtas, A. The use of nutritional supplements among recreational athletes in Athens, Greece. *Int. J. Sport Nutr. Exerc. Metab.* **2011**, *21*, 377–384. [CrossRef] [PubMed]
167. Vasilaki, F.; Tsitsimpikou, C.; Tsarouhas, K.; Germanakis, I.; Tzardi, M.; Kavvalakis, M.; Ozcagli, E.; Kouretas, D.; Tsatsakis, A.M. Cardiotoxicity in rabbits after long-term nandrolone decanoate administration. *Toxicol. Lett.* **2016**, *241*, 143–151. [CrossRef] [PubMed]
168. Baggish, A.L.; Weiner, R.B.; Kanayama, G.; Hudson, J.I.; Picard, M.H.; Hutter, A.M., Jr.; Pope, H.G., Jr. Long-term anabolic-androgenic steroid use is associated with left ventricular dysfunction. *Circ. Heart Fail.* **2010**, *3*, 472–476. [CrossRef] [PubMed]
169. Sattler, F.R.; Jaque, S.V.; Schroeder, E.T.; Olson, C.; Dube, M.P.; Martinez, C.; Briggs, W.; Horton, R.; Azen, S. Effects of pharmacological doses of nandrolone decanoate and progressive resistance training in immunodeficient patients infected with human immunodeficiency virus. *J. Clin. Endocrinol. Metab.* **1999**, *84*, 1268–1276. [CrossRef] [PubMed]

170. Shimada, Y.; Yoritaka, A.; Tanaka, Y.; Miyamoto, N.; Ueno, Y.; Hattori, N.; Takao, U. Cerebral Infarction in a Young Man Using High-dose Anabolic Steroids. *J. Stroke Cerebrovasc. Dis.* **2012**, *21*, 906-e9. [CrossRef] [PubMed]
171. D'Andrea, A.; Caso, P.; Salerno, G.; Scarafile, R.; De Corato, G.; Mita, C.; Di Salvo, G.; Severino, S.; Cuomo, S.; Liccardo, B.; et al. Left ventricular early myocardial dysfunction after chronic misuse of anabolic androgenic steroids: A Doppler myocardial and strain imaging analysis. *Br. J. Sports Med.* **2007**, *41*, 149–155. [CrossRef] [PubMed]
172. Garcia-Esperon, C.; Hervas-Garcia, J.V.; Jimenez-Gonzalez, M.; Perez de la Ossa-Herrero, N.; Gomis-Cortina, M.; Dorado-Bouix, L.; Lopez-Cancio Martinez, E.; Castano-Duque, C.H.; Millan-Torne, M.; Davalos, A. [Ingestion of anabolic steroids and ischaemic stroke. A clinical case report and review of the literature]. *Rev. Neurol.* **2013**, *56*, 327–331.
173. Low, M.S.; Vilcassim, S.; Fedele, P.; Grigoriadis, G. Anabolic androgenic steroids, an easily forgotten cause of polycythaemia and cerebral infarction. *Intern. Med. J.* **2016**, *46*, 497–499. [CrossRef]
174. Jouanjus, E.; Lapeyre-Mestre, M.; Micallef, J. Cannabis use: Signal of increasing risk of serious cardiovascular disorders. *J. Am. Heart Assoc.* **2014**, *3*, e000638. [CrossRef]

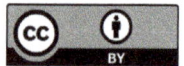

© 2019 by the authors. Licensee MDPI, Basel, Switzerland. This article is an open access article distributed under the terms and conditions of the Creative Commons Attribution (CC BY) license (http://creativecommons.org/licenses/by/4.0/).

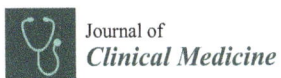

Article

Transient Laterality of Cerebral Oxygenation Changes in Response to Head-of-Bed Manipulation in Acute Ischemic Stroke

Naoki Katayama [1,2], Keiichi Odagiri [1,*], Akio Hakamata [1], Naoki Inui [1], Katsuya Yamauchi [3] and Hiroshi Watanabe [1]

1. Department of Clinical Pharmacology and Therapeutics, Hamamatsu University School of Medicine, 1-20-1 Handayama, Higashi-ku, Hamamatsu 431-3192, Japan; katayama_20@yahoo.co.jp (N.K.); hakamata@hama-med.ac.jp (A.H.); inui@hama-med.ac.jp (N.I.); hwat@hama-med.ac.jp (H.W.)
2. Department of Rehabilitation Medicine, Seirei Mikatahara General Hospital, 3453 Mikatahara-cho, Kita-ku, Hamamatsu 433-8558, Japan
3. Department of Rehabilitation Medicine, Hamamatsu University Hospital, 1-20-1 Handayama, Higashi-ku, Hamamatsu 431-3192, Japan; yamakatu@hama-med.ac.jp
* Correspondence: kodagiri@hama-med.ac.jp; Tel.: +81-53-435-2006

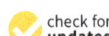

Received: 4 September 2019; Accepted: 18 October 2019; Published: 19 October 2019

Abstract: Background: Cerebral oxygenation monitoring provides important information for optimizing individualized management in patients with acute ischemic stroke (AIS). Although changes in cerebral oxygenation are known to occur in response to head-of-bed (HOB) elevation within 72 h after onset, changes in cerebral oxygenation during stroke recovery are unclear. We compared changes in total- (tHb), oxygenated- (HbO$_2$), and deoxygenated-hemoglobin (deoxyHb) concentrations in response to HOB manipulation between the timeframes within 72 h and 7–10 days after AIS onset. Methods: We measured forehead ΔtHb, ΔHbO$_2$, and ΔdeoxyHb in response to HOB elevation (30°) within 72 h (first measurement) and 7–10 days (second measurement) after AIS onset using time-resolved near-infrared spectroscopy. Results: We enrolled 30 participants (mean age 72.8 ± 11.3 years; 13 women) with a first AIS. There were no significant differences in ΔtHb, ΔHbO$_2$, or ΔdeoxyHb measurements on the infarct or contra-infarct side. At the first measurement, ΔtHb, ΔHbO$_2$, and ΔdeoxyHb measured on the contra-infarct side did not correlate with those measured on the infarct side: ΔtHb ($r = 0.114$, $p = 0.539$); ΔHbO$_2$ ($r = 0.143$, $p = 0.440$); ΔdeoxyHb ($r = 0.227$, $p = 0.221$). Notably, at the second measurement, correlation coefficients of ΔtHb and ΔHbO$_2$ between the contra-infarct and infarct sides were statistically significant: ΔtHb ($r = 0.491$, $p = 0.008$); ΔHbO$_2$ ($r = 0.479$, $p = 0.010$); ΔdeoxyHb ($r = 0.358$, $p = 0.054$). Conclusion. Although changes in cerebral oxygenation in response to HOB elevation had a laterality difference between hemispheres within 72 h of AIS onset, the difference had decreased, at least partially, 7–10 days after AIS onset.

Keywords: cerebral blood volume; hemodynamics; near-infrared spectroscopy; optical imaging; rehabilitation; stroke

1. Introduction

Acute ischemic stroke (AIS) is a significant cause of permanent disability [1]. Early rehabilitation for AIS patients—considered an important issue in poststroke functional outcomes—has been recommended in recent guidelines [2,3]. A large-scale clinical trial; however, provided evidence that early intervention was not associated with disability outcomes [4]. It is also recognized that supine AIS patients have improved cerebral blood flow (CBF) and oxygenation, although with an increased risk of aspiration pneumonia [5–8]. Another clinical trial revealed that a head-up position initiated within

24 h of AIS onset was not associated with a disability outcome or severe adverse effects, including pneumonia [9]. Thus, the optimal head position in patients with AIS is still unknown.

Near-infrared spectroscopy (NIRS) noninvasively measures hemoglobin (Hb) levels in the brain [10]. Compared with other technologies, such as transcranial Doppler (TCD) and positron emission tomography (PET), NIRS has several advantages: (1) it allows flexible measurements in sitting, standing, and moving subjects; (2) it is an irradiation-based, completely noninvasive technique that does not cause adverse effects on the body during repeated measurements, even in children; (3) it has high time resolution; and (4) it is compact and portable. Because of these advantages, the use of NIRS, such as cerebral oxygen monitors, is increasing in the medical field despite its drawbacks (e.g., possible interferences caused by attachment of optodes, shallow measurement depth, effects of drugs influencing cerebral blood flow or cutaneous blood flow, artifacts of cutaneous blood flow, and narrow measurement territory depending on the attachment site of optode). This increase is because these systems are simple but enable the observation of changes in brain activity over time via monitoring of Hb levels, which reflect fluctuations in regional cerebral blood flow. Indeed, NIRS can be useful to detect the intraindividual fluctuation and the interindividual difference of cerebral hemodynamic response in response to posture change [11]. Thus, well-known applications of NIRS include the monitoring of cerebral blood flow and hypoxic conditions in a variety of clinical settings [12–14]. During the last two decades, several studies have used the NIRS system to evaluate changes in cerebral oxygenation in upright AIS patients [7,15–17]. Their findings provided important information for optimal individualized management, based on cerebral oxygenation monitoring in AIS patients. Nevertheless, correlation of the total- (tHb), oxygenated- (HbO_2), and deoxygenated-hemoglobin (deoxyHb) concentrations in response to head-of-bed (HOB) elevation between the infarct and contra-infarct sides have never been assessed, leaving the changes in cerebral oxygenation during stroke recovery not well understood. In the current exploratory study, we therefore aim to compare the changes in tHb (ΔtHb), HbO_2 (ΔHbO_2), and deoxyHb (ΔdeoxyHb) in response to HOB manipulation between the timeframes within 72 h and 7–10 days after AIS onset.

2. Methods

2.1. Study Design and Participants

This study was designed as a single-center exploratory study to compare the changes in cerebral oxygenation in response to HOB manipulation between different time points in AIS patients, and it was conducted at Seirei Mikatahara General Hospital, Hamamatsu, Japan. Study participants were consecutively recruited from among acute cerebral infarction patients hospitalized at our hospital from September 2016 to March 2017. Eligible patients were those having a first-ever ischemic stroke and who had been hospitalized within 24 h of symptoms onset. Main exclusion criteria were a patient with infratentorial stroke; a history of cerebral disease (prior stroke, brain contusion, brain tumor, brain infections, intracerebral hemorrhage and trauma); orthostatic hypotension; taking antihypertensive agents after hospitalization; or unable to participate in this study (could not maintain a 30° passive sitting position; presence of a skin disease (not suitable for applying a probe to the forehead); unable to follow verbal instructions).

2.2. Ethics and Study Registration

This study protocol complied with the Helsinki Declaration. The institutional research review board of Seirei Mikatahara General Hospital and Hamamatsu University School of Medicine approved the study (Approved number 16-15 and 16-001). Written informed consent was provided by all participants. The study was registered at the UMIN Clinical Trials Registry (URL: http://www.umin.ac.jp/ctr/index.htm. Unique identifier: UMIN 000022904).

2.3. Cerebral Hemoglobin Concentration Measurement by Time-Resolved NIRS

We used a single-channel, time-resolved NIRS system (TRS-10; Hamamatsu Photonics K.K., Hamamatsu, Japan) to measure bilateral forehead cerebral (prefrontal cortex) hemoglobin concentration. The temporal profile obtained from TRS-10 measurement was fitted with that obtained from the theoretical solution of the photon diffusion equation (DE) [18], because the DE-fit method could provide information about the hemodynamic changes in the depth direction [19]. The TRS-10 system consists of three pulsed laser diodes with wavelengths of 759, 797, and 833 nm, having a duration of 100 ps and repetition frequency of 5 MHz. An optode, which includes infrared light irradiation and reception probes in a single device, was fixed on the participant's head with Velcro and a headband so the irradiated infrared light was positioned at Fp1 and Fp2 according to the International 10-20 system. This NIRS device can measure the tHb, HbO_2, and deoxyHb of tissues within a semicircular area between the irradiation and reception probes. The measurement depth increases with increased distance between the irradiation and reception probes (limit of 5 cm), because the farther the distance, the weaker the light reaching the reception probe. One study reporting simultaneous measurements with TRS-10 and PET found that TRS-10 measurements with irradiation and reception probes 3 cm apart significantly correlated with PET measurements around gray matter [20]. We therefore set the distance between the irradiation and reception probes at 3 cm outside the infrared reception port on the optode.

2.4. Cerebral Blood Hemoglobin Concentration Measurements Protocol

Based on previous studies [21–24], we measured forehead tHb, HbO_2, and deoxyHb within 72 h (first measurement) and 7–10 days (second measurement) after AIS onset. After placing probes on the forehead, the participant laid on his/her back. Data were collected every 10 s for 5 min at each HOB angle (0°, 30°, 0°) sequentially. At each HOB angle, the mean tHb, HbO_2, and deoxyHb values were calculated after discarding data obtained during the first minute, because it took 15 s to change the HOB position of the bed. Because the TRS-10 system has a single channel, two consecutive measurements were conducted in each participant. We first measured forehead tHb, HbO_2, and deoxyHb on the contra-infarct side and then on the infarct side. Systemic blood pressure and heart rate were also measured for 1 min in each position using an automatic hemodynamometer (HBP1300; Omron Corp., Tokyo, Japan).

2.5. Statistical Analysis

Values are expressed as means ± standard deviations (SD) or medians (interquartile range) (nonparametrically distributed values) of the indicated numbers or proportions (%). Changes in systemic blood pressure, heart rate, tHb, HbO_2, and deoxyHb were compared with the baseline (HOB 0°). These measurement values at HOB 30° were compared with those at HOB 0° using the Wilcoxon signed-rank test. Correlations between the infarct and contra-infarct sides for each measurement were assessed using Spearman's rank correlation coefficient. The significance of the difference between the two correlation coefficients was evaluated using the Fisher r-to-z transformation. $p < 0.05$ was regarded as indicating statistical significance. All statistical analyses were performed using PASW Statistics version 18.0.0 (IBM Co., Armonk, NY, USA) and Microsoft Excel 2016 (Microsoft Co., Redmond, WA, USA).

3. Results

3.1. Study Participants' Characteristics

Altogether, 32 AIS patients met the inclusion criteria and were enrolled. Two participants died before the second measurements and were excluded from the analyses. The participants' characteristics are shown in Table 1.

Table 1. Patients' characteristics.

Characteristic	Value
Age, year	72.8 ± 11.3
Female sex, n (%)	13 (43.3)
Height (cm)	158.0 ± 11.6
Body weight (kg)	56.0 ± 14.4
Body mass index (kg/m^2)	22.1 ± 3.1
Stroke side (right/left)	11/19
NIHSS score	7.6 ± 4.9
TOAST classification, n (%)	
Large-artery atherosclerosis	10 (33.3)
Small-vessel occlusion	10 (33.3)
Cardioembolism	6 (20.0)
Stroke of other determined etiology	4 (13.3)
Stroke of undetermined etiology	0 (0)
Vascular territorial segmentation, n (%)	
Anterior cerebral artery	6 (20.0)
Middle cerebral artery	17 (56.7)
Posterior cerebral artery	7 (20.3)
Medical history n (%)	
Hypertension	18 (60.0)
Diabetes mellitus	8 (26.7)
Dyslipidemia	22 (73.3)
Chronic atrial fibrillation	4 (13.3)
Tobacco use	12 (40.0)

Data are expressed as means ± Standard deviation unless otherwise stated; TOAST—Trial of Org 10172 in Acute Stroke Treatment; NIHSS—National Institutes of Health Stroke Scale.

3.2. Changes in Blood Pressure, Heart Rate, tHb, HbO$_2$, and deoxyHb with HOB Elevation

Table 2 shows the changes in systolic (SBP) and diastolic (DBP) blood pressures and the heart rate in response to HOB elevations from 0° to 30°. These HOB elevations did not affect any hemodynamic parameters. There were also no intraindividual differences in the SBP or heart rate at baseline measurements (HOB 0°) at each measurement session (first measurement: SBP ($p = 0.74$), DBP ($p = 0.87$), heart rate ($p = 0.94$); second measurement: SBP ($p = 0.83$), DBP ($p = 0.94$), heart rate ($p = 0.30$).

Table 2. Comparisons of the systemic blood pressure and heart rate in response to HOB manipulation.

Parameters	Item Measured	HOB 0°	HOB 30°	Difference	p
First Measurement					
Contra-infarct Side	sBP (mmHg)	137.6 ± 20.9	137.7 ± 19.8	0.1 ± 4.1	0.90
	dBP (mmHg)	75.9 ± 11.7	76.9 ± 10.6	1.0 ± 5.4	0.91
	HR (bpm)	73.5 ± 10.4	73.5 ± 9.7	0.0 ± 3.5	0.95
Infarct Side	sBP (mmHg)	137.9 ± 20.6	137.3 ± 19.8	−0.6 ± 3.7	0.39
	dBP (mmHg)	75.9 ± 11.2	76.4 ± 10.9	0.5 ± 4.6	0.63
	HR (bpm)	73.6 ± 11.0	73.4 ± 11.4	−0.2 ± 3.6	0.86
Second Measurement					
Contra-Infarct Side	sBP (mmHg)	128.9 ± 16.5	129.8 ± 15.0	0.9 ± 5.1	0.53
	dBP (mmHg)	71.0 ± 9.0	71.1 ± 8.6	0.0 ± 3.9	0.51
	HR (bpm)	75.6 ± 8.1	76.5 ± 7.8	0.9 ± 3.9	0.36
Infarct Side	sBP (mmHg)	129.5 ± 15.1	128.7 ± 15.6	−0.8 ± 5.3	0.10
	dBP (mmHg)	71.0 ± 8.4	70.3 ± 8.3	−0.7 ± 4.6	0.24
	HR (bpm)	74.8 ± 8.4	75.1 ± 7.7	0.3 ± 3.1	0.21

Data are expressed as means ± Standard deviation; HOB—head-of-bed, sBP—systolic blood pressure; dBP—diastolic blood pressure; HR—heart rate; bpm—beats per minute; mmHg—millimeters of mercury.

3.3. Changes in Cerebral Hemoglobin Concentrations with HOB Elevation

Figure 1 shows the time-series changes in the tHb in response to HOB manipulation. Changes in the tHb showed large interindividual differences, which were also observed in the changes in the HbO$_2$ and deoxyHb (Figure 2; Figure 3). There were no significant differences in the ΔtHb, ΔHbO$_2$, or ΔdeoxyHb on either the infarct or the contra-infarct side between the two measurements.

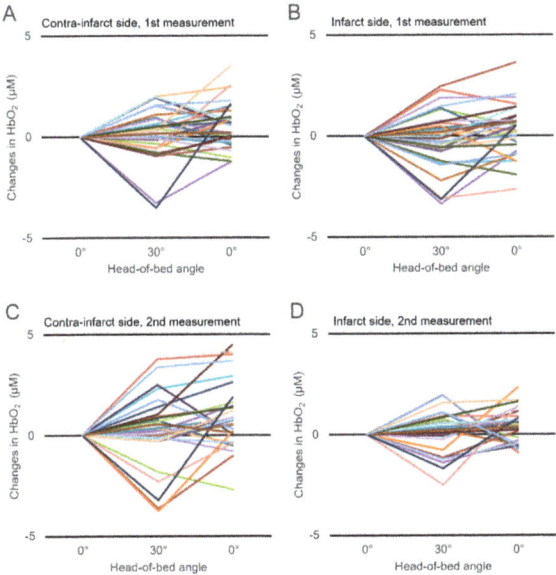

Figure 1. Time-series changes in the cerebral total hemoglobin (tHb) concentration in response to head-of-bed manipulation (from 0° to 30°) for 30 participants within 72 h of onset of acute ischemic stroke (AIS) (first measurement) on the contra-infarct (contralateral) side (**A**) and infarct side (**B**) and those measured 7–10 days after onset of AIS (second measurement) on the contra-infarct side (**C**) and infarct side (**D**).

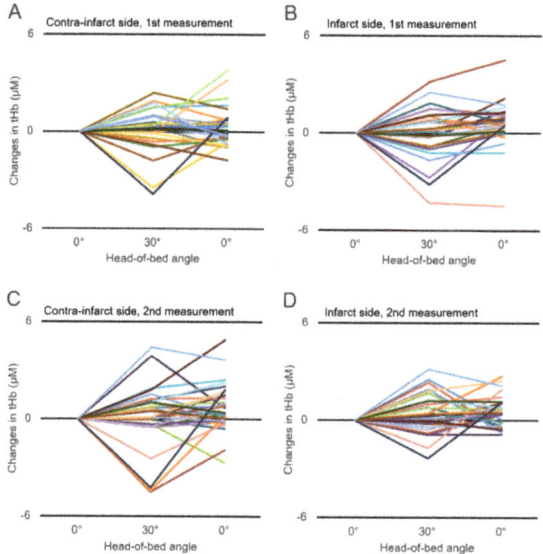

Figure 2. Time-series changes in the cerebral oxygenated-hemoglobin (HbO$_2$) concentration in response to head-of-bed manipulation for 30 participants within 72 h of AIS onset (first measurement) on the contra-infarct side (**A**) and infarct side (**B**) and those measured 7–10 days after AIS onset (second measurement) on the contra-infarct side (**C**) and infarct side (**D**).

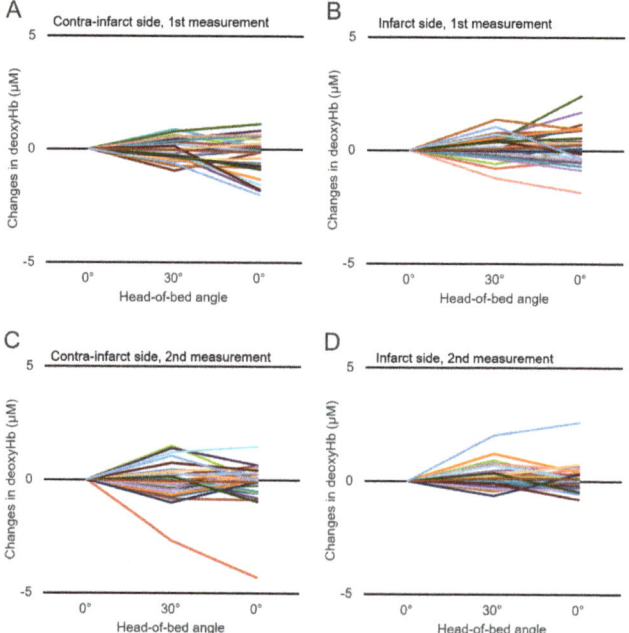

Figure 3. Time-series changes in the cerebral deoxygenated-hemoglobin (deoxyHb) concentration in response to head-of-bed manipulation for 30 participants within 72 h of AIS onset (first measurement) on the contra-infarct side (**A**) and infarct side (**B**) and those measured 7–10 days after onset of AIS (second measurement) on the contra-infarct side (**C**) and infarct side (**D**).

3.4. Correlations of Hemoglobin Concentration Changes with HOB Elevation between Measurements

Figure 4 shows the correlations of the ΔtHb, ΔHbO$_2$, and ΔdeoxyHb in response to HOB elevation between the first and second measurements for each hemisphere. The first measurements of the ΔtHb and ΔHbO$_2$ were significantly correlated with those at the second measurements for either hemisphere (ΔtHb: contra-infarct side ($r = 0.569$, $p = 0.020$), infarct side ($r = 0.408$, $p = 0.028$); ΔHbO$_2$: contra-infarct side ($r = 0.576$, $p = 0.020$), infarct side ($r = 0.378$, $p = 0.042$)). Although correlation coefficients in the contra-infarct side seemed to indicate a stronger relation than those in the infarct side, there were no statistically significant differences for ΔtHb or ΔHbO$_2$ (ΔtHb ($z = 0.772$, $p = 0.441$); ΔHbO$_2$ ($z = 0.955$, $p = 0.342$)), ΔdeoxyHb did not show a significant correlation between the first and second measurements (contra-infarct side ($z = 0.024$, $p = 0.896$); infarct side ($z = 0.176$, $p = 0.345$)).

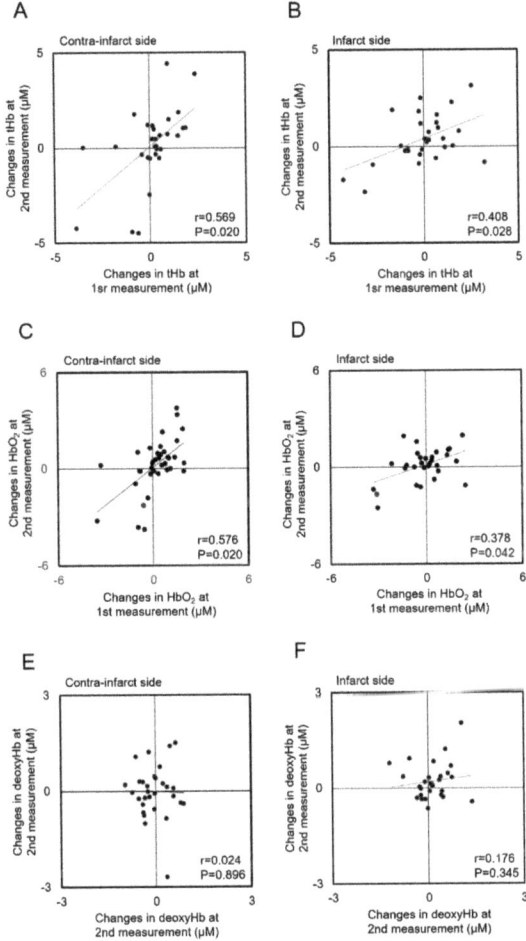

Figure 4. Scatterplots of the changes in total-hemoglobin (tHb) (**A** and **B**), oxygenated-hemoglobin (HbO$_2$) (**C** and **D**), and deoxygenated-hemoglobin (deoxyHb) (**E** and **F**) concentrations in response to head-of-bed elevation (from 0° to 30°) between the first and second measurements for each hemisphere.

3.5. Correlations of Hemoglobin Concentration Changes with HOB Elevation between Infarct and Contra-Infarct Sides

Figure 5 shows the correlations of ΔtHb, ΔHbO$_2$, and ΔdeoxyHb in response to HOB elevation between the infarct and contra-infarct sides. At the first measurement, ΔtHb, ΔHbO$_2$, and ΔdeoxyHb measured on the contra-infarct side did not correlate with those on the infarct side (ΔtHb (r = 0.114, p = 0.539), ΔHbO$_2$ (r = 0.143, p = 0.440); ΔdeoxyHb (r = 0.227, p = 0.221)) (Figure 5A–C). Notably, the correlation coefficients of ΔtHb, ΔHbO$_2$, and ΔdeoxyHb values between the infarct and contra-infarct sides at the second measurement were statistically significant, except for ΔdeoxyHb (ΔtHb (r = 0.491, p = 0.008); ΔHbO$_2$ (r = 0.479, p = 0.010); ΔdeoxyHb (r = 0.358, p = 0.054)) (Figure 5D–F).

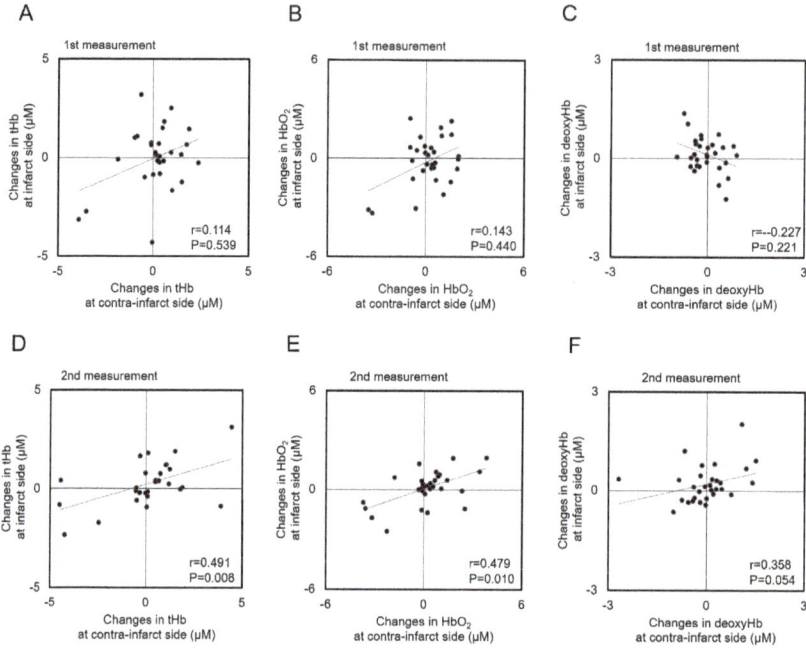

Figure 5. Scatterplots of the changes in total-hemoglobin (tHB), oxygenated-hemoglobin (HbO$_2$), and deoxygenated-hemoglobin (deoxyHb) concentrations in response to head-of-bed elevation (from 0° to 30°) at the first (**A–C**) and second (**D–F**) measurements for each hemisphere.

4. Discussion

We believe that this is the first study to assess the effect of gradual HOB manipulation (from 0° to 30°) of forehead hemoglobin concentration in AIS patients, revealed by two measurements using NIRS. There were three main findings of this investigation. (1) The HOB elevation from 0° to 30° did not affect systemic blood pressure or heart rate. ΔtHb, ΔHbO$_2$, and ΔdeoxyHb also did not change in response to HOB elevation, although large interindividual variabilities were observed. (2) ΔtHb and ΔHbO$_2$ in response to HOB elevation measured within 72 h of AIS onset showed significant correlations with those measured 7–10 days after AIS onset in both hemispheres. (3) Although ΔtHb, ΔHbO$_2$, and ΔdeoxyHb measured on the infarct side did not correlate with those measured on the contra-infarct side within 72 h of AIS onset, the correlation coefficients of these NIRS parameters were significantly correlated between the hemispheres 7–10 days after AIS onset.

It is known that CBF velocity (CBFV) and the total cerebral Hb concentration are reduced in head-up position of healthy subjects and chronic ischemic stroke patients. Furthermore, decreases in

CBVF and cerebral Hb concentration could be affected by a drop in systemic blood pressure [5,25–27]. In this study, the average blood pressure and heart rate did not change with HOB elevation from 0° to 30°. Neither were there changes in the cohort-averaged tHb, HbO_2, and deoxyHb concentrations for either hemisphere over two measurements. However, as shown in Figures 1–3, changes in tHb, HbO_2, and deoxyHb showed large differences among individuals. Approximately half of our study patients showed increased cerebral hemoglobin concentrations (the so-called paradoxical response) in response to HOB elevation for either hemisphere over the two measurements. This paradoxical response phenomenon was in line with previous reports that evaluated the effect of head-position changes on cerebral oxygenation in AIS patients [7,16,17]. Several previous studies reported that the paradoxical response was also seen in brain-injured patients but not healthy subjects, suggesting that it is pathological [11,28–30]. Although details of the mechanism of the paradoxical response are still unknown, an increasing intracranial pressure, the hemodynamic consequences of heart failure, and an autonomic disturbance have been proposed as causes [17]. Considerably varying individual cerebral oxygenation responses, including the paradoxical response, could explain why the cohort-averaged ΔtHb, ΔHbO_2, and ΔdeoxyHb concentrations did not change in response to HOB elevation.

Correlations of ΔtHb, ΔHbO_2, and ΔdeoxyHb concentrations in response to HOB elevation between the infarct and contra-infarct sides had not been reported prior to this study. Thus, we seem to be the first to show that the ΔtHb and ΔHbO_2 measurements within 72 h of AIS onset significantly correlated with those 7–10 days after AIS onset for either hemisphere. Notably, although the ΔtHb, ΔHbO_2, and ΔdeoxyHb, in response to HOB elevation, did not show a significant correlation between hemispheres within 72 h of AIS onset, correlations of the ΔtHb, ΔHbO_2, and ΔdeoxyHb 7–10 days after onset were statistically significant. Although we could not clarify the mechanism of this alteration, various possible explanations are assumed. Changes in cerebral oxygenation variables in response to HOB manipulation reflected CBF volume change. It could be related with gravitational force acting on passively contacted brain vessels in the ischemic territory [31]. It is also possible that systemic hemodynamics changes affect CBF; however, the HOB elevation from 0° to 30° did not affect systemic blood pressure or heart rate. A previous study, which measured cerebral mean flow velocity by TCD, suggested that the effect of BP change in response to head position change was equivocal [31–33]. In the current study, HOB elevations did not affect SBP, DBP, or HR, and no intraindividual differences in the SBP or heart rate at baseline measurements (HOB 0°) was observed at each measurement session. While cardiac output or stroke volume of the left ventricle was not measured, we thought that the effect of systemic hemodynamics changes could be limited. It is well-recognized that the brain edema is one of the lethal complications for AIS patients, and it causes a decrease in cerebral perfusion pressure through an increased intracranial pressure (ICP) [34]. Although we did not include AIS patients who received surgical decompression for severe brain edema (because of unsuitability of applying a probe to the forehead) and two participants who died before second measurement (suspected brain edema) were excluded from the analyses, the possibility that a raised ICP could affect the changes in ΔtHb, ΔHbO_2, and ΔdeoxyHb on the infarct side in response to HOB elevation could not be denied because we did not monitor the ICP in our participants. Development of collateral circulation also affected the changes in ΔtHb, ΔHbO_2, and ΔdeoxyHb on the infarct side in response to HOB elevation. Our study participants received magnetic resonance angiography (MRA) at the time of admission and 7–10 days after stroke onset. MRA often cannot provide information about the collateral circulation of AIS patients in clinical settings because of motion artifacts and its spatial resolution, whereas recent development of MRA can detect collateral circulation in research settings [35,36]. Furthermore, our study participants did not receive cerebral angiography because they had no indication of thrombolytic therapy at the time of admission. Thus, detailed information of collateral circulation is not available in the current study. Another possible mechanism is the alteration of cerebral autoregulation in AIS patients. Cerebral autoregulation is an inherent process of blood vessels that maintains CBF at a constant level over a wide range of changes in the systemic blood pressure or intracranial pressure. It has been generally accepted that cerebral autoregulation is impaired in patients with AIS [37,38]. Conventionally, TCD has often been used to measure the CBFV to assess cerebral autoregulation [39], and mean flow velocity index of dynamic autoregulation (Mx index) was established as a standard parameter [40,41]. Recent literature; however, has reported that cerebral oxygenation parameters measured by NIRS (e.g., cerebral oxygen saturation, cerebral oxygenation index) are considered surrogates of CBF [42–45]. In addition, it was reported that the NIRS-derived tHb signal reflects regional changes in cerebral blood volume (CBV), and HbO$_2$ correlates with cerebral capillary oxygen saturation [20,46–48]. Steiner, L. A. and colleagues demonstrated that tissue oxygen index of dynamic autoregulation (Tox) measured by NIRS (NIRO 200, Hamamatsu Photonics K.K.) significantly correlated with the Mx index [41]. Although NIRS is useful for cerebral autoregulation assessment, we could not make mention of the relationship between our results and cerebral autoregulation. We could not calculate the Tox index because we did not measure continuous blood pressure, and TRS-10 could not directly measure the tissue oxygen index. The literature suggests that AIS severity could influence the degree of spatiotemporal compromise of cerebral autoregulation [21,24,49]. Tutaj et al. reported that cerebral autoregulation was transiently impaired at an infarct hemisphere 1.3 ± 0.5 days after the onset of a large-vessel AIS, recovered at 9.75 ± 2.2 days—which could be in line with our findings [21]. Thus, we speculated the possibility that our findings might have been caused, at least in part, by transient changes in cerebral autoregulation. We need to conduct further studies to clarify whether current findings are induced by transient impairment of cerebral autoregulation.

This study has several limitations. The monitored systemic blood pressure and heart rate were not beat-to-beat measurements. Thus, we could not detect a transient drop in blood pressure in response to HOB manipulation. Lam et al. reported that the blood pressure may show a steep drop in response to gradual changes in head position (supine to 30°), although a blood pressure decline was observed in the head-up state [50]. Furthermore, the CBV paralleled blood pressure in the head-up position. These results supported our findings that neither blood pressure nor cerebral oxygenation parameters changed in response to HOB manipulation, at least according to the cohort-averaged assessment. Second, two consecutive NIRS measurements were needed for each participant because the TRS-10 system had only a single channel. Thus, we could not evaluate the cerebral oxygenation changes on the infarct and contra-infarct sides simultaneously. Furthermore, we could investigate forehead blood volume only within a narrow range of the prefrontal cortex. Multi-channel NIRS is currently in mainstream use and should be adopted in future studies to understand fluctuations in cerebral oxygenation in the entire brain in response to postural change. Third, we did not measure either endotidal carbon dioxide tension (EtCO$_2$) or partial pressure of carbon dioxide (pCO$_2$). It is known that CBF is influenced by CO$_2$, and hypercapnia dilates cerebral arteries and arterioles and increased blood flow, whereas hypocapnia causes vasoconstriction and decreased blood flow [51,52]. Indeed, Kim, Y.S. et al. reported that orthostatic manipulation decreases EtCO$_2$ from 40 mmHg to 35 mg in elder subjects [26]. Therefore, we cannot exclude that pCO$_2$ could also affect NIRS metrics. Fourth, we did not assess cerebral autoregulation or differences in the CBV responses among NIRS and other modalities (e.g., TCD, PET). Thus, we could not offer reasons why a statistically significant correlation of changes in cerebral oxygenation parameters between each hemisphere in response to HOB manipulation was found at 7–10 days after AIS onset but not within 72 h.

5. Conclusions

HOB manipulation from 0° to 30° did not affect cohort-averaged hemodynamic parameters. The cohort-averaged cerebral oxygenation parameters also did not change in response to HOB elevation, although large interindividual cerebral oxygenation changes were seen. Although changes in cerebral oxygenation in response to HOB elevation had a laterality difference between the hemispheres within 72 h of AIS onset, the difference decreased, at least partially, 7–10 days after AIS onset, and this could have suggested a sign of cerebral blood flow recovery. These findings suggest that HOB 30° within 72 h might not always be a preferred head position in AIS patients. Further studies are needed to establish the safety and efficacy of NIRS-guided neurological rehabilitation in AIS in the future.

Author Contributions: Conceptualization, N.K., K.O and A.H.; formal analysis, N.K.; investigation, N.K.; methodology, N.K. and K.O.; project administration, K.O.; resources, H.W.; supervision, N.I., K.Y. and H.W.; visualization, N.K.; writing—original draft preparation N.K.; writing—review and editing. K.O. and H.W.

Funding: This work was supported by grants from Daiichi-Sankyo Pharmaceuticals. The funding source had no role in the collection, analysis, interpretation, or report of the data.

Acknowledgments: We thank Nancy Schatken, BS, MT(ASCP), from Edanz Group (www.edanzediting.com/ac), for editing a draft of this manuscript.

Conflicts of Interest: The authors declare no conflict of interest.

References

1. Murray, C.J.; Vos, T.; Lozano, R.; Naghavi, M.; Flaxman, A.D.; Michaud, C.; Ezzati, M.; Shibuya, K.; Salomon, J.A.; Abdalla, S.; et al. Disability-adjusted life years (dalys) for 291 diseases and injuries in 21 regions, 1990-2010: A systematic analysis for the global burden of disease study 2010. *Lancet* **2012**, *380*, 2197–2223. [CrossRef]
2. Powers, W.J.; Rabinstein, A.A.; Ackerson, T.; Adeoye, O.M.; Bambakidis, N.C.; Becker, K.; Biller, J.; Brown, M.; Demaerschalk, B.M.; Hoh, B.; et al. 2018 guidelines for the early management of patients with acute ischemic stroke: A guideline for healthcare professionals from the american heart association/american stroke association. *Stroke* **2018**, *49*, e46–e110. [CrossRef] [PubMed]
3. Winstein, C.J.; Stein, J.; Arena, R.; Bates, B.; Cherney, L.R.; Cramer, S.C.; Deruyter, F.; Eng, J.J.; Fisher, B.; Harvey, R.L.; et al. Guidelines for adult stroke rehabilitation and recovery: A guideline for healthcare professionals from the american heart association/american stroke association. *Stroke* **2016**, *47*, e98–e169. [CrossRef] [PubMed]
4. AVERT Trial Collaboration group. Efficacy and safety of very early mobilisation within 24 h of stroke onset (avert): A randomised controlled trial. *Lancet* **2015**, *386*, 46–55.
5. Mehagnoul-Schipper, D.J.; Vloet, L.C.; Colier, W.N.; Hoefnagels, W.H.; Jansen, R.W. Cerebral oxygenation declines in healthy elderly subjects in response to assuming the upright position. *Stroke* **2000**, *31*, 1615–1620. [CrossRef]
6. Tyson, S.F.; Nightingale, P. The effects of position on oxygen saturation in acute stroke: A systematic review. *Clin. Rehabil.* **2004**, *18*, 863–871. [CrossRef]
7. Hargroves, D.; Tallis, R.; Pomeroy, V.; Bhalla, A. The influence of positioning upon cerebral oxygenation after acute stroke: A pilot study. *Age ageing* **2008**, *37*, 581–585. [CrossRef]
8. Olavarria, V.V.; Arima, H.; Anderson, C.S.; Brunser, A.M.; Munoz-Venturelli, P.; Heritier, S.; Lavados, P.M. Head position and cerebral blood flow velocity in acute ischemic stroke: A systematic review and meta-analysis. *Cerebrovasc. Dis.* **2014**, *37*, 401–408. [CrossRef]
9. Anderson, C.S.; Arima, H.; Lavados, P.; Billot, L.; Hackett, M.L.; Olavarria, V.V.; Munoz Venturelli, P.; Brunser, A.; Peng, B.; Cui, L.; et al. Cluster-randomized, crossover trial of head positioning in acute stroke. *N. Engl. J. Med.* **2017**, *376*, 2437–2447. [CrossRef]
10. Herold, F.; Wiegel, P.; Scholkmann, F.; Muller, N.G. Applications of functional near-infrared spectroscopy (fnirs) neuroimaging in exercise(-)cognition science: A systematic, methodology-focused review. *J. Clin. Med.* **2018**. [CrossRef]
11. Kim, M.N.; Edlow, B.L.; Durduran, T.; Frangos, S.; Mesquita, R.C.; Levine, J.M.; Greenberg, J.H.; Yodh, A.G.; Detre, J.A. Continuous optical monitoring of cerebral hemodynamics during head-of-bed manipulation in brain-injured adults. *Neurocrit. Care* **2014**, *20*, 443–453. [CrossRef] [PubMed]
12. Harrer, M.; Waldenberger, F.R.; Weiss, G.; Folkmann, S.; Gorlitzer, M.; Moidl, R.; Grabenwoeger, M. Aortic arch surgery using bilateral antegrade selective cerebral perfusion in combination with near-infrared spectroscopy. *Eur. J. Cardiothorac. Surg.* **2010**, *38*, 561–567. [CrossRef] [PubMed]
13. Ogino, H.; Ueda, Y.; Sugita, T.; Morioka, K.; Sakakibara, Y.; Matsubayashi, K.; Nomoto, T. Monitoring of regional cerebral oxygenation by near-infrared spectroscopy during continuous retrograde cerebral perfusion for aortic arch surgery. *Eur. J. Cardiothorac. Surg.* **1998**, *14*, 415–418. [CrossRef]
14. Weindling, A.M. Peripheral oxygenation and management in the perinatal period. *Semin. Fetal Neonatal. Med.* **2010**, *15*, 208–215. [CrossRef]

15. Aries, M.J.; Elting, J.W.; Stewart, R.; De Keyser, J.; Kremer, B.; Vroomen, P. Cerebral blood flow velocity changes during upright positioning in bed after acute stroke: An observational study. *BMJ Open* **2013**. [CrossRef] [PubMed]
16. Favilla, C.G.; Mesquita, R.C.; Mullen, M.; Durduran, T.; Lu, X.; Kim, M.N.; Minkoff, D.L.; Kasner, S.E.; Greenberg, J.H.; Yodh, A.G.; et al. Optical bedside monitoring of cerebral blood flow in acute ischemic stroke patients during head-of-bed manipulation. *Stroke* **2014**, *45*, 1269–1274. [CrossRef]
17. Durduran, T.; Zhou, C.; Edlow, B.L.; Yu, G.; Choe, R.; Kim, M.N.; Cucchiara, B.L.; Putt, M.E.; Shah, Q.; Kasner, S.E.; et al. Transcranial optical monitoring of cerebrovascular hemodynamics in acute stroke patients. *Opt. express* **2009**, *17*, 3884–3902. [CrossRef]
18. Patterson, M.S.; Chance, B.; Wilson, B.C. Time resolved reflectance and transmittance for the non-invasive measurement of tissue optical properties. *Appl. Opt.* **1989**, *28*, 2331–2336. [CrossRef]
19. Sato, C.; Yamaguchi, T.; Seida, M.; Ota, Y.; Yu, I.; Iguchi, Y.; Nemoto, M.; Hoshi, Y. Intraoperative monitoring of depth-dependent hemoglobin concentration changes during carotid endarterectomy by time-resolved spectroscopy. *Appl. Opt.* **2007**, *46*, 2785–2792. [CrossRef]
20. Ohmae, E.; Ouchi, Y.; Oda, M.; Suzuki, T.; Nobesawa, S.; Kanno, T.; Yoshikawa, E.; Futatsubashi, M.; Ueda, Y.; Okada, H.; et al. Cerebral hemodynamics evaluation by near-infrared time-resolved spectroscopy: Correlation with simultaneous positron emission tomography measurements. *NeuroImage* **2006**, *29*, 697–705. [CrossRef]
21. Tutaj, M.; Miller, M.; Krakowska-Stasiak, M.; Piatek, A.; Hebda, J.; Latka, M.; Strojny, J.; Szczudlik, A.; Slowik, A. Dynamic cerebral autoregulation is compromised in ischaemic stroke of undetermined aetiology only in the non-affected hemisphere. *Neurol. Neurochir. Pol.* **2014**, *48*, 91–97. [CrossRef] [PubMed]
22. Petersen, N.H.; Ortega-Gutierrez, S.; Reccius, A.; Masurkar, A.; Huang, A.; Marshall, R.S. Dynamic cerebral autoregulation is transiently impaired for one week after large-vessel acute ischemic stroke. *Cerebrovasc. Dis.* **2015**, *39*, 144–150. [CrossRef] [PubMed]
23. Panerai, R.B.; Jara, J.L.; Saeed, N.P.; Horsfield, M.A.; Robinson, T.G. Dynamic cerebral autoregulation following acute ischaemic stroke: Comparison of transcranial doppler and magnetic resonance imaging techniques. *J. Cereb. Blood Flow Metab.* **2016**, *36*, 2194–2202. [CrossRef] [PubMed]
24. Ma, H.; Guo, Z.N.; Jin, H.; Yan, X.; Liu, J.; Lv, S.; Zhang, P.; Sun, X.; Yang, Y. Preliminary study of dynamic cerebral autoregulation in acute ischemic stroke: Association with clinical factors. *Front Neurol.* **2018**, *9*, 1006. [CrossRef] [PubMed]
25. Novak, V.; Hu, K.; Desrochers, L.; Novak, P.; Caplan, L.; Lipsitz, L.; Selim, M. Cerebral flow velocities during daily activities depend on blood pressure in patients with chronic ischemic infarctions. *Stroke* **2010**, *41*, 61–66. [CrossRef] [PubMed]
26. Kim, Y.S.; Bogert, L.W.; Immink, R.V.; Harms, M.P.; Colier, W.N.; van Lieshout, J.J. Effects of aging on the cerebrovascular orthostatic response. *Neurobiol. Aging* **2011**, *32*, 344–353. [CrossRef] [PubMed]
27. Mehagnoul-Schipper, D.J.; Colier, W.N.; Jansen, R.W. Reproducibility of orthostatic changes in cerebral oxygenation in healthy subjects aged 70 years or older. *Clin. Physiol.* **2001**, *21*, 77–84. [CrossRef]
28. Chieregato, A.; Tanfani, A.; Compagnone, C.; Pascarella, R.; Targa, L.; Fainardi, E. Cerebral blood flow in traumatic contusions is predominantly reduced after an induced acute elevation of cerebral perfusion pressure. *Neurosurgery* **2007**, *60*, 115–123. [CrossRef]
29. Jaeger, M.; Schuhmann, M.U.; Soehle, M.; Nagel, C.; Meixensberger, J. Continuous monitoring of cerebrovascular autoregulation after subarachnoid hemorrhage by brain tissue oxygen pressure reactivity and its relation to delayed cerebral infarction. *Stroke* **2007**, *38*, 981–986. [CrossRef]
30. Gatto, R.; Hoffman, W.; Paisansathan, C.; Mantulin, W.; Gratton, E.; Charbel, F.T. Effect of age on brain oxygenation regulation during changes in position. *J. Neurosci. Methods* **2007**, *164*, 308–311. [CrossRef]
31. Wojner-Alexander, A.W.; Garami, Z.; Chernyshev, O.Y.; Alexandrov, A.V. Heads down: Flat positioning improves blood flow velocity in acute ischemic stroke. *Neurology* **2005**, *64*, 1354–1357. [CrossRef] [PubMed]
32. Wojner, A.W.; El-Mitwalli, A.; Alexandrov, A.V. Effect of head positioning on intracranial blood flow velocities in acute ischemic stroke: A pilot study. *Crit. Care Nurs. Q.* **2002**, *24*, 57–66. [CrossRef] [PubMed]
33. Hunter, A.J.; Snodgrass, S.J.; Quain, D.; Parsons, M.W.; Levi, C.R. Hoboe (head-of-bed optimization of elevation) study: Association of higher angle with reduced cerebral blood flow velocity in acute ischemic stroke. *Phys. Ther.* **2011**, *91*, 1503–1512. [CrossRef] [PubMed]

34. Bevers, M.B.; Kimberly, W.T. Critical care management of acute ischemic stroke. *Curr. Treat. Options Cardiovasc. Med.* **2017**, *19*, 41. [CrossRef]
35. Boujan, T.; Neuberger, U.; Pfaff, J.; Nagel, S.; Herweh, C.; Bendszus, M.; Mohlenbruch, M.A. Value of contrast-enhanced mra versus time-of-flight mra in acute ischemic stroke mri. *AJNR Am. J. Neuroradiol.* **2018**, *39*, 1710–1716. [CrossRef]
36. Bang, O.Y.; Goyal, M.; Liebeskind, D.S. Collateral circulation in ischemic stroke: Assessment tools and therapeutic strategies. *Stroke* **2015**, *46*, 3302–3309. [CrossRef]
37. Markus, H.S. Cerebral perfusion and stroke. *J. Neurol. Neurosurg. Psychiatry* **2004**, *75*, 353–361. [CrossRef]
38. Dohmen, C.; Bosche, B.; Graf, R.; Reithmeier, T.; Ernestus, R.I.; Brinker, G.; Sobesky, J.; Heiss, W.D. Identification and clinical impact of impaired cerebrovascular autoregulation in patients with malignant middle cerebral artery infarction. *Stroke* **2007**, *38*, 56–61. [CrossRef]
39. Aaslid, R.; Lindegaard, K.F.; Sorteberg, W.; Nornes, H. Cerebral autoregulation dynamics in humans. *Stroke* **1989**, *20*, 45–52. [CrossRef]
40. Czosnyka, M.; Smielewski, P.; Kirkpatrick, P.; Menon, D.K.; Pickard, J.D. Monitoring of cerebral autoregulation in head-injured patients. *Stroke* **1996**, *27*, 1829–1834. [CrossRef]
41. Steiner, L.A.; Pfister, D.; Strebel, S.P.; Radolovich, D.; Smielewski, P.; Czosnyka, M. Near-infrared spectroscopy can monitor dynamic cerebral autoregulation in adults. *Neurocrit. Care* **2009**, *10*, 122–128. [CrossRef] [PubMed]
42. Brady, K.M.; Lee, J.K.; Kibler, K.K.; Smielewski, P.; Czosnyka, M.; Easley, R.B.; Koehler, R.C.; Shaffner, D.H. Continuous time-domain analysis of cerebrovascular autoregulation using near-infrared spectroscopy. *Stroke* **2007**, *38*, 2818–2825. [CrossRef] [PubMed]
43. Brady, K.; Joshi, B.; Zweifel, C.; Smielewski, P.; Czosnyka, M.; Easley, R.B.; Hogue, C.W., Jr. Real-time continuous monitoring of cerebral blood flow autoregulation using near-infrared spectroscopy in patients undergoing cardiopulmonary bypass. *Stroke* **2010**, *41*, 1951–1956. [CrossRef]
44. Moerman, A.; De Hert, S. Recent advances in cerebral oximetry. Assessment of cerebral autoregulation with near-infrared spectroscopy: Myth or reality? *F1000Res* **2017**, *6*, 1615. [CrossRef]
45. Rivera-Lara, L.; Geocadin, R.; Zorrilla-Vaca, A.; Healy, R.; Radzik, B.R.; Palmisano, C.; Mirski, M.; Ziai, W.C.; Hogue, C. Validation of near-infrared spectroscopy for monitoring cerebral autoregulation in comatose patients. *Neurocrit. Care* **2017**, *27*, 362–369. [CrossRef] [PubMed]
46. Rostrup, E.; Law, I.; Pott, F.; Ide, K.; Knudsen, G.M. Cerebral hemodynamics measured with simultaneous pet and near-infrared spectroscopy in humans. *Brain Res.* **2002**, *954*, 183–193. [CrossRef]
47. Claassen, J.A.; Colier, W.N.; Jansen, R.W. Reproducibility of cerebral blood volume measurements by near infrared spectroscopy in 16 healthy elderly subjects. *Physiol. Meas.* **2006**, *27*, 255–264. [CrossRef]
48. Rasmussen, P.; Dawson, E.A.; Nybo, L.; van Lieshout, J.J.; Secher, N.H.; Gjedde, A. Capillary-oxygenation-level-dependent near-infrared spectrometry in frontal lobe of humans. *J. Cereb. Blood Flow Metab.* **2007**, *27*, 1082–1093. [CrossRef]
49. Xiong, L.; Tian, G.; Lin, W.; Wang, W.; Wang, L.; Leung, T.; Mok, V.; Liu, J.; Chen, X.; Wong, K.S. Is dynamic cerebral autoregulation bilaterally impaired after unilateral acute ischemic stroke? *J. Stroke Cerebrovasc. Dis.* **2017**, *26*, 1081–1087. [CrossRef]
50. Lam, M.Y.; Haunton, V.J.; Robinson, T.G.; Panerai, R.B. Does gradual change in head positioning affect cerebrovascular physiology? *Physiol. Rep.* **2018**. [CrossRef]
51. Kety, S.S.; Schmidt, C.F. The effects of altered arterial tensions of carbon dioxide and oxygen on cerebral blood flow and cerebral oxygen consumption of normal young men. *J. Clin. Invest.* **1948**, *27*, 484–492. [CrossRef] [PubMed]
52. Reivich, M. Arterial pco2 and cerebral hemodynamics. *Am. J. Physiol.* **1964**, *206*, 25–35. [CrossRef] [PubMed]

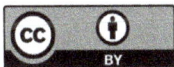 © 2019 by the authors. Licensee MDPI, Basel, Switzerland. This article is an open access article distributed under the terms and conditions of the Creative Commons Attribution (CC BY) license (http://creativecommons.org/licenses/by/4.0/).

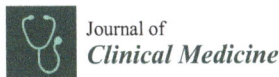

Review

Functional Role of Natriuretic Peptides in Risk Assessment and Prognosis of Patients with Mitral Regurgitation

Giovanna Gallo [1], Maurizio Forte [2], Rosita Stanzione [2], Maria Cotugno [2], Franca Bianchi [2], Simona Marchitti [2], Andrea Berni [1], Massimo Volpe [1,2] and Speranza Rubattu [1,2,*]

1. Department of Clinical and Molecular Medicine, School of Medicine and Psychology, Sapienza University of Rome, 00189 Rome, Italy; giovanna.gallo@uniroma1.it (G.G.); andrea.berni@uniroma1.it (A.B.); massimo.volpe@uniroma1.it (M.V.)
2. IRCCS Neuromed, 86077 Pozzilli (Isernia), Italy; maurizio.forte@neuromed.it (M.F.); stanzione@neuromed.it (R.S.); maria.cotugno@neuromed.it (M.C.); franca.bianchi@neuromed.it (F.B.); simona.marchitti@neuromed.it (S.M.)
* Correspondence: rubattu.speranza@neuromed.it; Tel.: +39-063377-59-79

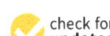

Received: 22 April 2020; Accepted: 1 May 2020; Published: 5 May 2020

Abstract: The management of mitral valve regurgitation (MR), a common valve disease, represents a challenge in clinical practice, since the indication for either surgical or percutaneous valve replacement or repair are guided by symptoms and by echocardiographic parameters which are not always feasible. In this complex scenario, the use of natriuretic peptide (NP) levels would serve as an additive diagnostic and prognostic tool. These biomarkers contribute to monitoring the progression of the valve disease, even before the development of hemodynamic consequences in a preclinical stage of myocardial damage. They may contribute to more accurate risk stratification by identifying patients who are more likely to experience death from cardiovascular causes, heart failure, and cardiac hospitalizations, thus requiring surgical management rather than a conservative approach. This article provides a comprehensive overview of the available evidence on the role of NPs in the management, risk evaluation, and prognostic assessment of patients with MR both before and after surgical or percutaneous valve repair. Despite largely positive evidence, a series of controversial findings exist on this relevant topic. Recent clinical trials failed to assess the role of NPs following the interventional procedure. Future larger studies are required to enable the introduction of NP levels into the guidelines for the management of MR.

Keywords: natriuretic peptides; mitral valve regurgitation; valve repair; valve replacement; risk prediction

1. Introduction

Mitral regurgitation (MR) represents one of the most frequent valve diseases with an indication for valve replacement or repair, both as surgical or transcatheter interventional management [1].

The etiology of mitral dysfunction, namely primary or secondary regurgitation, should be clearly identified. In primary or organic MR, the valve apparatus is directly affected as a consequence of a degenerative (i.e., fail leaflet or prolapse) or infective (i.e., endocarditis) process. In secondary or functional MR, the structure of the components of the valve apparatus, such as leaflets and chordae, is preserved, but an impaired left ventricular (LV) geometry is responsible of an altered balance between closing and tethering forces on the valve. In both abovementioned conditions, MR is responsible for or contributes to the development of LV and left atrial (LA) overload, leading to hemodynamic alterations.

According to the most recent European Guidelines [2], urgent surgery is recommended in cases of acute severe MR. In chronic primary MR, valve replacement or repair is indicated in symptomatic patients and, in the absence of symptoms, in the presence of LV ejection fraction (LVEF) <60%, LV end-systolic diameter (LVESD) ≥45 mm, atrial fibrillation (AF), and systolic pulmonary pressure ≥50 mmHg. Valve repair should be preferred if feasible and able to achieve a durable result with a low risk of re-intervention, such as in segmental valve prolapse. Rheumatic lesions, leaflets, or extensive annular calcifications more often require valvular replacement, preferably preserving sub-valvular apparatuses. In patients with high surgical risk, percutaneous edge-to-edge mitral repair is currently widely adopted and recommended by international Guidelines [2,3].

In secondary MR, due to significant operative mortality, high rates of recurrent MR, and the absence of a definite survival benefit, surgery is indicated when concomitant coronary revascularization is required. Even in this circumstance, percutaneous edge-to-edge repair may represent an efficacious option [4,5].

Although a "watchful waiting" strategy is considered safe and is accepted in asymptomatic patients, the assessment of correct and univocal timing of surgeries still remains a challenge. The identification of symptoms may be difficult due to its subjective nature and to the risk that patients could minimize their clinical manifestations in order to delay surgery, or could progressively reduce their activities as a consequence of an impaired functional capacity. In addition, symptoms may become clear when LV dysfunction is irreversible [6].

In this complex scenario, one of the unmet needs is a more accurate risk stratification, in which biomarkers may represent a useful tool to identify patients with a possibly unfavorable prognosis under conservative management or after mitral valve (MV) surgery.

Among several biomarkers available in clinical practice, natriuretic peptides (NPs) have a well-established role in cardiovascular diseases and, particularly, in heart failure (HF) where they reflect cardiac overload, LV systolic and diastolic dysfunctions, and are associated to cardiovascular outcomes [7].

Atrial natriuretic peptide (ANP), brain natriuretic peptide (BNP), and their inactive N-terminal portions (NT-proANP and NT-proBNP) are released in response to increased myocardial stretch, as a consequence of volume or pressure overload. NPs exert several cardiovascular and renal actions mediated by the type A natriuretic peptide receptor through the second messenger cGMP. The effects of NPs are able to counterbalance hemodynamic congestion through the regulation of electrolytes, water balance, and permeability of systemic vasculature. Moreover, they inhibit the renin–angiotensin–aldosterone system and the sympathetic nervous system. At the cellular level, a modulatory role on cellular growth and proliferation is recognized [8–10]. Some differences exist among NPs. ANP is stored in granules as a previously synthesized pool within the atrial cardiomyocytes and is quickly released upon request. BNP production is regulated by gene expression in ventricular cardiomyocytes, secreted as a prohormone, then cleaved into the active peptide and the NT-proBNP. As compared to ANP, BNP has a longer half-life (1–2 hours compared to approximately 22 minutes) and greater plasma concentrations (about 10-fold higher) [11,12]. Moreover, it has been proposed that NPs' responses may depend on the specific pathophysiology of the underlying cardiac stress, suggesting that ANP may be more sensitive in the case of subclinical damage, whereas the BNP level shows a greater increase in acute conditions [13,14].

The aim of our review is to analyze the current available evidence on the role of NPs in the management, risk evaluation, and prognostic assessment of patients with MR before and after surgical or percutaneous valve repair.

2. NPs and Risk Assessment in MR

Several studies have investigated the association between increased levels of NPs in patients with MR, parameters of LV dysfunction, and cardiovascular outcomes.

An analysis of data obtained in 1399 patients from 15 studies found a positive relationship between levels of NPs and LV end-systolic parameters, such as the LV end-systolic index (LVESI) and LVESD [15]. BNP level was also associated with the myocardial performance index (MPI), an echocardiographic index of systolic and diastolic function [16]. Mayer and colleagues documented that patients with severe MR and BNP values >409 pg/mL had a mean LVESD of 40 mm [17], which represents a criterion for surgery according to U.S. Guidelines [3]. A linear relationship between the LVESD value of 40 mm and NT-proBNP level >292 pg/mL was identified by Potocki et al. [18]. An elevated BNP level has been documented in patients with pulmonary artery pressure >50 mmHg [18], this parameter being another indication for valve replacement or repair [2,3]. NT-proBNP values were directly related to HF functional classes in MR, with mean levels of 97 pg/mL for New York Heart Association (NYHA) class I, 170 pg/mL for class II, and 458 pg/mL for class III [19]. The addition of BNP to the Society of Thoracic Surgeons (STS) score improved the risk stratification in patients with primary MR and preserved LVEF [20].

In a prospective study conducted in 124 patients with chronic primary MR, Detaint and colleagues analyzed the relationship between BNP level, MR degree, LV and LA remodeling, and prognosis [21]. BNP level was associated to the LV end-systolic volume index, LA volume, and symptoms, and it was able to predict prognosis independently from age, sex, functional class, MR severity, and LVEF. At the 5-year follow-up, survival was significantly worse in patients with BNP level >31 pg/mL, showing a higher incidence of the combined end-point of death and HF [21].

In another study, BNP level >105 pg/mL had stronger predictive power compared to the most common parameters of MR severity, such as an effective orifice regurgitant area (EROA) and LVESD [22]. In 49 patients with MR and preserved ejection fraction (>55%), BNP > 41 pg/mL and NT-proBNP > 173 pg/mL showed the best accuracy in predicting the development of symptoms [23]. In 87 patients with severe MR, BNP below 80 pg/mL and NT-proBNP lower than 200 pg/mL showed the greatest negative predictive value of 98% for the development of symptoms or LV dysfunction during follow-up [24].

The prognostic role of BNP level in the management of MR has also been examined during exercise. Exercise BNP level was strongly correlated with those measured at rest [25]. Patients with higher BNP values showed more severe MR, greater LA volume, more elevated systolic pulmonary pressure, and LV filling pressure estimated as an E/e' ratio. Moreover, detected exercise BNP levels were higher in patients who developed symptoms and had an increased incidence of cardiac events, independently from age, gender, and body mass index. In patients with moderate MR, only the exercise LV global longitudinal strain, but neither resting nor exercise LVEF, was an independent determinant of exercise BNP level. A plausible explanation of these findings is that the BNP level has been assessed in patients with degenerative MR and not in MR secondary to LV dilatation, in which levels of NPs were measured before the development of LV systolic dysfunction [25]. A cut-off of 64 pg/mL was identified as the best cut-off value for exercise BNP level to behave as an independent predictor of worse cardiovascular outcomes [25]. Other studies have consistently demonstrated that an increase in BNP level during exercise is related to the development of HF, to subclinical LV dysfunction, and to reduced performance capacity [26,27].

According to the abovementioned results, BNP level may be used in clinical practice as a complementary tool for echocardiographic exams and exercise tests in order to identify those patients who are more likely to experience death from cardiovascular causes, and HF and cardiac hospitalizations, thus requiring surgical management, rather than a conservative approach. In addition, NPs may represent an essential tool to monitor the progression of the valve disease before the development of hemodynamic consequences in a preclinical stage of myocardial damage.

However, some controversial aspects deserve to be better-clarified. First of all, as documented by the abovementioned studies, it is still difficult to establish a univocal cut-off level able to identify MR patients at elevated cardiovascular risk, since different levels of NPs have been identified in the different studies. To overcome this problem, Clavel et al. introduced the BNP ratio, which is derived from a measured BNP value divided by the expected value related to the age and sex of each patient [26].

This parameter behaves as a significant independent prognostic marker of outcomes in valve heart disease patients, including MR patients under medical treatment [28,29]. However, it failed to maintain its role after surgery [28]. Interestingly, the BNP/ANP ratio revealed a prognostic role in one study, being significantly higher in the presence of clinical and echocardiographic criteria used for surgery recommendation, such as LVESD ≥ 45 mm, LVEF ≤ 60%, NYHA class II or greater, and AF [30].

Other critical issues relate to the appropriate time interval that should be considered for the subsequent measurements of the NP level, and the magnitude of changes of NP values between baseline and subsequent assessments, which may be related to a poor clinical outcome. In addition, age, AF, renal function, and body weight are known modulators of NP levels, thus representing potential confounders [31]. Finally, since a high BNP level may also be detected in patients with moderate MR, it cannot be used as a surrogate for MR quantification. On the other hand, it should be pointed out that, in the presence of good hemodynamic compensation with a normal NP level, regardless of LV dimension, the need for an interventional strategy may be missed.

3. The Role of NPs to Predict Outcome after MV Surgery or Percutaneous Repair

During the last few years, percutaneous edge-to-edge MV repair with the MitraClip (Abbott Vascular, CA USA) device has acquired increasing importance as a treatment option, especially in patients with HF with an elevated surgical risk. However, many patients are still being treated with the surgical MV repair or replacement, which represents the gold-standard procedure. Apart from the reduction of MR, both percutaneous and surgical interventions may produce several hemodynamic benefits, reducing LV and LA pressure and volume overload and, as a consequence, the myocardial wall stretch [2,3].

In this context, several studies have assessed the role of NPs in the management of patients treated with MV repair or replacement, investigating the sensibility of these biomarkers in identifying subjects with a worse response to the performed interventional procedure and with a lower chance of survival.

In a study involving 65 patients treated with edge-to-edge valve repair, a low NT-proBNP level, measured 6 months after the procedure, was associated with a significant reduction in LV end-diastolic volume (LVEDV) and end-systolic volume (LVESV) and to an improvement in LV and LA longitudinal strain [32]. Worse renal function, larger LVEDV, and a higher transmitral gradient after MitraClip (Abbott Vascular, CA USA) implantation were independently associated with a higher level of NT-proBNP at follow-up. Patients with low and medium NT-proBNP tertiles experienced a significantly greater reduction in NYHA functional class symptoms and quality of life score compared to those with a higher NT-proBNP level. At the 6-month follow-up, successful MR reduction was observed in a higher number of patients with low and medium NT-proBNP tertiles, whereas severe MR more often persisted in the high NT-proBNP tertile group (43%) [32].

After percutaneous valve repair, improvements in 6-minute walking distances and a decrease in LV volumes were paralleled by a significant reduction of NT-proBNP level [33].

Hwang and colleagues identified a BNP cut-off level of 125 pg/mL associated with a higher risk of cardiac death and re-hospitalization for cardiac causes in 117 patients who underwent surgical MV replacement [34]. Interestingly, a study conducted with 44 patients treated with transcatheter valve repair, as well as baseline levels of mid-regional proANP and NT-proBNP were significantly higher in those who experienced death or re-hospitalization for HF during a median follow-up of 211 days [35]. In a cohort of 174 retrospectively examined patients, the NT-proBNP level was significantly associated to survival at univariate analysis, but the independent predictive power of NT-proBNP was not confirmed at multivariate analysis [36]. However, the post-operative NT-proBNP level maintained its predictive role for a clinical outcome at multivariate analysis in other studies [37–39].

As for the pre-operative level, controversial findings were frequently reported with regard to the post-operative level. In 59 patients who underwent percutaneous MV repair, achieving a reduction of MR, an improvement of functional class, and structural reverse cardiac remodeling (reduced LA volume and LVESD and increased LVEF), the NT-proBNP level did not decrease significantly [40].

Similar findings were provided by Yoon et al. in a cohort of 144 patients successfully treated with edge-to-edge repair, in which the NT-proBNP level did not significantly decrease after MV clipping. In addition, NT-proBNP changes were not related to baseline LVEF and LV diameter and were not able to predict cardiovascular outcomes during a 6-month follow-up [41]. Furthermore, in a study which enrolled 194 patients treated with percutaneous valve repair, the NT-proBNP level remained elevated (≥10,000 pg/mL) in those patients who achieved a reduction of MR to grade ≤2 (21%) [42]. These controversial results may be explained by differences in the sample size of the enrolled populations, in the characteristics of the included patients (baseline LVEF, pulmonary artery pressure, LV diameter and diastolic function), in the duration of the follow-up, and also the rhythm status (i.e., sinus rhythm or AF) [43].

Finally, as for the pre-surgical management, it has not been clearly established which biomarker should be chosen, which cut-off value should be considered for the risk assessment of the patients, and which interval for serial monitoring of NPs has the best accuracy.

4. NPs Levels in MITRA-FR and COAPT Trials

Two recent trials have become available in patients subjected to MV repair. The MITRA-FR (Percutaneous Repair with the MitraClip Device (Abbott Vascular, CA USA) for Severe Functional/Secondary Mitral Regurgitation) trial, conducted in patients with severe secondary MR, showed that percutaneous MV repair added to standard pharmacological therapy was unable to reduce the rate of death or unplanned hospitalizations for HF at 1 year compared to those who received medical therapy alone [44].

The Cardiovascular Outcomes Assessment of the MitraClip Percutaneous Therapy for Heart Failure Patients with Functional Mitral Regurgitation (COAPT) study demonstrated that the transcatheter MV repair reduced the rate of hospitalizations for HF and all-cause mortality within 12 and 24 months of follow-up [45]. Although the MITRA-FR and COAPT trials enrolled comparable populations of patients with secondary MR, they obtained diametrically opposed results [44,45].

Several possible mechanisms have been proposed to explain the discrepant findings, mostly focusing on the different echocardiographic characteristics of the subjects included in the two trials [46,47]. The COAPT excluded patients with very severe LV dilation (LVESD < 70 mm), whereas LV diameter did not represent an exclusion criterion in MITRA-FR. This resulted in a significant difference in the documented mean LV volume (LVEDV 135 ± 35 mL/m^2 in MITRA-FR vs. 101 ± 34 mL/m^2 in COAPT) [44–47]. More interestingly, the two populations had a different degree of MR, the EROA being significantly greater in COAPT as compared with MITRA-FR (41 ± 15 mm^2 vs. 31 ± 10 mm^2, respectively) [44–47]. According to these considerations, it has been supposed that the underlying cardiac disease was probably the main cause of HF and the determinant of prognosis in MITRA-FR, with MR being a marker of adverse LV remodeling. In contrast, the LV dysfunction was more related to MR severity in COAPT, which also represented the main contributor to outcomes [48]. In such a context, it has been proposed that the degree of MR was "proportionate" to the degree of LV dilatation in MITRA-FR, whereas it was "disproportionate" in COAPT, and this parameter may have influenced the different clinical response to the percutaneous repair procedure [46,47].

In this complex scenario, the differences in the baseline NP levels between the two studies may mirror the different pathophysiological mechanisms. In the COAPT trial, both NT-proBNP and BNP levels were significantly higher than in MITRA-FR (median NT-proBNP > 5100 vs. 3200 pg/mL and median BNP >1000 vs. >760 pg/mL, respectively), and it may be argued that they were more related to MR severity than to either LVEF or LV diameter [44,45]. In fact, a higher degree of MR may have produced an increase in atrial and ventricular loading conditions, leading to a higher NP level. Unfortunately, precise data about the LA dimension, diastolic function (i.e., assessed with E/e' ratio), and systolic pulmonary pressure were not provided in the two trial populations. Furthermore, the two studies did not obtain any information about overtime changes in NPs levels after the transcatheter

MV repair procedure. Therefore, their potential relationship to echocardiographic parameters and to clinical outcomes could not be assessed in these trials.

5. NPs and Other Biomarkers

The most plausible pathophysiological explanation for the better association of NPs with pre- and post-procedural outcomes may be their optimal capacity to reflect cardiac performance in different hemodynamic conditions. Of note, lack of a sufficient number of studies using ANP as a marker in the management of MR does not currently allow to make a robust comparison with BNP.

Several efforts have been made over the last few years to investigate the role of other biomarkers in the MR condition, and have been previously reviewed [49]. More recently, other biomarkers have been investigated with some interesting insights.

The neutrophil gelatinase-associated lipocalin (NGAL) and cystatin C, both markers of functional and structural kidney damage, were shown to predict mortality in high-risk patients undergoing percutaneous MV repair [50]. However, they had low accuracy, probably due to a lack of relationship with the hemodynamic balance [35]. Similarly, the highly sensitive C-reactive protein (hsCRP), a biomarker able to improve risk prediction for cardiovascular diseases, showed low performance in the prognostic assessment of the MR patients [35]. On the other hand, the pre-operative level of soluble ST-2, a member of the interleukin-1 receptor family previously described as a stronger biomarker of myocardial stretch in HF, was correlated with LV function and structure after MV repair, thus providing complementary prognostic information to NT-proBNP level [35]. The level of galectin-3, a well-established marker of LV fibrosis, has been associated with worse cardiovascular outcomes after MV repair [35]. Interestingly, low galectin-3 and ST2 plasma levels were predictors of therapeutic success in 210 patients treated with percutaneous MV repair (PMVR) [51]. Of note, a lower galectin-3 level was a predictor of MR improvement after cardiac resynchronization therapy (CRT) [52]. In addition, biomarkers reflecting inflammation (hsCRP, interleukin-6) and cardiac remodeling processes (matrix metalloproteinases (MMP-2 and MMP-9)) were associated with a higher risk of mortality following the procedure [53]. The highly sensitive troponin T showed strong prognostic power in predicting survival after transcatheter MV repair, with an accuracy comparable to that of a mid-regional proANP level [35].

Of note, some evidence of the role of other parameters in the outcome prediction of MR patients has been collected. For instance, it was found that abnormalities of the calcium-phosphate metabolism may influence the health-related quality of life in patients with severe MR [54]. Amelioration of oxidative stress and endothelial dysfunction may be indicators of successful MV repair in patients with MV prolapse [55].

Finally, one study reported the negative prognostic impact of pre-procedural anemia in patients who underwent PMVR with a higher baseline NT-proBNP level [56].

Based on the evidence collected so far, markers of mechanisms involved in the cardiac remodeling process may be considered as complementary prognostic tools to the NP level.

6. Conclusions

The management of MR still represents a real challenge for physicians, since the assessment of symptoms is difficult and the recommended diagnostic exams, such as the echocardiogram, are often not accurately performed. It is well-known that NP secretion occurs in the presence of atrial and ventricular stretch, as a consequence of pressure and volume overload, and that NPs are independent predictors of mortality and morbidity in patients with severe MR. Due to their feasible measurement and to their significant association with echocardiographic parameters of LV dysfunction and of impaired filling, these biomarkers may represent an important tool to identify patients at elevated risk of adverse clinical outcomes, in which early surgical or percutaneous intervention should be considered (Figures 1 and 2).

Moreover, the NP level has also been documented to be a powerful independent predictor of reduced cardiac event-free survival in patients treated with surgical or transcatheter valve repair or replacement, thus representing potential instruments to significantly improve the evaluation of a short- and long-term prognosis after these procedures.

Although some controversies still exist, the majority of findings discussed in our review article are encouraging, and indicate NPs as potentially useful biomarkers for the clinical management of MR. Further larger studies are needed to solve key issues, that is, to better define which biomarker should preferably be used among NPs, which rest and eventually stress cut-off levels could clearly identify high-risk patients, and which degree of variation between serial measurements may have the best clinical accuracy. It is hoped that these future studies will allow the introduction of NP levels into the guidelines for the management of MR.

Figure 1

- NPs level is related to cardiac remodeling in MR.
- NPs level may be used to monitor the progression of MR, before the development of hemodynamic consequences.
- NPs may represent an important tool in the risk stratification of patients with severe MR.
- NPs level may contribute to identify patients who are more likely to have a poor clinical outcome and who should benefit from an invasive management rather than a conservative approach.
- NPs levels may predict adverse LV remodeling and higher CV risk after MV surgery or percutaneous repair.
- Most accurate cut-off values and intervals for serial monitoring of NPs should be better defined by further studies.

Figure 1. Summary of the main topics discussed in this review. Abbreviation legends: CV = cardiovascular; MR = mitral regurgitation; MV = mitral valve; NPs = natriuretic peptides.

Figure 2

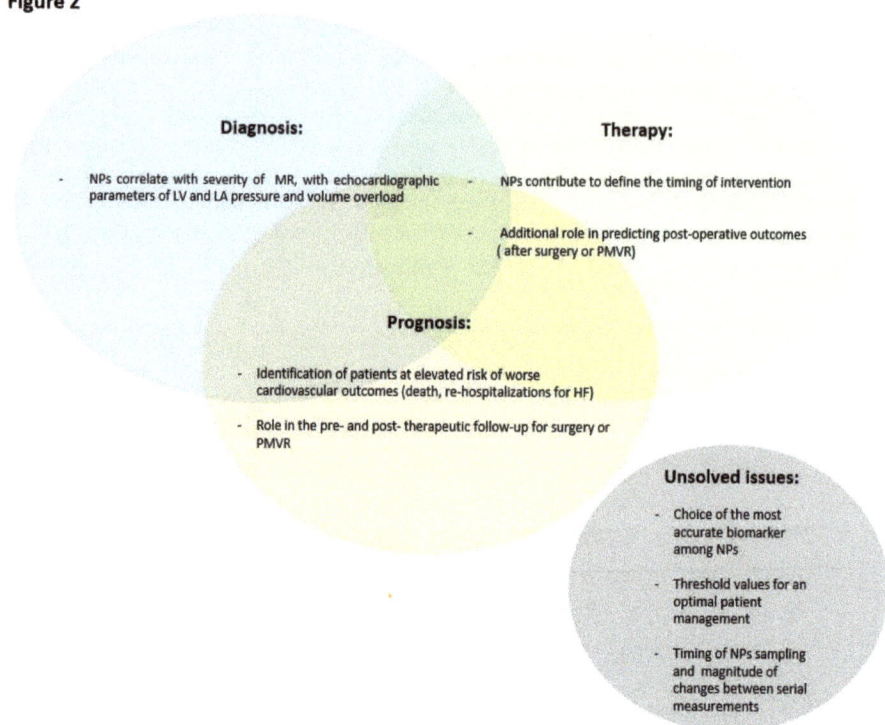

Figure 2. Main clinical implications of NPs in MR. Abbreviation legends: HF = Heart failure; LA = left atrium; LV = left ventricle; NPs = natriuretic peptides; PMVR = percutaneous mitral valve repair.

Author Contributions: Conceptualization, G.G. and S.R.; methodology, G.G., M.F., R.S., M.C., F.B., S.M. and S.R.; formal analysis, G.G., M.F., R.S., M.C., F.B., S.M. and S.R.; investigation, G.G., M.F., R.S., M.C., F.B., S.M. and S.R.; resources, S.R. and M.V.; data curation, G.G., M.F., R.S., M.C., F.B., S.M. and S.R.; writing—original draft preparation, G.G. and S.R.; writing—review and editing, S.R., A.B. and M.V.; visualization, G.G. and S.R.; supervision, S.R.; project administration, S.R.; funding acquisition, S.R. and M.V. All authors have read and agreed to the published version of the manuscript.

Funding: This research and the APC are funded by a grant from the Italian Ministry of Health.

Conflicts of Interest: The authors declare no conflict of interest. The funders had no role in the design of the study; in the collection, analyses, or interpretation of data; in the writing of the manuscript, or in the decision to publish the results.

References

1. Iung, B.; Baron, G.; Butchart, E.G.; Delahaye, F.; Gohlke-Bärwolf, C.; Levang, O.W.; Tornos, P.; Vanoverschelde, J.L.; Vermeer, F.; Boersma, E.; et al. A prospective survey of patients with valvular heart disease in Europe: The Euro Heart Survey on Valvular Heart Disease. *Eur. Heart J.* **2003**, *24*, 1231–1243. [CrossRef]
2. Baumgartner, H.; Falk, V.; Bax, J.J.; De Bonis, M.; Hamm, C.; Holm, P.J.; Iung, B.; Lancellotti, P.; Lansac, E.; Muñoz, D.R.; et al. ESC/EACTS Guidelines for the management of valvular heart disease. *Eur. Heart J.* **2017**, *38*, 2739–2791. [CrossRef] [PubMed]

3. Nishimura, R.A.; Otto, C.M.; Bonow, R.O.; Carabello, B.A.; Erwin, J.P. III; Fleisher, L.A.; Jneid, H.; Mack, M.J.; McLeod, C.J.; O'Gara, P.T.; et al. AHA/ACC Focused Update of the 2014 AHA/ACC Guideline for the Management of Patients With Valvular Heart Disease: A Report of the American College of Cardiology/American Heart Association Task Force on Clinical Practice Guidelines. *Circulation* **2017**, *135*, e1159–e1195. [CrossRef] [PubMed]
4. Feldman, T.; Kar, S.; Elmariah, S.; Smart, S.C.; Trento, A.; Siegel, R.J.; Apruzzese, P.; Fail, P.; Rinaldi, M.J.; Smalling, R.W.; et al. EVEREST II Investigators. *J. Am. Coll. Cardiol.* **2015**, *66*, 2844–2854. [CrossRef] [PubMed]
5. Arnold, S.V.; Stone, G.W.; Mack, M.J.; Chhatriwalla, D.K.; Austin, B.A.; Zhang, Z.; Ben-Yehuda, O.; Kar, S.; Lim, D.S.; Lindenfeld, J.A.; et al. COAPT Investigators Health Status Changes and Outcomes in Patients with Heart Failure and Mitral Regurgitation: From COAPT. *J. Am. Coll. Cardiol.* **2020**, *75*, 2099–2106. [CrossRef] [PubMed]
6. Magne, J.; Lancellotti, P.; Piérard, L.A. Exercise-induced changes in degenerative mitral regurgitation. *J. Am. Coll. Cardiol.* **2010**, *56*, 300–309. [CrossRef]
7. Flint, N.; Raschpichler, M.; Rader, F.; Shmueli, H.; Siegel, R.J. Asymptomatic Degenerative Mitral Regurgitation: A Review. *JAMA Cardiol.* **2020**. [CrossRef]
8. Natriuretic Peptides Studies Collaboration; Willeit, P.; Kaptoge, S.; Welsh, P.; Butterworth, A.S.; Chowdhury, R.; Spackman, S.A.; Pennells, L.; Gao, P.; Burgess, S.; et al. Natriuretic peptides and integrated risk assessment for cardiovascular disease: An individual-participant-data meta-analysis. *Lancet Diabetes Endocrinol.* **2016**, *4*, 840–849. [CrossRef]
9. Volpe, M.; Battistoni, A.; Rubattu, S. Natriuretic peptides in heart failure: Current achievements and future perspectives. *Int. J. Cardiol.* **2019**, *281*, 186–189. [CrossRef]
10. Rubattu, S.; Volpe, M. Natriuretic Peptides in the Cardiovascular System: Multifaceted Roles in Physiology, Pathology and Therapeutics. *Int. J. Mol. Sci.* **2019**, *20*, 3991. [CrossRef]
11. Yasue, H.; Yoshimura, H.; Sumida, H.; Kikuta, K.; Kugiyama, K.; Jougasaki, M.; Ogawa, H.; Okumura, K.; Mukoyama, M.; Nakao, K. Localization and mechanism of secretion of B-type natriuretic peptide in comparison with those of A-type natriuretic peptide in normal subjects and patients with heart failure. *Circulation* **1994**, *90*, 195–203. [CrossRef] [PubMed]
12. Xu-Cai, Y.O.; Wu, Q. Molecular forms of natriuretic peptides in heart failure and their implications. *Heart* **2010**, *96*, 419–424. [CrossRef] [PubMed]
13. Karakas, M.; Jaensch, A.; Breitling, L.P.; Brenner, H.; Koenig, W.; Rothenbacher, D. Prognostic value of midregional pro-A-type natriuretic peptide and N-terminal pro-B-type natriuretic peptide in patients with stable coronary heart disease followed over 8 years. *Clin. Chem.* **2014**, *60*, 1441–1449. [CrossRef] [PubMed]
14. Lugnier, C.; Meyer, A.; Charloux, A.; Andrès, E.; Gény, B.; Talha, S. The Endocrine Function of the Heart: Physiology and Involvements of Natriuretic Peptides and Cyclic Nucleotide Phosphodiesterases in Heart Failure. *J. Clin. Med.* **2019**, *8*, 1746. [CrossRef] [PubMed]
15. Johl, M.M.; Malhotra, P.; Kehl, D.W.; Rader, F.; Siegel, R.J. Natriuretic peptides in the evaluation and management of degenerative mitral regurgitation: A systematic review. *Heart* **2017**, *103*, 738–744. [CrossRef] [PubMed]
16. Sayar, N.; Lütfullah Orhan, A.; Cakmak, N.; Yılmaz, H.; Atmaca, H.; Tangürek, B.; Hasdemir, H.; Nurkalem, Z.; Ergelen, M.; Aksu, H.; et al. Correlation of the myocardial performance index with plasma B-type natriuretic peptide levels in patients with mitral regurgitation. *Int. J. Cardiovasc. Imag.* **2008**, *24*, 151–157. [CrossRef]
17. Mayer, S.A.; De Lemos, J.A.; Murphy, S.A.; Brooks, S.; Roberts, B.J.; Paul, A.; Grayburn, P.A. Comparison of B-type natriuretic peptide levels in patients with heart failure with versus without mitral regurgitation. *Am. J. Cardiol.* **2004**, *93*, 1002–1006. [CrossRef]
18. Potocki, M.; Mair, J.; Weber, M.; Hamm, C.; Burkard, T.; Hiemetzberger, R.; Peters, K.; Jander, N.; Cron, T.A.; Hess, N.; et al. Relation of N-terminal pro-B-type natriuretic peptide to symptoms, severity, and left ventricular remodeling in patients with organic mitral regurgitation. *Am. J. Cardiol.* **2009**, *104*, 559–564. [CrossRef]
19. Yusoff, R.; Clayton, N.; Keevil, B.; Morris, J.; Ray, S. Utility of plasma N-terminal brain natriuretic peptide as a marker of functional capacity in patients with chronic severe mitral regurgitation. *Am. J. Cardiol.* **2006**, *97*, 1498–1501. [CrossRef]

20. Mentias, A.; Patel, K.; Patel, H.; Gillinov, A.M.; Rodriguez, L.L.; Svensson, L.G.; Mihaljevic, T.; Sabik, J.F.; Griffin, B.P.; Desai, M.Y. Prognostic Utility of Brain Natriuretic Peptide in Asymptomatic Patients With Significant Mitral Regurgitation and Preserved Left Ventricular Ejection Fraction. *Am. J. Cardiol.* **2016**, *117*, 258–263. [CrossRef]
21. Detaint, D.; Messika-Zeitoun, D.; Avierinos, J.F.; Scott, C.; Chen, H.; Burnett, C.J., Jr.; Enriquez-Sarano, M. B-type natriuretic peptide in organic mitral regurgitation: Determinants and impact on outcome. *Circulation* **2005**, *111*, 2391–2397. [CrossRef]
22. Magne, J.; Mahjoub, H.; Pierard, L.A.; O'Connor, K.; Pirlet, C.; Pibarot, P.; Lancellotti, P. Prognostic importance of brain natriuretic peptide and left ventricular longitudinal function in asymptomatic degenerative mitral regurgitation. *Heart* **2012**, *98*, 584–591. [CrossRef] [PubMed]
23. Sutton, T.M.; Stewart, R.A.; Gerber, I.L.; West, T.M.; Richards, A.M.; Yandle, T.G.; Kerr, A.J. Plasma natriuretic peptide levels increase with symptoms and severity of mitral regurgitation. *J. Am. Coll. Cardiol.* **2003**, *41*, 2280–2287. [CrossRef]
24. Klaar, U.; Gabriel, H.; Bergler-Klein, J.; Pernicka, E.; Heger, M.; Mascherbauer, J.; Rosenhek, R.; Binder, T.; Maurer, G.; Baumgartner, H. Prognostic value of serial B-type natriuretic peptide measurement in asymptomatic organic mitral regurgitation. *Eur. J. Heart Fail.* **2011**, *13*, 163–169. [CrossRef]
25. Magne, J.; Mahjoub, H.; Pibarot, P.; Pirlet, C.; Pierard, L.A.; Lancellotti, P. Prognostic importance of exercise brain natriuretic peptide in asymptomatic degenerative mitral regurgitation. *Eur. J. Heart Fail.* **2012**, *14*, 1293–1302. [CrossRef] [PubMed]
26. Pascual-Figal, D.A.; Peñafiel, P.; de la Morena, G.; Redondo, B.; Nicolás, F.; Casas, T.; Valdés, M. Relation of B-type natriuretic peptide levels before and after exercise and functional capacity in patients with idiopathic dilated cardiomyopathy. *Am. J. Cardiol.* **2007**, *99*, 1279–1283. [CrossRef]
27. Kato, M.; Kinugawa, T.; Ogino, K.; Redondo, B.; Nicolás, F.; Casas, T.; Valdés, M. Augmented response in plasma brain natriuretic peptide to dynamic exercise in patients with left ventricular dysfunction and congestive heart failure. *J. Intern. Med.* **2000**, *248*, 309–315. [CrossRef]
28. Clavel, M.A.; Tribouilloy, C.; Vanoverschelde, J.L.; Pizarro, R.; Suri, R.M.; Szymanski, C.; Lazam, S.; Oberti, P.; Michelena, H.I.; Jaffe, A.; et al. Association of B-Type Natriuretic Peptide With Survival in Patients With Degenerative Mitral Regurgitation. *J. Am. Coll. Cardiol.* **2016**, *68*, 1297–1307. [CrossRef]
29. Zhang, B.; Xu, H.; Zhang, H.; Liu, Q.; Ye, Y.; Hao, J.; Zhao, Q.; Qi, X.; Liu, S.; Zhang, E.; et al. CHINA-DVD CollaboratorsPrognostic Value of N-Terminal Pro-B-Type Natriuretic Peptide in Elderly Patients With Valvular Heart Disease. *J. Am. Coll. Cardiol.* **2020**, *75*, 1659–1672. [CrossRef]
30. Shimamoto, K.; Kusumoto, M.; Sakai, R.; Watanabe, H.; Ihara, S.; Koike, N.; Kawana, M. Usefulness of the brain natriuretic peptide to atrial natriuretic peptide ratio in determining the severity of mitral regurgitation. *Can. J. Cardiol.* **2007**, *23*, 295–300. [CrossRef]
31. Kaneko, H.; Neuss, M.; Schau, T.; Weissenborn, J.; Butter, C. Interaction between renal function and percutaneous edge-to-edge mitral valve repair using MitraClip. *J. Cardiol.* **2017**, *69*, 476–482. [CrossRef]
32. Van Wijngaarden, S.E.; Kamperidis, V.; Al-Amri, I.; van der Kley, F.; Schalij, M.J.; Ajmone Marsan, N.; Bax, J.J.; Delgado, V. Effects of Transcatheter Mitral Valve Repair With MitraClip on Left Ventricular and Atrial Hemodynamic Load and Myocardial Wall Stress. *J. Card. Fail.* **2018**, *24*, 137–145. [CrossRef]
33. Franzen, O.; van der Heyden, J.; Baldus, S.; Schlüter, M.; Schillinger, W.; Butter, C.; Hoffmann, R.; Corti, R.; Pedrazzini, G.; Swaans, M.J.; et al. MitraClip®therapy in patients with end-stage systolic heart failure. *Eur. J. Heart Fail.* **2011**, *13*, 569–576. [CrossRef] [PubMed]
34. Hwang, I.C.; Kim, Y.J.; Kim, K.H.; Lee, S.P.; Kim, Y.K.; Sohn, D.W.; Oh, B.H.; Parket, Y.B. Prognostic value of B-type natriuretic peptide in patients with chronic mitral regurgitation undergoing surgery: Mid-term follow-up results. *Eur. J. Cardiothorac. Surg.* **2013**, *43*, e1–e6. [CrossRef] [PubMed]
35. Wöhrle, J.; Karakas, M.; Trepte, U.; Seeger, J.; Gonska, B.; Koenig, W.; Rottbauer, W. Midregional-proAtrial Natriuretic Peptide and High Sensitive Troponin T Strongly Predict Adverse Outcome in Patients Undergoing Percutaneous Repair of Mitral Valve Regurgitation. *PLoS ONE* **2015**, *10*, e0137463. [CrossRef] [PubMed]
36. Kreusser, M.M.; Geis, N.A.; Berlin, N.; Greiner, S.; Pleger, S.T.; Bekeredjian, R.; Katus, K.A.; Raake, P.W. Invasive hemodynamics and cardiac biomarkers to predict outcomes after percutaneous edge-to-edge mitral valve repair in patients with severe heart failure. *Clin. Res. Cardiol.* **2019**, *108*, 375–387. [CrossRef]

37. Triantafyllis, A.S.; Kortlandt, F.; Bakker, A.L.; Swaans, M.J.; Eefting, F.D.; van der Heyden, J.A.S.; Post, M.C.; Rensing, B.W.J.M. Long-term survival and preprocedural predictors of mortality in high surgical risk patients undergoing percutaneous mitral valve repair. *Catheter Cardiovasc. Interv.* **2016**, *87*, 467–475. [CrossRef]
38. Toggweiler, S.; Zuber, M.; Sürder, D.; Biaggi, P.; Gstrein, C.; Moccetti, T.; Pasotti, E.; Gaemperli, O.; Faletra, F.; Petrova-Slater, I.; et al. Two-year outcomes after percutaneous mitral valve repair with the MitraClip system: Durability of the procedure and predictors of outcome. *Open Heart* **2014**, *1*, e000056. [CrossRef]
39. Perreas, K.; Samanidis, G.; Dimitriou, S.; Athanasiou, A.; Balanika, M.; Smirli, A.; Antzaka, C.; Politis, K.; Khoury, M.; Michalis, A. NT-proBNP in the mitral valve surgery. *Critl. Pathw. Cardiol.* **2014**, *13*, 55–61. [CrossRef]
40. Pleger, S.T.; Schulz-Schönhagen, M.; Geis, N.; Chorianopoulos, E.; Antaredja, M.; Lewening, M.; Katus, H.A.; Bekeredjian, R. One year clinical efficacy and reverse cardiac remodelling in patients with severe mitral regurgitation and reduced ejection fraction after MitraClip implantation. *Eur. J. Heart Fail.* **2013**, *15*, 919–927. [CrossRef]
41. Yoon, J.N.; Frangieh, A.H.; Attinger-Toller, A.; Gruner, C.; Tanner, F.C.; Taramasso, M.; Corti, R.; Lüscher, T.F.; Ruschitzka, F.; Bettex, D.; et al. Changes in serum biomarker profiles after percutaneous mitral valve repair with the MitraClip system. *Cardiol. J.* **2016**, *23*, 384–392. [CrossRef] [PubMed]
42. Schau, T.; Isotani, A.; Neuss, M.; Schöpp, M.; Seifert, M.; Höpfner, C.; Burkhoff, D.; Butter, C. Long-term survival after Mitraclip therapy in patients with severe mitral regurgitation and severe congestive heart failure: A comparison among survivals predicted by heart failure models. *J. Cardiol.* **2016**, *67*, 287–294. [CrossRef] [PubMed]
43. Hwang, I.C.; Kim, D.H.; Kim, Y.J.; Kim, K.H.; Lee, S.P.; Kim, Y.K.; Sohn, D.W.; Oh, B.H.; Park, Y.B. Change of B-type natriuretic peptide after surgery and its association with rhythm status in patients with chronic severe mitral regurgitation. *Can. J. Cardiol.* **2013**, *29*, 704–711. [CrossRef] [PubMed]
44. Obadia, J.F.; Messika-Zeitoun, D.; Leurent, G.; Iung, B.; Bonnet, G.; Piriou, N.; Lefèvre, T.; Piot, C.; Rouleau, F.; Carrié, D.; et al. MITRA-FR Investigators.Percutaneous Repair or Medical Treatment for Secondary Mitral Regurgitation. *N. Engl. J. Med.* **2018**, *379*, 2297–2306. [CrossRef]
45. Stone, G.W.; Lindenfeld, J.; Abraham, W.T.; Kar, S.; Lim, D.S.; Mishell, J.M.; Whisenant, B.; Grayburn, P.A.; Rinaldi, M.; Kapadia, S.R.; et al. COAPT Investigators.Transcatheter Mitral-Valve Repair in Patients with Heart Failure. *N. Engl. J. Med.* **2018**, *379*, 2307–2318. [CrossRef]
46. Pibarot, P.; Delgado, V.; Bax, J.J. MITRA-FR vs. COAPT: Lessons from two trials with diametrically opposed results. *Eur. Heart J. Cardiovasc. Imag.* **2019**, *20*, 620–624. [CrossRef]
47. Hagendorff, A.; Doenst, T.; Falk, V. Echocardiographic assessment of functional mitral regurgitation: Opening Pandora's box? *ESC Heart Fail.* **2019**, *6*, 678–685. [CrossRef]
48. Grayburn, P.A.; Sannino, A.; Packer, M. Proportionate and Disproportionate Functional Mitral Regurgitation: A New Conceptual Framework That Reconciles the Results of the MITRA-FR and COAPT Trials. *JACC Cardiovasc. Imag.* **2019**, *12*, 353–362. [CrossRef]
49. Bäck, M.; Pizarro, R.; Clavel, M.A. Biomarkers in Mitral Regurgitation. *Prog. Cardiovasc. Dis.* **2017**, *60*, 334–341. [CrossRef]
50. Dörr, O.; Walther, C.; Liebetrau, C.; Keller, T.; Ortlieb, R.M.; Boeder, N.; Bauer, P.; Möllmann, H.; Gaede, L.; Troidl, C.; et al. Evaluation of cystatin C and neutrophil gelatinase-associated lipocalin as predictors of mortality in patients undergoing percutaneous mitral valve repair (MitraClip). *Clin. Cardiol.* **2018**, *41*, 1474–1479. [CrossRef]
51. Dörr, O.; Walther, C.; Liebetrau, C.; Keller, T.; Ortlieb, R.M.; Boeder, N.; Bauer, P.; Möllmann, H.; Gaede, L.; Troidl, C.; et al. Galectin-3 and ST2 as predictors of therapeutic success in high-risk patients undergoing percutaneous mitral valve repair (MitraClip). *Clin. Cardiol.* **2018**, *41*, 1164–1169. [CrossRef] [PubMed]
52. Beaudoin, J.; Singh, J.P.; Szymonifka, J.; Zhou, Q.; Levine, R.A.; Januzzi, J.L.; Truong, Q.A. Novel Heart Failure Biomarkers Predict Improvement of Mitral Regurgitation in Patients Receiving Cardiac Resynchronization Therapy-The BIOCRT Study. *Can. J. Cardiol.* **2016**, *32*, 1478–1484. [CrossRef] [PubMed]
53. Dörr, O.; Walther, C.; Liebetrau, C.; Keller, T.; Ortlieb, R.M.; Boeder, N.; Bauer, P.; Möllmann, H.; Gaede, L.; Troidl, C.; et al. Specific biomarkers of myocardial inflammation and remodeling processes as predictors of mortality in high-risk patients undergoing percutaneous mitral valve repair (MitraClip). *Clin. Cardiol.* **2018**, *41*, 481–487. [CrossRef] [PubMed]

54. Mozenska, O.; Bil, J.; Segiet, A.; Kosior, D.A. The influence of calcium-phosphate metabolism abnormalities on the quality of life in patients with hemodynamically significant mitral regurgitation. *BMC Cardiovasc. Disord.* **2019**, *19*, 116. [CrossRef] [PubMed]
55. Porro, B.; Songia, P.; Myasoedova, V.A.; Valerio, V.; Moschetta, D.; Gripari, P.; Fusini, L.; Cavallotti, L.; Canzano, P.; Turnu, L.; et al. Endothelial Dysfunction in Patients with Severe Mitral Regurgitation. *J. Clin. Med.* **2019**, *8*, 835. [CrossRef] [PubMed]
56. Kaneko, H.; Neuss, M.; Okamoto, M.; Weissenborn, J.; Butter, C. Impact of Preprocedural Anemia on Outcomes of Patients with Mitral Regurgitation Who Underwent MitraClip Implantation. *Am. J. Cardiol.* **2018**, *122*, 859–865. [CrossRef]

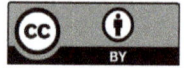

© 2020 by the authors. Licensee MDPI, Basel, Switzerland. This article is an open access article distributed under the terms and conditions of the Creative Commons Attribution (CC BY) license (http://creativecommons.org/licenses/by/4.0/).

Increased Citrullinated Histone H3 Levels in the Early Post-Resuscitative Period Are Associated with Poor Neurologic Function in Cardiac Arrest Survivors—A Prospective Observational Study

Lisa-Marie Mauracher [1], Nina Buchtele [1,2], Christian Schörgenhofer [2], Christoph Weiser [3], Harald Herkner [3], Anne Merrelaar [3], Alexander O. Spiel [3], Lena Hell [1], Cihan Ay [1,4], Ingrid Pabinger [1], Bernd Jilma [2] and Michael Schwameis [3,*]

1. Clinical Division of Hematology and Hemostaseology, Department of Medicine I, Medical University of Vienna, 1090 Vienna, Austria; lisa-marie.mauracher@meduniwien.ac.at (L.-M.M.); nina.buchtele@meduniwien.ac.at (N.B.); lena.hell@meduniwien.ac.at (L.H.); cihan.ay@meduniwien.ac.at (C.A.); ingrid.pabinger@meduniwien.ac.at (I.P.)
2. Department of Clinical Pharmacology, Medical University of Vienna, 1090 Vienna, Austria; christian.schoergenhofer@meduniwien.ac.at (C.S.); bernd.jilma@meduniwien.ac.at (B.J.)
3. Department of Emergency Medicine, Medical University of Vienna, 1090 Vienna, Austria; christoph.weiser@meduniwien.ac.at (C.W.); Harald.herkner@meduniwien.ac.at (H.H.); anne.merrelaar@meduniwien.ac.at (A.M.); alexander.spiel@meduniwien.ac.at (A.O.S.)
4. I.M. Sechenov First Moscow State Medical University (Sechenov University), 119146 Moscow, Russia
* Correspondence: michael.schwameis@meduniwien.ac.at; Tel.: +43-1-40400-19640

Received: 29 August 2019; Accepted: 24 September 2019; Published: 1 October 2019

Abstract: The exact contribution of neutrophils to post-resuscitative brain damage is unknown. We aimed to investigate whether neutrophil extracellular trap (NET) formation in the early phase after return of spontaneous circulation (ROSC) may be associated with poor 30 day neurologic function in cardiac arrest survivors. This study prospectively included adult (≥18 years) out-of-hospital cardiac arrest (OHCA) survivors with cardiac origin, who were subjected to targeted temperature management. Plasma levels of specific (citrullinated histone H3, H3Cit) and putative (cell-free DNA (cfDNA) and nucleosomes) biomarkers of NET formation were assessed at 0 and 12 h after admission. The primary outcome was neurologic function on day 30 after admission, which was assessed using the five-point cerebral performance category (CPC) score, classifying patients into good (CPC 1–2) or poor (CPC 3–5) neurologic function. The main variable of interest was the effect of H3Cit level quintiles at 12 h on 30 day neurologic function, assessed by logistic regression. The first quintile was used as a baseline reference. Results are given as crude odds ratio (OR) with 95% confidence interval (95% CI). Sixty-two patients (79% male, median age: 57 years) were enrolled. The odds of poor neurologic function increased linearly, with 0 h levels of cfNDA (crude OR 1.8, 95% CI: 1.2–2.7, $p = 0.007$) and nucleosomes (crude OR 1.7, 95% CI: 1.0–2.2, $p = 0.049$), as well as with 12 h levels of cfDNA (crude OR 1.6, 95% CI: 1.1–2.4, $p = 0.024$), nucleosomes (crude OR 1.7, 95% CI: 1.1–2.5, $p = 0.020$), and H3Cit (crude OR 1.6, 95% CI: 1.1–2.3, $p = 0.029$). Patients in the fourth (7.9, 95% CI: 1.1–56, $p = 0.039$) and fifth (9.0, 95% CI: 1.3–63, $p = 0.027$) H3Cit quintile had significantly higher odds of poor 30 day neurologic function compared to patients in the first quintile. Increased plasma levels of H3Cit, 12 h after admission, are associated with poor 30 day neurologic function in adult OHCA survivors, which may suggest a contribution of NET formation to post-resuscitative brain damage and therefore provide a therapeutic target in the future.

Keywords: neutrophil extracellular traps; citrullinated histone H3; cardiac arrest; neurologic function

1. Introduction

In cardiac arrest survivors good neurologic outcome remains difficult to achieve [1]. Brain injury does not occur solely during circulatory interruption, but may progress during the reperfusion period after sustained return of spontaneous circulation (ROSC) [2]. Ischemic reperfusion is considered a main trigger of a complex cascade of pro-inflammatory and pro-thrombotic events occurring hours to days after resuscitation, which may impair cerebral microvascular perfusion despite restoration of macrovascular flow [3,4]. Recent data suggest that the response of neutrophils to hypoxia could be an early and critical mediator of ischemic reperfusion injury [5]. This is consistent with previous studies reporting substantial mortality and neurologic morbidity in resuscitated cardiac arrest patients with an elevated number of blood neutrophils in relation to other leukocyte counts [6–8]. The mechanisms by which neutrophils may contribute to post-resuscitative brain damage have, however, not yet been elucidated.

In recent years, neutrophil extracellular traps (NETs) have emerged as a central player in inflammation, thrombogenesis, and cardiovascular disease [9–14]. NETs are chromatin fibers consisting of histones, cell free DNA (cfDNA), and granular proteins, and are released within minutes [15] to hours [16] following activation by various stimuli including ischemia and reperfusion [17]. While NETs have primarily been recognized as mediators of antimicrobial host defense, they may exert detrimental inflammatory and procoagulant effects causing endothelial damage, platelet activation, microvessel occlusions, and ultimately tissue malperfusion [18]. In particular, neutrophil histones and DNA are considered cytotoxic and procoagulant components of NETs [19], and have been implicated in organ damage in various noninfectious conditions [20,21]. Citrullination of histone H3 (H3Cit) by peptidylarginine deiminase 4 (PAD4) is a key signal for chromatin decondensation and NET formation [22]. H3Cit is commonly accepted as a NET biomarker, and has been measured in various studies to investigate NET formation. Despite this, the role of NETs in cardiac arrest has not yet been investigated. Pro-inflammatory and pro-thrombotic properties, however, render them possible mediators of neutrophil-borne brain injury after successful resuscitation.

We hypothesized that neutrophil extracellular trap (NET) formation may be associated with poor neurologic function after cardiac arrest. This study aimed to assess plasma levels of NET biomarkers in the early phase after ROSC and investigate its association with short-term neurologic function in a selected cohort of out-of-hospital cardiac arrest (OHCA) survivors.

2. Methods

This prospective single-center observational cohort study was conducted at the Emergency Department at the Medical University of Vienna. Adult (≥18 years) OHCA survivors with cardiac origin who received in-hospital targeted temperature management (33 ± 0.5 °C) were enrolled. Exclusion criteria included current oral anticoagulation therapy, thrombolytic therapy, intravascular cooling, and application of extracorporeal assist devices (Figure S1). A waiver for written informed consent was obtained from the local ethics committee. The informed consent was permanently waived if the patient did not regain consciousness. Patients who regained consciousness were informed of their participation as soon as they were able to understand the purpose of the study. Post-resuscitation care was performed in accordance with the International Liaison Committee on resuscitation guidelines [23]. The primary outcome was neurologic function on day 30 after admission, which was assessed by independent study fellows blinded to levels of NET-related biomarker measurement. For primary outcome assessment, the five-point cerebral performance category (CPC) score was used, which classifies patients into good (CPC 1–2) and poor neurologic function (CPC 3–5; 3 = severe cerebral disability, 4 = coma or vegetative state, 5 = death) [24].

Resuscitation-related parameters were collected via structured telephone interviews with the dispatch center, the emergency physicians, and paramedics at the scene, as well as the bystander who made the emergency call. These parameters included location of cardiac arrest (home vs. public), initial rhythm (non-shockable vs. shockable), witness status, basic life support, downtime (interval from collapse to ROSC), the amount of epinephrine administered, and the administration of heparin by the emergency medical service (EMS). Demographics and chronic health conditions that existed pre-arrest were collected by review of past medical reports and interviews with relatives and the general practitioner if available.

The study was approved by the ethics committee of the Medical University of Vienna (EC Number 1674/2013) and conducted in accordance with Helsinki declarations.

2.1. Blood Sampling

Whole blood was obtained on admission immediately after vascular access was available and again 12 h later and stored in blood collection tubes containing 3.8% trisodium citrate (Greiner BioOne, Kremsmünster, Austria). Immediately thereafter, samples were centrifuged for 10 min at 3000 g and platelet poor plasma was stored at −80 °C until final analysis.

2.2. Laboratory Analysis of NET Related Biomarker

Citrullinated histone H3 (H3Cit), nucleosome, and cell free DNA (cfDNA) levels were obtained from plasma samples as previously described [12]. Briefly, cfDNA was measured using Quant-iT PicoGreen dsDNA Assay Kit (Thermo Fisher Scientific, Waltham, MA, USA) according to the manufacturer's instructions. Nucleosomes were measured using Cell Death Detection ELISAPLUS (Roche Diagnostics, Mannheim, Germany) and the resultant values were compared to a plasma pool from male healthy controls. H3Cit levels were obtained by using a Cell Death Detection ELISA Kit (Sigma Aldrich, St. Louis, MO, USA). After overnight coating with anti-histone antibody at 4 °C, the 96-well plate (Nunc MicroWell 96-well microplates, Thermo Fisher Scientific, Waltham, MA, USA) was blocked with incubation buffer. After washing with phosphate buffered saline (PBS)-Tween, self-made H3Cit standards as well as plasma samples were incubated for 1.5 h at room temperature and washed again. Anti-H3Cit antibody (1:1000 ab5103, Abcam, Cambridge, MA, USA) was applied and incubated for 1.5 h at room temperature. After another washing step, secondary antibody (1:5000 goat anti-rabbit IgG horseradish peroxidase (HRP), Biorad, Hertfordshire, U.K.) was incubated for 1 h at room temperature and washed again. Incubation with TMB (3,3′, 5,5′-tetramethylbenzidine, Sigma Aldrich, St. Louis, MO, USA) for 25 min and the addition of 2% sulfuric acid resulted in a colorimetric change, readable at 450 nm. Measurement of NET biomarkers was performed without an awareness of neurologic assessment outcome. NET-related biomarkers were obtained in duplicate, and the respective mean value was used for the final statistical analysis. Resulted values are given in ng/mL, multiple-of-the-mean (MoM), and ng/mL for cfDNA, nucleosomes, and H3Cit respectively.

2.3. Statistical Methods

Categorical data are presented as absolute count numbers (n) and relative frequencies (%), continuous data as medians and 25–75% interquartile ranges. The patients were analyzed according to their neurologic function on day 30 (CPC 3–5/poor vs. 1–2/good). For between-group comparisons we used the Mann–Whitney U test for continuous variables and the Fisher's exact test for categorical variables. We used a score test to assess a trend of increasing biomarker levels at specific time points for neurologic outcome and logistic regression models, including each relevant co-variable separately, to estimate the effect of NET biomarkers on neurologic function. A subgroup analysis of the effect of H3Cit on the primary outcome included only patients with a CPC of 1–4 on day 30 after admission. The score test is a nonparametric test for a trend across ordered groups as an extension of the Wilcoxon rank-sum test [25]. Results are given as crude odds ratio (OR) with 95% confidence interval (95% CI). NET biomarker levels were categorized into quintiles prior to analysis. The first quintile of each biomarker level distribution was used as a baseline reference. Covariables judged to be clinically plausible included age, sex, location of cardiac arrest (place of residence vs. public place), initial rhythm (non-shockable vs. shockable), witnessed status, basic life support, downtime (interval from collapse to ROSC equaling the sum of no-flow and low-flow time), amount of epinephrine administered, and d-dimer and lactate levels. D-dimer and lactate levels were log transformed to normalize data distribution. The likelihood ratio test was performed to assess deviations from linearity. The Spearman method was used to assess the correlation between plasma levels of cfDNA, nucleosomes, and H3cit. No data-imputation was applied for missing data. We used Stata Statistical Software (Release 14, StataCorp LLC, College Station, TX, USA) for data analysis and GraphPad Prism Version 8.0.2 for Windows (GraphPad Software, La Jolla, CA, USA) to draw figures. Generally, we considered a two-sided p-value < 0.05 as statistically significant.

3. Results

Between January 2014 and January 2017, 62 patients (79% male, median age: 57 years, 46–67) with OHCA who had achieved ROSC on admission were enrolled. In total, 52% of patients ($n = 32$) had a poor 30 day neurologic function. The number of patients with acute coronary syndrome was similar between patients with good and those with poor 30 day neurologic function (77% vs. 66%, $p = 0.338$). The time interval between collapse and study-related blood sampling was longer in patients with poor outcome (65 min vs. 56 min, $p = 0.033$). At 12 h, both the neutrophil count (11.8 vs. 9.9 G/L, $p = 0.051$) and the neutrophil-to-lymphocyte ratio (11.6 vs. 6.8, $p = 0.046$) were higher in patients with poor function compared with those with good neurologic function. The characteristics of the study patients, including median levels of NET-related biomarkers at 0 and 12 h, are shown in Table 1. Across all patients, there was no association between H3Cit and cfDNA (0 h: rho = 0.05, $p = 0.718$; 12 h: rho = 0.18, $p = 0.189$) or nucleosome levels (0 h: rho = 0.06, $p = 0.669$; 12 h: rho = 0.13, $p = 0.328$), neither on admission nor 12 h later. In contrast, cfDNA levels correlated with nucleosome levels at both time points (0 h: rho = 0.64, $p < 0.001$; 12 h: rho = 0.53; $p < 0.001$).

Table 1. Patient characteristics according to neurologic function on day 30. Data are n (%) or median (25–75% interquartile range).

Variable	Total ($n = 62$)	Good Function CPC 1–2 ($n = 30$)	Poor Function CPC 3–5 ($n = 32$)	p-Value
Male sex	49 (79)	25 (83)	24 (75)	0.421
Age, years	57 (46–67)	52 (44–61)	61 (53–70)	0.030 *
Cause of cardiac arrest				0.338
Acute coronary syndrome	44 (71)	23 (77)	21 (66)	
Primary arrhythmia	18 (29)	7 (23)	11 (34)	
PCI with stenting	42 (68)	22 (73)	20 (63)	0.362
Resuscitation characteristics				
CPC prior to cardiac arrest				
CPC 1	61 (98)	30 (100)	31 (95)	1.0
CPC 2	1 (2)	0	1 (5)	
Location of cardiac arrest				
Place of residence	35 (57)	19 (63)	16 (50)	0.290
Public place	27 (43)	11 (37)	16 (50)	
Witnessed	54 (87)	28 (93)	26 (81)	0.258
Basic life support	44 (71)	23 (77)	21 (66)	0.338
Shockable rhythm	46 (77)	27 (93)	19 (61)	0.004 *
Administration of heparin by EMS	28 (45.2)	14 (47)	14 (44)	0.795
Epinephrine, mg	3 (1–4)	1 (0–4)	3 (2–5)	0.004 *
Down time, min	29 (19–47)	23 (11–36)	38 (24–50)	0.011 *
Temp at admission, °C	35.3 (34.8–35.7)	35.4 (35.0–35.6)	35.1 (34.7–36)	0.676
Time from collapse to blood sampling, min	60 (49–72)	65 (52–87)	56 (43–65)	0.033 *
Laboratory values				
Lactate, mmol/L 0 h	7 (5–10)	6 (3–7)	10 (6–12)	0.001 *
D-dimer, µg/mL 0 h	8 (3–17)	4 (2–8)	14 (8–21)	0.003 *
D-dimer, µg/mL 12 h	4 (2–6)	2 (1–4)	6 (3–8)	0.009 *
Aptt, s 0 h	47 (36–121)	48 (33–129)	46 (37–119)	0.444
Aptt, s 12 h	37 (34–42)	37 (34–42)	38 (34–45)	0.487
Prothrombin time, % 0 h	79 (67–61)	79 (64–88)	78 (71–91)	0.418

Table 1. Cont.

Variable	Total (n = 62)	Good Function CPC 1–2 (n = 30)	Poor Function CPC 3–5 (n = 32)	p-Value
Prothrombin time, % 12 h	77 (66–87)	80 (68–88)	76 (63–86)	0.549
Fibrinogen, mg/dL 0 h	290 (242–322)	297 (246–317)	283 (240–343)	0.983
Fibrinogen, mg/dL 12 h	297 (258–350)	295 (260–346)	308 (241–359)	0.502
Platelet count, G/L 0 h	204 (163–245)	204 (163–235)	204 (164–251)	0.972
Platelet count, G/L 12h	193 (141–240)	193 (141–239)	193 (150–252)	0.490
CRP, mg/dL 0 h	0.2 (0.1–0.6)	0.2 (0.1–0.4)	0.3 (0.1–0.7)	0.410
CRP, mg/dL 12 h	1.6 (0.7–3.1)	1.0 (0.3–2.8)	1.7 (1.0–3.3)	0.057
Neutrophils 0 h, G/L	8.5 (6.2–12.8)	7.8 (6.0–12.8)	9.6 (6.4–13.2)	0.443
Neutrophils 12 h, G/L	10.9 (8.5–14.6)	9.9 (7.7–12.2)	11.8 (8.8–16)	0.051
NLR 0 h	2.5 (1.4–4.4)	2.6 (1.4–4.7)	2.4 (1.3–3.8)	0.375
NLR 12 h	10.3 (6.1–14.8)	6.8 (5.7–11.5)	11.6 (7–18)	0.046 *
cfDNA 0h, ng/mL	1481 (948–2176)	1197 (835–1544)	1898 (1148–2377)	0.007 *
cfDNA 12 h, ng/mL	555 (436–721)	489 (404–634)	593 (516–807)	0.016 *
Nucleosomes 0 h, MoM	4.4 (2.4–7.1)	3.8 (1.6–4.9)	5.6 (2.8–9.7)	0.032 *
Nucleosomes 12 h, MoM	0.7 (0.3–1.8)	0.4 (0.2–1.1)	1.1 (0.5–2.4)	0.036 *
H3Cit 0 h, ng/mL	447 (228–772)	447 (229–744)	434 (205–899)	0.755
H3Cit 12 h, ng/mL	386 (207–968)	299 (146–789)	667 (300–1201)	0.047 *

cfDNA, cell-free DNA; CPC, cerebral performance category; CRP, C-reactive protein; EMS, emergency medical service; H3Cit, citrullinated histones H3; MoM, multiple-of-the-mean; NLR, neutrophil-to-lymphocyte ratio; PCI, percutaneous coronary intervention; Temp, temperature; TnT, troponin. * indicates significance.

The poor neurologic function group had higher on-admission levels of cfDNA (1898 vs. 1197 ng/mL, $p = 0.007$) and nucleosomes (5.6 vs. 3.8 MoM, $p = 0.032$), but similar levels of H3Cit (434 vs. 447 ng/mL, $p = 0.755$) compared to patients with good neurologic function. While median levels of cfDNA and nucleosomes decreased in both groups from admission to 12 h, median levels of H3Cit increased in patients with poor 30 day neurologic function (Figure 1). At 12 h, all three biomarkers were higher in patients with poor 30 day neurologic function (cfDNA, 589 vs. 493 ng/mL, $p = 0.016$; nucleosomes, 1.1 vs. 0.4 MoM, $p = 0.036$; H3Cit, 667 vs. 299 ng/mL, $p = 0.043$). The score test showed a consistent trend towards poor neurologic function with increasing NET biomarker levels ($p < 0.05$) on admission ($p > 0.85$). This did not apply to H3Cit levels (Table S2).

In crude regression analysis, the odds of poor neurologic function on day 30 increased with increasing levels of NET-related biomarkers at both time points (Figure 2). In this, 0 h levels of cfDNA and nucleosomes were associated with 1.8 (crude OR, 95% CI: 1.2–2.7, $p = 0.007$) and 1.7 (crude OR, 95% CI: 1.0–2.2, $p = 0.049$) times higher odds of poor neurologic function. 12 h levels of cfDNA, nucleosomes, and H3Cit were associated with 1.6 (crude OR, 95% CI: 1.1–2.4, $p = 0.024$), 1.7 (crude OR, 95% CI: 1.1–2.5; $p = 0.02$), and 1.6 (crude OR, 95% CI: 1.1–2.3; $p = 0.029$) times higher odds of poor neurologic function. In patients with a CPC of 1–4 (n = 50), the odds of poor neurologic function on day 30 likewise increased with increasing 12 h levels of H3Cit (crude OR 1.7, 95% CI 1.0–3.0). The test for deviation from linearity indicated a linear association for all these biomarkers. The effect remained unchanged after adjustment for covariables (Table S1).

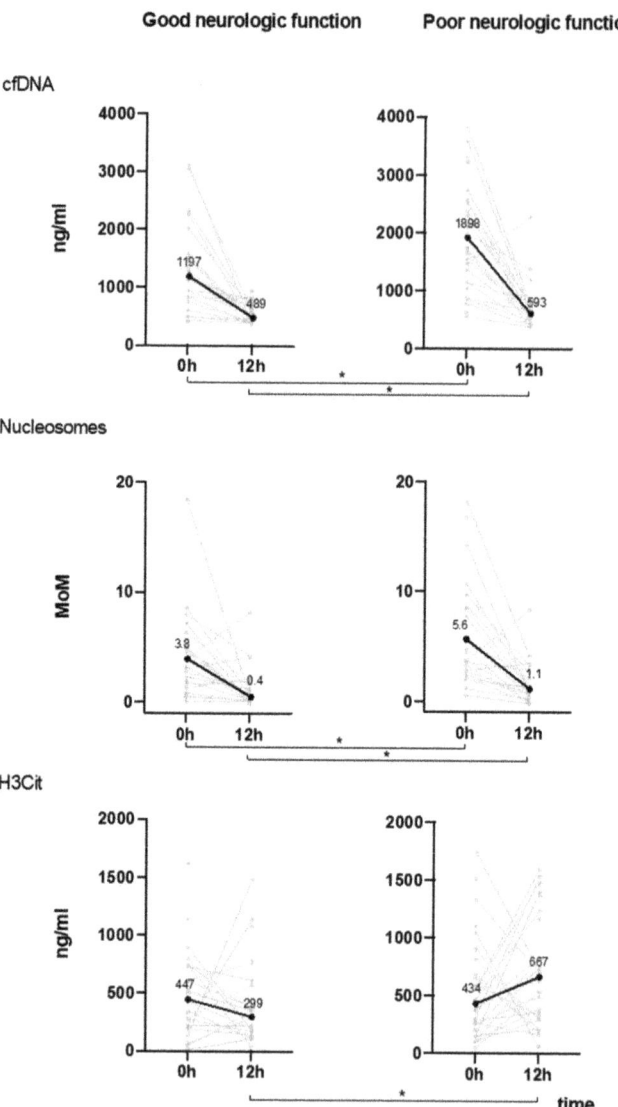

Figure 1. Plasma levels of neutrophil extracellular trap (NET) components (*y*-axis) on admission (0 h) and at 12 h (*x*-axis) in patients with good (left) and poor (right) 30 day neurologic function. Median levels of cfDNA and nucleosomes decreased in both groups from 0 to 12 h, while median H3Cit levels increased only in patients with poor 30 day neurologic function. Grey lines indicate individual data points, black lines represent median levels of NET-related biomarkers. * indicates significant difference. Individual and median d-dimer levels at 0 h and 12 h in the poor outcome group are available in the Supplementary Materials (Figure S2).

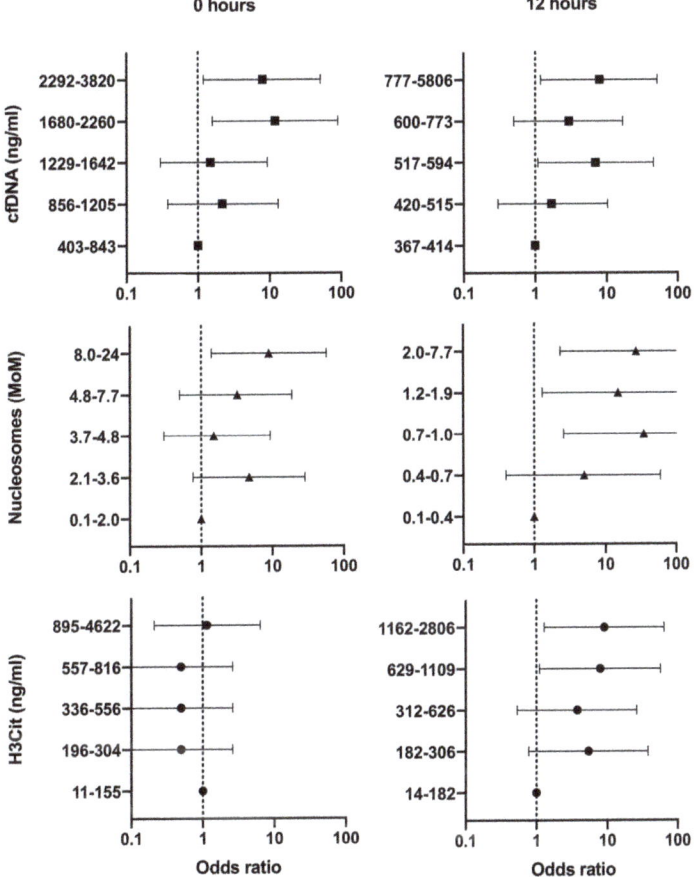

Figure 2. The crude odds of poor 30 day neurologic function (x-axis; crude odds ratio, log scale) according to plasma level quintiles of NET components (y-axis) on admission (left) and at 12 h (right). Confidence bands represent 95% confidence intervals. MoM, multiple-of-the-mean.

4. Discussion

Neurologic disability causes a high degree of morbidity in cardiac arrest survivors. This study investigated whether early plasma NET formation is associated with poor neurologic 30 day function following successful out-of-hospital resuscitation. The study was built on previous data suggesting a possible role of neutrophils in the development of post-resuscitative organ damage and was driven by the hypothesis that excessive NET release upon ischemic reperfusion may contribute to cerebral micro-circulatory compromise and thus neurologic disability in cardiac arrest survivors [5–8].

Previous studies reported increased mortality and neurologic morbidity in resuscitated cardiac arrest patients presenting with markers of neutrophil inflammation or elevated neutrophil counts in proportion to other leucocytes [6–8,26–28]. However, it has not been investigated whether these findings simply reflect stress response or whether neutrophils might be causally involved in the progression of organ injury following successful resuscitation.

This study provides a first indication that components of NETs may be involved in post-resuscitative brain damage. We found that NET-related biomarkers were already markedly elevated in cardiac arrest survivors at the time of admission, with these being even higher than levels measured in patients with cancer [12]. Although median levels of cfDNA and nucleosomes decreased over time, median levels of H3Cit increased in patients with poor neurologic function and were 30-fold higher at 12 h compared to those with good neurologic function on day 30.

cfDNA and nucleosomes are structural components of NETs but may have various sources and do not necessarily indicate their formation. Both are unspecific markers of cell death and cell turnover and may be interpreted as a measure of disease burden, but do not necessarily reflect the mechanism or source of disease. In this context, cfDNA levels have previously been shown to correlate with hospital mortality in cardiac arrest survivors [29]. H3Cit, in contrast, is considered a specific indicator of NET formation. Consistently, in this study, levels of cfDNA and nucleosomes on admission were significantly higher in patients with poor 30 day neurologic function, but decreased after successful resuscitation. In contrast, median H3Cit increased to significant levels at 12 h only in patients with poor 30 day neurologic function. It is likely that H3Cit are not detectable immediately upon admission, but take time to be formed, while less-specific markers originating from ischemic cell damage fall after ROSC. The lack of correlation between cfDNA and nucleosomes and H3Cit levels in our patients may further suggest that the biomarkers have different origins, and this is consistent with previous data on NET formation in patients with cancer [12], in whom H3Cit levels were likewise associated with an increased risk of mortality [30].

Although links in the chain of survival have substantially improved over the past decades, neurologic outcomes remain poor [31]. This is mainly attributable to the fact that several outcome-success factors cannot be influenced, such as witness status or a bystander's capability to provide basic life support. It might, however, highlight the lack of knowledge of the mechanisms driving post-resuscitative organ damage, limiting current post-resuscitation care to targeted temperature management [32].

The potential of post-resuscitation care to improve neurologic outcome is yet to be realized. Timely targeted interventions may offer the opportunity to alleviate or even interrupt early organ damage cascades triggered by ischemic reperfusion. Our data show that NETs may be associated with poor neurologic function 30 days after successful resuscitation. In contrast to previously identified coagulation makers associated with poor outcome after cardiac arrest [33,34], NET components may have the potential to serve as therapeutic target structures. NET-targeting agents administered soon after or even during resuscitation could contribute to preventing secondary brain injury and improving neurologic function. Supporting evidence comes from a recent mouse model study that shows the critical involvement of high mobility group box 1 formation in NET formation [35]. High mobility group box 1 is released by neutrophils [36], and the inhibition of high mobility group box 1 formation upon ischemic reperfusion successfully attenuated post-resuscitative brain injury in a rat model study [37].

However, it remains to be determined which step of NET formation should be targeted for therapy and which component of NETs is most appropriate to serve as a target structure. From our data we are able to infer that the early inhibition of histone H3 citrullination by selective peptidylarginine deiminase 4 (PAD 4) inhibitors might be a promising approach. This has already proven effective in disrupting in vitro NET formation in mouse and human neutrophils as well as in vivo [38,39]. Therapeutic degradation of formed NETs by DNase 1 may be an alternative or additional approach, one that has already been successfully used in mouse models to prevent thromboembolic disease [40]. In septic mice, infusion of DNase 1 resulted in significantly lower quantities of intravascular thrombin activity, reduced platelet aggregation, and ultimately improved microvascular perfusion.

The use of DNase 1 might be particularly beneficial in cardiac arrest patients with myocardial infarction, as coronary DNase activity has been found to negatively correlate with coronary NET burden and also with infarct size [11]. In this study, we analyzed a group of patients who had cardiac arrest of cardiac etiology. These patients commonly receive early antithrombotic and anticoagulant therapy and may thus be prone to experiencing hemorrhagic complications. A possible advantage of PAD 4 inhibitors and DNase 1 may be that both are considered to preserve physiological coagulation and thus should not cause additional bleeding risk [40]. Until advancements are made in human clinical testing, we can only speculate on the safety of these substances in humans. If further studies confirm our results, however, interventional trials investigating the safety and efficacy of NET-targeting agents in resuscitated animals may be warranted.

Limitations

The study was mainly limited by its sample size, resulting in large confidence intervals and the limited outcome events rate. We attempted to compensate for possible confounding by adjustment for clinically plausible covariables. Multivariable analyses including each relevant co-variable separately did not indicate relevant confounding. We included and analyzed a highly selected sample of patients with cardiac arrest of cardiac etiology who had achieved ROSC prior to hospital admission. Appropriate caution needs to be taken when interpreting our results. Furthermore, it must be mentioned that single patients with poor 30 day neurologic function did not show an increase in H3Cit levels from 0 to 12 h, while H3Cit levels did increase in some individuals with good neurologic outcome. Larger sampled studies investigating a more heterogeneous sample of cardiac arrest patients over a prolonged period of time may expand our results and aim at identifying specific patient characteristics, which allow for reliable prediction of NET formation in the individual patient in the early post-resuscitative stage.

Furthermore, a gold standard method for reliable measurement of NET formation in plasma is not available. We assessed three established NET-related biomarkers including H3Cit, which is considered a specific indicator of NET formation in plasma. It is, however, conceivable, that the assessment of additional NET components may gain test specificity and ultimately provide different results. The most reliable measure would perhaps be direct visualization of tissue NET formation, which may be investigated once a validated method becomes available.

Finally, we analyzed NET biomarker levels at only two time points, on admission and 12 h later. A more precise assessment of the time course of NET formation after cardiac arrest, however, may be of interest, because any NET-targeted therapy should likely be administered as early as possible to achieve the maximum beneficial effect.

5. Conclusions

We found that plasma levels of NET biomarkers assessed at an early post-resuscitative stage are associated with poor 30 day neurologic function in successfully resuscitated adults with OHCA. Further studies may assess whether NETs are causally involved in the pathophysiology of post-resuscitative brain damage, as well as discovering which components of NETs may have the potential to serve as therapeutic target structures to improve neurologic outcomes in cardiac arrest survivors in the future.

Supplementary Materials: The following are available online at http://www.mdpi.com/2077-0383/8/10/1568/s1, Table S1: Logistic regression. Table S2: Score test for trend. Figure S1: Study flow chart showing the selection process of study patients. Figure S2: Plasma levels at 0 h and 12 h for d dimer and H3Cit in patients with poor 30 day neurologic function.

Author Contributions: Conceptualization, L.-M.M., N.B., B.J. and M.S.; data curation, N.B., C.S., C.W., A.M., A.O.S. and M.S.; formal analysis, L.-M.M., H.H. and M.S.; funding acquisition, I.P. and B.J.; methodology, L.-M.M., L.H., C.A. and I.P.; Writing—Original draft, L.-M.M., N.B. and M.S.; Writing—Review and editing, C.S., C.W, H.H., A.M., A.O.S., L.H., C.A., I.P. and B.J. The manuscript has been seen and approved by all authors, has not been previously published, and is not under consideration for publication in the same or substantially similar form in any other peer-reviewed media.

Funding: L.-M.M., N.B., and L.H. are funded by the Austrian Science Fund (Fonds zur Förderung der wissenschaftlichen Forschung, FWF) grant SFB54/APF05404FW.

Acknowledgments: The authors thank Gerhard Ruzicka and study fellows for their valuable support. Open Access Funding by the Austrian Science Fund (Fonds zur Förderung der wissenschaftlichen Forschung, FWF).

Conflicts of Interest: The authors declare no conflict of interest. The funders had no role in the design of the study; in the collection, analyses, or interpretation of data; in the writing of the manuscript, or in the decision to publish the results.

References

1. Lilja, G.; Nielsen, N.; Friberg, H.; Horn, J.; Kjaergaard, J.; Nilsson, F.; Pellis, T.; Wetterslev, J.; Wise, M.P.; Bosch, F.; et al. Cognitive function in survivors of out-of-hospital cardiac arrest after target temperature management at 33 degrees C versus 36 degrees C. *Circulation* **2015**, *131*, 1340–1349. [CrossRef] [PubMed]
2. Sugita, A.; Kinoshita, K.; Sakurai, A.; Chiba, N.; Yamaguchi, J.; Kuwana, T.; Sawada, N.; Hori, S. Systemic impact on secondary brain aggravation due to ischemia/reperfusion injury in post-cardiac arrest syndrome: A prospective observational study using high-mobility group box 1 protein. *Crit. Care* **2017**, *21*, 247. [CrossRef] [PubMed]
3. Mongardon, N.; Dumas, F.; Ricome, S.; Grimaldi, D.; Hissem, T.; Pene, F.; Cariou, A. Postcardiac arrest syndrome: From immediate resuscitation to long-term outcome. *Ann. Intensive Care* **2011**, *1*, 45. [CrossRef] [PubMed]
4. Wada, T. Coagulofibrinolytic Changes in Patients with Post-cardiac Arrest Syndrome. *Front. Med. (Lausanne)* **2017**, *4*, 156. [CrossRef]
5. Cho, Y.D.; Park, S.J.; Choi, S.H.; Yoon, Y.H.; Kim, J.Y.; Lee, S.W.; Lim, C.S. The inflammatory response of neutrophils in an in vitro model that approximates the postcardiac arrest state. *Ann. Surg. Treat. Res.* **2017**, *93*, 217–224. [CrossRef]
6. Weiser, C.; Schwameis, M.; Sterz, F.; Herkner, H.; Lang, I.M.; Schwarzinger, I.; Spiel, A.O. Mortality in patients resuscitated from out-of-hospital cardiac arrest based on automated blood cell count and neutrophil lymphocyte ratio at admission. *Resuscitation* **2017**, *116*, 49–55. [CrossRef]
7. Patel, V.H.; Vendittelli, P.; Garg, R.; Szpunar, S.; LaLonde, T.; Lee, J.; Rosman, H.; Mehta, R.H.; Othman, H. Neutrophil-lymphocyte ratio: A prognostic tool in patients with in-hospital cardiac arrest. *World J. Crit. Care Med.* **2019**, *8*, 9–17. [CrossRef]
8. Kim, H.J.; Park, K.N.; Kim, S.H.; Lee, B.K.; Oh, S.H.; Moon, H.K.; Jeung, K.W.; Choi, S.P.; Cho, I.S.; Youn, C.S. Association between the neutrophil-to-lymphocyte ratio and neurological outcomes in patients undergoing targeted temperature management after cardiac arrest. *J. Crit. Care* **2018**, *47*, 227–231. [CrossRef]
9. Boeltz, S.; Amini, P.; Anders, H.J.; Andrade, F.; Bilyy, R.; Chatfield, S.; Cichon, I.; Clancy, D.M.; Desai, J.; Dumych, T.; et al. To NET or not to NET:current opinions and state of the science regarding the formation of neutrophil extracellular traps. *Cell Death Differ.* **2019**, *26*, 395–408. [CrossRef]
10. Kimball, A.S.; Obi, A.T.; Diaz, J.A.; Henke, P.K. The Emerging Role of NETs in Venous Thrombosis and Immunothrombosis. *Front. Immunol.* **2016**, *7*, 236. [CrossRef]
11. Mangold, A.; Alias, S.; Scherz, T.; Hofbauer, T.; Jakowitsch, J.; Panzenbock, A.; Simon, D.; Laimer, D.; Bangert, C.; Kammerlander, A.; et al. Coronary neutrophil extracellular trap burden and deoxyribonuclease activity in ST-elevation acute coronary syndrome are predictors of ST-segment resolution and infarct size. *Circ. Res.* **2015**, *116*, 1182–1192. [CrossRef] [PubMed]
12. Mauracher, L.M.; Posch, F.; Martinod, K.; Grilz, E.; Daullary, T.; Hell, L.; Brostjan, C.; Zielinski, C.; Ay, C.; Wagner, D.D.; et al. Citrullinated histone H3, a biomarker of neutrophil extracellular trap formation, predicts the risk of venous thromboembolism in cancer patients. *J. Thromb. Haemost.* **2018**, *16*, 508–518. [CrossRef] [PubMed]
13. Papayannopoulos, V. Neutrophil extracellular traps in immunity and disease. *Nat. Rev. Immunol.* **2018**, *18*, 134–147. [CrossRef] [PubMed]
14. Pertiwi, K.R.; van der Wal, A.C.; Pabittei, D.R.; Mackaaij, C.; van Leeuwen, M.B.; Li, X.; de Boer, O.J. Neutrophil Extracellular Traps Participate in All Different Types of Thrombotic and Haemorrhagic Complications of Coronary Atherosclerosis. *Thromb. Haemost.* **2018**, *118*, 1078–1087. [CrossRef]
15. Yipp, B.G.; Petri, B.; Salina, D.; Jenne, C.N.; Scott, B.N.; Zbytnuik, L.D.; Pittman, K.; Asaduzzaman, M.; Wu, K.; Meijndert, H.C.; et al. Infection-induced NETosis is a dynamic process involving neutrophil multitasking in vivo. *Nat. Med.* **2012**, *18*, 1386–1393. [CrossRef]
16. Fuchs, T.A.; Abed, U.; Goosmann, C.; Hurwitz, R.; Schulze, I.; Wahn, V.; Weinrauch, Y.; Brinkmann, V.; Zychlinsky, A. Novel cell death program leads to neutrophil extracellular traps. *J. Cell Biol.* **2007**, *176*, 231–241. [CrossRef]
17. Ge, L.; Zhou, X.; Ji, W.J.; Lu, R.Y.; Zhang, Y.; Zhang, Y.D.; Ma, Y.Q.; Zhao, J.H.; Li, Y.M. Neutrophil extracellular traps in ischemia-reperfusion injury-induced myocardial no-reflow: Therapeutic potential of DNase-based reperfusion strategy. *Am. J. Physiol. Heart Circ. Physiol.* **2015**, *308*, H500–H509. [CrossRef]

18. Gould, T.J.; Lysov, Z.; Liaw, P.C. Extracellular DNA and histones: Double-edged swords in immunothrombosis. *J. Thromb. Haemost.* **2015**, *13*, S82–S91. [CrossRef]
19. Noubouossie, D.F.; Whelihan, M.F.; Yu, Y.B.; Sparkenbaugh, E.; Pawlinski, R.; Monroe, D.M.; Key, N.S. In vitro activation of coagulation by human neutrophil DNA and histone proteins but not neutrophil extracellular traps. *Blood* **2017**, *129*, 1021–1029. [CrossRef]
20. Silk, E.; Zhao, H.; Weng, H.; Ma, D. The role of extracellular histone in organ injury. *Cell Death Dis.* **2017**, *8*, e2812. [CrossRef]
21. Jorch, S.K.; Kubes, P. An emerging role for neutrophil extracellular traps in noninfectious disease. *Nat. Med.* **2017**, *23*, 279–287. [CrossRef] [PubMed]
22. Li, P.; Li, M.; Lindberg, M.R.; Kennett, M.J.; Xiong, N.; Wang, Y. PAD4 is essential for antibacterial innate immunity mediated by neutrophil extracellular traps. *J. Exp. Med.* **2010**, *207*, 1853–1862. [CrossRef]
23. Nolan, J.P.; Hazinski, M.F.; Aickin, R.; Bhanji, F.; Billi, J.E.; Callaway, C.W.; Castren, M.; de Caen, A.R.; Ferrer, J.M.; Finn, J.C.; et al. Part 1: Executive summary: 2015 International Consensus on Cardiopulmonary Resuscitation and Emergency Cardiovascular Care Science with Treatment Recommendations. *Resuscitation* **2015**, *95*, e1–e31. [CrossRef]
24. Edgren, E.; Hedstrand, U.; Kelsey, S.; Sutton-Tyrrell, K.; Safar, P. Assessment of neurological prognosis in comatose survivors of cardiac arrest. BRCT I Study Group. *Lancet* **1994**, *343*, 1055–1059. [CrossRef]
25. Cuzick, J. A Wilcoxon-type test for trend. *Stat. Med.* **1985**, *4*, 87–90. [CrossRef]
26. Peberdy, M.A.; Andersen, L.W.; Abbate, A.; Thacker, L.R.; Gaieski, D.; Abella, B.S.; Grossestreuer, A.V.; Rittenberger, J.C.; Clore, J.; Ornato, J.; et al. Inflammatory markers following resuscitation from out-of-hospital cardiac arrest-A prospective multicenter observational study. *Resuscitation* **2016**, *103*, 117–124. [CrossRef] [PubMed]
27. Bro-Jeppesen, J.; Kjaergaard, J.; Wanscher, M.; Nielsen, N.; Friberg, H.; Bjerre, M.; Hassager, C. The inflammatory response after out-of-hospital cardiac arrest is not modified by targeted temperature management at 33 degrees C or 36 degrees C. *Resuscitation* **2014**, *85*, 1480–1487. [CrossRef] [PubMed]
28. Bro-Jeppesen, J.; Kjaergaard, J.; Stammet, P.; Wise, M.P.; Hovdenes, J.; Aneman, A.; Horn, J.; Devaux, Y.; Erlinge, D.; Gasche, Y.; et al. Predictive value of interleukin-6 in post-cardiac arrest patients treated with targeted temperature management at 33 degrees C or 36 degrees C. *Resuscitation* **2016**, *98*, 1–8. [CrossRef]
29. Arnalich, F.; Menendez, M.; Lagos, V.; Ciria, E.; Quesada, A.; Codoceo, R.; Vazquez, J.J.; Lopez-Collazo, E.; Montiel, C. Prognostic value of cell-free plasma DNA in patients with cardiac arrest outside the hospital: An observational cohort study. *Crit. Care* **2010**, *14*, R47. [CrossRef]
30. Grilz, E.; Mauracher, L.M.; Posch, F.; Konigsbrugge, O.; Zochbauer-Muller, S.; Marosi, C.; Lang, I.; Pabinger, I.; Ay, C. Citrullinated histone H3, a biomarker for neutrophil extracellular trap formation, predicts the risk of mortality in patients with cancer. *Br. J. Haematol.* **2019**, *186*, 311–320. [CrossRef] [PubMed]
31. Sulzgruber, P.; Sterz, F.; Schober, A.; Uray, T.; Van Tulder, R.; Hubner, P.; Wallmuller, C.; El-Tattan, D.; Graf, N.; Ruzicka, G.; et al. Editor's Choice-Progress in the chain of survival and its impact on outcomes of patients admitted to a specialized high-volume cardiac arrest center during the past two decades. *Eur. Heart J. Acute Cardiovasc. Care* **2016**, *5*, 3–12. [CrossRef] [PubMed]
32. Arrich, J.; Holzer, M.; Havel, C.; Mullner, M.; Herkner, H. Hypothermia for neuroprotection in adults after cardiopulmonary resuscitation. *Cochrane Database Syst. Rev.* **2016**, *2*, CD004128. [CrossRef] [PubMed]
33. Adrie, C.; Monchi, M.; Laurent, I.; Um, S.; Yan, S.B.; Thuong, M.; Cariou, A.; Charpentier, J.; Dhainaut, J.F. Coagulopathy after successful cardiopulmonary resuscitation following cardiac arrest: Implication of the protein C anticoagulant pathway. *J. Am. Coll. Cardiol.* **2005**, *46*, 21–28. [CrossRef] [PubMed]
34. Buchtele, N.; Schober, A.; Schoergenhofer, C.; Spiel, A.O.; Mauracher, L.; Weiser, C.; Sterz, F.; Jilma, B.; Schwameis, M. Added value of the DIC score and of D-dimer to predict outcome after successfully resuscitated out-of-hospital cardiac arrest. *Eur. J. Intern. Med.* **2018**, *57*, 44–48. [CrossRef]
35. Tadie, J.M.; Bae, H.B.; Jiang, S.; Park, D.W.; Bell, C.P.; Yang, H.; Pittet, J.F.; Tracey, K.; Thannickal, V.J.; Abraham, E.; et al. HMGB1 promotes neutrophil extracellular trap formation through interactions with Toll-like receptor 4. *Am. J. Physiol. Lung Cell. Mol. Physiol.* **2013**, *304*, L342–L349. [CrossRef] [PubMed]
36. Ito, I.; Fukazawa, J.; Yoshida, M. Post-translational methylation of high mobility group box 1 (HMGB1) causes its cytoplasmic localization in neutrophils. *J. Biol. Chem.* **2007**, *282*, 16336–16344. [CrossRef] [PubMed]

37. Shi, X.; Li, M.; Huang, K.; Zhou, S.; Hu, Y.; Pan, S.; Gu, Y. HMGB1 binding heptamer peptide improves survival and ameliorates brain injury in rats after cardiac arrest and cardiopulmonary resuscitation. *Neuroscience* **2017**, *360*, 128–138. [CrossRef]
38. Lewis, H.D.; Liddle, J.; Coote, J.E.; Atkinson, S.J.; Barker, M.D.; Bax, B.D.; Bicker, K.L.; Bingham, R.P.; Campbell, M.; Chen, Y.H.; et al. Inhibition of PAD4 activity is sufficient to disrupt mouse and human NET formation. *Nat. Chem. Biol.* **2015**, *11*, 189–191. [CrossRef]
39. Martinod, K.; Demers, M.; Fuchs, T.A.; Wong, S.L.; Brill, A.; Gallant, M.; Hu, J.; Wang, Y.; Wagner, D.D. Neutrophil histone modification by peptidylarginine deiminase 4 is critical for deep vein thrombosis in mice. *Proc. Natl. Acad. Sci. USA* **2013**, *110*, 8674–8679. [CrossRef]
40. Martinod, K.; Wagner, D.D. Thrombosis: Tangled up in NETs. *Blood* **2014**, *123*, 2768–2776. [CrossRef]

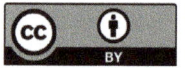 © 2019 by the authors. Licensee MDPI, Basel, Switzerland. This article is an open access article distributed under the terms and conditions of the Creative Commons Attribution (CC BY) license (http://creativecommons.org/licenses/by/4.0/).

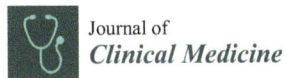

Article

Resistin and Cardiac Arrest—A Prospective Study

Raluca M. Tat [1,†], Adela Golea [2,†], Rodica Rahaian [3], Ștefan C. Vesa [4,*] and Daniela Ionescu [1,5]

1. Department of Anesthesia and Intensive Care I, "Iuliu Hațieganu" University of Medicine and Pharmacy, 400012 Cluj-Napoca, Romania; tatralu@yahoo.com
2. Surgical Department of "Iuliu Hațieganu" University of Medicine and Pharmacy, 400012 Cluj-Napoca, Romania; adeg2810@gmail.com
3. Department of Immunology Laboratory, County Emergency Hospital, 400006 Cluj-Napoca, Romania; rodirahaian@yahoo.com
4. Department of Pharmacology, Toxicology and Clinical Pharmacology, "Iuliu Hațieganu" University of Medicine and Pharmacy, 400012 Cluj-Napoca, Romania
5. Outcome Research Consortium, Cleveland, OH 44195, USA; dionescuati@yahoo.com
* Correspondence: stefanvesa@gmail.com; Tel.: +40-074-0125-980
† Authors with equal contributions.

Received: 6 November 2019; Accepted: 24 December 2019; Published: 25 December 2019

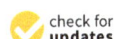

Abstract: The systemic response to ischemia-reperfusion that occurs after a cardiac arrest (CA) followed by the return of spontaneous circulation leads to endothelial toxicity and cytokine production, both responsible for the subsequent occurrence of severe cardiocirculatory dysfunction and early death. Resistin is emerging as a biomarker of proinflammatory status and myocardial ischemic injury and as a mediator of endothelial dysfunction. The study aimed to analyze the possible associations between several clinical and biological variables and the serum levels of resistin in CA survivors. Forty patients with out-of-hospital resuscitated CA, were enrolled in the study. Demographic, clinical and laboratory data (including serum resistin measurements at admission and at 6, 12, 24, 48 and 72 h) were recorded. For resistin, we calculated the area under the curve (AUC) using the trapezoidal method with measurements from 0 to 12 h, 0 to 24 h, 0 to 48 h and 0 to 72 h. Fifteen (37.5%) patients died in the first 72 h after CA. Cardiovascular comorbidities were present in 65% of patients. The majority of patients had post-CA shock (29 (72.5%)). Resistin serum levels rose in the first 12–24 h and decreased in the next 48–72 h. In univariate analysis, advanced age, longer duration of resuscitation, high sequential organ failure assessment score, high lactate levels, presence of cardiovascular comorbidities and the post-CA shock were associated with higher resistin levels. In multivariate analysis, post-CA shock or cardiovascular comorbidities were independently associated with higher AUCs for resistin for 0–12 h and 0–24 h. The only identified variable to independently predict higher AUCs for resistin for 0–48 h and 0–72 h was the presence of post-CA shock. Our data demonstrate strong independent correlation between high serum resistin levels, cardiac comorbidities and post-CA shock. The impact of the post-CA shock on serum concentration of resistin was greater than that of cardiac comorbidities.

Keywords: cardiac arrest; resistin; post-cardiac-arrest shock

1. Introduction

One of the relatively common presentations in the emergency department (ED) is that of a patient who suffered an out-of-hospital cardiac arrest (OHCA). Regardless of the etiology of cardiac arrest (CA), the physicians' efforts are centered on the early control of all consequences secondary to the interruption of blood flow to organs and return of spontaneous circulation (ROSC). They are known under the term of post-cardiac-arrest syndrome (PCAS)—which is responsible for the high mortality of post-resuscitation patients [1,2]. In PCAS, four components have been described: post-cardiac-arrest brain injury, post-cardiac-arrest myocardial dysfunction, systemic response to ischemia/reperfusion and persistent precipitating pathology [2]. Although post-cardiac-arrest brain injury remains an important cause of mortality and morbidity among CA patients, the other elements of PCAS (like systemic response to ischemia/reperfusion) also lead to multiple organ failure and early death [2,3].

The pathophysiology of PCAS is very complex and involves ischemia-reperfusion injury and activation of nonspecific mechanisms of systemic inflammatory response. Summarizing the process, the oxygen supply during ischemia is reduced and the cellular metabolism is affected, ultimately resulting in an increase in the intracytoplasmic calcium concentration responsible for the first cellular and tissue lesions. During the reperfusion phase, following restoration of the blood flow, reactive oxygen species formed during the ischemic phase induce cell death through their cytotoxic effect (inactivation of cytochromes, alteration of membrane transport proteins, inducing lipid peroxidation of the membrane). The pro-oxidant state that occurs inside the cells marks the transition to the next stage, characterized by aggressive endothelial toxicity. The onset of vascular endothelial lesions paves the way to systemic inflammation via the ischemia-reperfusion mechanisms: cytokine production, complement activation, arachidonic acid synthesis, leukocyte adhesion to endothelial cells and triggering of activation and chemotaxis of polymorphonuclear neutrophils at the origin of the inflammatory response. All of these are responsible for the subsequent development of multiple organ failure. Of note, the activation of the systemic inflammatory response is also associated with changes in coagulation (intravascular coagulation dissemination), which generate additional endothelial lesions. This creates a vicious circle where inflammatory lesions and coagulation abnormalities induce further organ damage by accentuating pre-existing lesions and enhancing the persistence of the precipitating pathology of CA, more likely in close dependence with the duration of resuscitation and the rhythm of CA [4–7].

In the past few years, the research community has been focused on identifying biomarkers able to adequately predict the severity of the lesions that underline the pathophysiological processes in CA.

Resistin is a cysteine-rich, adipose-derived peptide hormone encoded by the *RETN* gene that is highly expressed in circulating monocytes, macrophages and vascular endothelium [8–10]. It is involved in numerous pathological processes (obesity, disorders of glucose and insulin metabolism, atherosclerosis, malignancies, rheumatic diseases, chronic kidney disease, etc.) [11–14]. Resistin has been suggested as a marker of the severity of myocardial ischemic lesion [8,12] and proposed as a mediator of endothelial dysfunction [8,12,15–17]. Moreover, resistin has been potentially introduced as a marker of proinflammatory status (cytokine-like) in relation to sepsis and in other nonseptic critical pathologies [8,12–14]. In a previous study, we investigated the role of resistin as a biomarker for predicting mortality after CA. The results showed that elevated serum resistin levels were highly predictive of mortality in critically ill patients who survived a CA [14,18].

Taking into account the proposed mechanisms of action of resistin and the pathophysiology of CA, the aim of our study was to investigate the clinical and biological variables that correlate with serum resistin levels in CA survivors.

2. Materials and Methods

A prospective, analytical, longitudinal, observational cohort study included consecutive patients resuscitated after the OHCA and admitted to the ED of County Emergency Hospital Cluj-Napoca between May 2016 and October 2017. Informed consent for inclusion in the study was obtained from patients' proxies in all cases. The study was conducted in accordance with the Declaration of Helsinki, and the protocol was approved by the Ethics Committee of "Iuliu Hațieganu" University of Medicine and Pharmacy, with registration number 59/14.03.2016.

The inclusion criteria were as follows: age between 18–85 years and resuscitated OHCA. The exclusion criteria were as follows: ages under 18 or over 85 years, pregnancy, re-arrest with unsuccessful resuscitation within 6 h from hospital arrival, inmates, absence of informed consent and CA due to trauma, acute bleeding from nontraumatic condition, hypothermia or terminal neoplastic disease.

2.1. Study Protocol and Laboratory Assays

The management protocol of the patients admitted to the study, the post-CA shock definition and the lab protocols were previously described [18].

Each patient with out-of-hospital CA admitted to the study was resuscitated by emergency medical team members according to the recommendations of the European Resuscitation Council 2015 [19,20]. Fluids infusion and vasoactive drugs (adrenaline, noradrenaline, dopamine, dobutamine), alone or in combination, were administered in order to maintain mean arterial pressure ≥65 mmHg and urine output ≥0.5 mL/kg/h. For patients remaining comatose after successful resuscitation, able to maintain a systolic blood pressure above 90 mmHg (mean arterial pressure—MAP ≥65 mmHg) and without sepsis, controlled therapeutic hypothermia was administered in the first 24 h, in order to maintain a central temperature with a target between 34–35°C, using ice bags and cooling blanket. Reheating was slow, at a rate of 0.25–0.5 °C/h. According to local protocols which follow current guidelines, hyperthermia, seizures and hyperglycemia were avoided and immediately treated [21,22].

Blood samples were drawn from a peripheral vein where no medication was administered, at 0-time interval (emergency admission), 6, 12, 24, 48 and 72 h following resuscitation. Five-milliliter biochemistry vacutainers with serum separator clot activator were used for blood sample collection. To collect blood samples, we used 5 mL biochemistry vacutainers with serum separator clot activator. The identified hemolyzed samples were excluded and blood samples were immediately repeated. Samples were centrifuged at 3000 rotation/minutes during the first 60 min after collection and were stored at −70 °C. Subsequently, serum concentrations of biomarkers (resistin, S-100B and NSE) were analyzed using a quantitative sandwich immunoassay technique (ELISA; BioVendor, LM, Czech Republic) according to the manufacturer's instructions. After processing, defrosted blood samples were no longer used and underwent destruction.

For every patient, the following data were recorded: demographic (age, gender), clinical (presence of cardiovascular diseases and/or strong risk factors for cardiovascular disease (arterial hypertension, coronary artery disease, valvular heart disease, congestive heart failure, history of stroke, diabetes mellitus and obesity), the rhythm of OHCA, duration of resuscitation, body mass index (BMI), presence of post-CA shock), sequential organ failure assessment (SOFA) score at admission and laboratory data (lactate and glycemia at admission; resistin at 6, 12, 24, 48 and 72 h). Obesity was defined by a body mass index (BMI) ≥30 kg/m^2. The overweight was classified at a BMI between 25 and 29.9 kg/m^2. Post-CA shock was defined as the need to administer vasoactive/inotropic therapy to maintain a MAP >65 mmHg for at least 6 h immediate after return of spontaneous circulation, although fluid therapy was adequate.

2.2. Statistical Analysis

Statistical analysis was performed using the MedCalc Statistical Software version 18.11.3 (MedCalc Software bvba, Ostend, Belgium; https://www.medcalc.org; 2019). Quantitative data normality was assessed using the Shapiro–Wilk test, measures of skewness and kurtosis and histograms. Quantitative data were expressed as median and interquartile range (IQR). Qualitative data were characterized by frequency and percentage. For resistin, we calculated the area under the curve (AUC) using the trapezoidal method with measurements from 0 to 12 h, 0 to 24 h, 0 to 48 h and 0 to 72 h. The sample size was calculated from a pilot study (13 patients with post-CA shock and 4 patients without post-CA shock). Calculated AUC for resistin, for 0–12 h measurements, showed a 24 ng × h/mL mean difference between the two groups. For a type 1 (a) error of 0.01 and a type 2 (b) error of 0.05, we calculated a sample size of 34 patients. The power of the study was calculated as 95%. Correlations between quantitative variables were assessed using the Spearman's rank correlation coefficient. The differences between groups were verified with Mann–Whitney test. In order to find out which variables can be independently linked to resistin, we constructed several models using multiple linear regressions. Due to the fact that the resistin values followed a non-normal distribution, we performed a logarithmic transformation. We introduced the variables that were significantly associated with the AUCs for resistin during the univariate analysis. A *p*-value of less than 0.05 was considered statistically significant.

3. Results

Forty patients admitted to ED who met the inclusion criteria were included in the study. Patient characteristics are described in Table 1. On the first and second day, 12 (30%) patients died, and by the third day there were another three (7.5%) deaths. The 25 survivors after 72 h were followed for 30 days, and we recorded the deaths of 13 of them in this interval. Most of the recorded CA rhythm was asystole. Of the total number of patients admitted in our study, only 11 (28.5%) patients did not develop immediate post-resuscitation shock. Of the total admitted patients, 14 (35%) were obese and 20 (50%) were overweight.

Table 1. Baseline characteristics of the study group.

Characteristics		Eligible Patients with CA (*n* = 40)
Age, years, median (IQR)		67 (59.2 to 76.0)
Gender, *n* (%)	Female	12 (30.0)
	Male	28 (70.0)
Presenting rhythm, *n* (%)	Asystole	23 (57.5)
	PEA	5 (12.5)
	VF	11 (27.5)
	VT without pulse	1 (2.5)
Duration of CPR, minutes, median (IQR)		15 (7.7 to 28.7)
Current smoking, *n* (%)		4 (10)
Chronic alcohol consumer, *n* (%)		5 (12.5)
Medical history, *n* (%)	Non-cardiovascular comorbidities	18 (45.0)
	Cardiovascular comorbidities	26 (65.0)
	Arterial hypertension	23 (57.5)
	Coronary artery disease	17 (42.5)
	Valvular heart disease	8 (20%)
	Congestive heart failure	15 (37.5)
	Stroke	3 (7.5)
	Diabetes mellitus	7 (17.5)
BMI, median (IQR)		28 (26.0 to 31.0)
Obesity, *n* (%)		14 (35)
SOFA score, median (IQR)		15 (12.0 to 16.0)
Patients with post-CA shock, *n* (%)		29 (72.5)
Lactate (mmol/L), median (IQR)		10.42 (7.6 to 12.9)
Blood glucose (mg/dL), median (IQR)		249.0 (156.0 to 330.0)

IQR = interquartile range; PEA = pulseless electrical activity; VF = ventricular fibrillation; VT = ventricular tachycardia; CPR = cardiopulmonary resuscitation; BMI = body mass index; SOFA = sequential organ failure assessment score; CA = cardiac arrest.

For serum resistin levels we calculated the AUCs using the trapezoidal method with measurements from 0 to 24 h, 0 to 48 h and 0 to 72 h. Resistin levels and AUCs showed an increase in the first 12 h after admission, followed by a gradual decrease in the next 60 h (Table 2).

Table 2. Median serum levels of resistin and the AUC for resistin during the first 72 h.

Variable		Median (IQR)
Resistin, (ng/mL)	at 0 h	7.1 (4.6 to 11.8)
	at 6 h	9.8 (4.4 to 17.7)
	at 12 h	13.5 (5.5 to 21.0)
	at 24 h	12.3 (6.7 to 21.0)
	at 48 h	7.2 (3.5 to 14.6)
	at 72 h	7.4 (3.6 to 11.9)
AUC resistin, (ng × h/mL)	in the first 12 h	26.0 (11.5 to 43.2)
	in the first 24 h	25.8 (15.2 to 44.7)
	in the first 48 h	16.6 (10.4 to 35.1)
	in the first 72 h	34.6 (17.9 to 46.5)

AUC = area under the curve; IQR = interquartile range.

We found that SOFA score and serum lactate values at admission were the most important clinical and laboratory parameters associated with serum resistin levels (strong positive correlation to all repeated measurements) (Table 3). The serum resistin levels were not influenced by BMI.

Table 3. Correlations between the AUCs for resistin and the study quantitative variables.

Variable	AUC for 0–12 h		AUC for 0–24 h		AUC for 0–48 h		AUC for 0–72 h	
	r	p	r	p	r	p	r	p
Age, years	0.316	0.04	0.360	0.03	0.467	0.01	0.356	0.08
Duration of CPR, minutes	0.364	0.02	0.386	0.02	0.414	0.02	0.357	0.08
BMI	0.039	0.8	−0.148	0.4	−0.183	0.3	−0.141	0.5
SOFA score	0.586	<0.001	0.579	<0.001	0.510	0.006	0.529	0.007
Lactate (mmol/L)	0.499	<0.001	0.592	<0.001	0.501	0.007	0.509	0.009
Blood glucose (mg/dL)	0.185	0.2	0.417	0.01	0.176	0.3	−0.023	0.9

AUC = area under the curve; CPR = cardiopulmonary resuscitation; BMI = body mass index; SOFA = sequential organ failure assessment score; r = correlation coefficient.

The AUCs for resistin were higher in patients who presented asystole or PEA rhythm of CA (especially), cardiovascular comorbidities, history of congestive heart failure, arterial hypertension or post-CA shock (Table 4). We found no associations between AUCs for resistin and history of coronary artery disease, stroke, diabetes mellitus, obesity, smoking or alcoholic beverages.

Several models based on multiple linear regression were used in order to determine the independent association between clinical/laboratory data and the AUCs for resistin. The variables that were significantly linked to the AUCs in the univariate analysis were introduced in the models. Due to the fact that the resistin values followed a non-normal distribution, we performed a logarithmic transformation. When we introduced the history of congestive heart failure or arterial hypertension as separate variables, we found no statistically significant association with the log AUCs for resistin. Post-CA shock or cardiovascular comorbidities were independently associated with the log AUC for resistin for 0–12 h and 0–24 h. The only identified variable independently linked to the log AUC for resistin for 0–48 h and 0–72 h was the presence of post-CA shock (Table 5).

Table 4. Associations between the AUC for resistin and the qualitative variables studied.

Variable		AUC for 0–12 h		AUC for 0–24 h		AUC for 0–48 h		AUC for 0–72 h	
		Median (IQR)	p	Median (IQR)	p	Median (IQR)	p	Median (IQR)	p
Gender	Female	26.5 (23.0 to 42.5)	0.4	30.0 (17.4 to 44.1)	0.8	20.6 (13.3 to 49.2)	0.3	25.0 (17.1 to 74.0)	0.7
	Male	23.0 (10.2 to 43.2)		25.2 (13.8 to 44.7)		15.9 (9.3 to 33.8)		35.3 (18.7 to 46.1)	
Presenting rhythm of CA	Asystole/PEA	30.5 (22.0 to 47.7)	0.002	30.3 (19.9 to 51.4)	0.002	23.5 (14.5 to 38.7)	0.009	37.8 (25.0 to 69.8)	0.01
	VF/VT without pulse	10.5 (4.2 to 22.5)		14.3 (8.0 to 24.1)		12.4 (4.8 to 16.0)		23.4 (13.8 to 31.9)	
Cardiovascular comorbidities	present	29.0 (22.0 to 45.5)	0.03	37.2 (18.3 to 50.2)	0.01	22.7 (14.2 to 38.1)	0.06	37.4 (23.6 to 64.0)	0.08
	absent	16.5 (4.7 to 31.5)		18.8 (11.1 to 25.8)		13.7 (5.3 to 28.4)		27.6 (15.0 to 36.7)	
History of arterial hypertension	present	28 (22 to 45)	0.1	37.2 (18.2 to 49.1)	0.05	22 (14.1 to 39)	0.1	37.8 (22.2 to 67.3)	0.1
	absent	18 (7 to 37)		19.9 (14.3 to 26.4)		14.5 (5.8 to 27.3)		29.3 (15.4 to 36.9)	
History of congestive heart failure	present	30.5 (23 to 46.5)	0.04	38 (29.9 to 49.7)	0.02	34.8 (19.6 to 46.4)	0.02	52.8 (23.5 to 92)	0.04
	absent	18.5 (7.5 to 32.7)		19.3 (9.8 to 31.6)		14.5 (9.2 to 23.9)		27.6 (16.9 to 36.8)	
Post-CA shock	present	31.0 (24.0 to 47.5)	<0.001	30.3 (24.1 to 51.4)	<0.001	30.8 (15.9 to 38.7)	0.002	41.8 (23.4 to 70.8)	0.01
	absent	10.0 (4.0 to 15.0)		13.4 (8.0 to 18.8)		12.4 (4.8 to 15.8)		27.5 (12.1 to 34.6)	

AUC = area under the curve; IQR = interquartile range; PEA = pulseless electrical activity; VF = ventricular fibrillation; VT = ventricular tachycardia; CA = cardiac arrest.

Table 5. Multiple linear regression for the AUCs for resistin.

Variables for the log of AUC for 0–12 h	B	p	95.0% CI for B	
			Min	Max
(Constant)	0.784	<0.001	0.581	0.988
Post-CA shock	0.528	<0.001	0.309	0.747
Cardiovascular comorbidities	0.214	0.04	0.009	0.419
Variables for the log of AUC for 0–24 h	**B**	**p**	**95.0% CI for B**	
			Min	Max
(Constant)	0.954	<0.001	0.768	1.140
Post-CA shock	0.415	<0.001	0.211	0.619
Cardiovascular comorbidities	0.201	0.04	0.004	0.397
Variables for the log of AUC for 0–48 h	**B**	**p**	**95.0% CI for B**	
			Min	Max
(Constant)	0.939	<0.001	0.739	1.139
Post-CA shock	0.470	0.001	0.212	0.727
Variables for the log of AUC for 0–72 h	**B**	**p**	**95.0% CI for B**	
			Min	Max
(Constant)	1.321	<0.001	1.154	1.488
Post-CA shock	0.303	0.01	0.079	0.526

AUC = area under the curve; B = standardized beta coefficient; CA = cardiac arrest.

4. Discussions

CA involves the most severe form of circulatory failure. The complex changes produced by disruption of cell morpho-functional integrity during the general ischemia phase do not stop with the return of spontaneous circulation and are subsequently supplemented by those appearing during the reperfusion phase. The release of proinflammatory cytokines with the onset of systemic inflammatory response syndrome and endothelial damage (with coagulation/anticoagulation and fibrinogenesis/fibrinolysis imbalance) are intricate mechanisms that ultimately contribute to organ failures with negative impact prognosis of resuscitated patients [6,8,13,14,23].

In our previous study, we investigated for the first time the serum levels of resistin as a possible predictor of mortality after CA. Our results were promising, showing that high serum values of resistin accurately predicted death at 30 days, making resistin a marker with a high predictive value of survival [14,18].

However, resistin levels can be influenced by a variety of factors, such as the presence of atherosclerosis, obesity or sepsis. In light of this, we investigated the possible correlations of several clinical and biochemical factors with the serum concentration of resistin in patients with CA, for a better understanding of its role in CA [18].

Initially described in 1994 as a way of quantifying organ dysfunction by evaluating respiratory, cardiovascular, hepatic, renal, neurological and coagulation systems [24], the SOFA score remained useful over the years and is now being used with accuracy in quantifying the prognosis of critically ill patients [25]. The ischemia-reperfusion lesion is one of the most important mechanisms that link CA to multiple organ failures, including circulatory and cardiac dysfunction. Our results showed that there is a strong correlation between the severity of the disease (quantified by the SOFA score) and serum levels of resistin, a potential marker that may correctly reflect organ failures.

Over time, elevated levels of resistin have been associated with increased risk of coronary heart disease, especially with myocardial infarction (but not with stroke) [26] and with the degree of heart failure, both responsible for increasing the rate of cardiac events, including the risk of death [26,27]. At the same time, obesity, diabetes, high carbohydrate and unsaturated fat diet and chronic alcohol consumption, but not smoking, were described as cardiovascular risk factors correlated with elevated human serum resistin levels [28–31]. In our study, we found no associations between resistin levels in patients with CA and history of coronary artery disease, stroke, diabetes mellitus, obesity, smoking or alcoholic beverages. This reinforces the idea that in an acute critical illness high levels of resistin (or other adipokines) are mostly due to inflammatory status and not to adipose tissue mass or pre-existing unhealthy lifestyle [32].

At multivariate analysis, we found that the presence of post-CA shock and cardiovascular comorbidities were independently associated with serum resistin levels in the first 24 h after CA.

In fact, the presence of post-CA shock was the only independent variable associated with serum resistin levels at 48 and 72 h following CA. These results show that the elevated serum concentrations of resistin might be influenced by the post-CA shock, rather than by pre-CA cardiovascular comorbidities. The shock that occurs after CA is the result of myocardial dysfunction, vasoplegic shock and systemic inflammatory response [25]. Part of a complex vicious circle, as this shock becomes more refractory to treatment, cardiocirculatory dysfunction evolves in turn into a more severe form, resulting in multiple organ failures responsible for early death. The strong association of resistin with post-CA shock and with the presence of cardiovascular comorbidities may support the theory that serum resistin levels correlate equally with both the amplitude of the inflammatory process and cardiac dysfunction after resuscitation.

In previous studies, increased serum levels of lactate upon admission to the emergency department and intensive care units were associated with the negative prognosis of patients with acute critical illness [18]. Our data revealed that high serum levels of lactate at admission correlate strongly with serum resistin levels. This may support the idea that resistin is directly involved in the process of systemic inflammation in CA pathogenesis, seeing as elevated lactate levels are in fact associated with severe cardiocirculatory dysfunction [33]. However, at multivariate analysis, the aforementioned correlation did not remain statistically significant, suggesting that there were other important factors that interfere in the CA physiopathological sequence.

To our knowledge, this is the first study that evaluated the factors that influence the kinetics of resistin after CA. These results were obtained on a small number of patients, although statistically significant. The high number of measurements present an accurate kinetics of resistin after a CA, with a peak at 12–24 h and a rapid decrease to admission values after 48 h. This is important for future studies on acute events, as it shows that the focus on resistin should be especially in the first 24 h.

In order to strengthen our hypothesis, it is essential that we develop further/future studies on larger groups of patients. Also, they must include other markers of acute inflammation, with a special interest for those reportedly correlated with resistin during acute cardiovascular events: tumor necrosis factor α (TNF-α), interleukin-6 (IL-6), high-sensitivity C-reactive protein (hs-CRP) and other proinflammatory cytokines [34]. Resistin promotes the production of TNF-α, IL-1β, IL-6 and other cytokines [12,35]. There are several drugs that have been shown to reduce the levels of resistin in chronic administration: statins, anti-TNF-α monoclonal antibodies and folic acid [36–38]. Experimental animal or in vitro studies in acute situations with drugs that lower resistin concentration are worth considering.

Other markers that could provide insights into the functions and pathophysiological implications of resistin are the microvesicles (large extracellular vesicles that appear from different cells after apoptosis) [39]. Platelet-derived microvesicles are a source of TNF-α and IL-6, while endothelial-derived microvesicles are stimulated by TNF-α [40]. Elevated levels of endothelial-derived microvesicles were found in acute coronary syndrome patients, but they were not evaluated in patients that survived a CA; one can speculate that investigating this class of micro-vesicles will offer valuable data [41,42].

Markers that evaluate post-cardiac-arrest myocardial dysfunction should be studied in any future research on patients after a successfully resuscitated CA. Left ventricular systolic dysfunction is present in almost 60% of patients resuscitated after CA [33]. The assessment of left ventricle ejection fraction, biomarkers of ventricular dysfunction and the correlation with proinflammatory markers will generate a better understanding of the complexity of PCAS. The N-terminal pro-B-type natriuretic peptide

(NT-proBNP) and marinobufagenin are reliable indicators of ventricular dysfunction and, as such, can serve as excellent candidates for future studies on OHCA [43,44].

Even though the multivariate analysis showed that the post-CA shock was independently associated with higher levels of resistin, an important bias could be the presence of cardiovascular comorbidities. The myocardial systolic and diastolic dysfunctions appear in post-CA shock, even if the patient does not have a prior coronary disease [45]. Future studies should include patients with noncardiac causes of CA, because the presence of cardiac diseases aggravates the left ventricular dysfunction. Other diseases that were proven to have an influence on the resistin concentrations should be excluded (nonalcoholic fatty liver disease, asthma, autoimmune disease, chronic kidney disease) [46]. That could provide a clearer picture about the association between post-CA shock and resistin kinetics.

5. Conclusions

Our findings demonstrate strong independent correlation between high serum resistin levels, cardiac comorbidities and post-CA shock. The impact of the post-CA shock on serum concentration of resistin was greater than that of cardiac comorbidities.

Author Contributions: Conceptualization, R.M.T., Ş.C.V. and D.I.; Data curation, R.M.T., A.G. and R.R.; Formal analysis, R.R., Ş.C.V. and D.I.; Funding acquisition, R.M.T.; Investigation, R.M.T. and A.G.; Methodology, R.M.T. and Ş.C.V.; Supervision, D.I.; Writing—original draft, R.M.T., A.G., Ş.C.V. and D.I. All authors have read and agreed to the published version of the manuscript.

Funding: "Iuliu Haţieganu" University of Medicine and Pharmacy: 7690/42/15.04.2016.

Acknowledgments: The study was partially funded by "Iuliu Haţieganu" University of Medicine and Pharmacy, Cluj-Napoca, through the Doctoral Research Project-2015[No. 7690/42/15.04.2016]. The financial support allocated from the grant was used for the acquisition of biomarkers and laboratory supplies.

Conflicts of Interest: The authors declare no conflict of interest.

References

1. Nolan, J.P.; Soar, J.; Cariou, A.; Cronberg, T.; Moulaert, V.R.; Deakin, C.D.; Bottiger, B.W.; Friberg, H.; Sunde, K.; Sandroni, C. European Resuscitation Council and European Society of Intensive Care Medicine Guidelines for Post-resuscitation Care. *Intensive Care Med.* **2015**, *41*, 2039–2056. [CrossRef] [PubMed]
2. Nolan, J.P.; Neumar, R.W.; Adrie, C.; Aibiki, M.; Berg, R.A.; Bottiger, B.W.; Callaway, C.; Clark, R.S.; Geocadin, R.G.; Jauch, E.C.; et al. Post-cardiac arrest syndrome: Epidemiology, pathophysiology, treatment, and prognostication. A Scientific Statement from the International Liaison Committee on Resuscitation; the American Heart Association Emergency Cardiovascular Care Committee; the Council on Cardiovascular Surgery and Anesthesia; the Council on Cardiopulmonary, Perioperative, and Critical Care; the Council on Clinical Cardiology; the Council on Stroke. *Resuscitation* **2008**, *79*, 350–379. [PubMed]
3. Mongardon, N.; Dumas, F.; Ricome, S.; Grimaldi, D.; Hissem, T.; Pène, F.; Cariou, A. Postcardiac arrest syndrome: From immediate resuscitation to long-term outcome. *Ann. Intensive Care* **2011**, *1*, 45. [CrossRef] [PubMed]
4. Huet, O.; Dupic, L.; Batteux, F.; Matar, C.; Conti, M.; Chereau, C.; Lemiale, V.; Harrois, A.; Mira, J.P.; Vicaut, E.; et al. Postresuscitation syndrome: Potential role of hydroxyl radical-induced endothelial cell damage. *Crit. Care Med.* **2011**, *39*, 1712–1720. [CrossRef]
5. Gando, S.; Nanzaki, S.; Morimoto, Y.; Kobayashi, S.; Kemmotsu, O. Out-of-hospital cardiac arrest increases soluble vascular endothelial adhesion molecules and neutrophil elastase associated with endothelial injury. *Intensive Care Med.* **2000**, *26*, 38–44. [CrossRef]
6. Jou, C.; Shah, R.; Figueroa, A.; Patel, J.K. The role of inflammatory cytokines in cardiac arrest. *J. Intensive Care Med.* **2018**, 885066618817518. [CrossRef]
7. Adrie, C.; Monchi, M.; Laurent, I.; Um, S.; Yan, S.B.; Thuong, M.; Cariou, A.; Charpentier, J.; Dhainaut, J.F. Coagulopathy after successful cardiopulmonary resuscitation following cardiac arrest: Implication of the protein C anticoagulant pathway. *J. Am. Coll. Cardiol.* **2005**, *46*, 21–28. [CrossRef]

8. Mocan Hognogi, L.D.; Goidescu, C.M.; Farcaș, A.D. Usefulness of the adipokines as biomarkers of ischemic cardiac dysfunction. *Dis. Markers* **2018**, *2018*, 8. [CrossRef]
9. Patel, L.; Buckels, A.C.; Kinghorn, I.J.; Murdock, P.R.; Holbrook, J.D.; Plumpton, C.; Macphee, C.H.; Smith, S.A. Resistin is expressed in human macrophages and directly regulated by PPAR gamma activators. *Biochem. Biophys. Res. Commun.* **2003**, *300*, 472–476. [CrossRef]
10. Wang, H.; Chu, W.S.; Hemphill, C.; Elbein, S.C. Human resistin gene: Molecular scanning and evaluation of association with insulin sensitivity and type 2 diabetes in Caucasians. *J. Clin. Endocrinol. Metab.* **2002**, *87*, 2520–2524. [CrossRef]
11. Vlaicu, S.I.; Tatomir, A.; Boodhoo, D.; Vesa, S.; Mircea, P.A.; Rus, H. The role of complement system in adipose tissue-related inflammation. *Immunol. Res.* **2016**, *64*, 653–664. [CrossRef] [PubMed]
12. Filkova, M.; Haluzik, M.; Gay, S.; Senolt, L. The role of resistin as a regulator of inflammation: Implications for various human pathologies. *Clin. Immunol.* **2009**, *133*, 157–170. [CrossRef] [PubMed]
13. Macdonald, S.P.; Stone, S.F.; Neil, C.L.; van Eeden, P.E.; Fatovich, D.M.; Arendts, G.; Brown, S.G. Sustained elevation of resistin, NGAL and IL-8 are associated with severe sepsis/septic shock in the emergency department. *PLoS ONE* **2014**, *9*, e110678. [CrossRef] [PubMed]
14. Koch, A.; Gressner, O.A.; Sanson, E.; Tacke, F.; Trautwein, C. Serum resistin levels in critically ill patients are associated with inflammation, organ dysfunction and metabolism and may predict survival of non-septic patients. *Crit Care* **2009**, *13*, R95. [CrossRef]
15. Chen, C.; Jiang, J.; Lu, J.M.; Chai, H.; Wang, X.; Lin, P.H.; Yao, Q. Resistin decreases expression of endothelial nitric oxide synthase through oxidative stress in human coronary artery endothelial cells. *Am. J. Physiol. Heart Circ. Physiol.* **2010**, *299*, H193–H201. [CrossRef]
16. Hsu, W.Y.; Chao, Y.W.; Tsai, Y.L.; Lien, C.C.; Chang, C.F.; Deng, M.C.; Ho, L.T.; Kwok, C.F.; Juan, C.C. Resistin induces monocyte-endothelial cell adhesion by increasing ICAM-1 and VCAM-1 expression in endothelial cells via p38MAPK-dependent pathway. *J. Cell Physiol.* **2011**, *226*, 2181–2188. [CrossRef]
17. Ciobanu, D.M.; Mircea, P.A.; Bala, C.; Rusu, A.; Vesa, S.; Roman, G. Intercellular adhesion molecule-1 (ICAM-1) associates with 24-h ambulatory blood pressure variability in type 2 diabetes and controls. *Cytokine* **2019**, *116*, 134–138. [CrossRef]
18. Tat, R.M.; Golea, A.; Vesa, S.C.; Ionescu, D. Resistin-Can it be a new early marker for prognosis in patients who survive after a cardiac arrest? A pilot study. *PLoS ONE* **2019**, *14*, e0210666. [CrossRef]
19. Perkins, G.D.; Handley, A.J.; Koster, R.W.; Castrén, M.; Smyth, M.A.; Olasveengen, T.; Monsieurs, K.G.; Raffay, V.; Gräsner, J.T.; Wenzel, V.; et al. European Resuscitation Council Guidelines for Resuscitation 2015: Section 2. Adult basic life support and automated external defibrillation. *Resuscitation* **2015**, *95*, 81–99. [CrossRef]
20. Soar, J.; Nolan, J.P.; Bottiger, B.W.; Perkins, G.D.; Lott, C.; Carli, P.; Pellis, T.; Sandroni, C.; Skrifvars, M.B.; Smith, G.B.; et al. European Resuscitation Council Guidelines for Resuscitation 2015: Section 3. Adult advanced life support. *Resuscitation* **2015**, *95*, 100–147. [CrossRef]
21. Nolan, J.P.; Soar, J.; Cariou, A.; Cronberg, T.; Moulaert, V.R.; Deakin, C.D.; Bottiger, B.W.; Friberg, H.; Sunde, K.; Sandroni, C. European Resuscitation Council and European Society of Intensive Care Medicine Guidelines for Post-resuscitation Care 2015: Section 5 of the European Resuscitation Council Guidelines for Resuscitation 2015. *Resuscitation* **2015**, *95*, 202–222. [CrossRef] [PubMed]
22. Callaway, C.W.; Soar, J.; Aibiki, M.; Böttiger, B.W.; Brooks, S.C.; Deakin, C.D.; Donnino, M.W.; Drajer, S.; Kloeck, W.; Morley, P.T. Part 4: Advanced Life Support: 2015 International Consensus on Cardiopulmonary Resuscitation and Emergency Cardiovascular Care Science With Treatment Recommendations. *Circulation* **2015**, *132*, S84–S145. [CrossRef] [PubMed]
23. Fain, J.N.; Cheema, P.S.; Bahouth, S.W.; Lloyd Hiler, M. Resistin release by human adipose tissue explants in primary culture. *Biochem. Biophys. Res. Commun.* **2003**, *300*, 674–678. [CrossRef]
24. Vincent, J.L.; Moreno, R.; Takala, J.; Willatts, S.; De Mendonca, A.; Bruining, H.; Reinhart, C.K.; Suter, P.; Thijs, L.G. The SOFA (Sepsis-related Organ Failure Assessment) score to describe organ dysfunction/failure. On behalf of the Working Group on Sepsis-Related Problems of the European Society of Intensive Care Medicine. *Intensive Care Med.* **1996**, *22*, 707–710. [CrossRef]
25. Raith, E.P.; Udy, A.A.; Bailey, M.; McGloughlin, S.; MacIsaac, C.; Bellomo, R.; Pilcher, D.V. Prognostic accuracy of the SOFA score, SIRS criteria, and qSOFA score for in-hospital mortality among adults with suspected infection admitted to the intensive care unit. *JAMA* **2017**, *317*, 290–300. [CrossRef]

26. Gencer, B.; Auer, R.; De Rekeneire, N.; Butler, J.; Kalogeropoulos, A.; Bauer, D.C.; Kritchevsky, S.B.; Miljkovic, I.; Vittinghoff, E.; Harris, T.; et al. Association between resistin levels and cardiovascular desease events in older adults: The health, aging and body composition study. *Atherosclerosis* **2016**, *245*, 181–186. [CrossRef]
27. Takeishi, Y.; Niizeki, T.; Arimoto, T.; Nozaki, N.; Hirono, O.; Nitobe, J.; Watanabe, T.; Takabatake, N.; Kubota, I. Serum resistin is associated with high risk in patients with congestive heart failure. *Circ. J.* **2007**, *71*, 460–464. [CrossRef]
28. Lemming, E.W.; Byberg, L.; Stattin, K.; Ahmad, S.; Lind, L.; Elmståhl, S.; Larsson, S.C.; Wolk, A.; Michaëlsson, K. Dietary Pattern Specific Protein Biomarkers for Cardiovascular Disease: A Cross-Sectional Study in 2 Independent Cohorts. *J. Am. Heart Assoc.* **2019**, *8*, e011860.
29. McTernan, P.G.; Fisher, F.M.; Valsamakis, G.; Chetty, R.; Harte, A.; McTernan, C.L.; Clark, P.M.; Smith, S.A.; Barnett, A.H.; Kumar, S. Resistin and type 2 diabetes: Regulation of resistin expression by insulin and rosiglitazone and the effects of recombinant resistin on lipid and glucose metabolism in human differentiated adipocytes. *J. Clin. Endocrinol. Metab.* **2003**, *88*, 6098–6106. [CrossRef]
30. Steppan, C.M.; Bailey, S.T.; Bhat, S.; Brown, E.J.; Banerjee, R.R.; Wright, C.M.; Patel, H.R.; Ahima, R.S.; Lazar, M.A. The hormone resistin links obesity to diabetes. *Nature* **2001**, *409*, 307–312. [CrossRef]
31. Shuldiner, A.R.; Yang, R.; Gong, D.W. Resistin, obesity, and insulin resistance—The emerging role of the adipocyte as an endocrine organ. *N. Engl. J. Med.* **2001**, *345*, 1345–1346. [CrossRef] [PubMed]
32. Koch, A.; Weiskirchen, R.; Krusch, A.; Bruensing, J.; Buendgens, L.; Herbers, U.; Yagmur, E.; Koek, G.H.; Trautwein, C.; Tacke, F. Visfatin serum levels predict mortality in critically ill patients. *Dis. Markers* **2018**, *2018*, 7315356. [CrossRef] [PubMed]
33. Jentzer, J.C.; Chonde, M.D.; Dezfulian, C. Myocardial dysfunction and shock after cardiac arrest. *Biomed. Res. Int.* **2015**, *2015*, 314796. [CrossRef] [PubMed]
34. Liu, X.; Zheng, X.; Su, X.; Tian, W.; Hu, Y.; Zhang, Z. Plasma Resistin Levels in Patients with Acute Aortic Dissection: A Propensity Score-Matched Observational Case-Control Study. *Med. Sci. Monit.* **2018**, *24*, 6431–6437. [CrossRef]
35. Silswal, N.; Singh, A.K.; Aruna, B.; Mukhopadhyay, S.; Ghosh, S.; Ehtesham, N.Z. Human resistin stimulates the pro-inflammatory cytokines TNF-alpha and IL-12 in macrophages by NF-kappaB-dependent pathway. *Biochem. Biophys. Res. Commun.* **2005**, *334*, 1092–1101. [CrossRef]
36. Shyu, K.G.; Chua, S.K.; Wang, B.W.; Kuan, P. Mechanism of inhibitory effect of atorvastatin on resistin expression induced by tumor necrosis factor-alpha in macrophages. *J. Biomed. Sci.* **2009**, *16*, 50. [CrossRef]
37. Gonzalez-Gay, M.A.; Garcia-Unzueta, M.T.; Gonzalez-Juanatey, C.; Miranda-Filloy, J.A.; Vazquez-Rodriguez, T.R.; De Matias, J.M.; Martin, J.; Dessein, P.H.; Llorca, J. Anti-TNF-alpha therapy modulates resistin in patients with rheumatoid arthritis. *Clin. Exp. Rheumatol.* **2008**, *26*, 311–316.
38. Seto, S.W.; Lam, T.Y.; Or, P.M.; Lee, W.Y.; Au, A.L.; Poon, C.C.; Li, R.W.S.; Chan, S.W.; Yeung, J.H.K.; Leung, G.P.H.; et al. Folic acid consumption reduces resistin level and restores blunted acetylcholine-induced aortic relaxation in obese/diabetic mice. *J. Nutr. Biochem.* **2010**, *21*, 872–880. [CrossRef]
39. Słomka, A.; Urban, S.K.; Lukacs-Kornek, V.; Żekanowska, E.; Kornek, M. Large Extracellular Vesicles: Have We Found the Holy Grail of Inflammation? *Front. Immunol.* **2018**, *9*, 2723. [CrossRef]
40. Balvers, K.; Curry, N.; Kleinveld, D.J.; Böing, A.N.; Nieuwland, R.; Goslings, J.C.; Juffermans, N.P. Endogenous microparticles drive the proinflammatory host immune response in severely injured trauma patients. *Shock* **2015**, *43*, 317–321. [CrossRef]
41. Alexy, T.; Rooney, K.; Weber, M.; Gray, W.D.; Searles, C.D. TNF-α alters the release and transfer of microparticle-encapsulated miRNAs from endothelial cells. *Physiol. Genom.* **2014**, *46*, 833–840. [CrossRef] [PubMed]
42. Morel, O.; Pereira, B.; Averous, G.; Faure, A.; Jesel, L.; Germain, P.; Grunebaum, L.; Ohlmann, P.; Freyssinet, J.M.; Bareiss, P.; et al. Increased levels of procoagulant tissue factor-bearing microparticles within the occluded coronary artery of patients with ST-segment elevation myocardial infarction: Role of endothelial damage and leukocyte activation. *Atherosclerosis* **2009**, *204*, 636–641. [CrossRef] [PubMed]
43. Fridman, A.I.; Matveev, S.A.; Agalakova, N.I.; Fedorova, O.V.; Lakatta, E.G.; Bagrov, A.Y. Marinobufagenin, an endogenous ligand of alpha-1 sodium pump, is a marker of congestive heart failure severity. *J. Hypertens.* **2002**, *20*, 1189–1194. [CrossRef] [PubMed]

44. Myhre, P.L.; Tiainen, M.; Pettilä, V.; Vaahersalo, J.; Hagve, T.A.; Kurola, J. NT-proBNP in patients with out-of-hospital cardiac arrest: Results from the FINNRESUSCI Study. *Resuscitation* **2016**, *104*, 12–18. [CrossRef] [PubMed]
45. Laurent, I.; Monchi, M.; Chiche, J.D.; Joly, L.M.; Spaulding, C.; Bourgeois, B.; Cariou, A.; Rozenberg, A.; Carli, P.; Weber, S.; et al. Reversible myocardial dysfunction in survivors of out-of-hospital cardiac arrest. *J. Am. Coll. Cardiol.* **2002**, *40*, 2110–2116. [CrossRef]
46. Jamaluddin, M.S.; Weakley, S.M.; Yao, O.; Chen, C. Resistin: Functional Roles and Therapeutic Considerations for Cardiovascular Disease. *Br. J. Pharmacol.* **2012**, *165*, 622–632. [CrossRef]

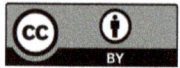

© 2019 by the authors. Licensee MDPI, Basel, Switzerland. This article is an open access article distributed under the terms and conditions of the Creative Commons Attribution (CC BY) license (http://creativecommons.org/licenses/by/4.0/).

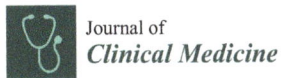

Article

We are What We Eat: Impact of Food from Short Supply Chain on Metabolic Syndrome

Gaetano Santulli [1,2,3,*], Valeria Pascale [4], Rosa Finelli [4], Valeria Visco [4], Rocco Giannotti [4], Angelo Massari [5], Carmine Morisco [2], Michele Ciccarelli [4], Maddalena Illario [6,7], Guido Iaccarino [2,3,*] and Enrico Coscioni [5]

1. Dept. of Medicine, Division of Cardiology, and Dept. of Molecular Pharmacology, Montefiore University Hospital, Fleischer Institute for Diabetes and Metabolism (FIDAM), Albert Einstein College of Medicine (AECOM), New York, NY 10461, USA
2. Dept. of Advanced Biomedical Science, Federico II University, 80131 Naples, Italy; carmine.morisco@unina.it
3. International Translational Research and Medical Education Consortium (ITME), 80131 Naples, Italy
4. Dept. of Medicine, Surgery and Dentistry, University of Salerno, 8408 Baronissi, Italy; pascalevaleria@gmail.com (V.P.); rosafinelli1@gmail.com (R.F.); valeriavisco1991@libero.it (V.V.); tintorangocico@live.it (R.G.); mciccarelli@unisa.it (M.C.)
5. "San Giovanni di Dio e Ruggi d'Aragona" University Hospital, 84131 Salerno, Italy; angelo.massari@sangiovannieruggi.it (A.M.); enrico.coscioni@regione.campania.it (E.C.)
6. Health's Innovation, Campania Regional Government, 80132 Naples, Italy; illario@unina.it
7. Dept. of Public Health, Federico II University, 80131 Naples, Italy
* Correspondence: gaetano.santulli@einsteinmed.org or gsantulli001@gmail.com (G.S.); guiaccar@unina.it (G.I.)

Received: 21 October 2019; Accepted: 19 November 2019; Published: 23 November 2019

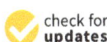

Abstract: Food supply in the Mediterranean area has been recently modified by big retail distribution; for instance, industrial retail has favored shipments of groceries from regions that are intensive producers of mass food, generating a long supply chain (LSC) of food that opposes short supply chains (SSCs) that promote local food markets. However, the actual functional role of food retail and distribution in the determination of the risk of developing metabolic syndrome (MetS) has not been studied hitherto. The main aim of this study was to test the effects of food chain length on the prevalence of MetS in a population accustomed to the Mediterranean diet. We conducted an observational study in Southern Italy on individuals adhering to the Mediterranean diet. We examined a total of 407 subjects (41% females) with an average age of 56 ± 14.5 years (as standard deviation) and found that being on the Mediterranean diet with a SSC significantly reduces the prevalence of MetS compared with the LSC (SSC: 19.65%, LSC: 31.46%; p: 0.007). Our data indicate for the first time that the length of food supply chain plays a key role in determining the risk of MetS in a population adhering to the Mediterranean diet.

Keywords: mediterranean diet; supply chain of food; metabolic syndrome; food retail; cardiovascular risk

1. Introduction

Several studies have demonstrated that the Mediterranean diet significantly reduces the risk of developing metabolic syndrome (MetS) [1–4], a cluster of clinical conditions that occur together and increase the risk of heart disease, stroke, and type 2 diabetes [5–7]. However, the exact role of food retail and distribution in the risk of developing MetS has not yet been fully determined.

Recently, the development of big retail food distribution has deeply modified food supply in the Mediterranean area [8,9]. Indeed, industrial retail has favored shipments of groceries from regions that are intensive producers of mass foods, generating the long supply chain (LSC) of food [10]; on the other hand, short supply chains (SSCs) involve local self-producers that promote local food markets [8]. The origin of food, the long period of time elapsing from production to consumption, the need to add preservatives, as well as the loss of perishable nutrients such as vitamins, can all contribute to reducing the quality of food. Nevertheless, whether food quality loss has an impact on the health of the population remains to be determined.

The increasing availability of foods from big retail is a revolutionary event that has impacted health on a population-size level. In particular, the adherence to the Mediterranean diet is decreasing even within those regions where it was first discovered [11,12], and such a change in the alimentary habit is generally seen as one of the potential causes of the obesity epidemic [13], especially among adolescents [14].

The overarching aim of our study was to test the effects of food chain length on metabolic alterations in a population accustomed to the Mediterranean diet. Specifically, we compared SSCs of food—in which aliments are produced *in loco*, usually with traditional and low-technology methodologies—to the LSC of food.

2. Methods

2.1. Subjects

We conducted an observational, cross-sectional study on the general population of Salerno (population: 138,000 inhabitants) and of five nearby villages (population <6000 inhabitants): Castelnuovo Cilento, Polla, Sapri, San Gregorio Magno, and Satriano di Lucania. In order to be considered eligible, subjects had to be currently and stably (for at least 10 years) living in the cities indicated, and to have signed the informed consent.

2.2. Study Approval

The study was approved by the Institutional Ethical Committee of Salerno University Hospital. Written informed consent was obtained from all participants. The study is registered in the ClincalTrial.gov database (Trial number: NCT03305276).

2.3. Data Acquisition

On the occasion of 2015–2017 World Hypertension Day (May 17th), booths were organized in the major squares of the mentioned villages, harnessing a collaborative effort of the Medical School of Salerno and local authorities [15]. The event was successfully publicized with a 15-day notice via local media advertisements, and we had the partnership of local authorities and patient associations, as well as parishes. The population was instructed to show up on the day of the event at the booths, where subjects were asked to sign the informed consent to participate in the survey and to donate blood samples for analysis. Anamnesis and anthropometric parameters were obtained including weight, height, waist and hip circumferences, and BMI. Blood pressure was detected according to the Guidelines of the European Society of Cardiology and European Society of Hypertension (ESC/ESH) [16]. Current smokers were defined as those reporting having smoked at least 100 cigarettes during their lifetime and currently smoking every day or some days [17]. Dietary habits were collected by means of a questionnaire previously described by Trichopoulou et al. [18]. This nine-question questionnaire allows a score (Trichopoulou score) to be attributed to each subject. To determine the use of SSCs or the LSC, we formulated a questionnaire that included the following eight questions: (1) "Do the vegetables you consume come mainly from your vegetable garden?" (Yes = 1); (2) "Do you buy fruit grown in your area?" (Yes = 1); (3) "Do you eat seasonal fruit?" (Yes = 1); (4) "Does the meat you consume come mainly from local farms or from butchers in your area?" (Yes = 1); (5) "Do you eat mostly fresh, unpackaged food?" (Yes = 1); (6) "Do you eat cookies, snacks, and/or sweets more than once a week?" (No = 1); (7) "Do you use canned or frozen food?" (No = 1); and (8) "Do you drink carbonated or sweetened drinks?" (No = 1). These questions were derived from preliminary interviews performed by experienced personnel to relatives and families of volunteers in order to verify the kinds of food that are more frequently acquired from small business stores, as well as the ones mostly purchased from big food retail shops. According to this survey, fruits, vegetables, and meats were purchased more often from small business shops, whereas preserved and canned foods, as well as frozen food, sodas, cookies, and snacks, were mainly obtained from big resellers. In a second phase, we asked one big food retailer from the city of Salerno and two small business of the city of San Gregorio Magno to provide us with the suppliers of the listed products, so as to substantiate the actual length of the supply chain of food. The optimal cut-off of the score (5) was determined by receiver operating characteristic (ROC) curves (see Supplementary Figure S1), applying Youden's index [19,20]; with a score ≥5, the subject was included in the SSC group, whereas with a score <5 the subject was included in the LSC group. MetS was diagnosed according to the 2009 Harmonized Criteria, implementing the criteria of the International Diabetes Federation (IDF) to evaluate abdominal obesity [7,21].

2.4. Blood Sample Laboratory Analysis

A venous blood sample was collected from the antecubital vein in a dedicate booth from experienced volunteer nurses in two tubes of 5.0 mL and centrifuged the same day. The time of the last meal was recorded during data collection. We measured blood glucose, insulin, total cholesterol, HDL cholesterol, LDL cholesterol, and triglycerides. The homeostatic model assessment (HOMA) index was calculated as previously described, based on an adequate fasting time (6 h) [22].

2.5. Statistical Analysis

Continuous data are presented as mean ± SE. Categorical data are presented as absolute values and/or frequencies. To observe a change of one quartile in frequency with an α cut-off of 5% and a β cut-off of 20%, and given an estimated incidence of MetS of 26% in our population [23], we calculated that a $n = 398$ would have been necessary to reach statistical significance. A Kolmogorov–Smirnov test was used to verify the normality of distributions of continuous variables. A chi-square (χ^2) test was used to compare frequencies. Independent sample t-tests were used for between-group comparisons. In all the above-mentioned tests, $p < 0.05$ was considered statistically significant. Statistical analysis was performed with SPSS (Statistical Package for the Social Sciences) 24.0 (IBM, Armonk, NY, USA) and Prism 7 (GraphPad Software, San Diego, CA, USA).

3. Results

3.1. Clinical Features of Study Population

A total of 808 subjects (45% male and 55% female, 14–85 years) were recruited during the XI, XII, and XIII editions of World Hypertension Day, which is celebrated every year on 17 May. We excluded from the analysis patients younger than 30 ($n = 70$) and older than 80 years ($n = 30$) because of the previously reported relatively low adherence to the Mediterranean diet by populations at those ages [12,24–26]. We also excluded those with an incomplete database, thereby precluding the calculation of adherence to the Mediterranean diet, SSCs or the LSC, or the HOMA index ($n = 269$), as well as 28 outliers (3 SD over/below mean) in MetS determinants.

The main characteristics of our population (407 subjects, 41% females, with an average age of ~56 years) are depicted in Table 1.

3.2. Effects of SSCs on Clinical Features

We divided the population according to the eight-point questionnaire indicated above, using the score of 5 as a cutoff to indicate adherence to SSCs (≥5) or the LSC (<5). Data are indicated in Table 1.

Table 1. Impact of SSCs and the LSC on anthropometric and clinical characteristics.

	Total	LSC	SSC	p
N	407	178	229	-
Age (years)	55.9 ± 0.58	56.4 ± 0.8	55.52 ± 0.8	0.422
Sex (M, %)	59	60	58	0.765
Weight (Kg)	73.8 ± 0.82	72.2 ± 1.2	75.1 ± 1.08	0.085
Height (cm)	163.7 ± 0.6	164.2 ± 0.6	163.3 ± 0.91	0.399
Waist (cm)	96.3 ± 0.74	96.4 ± 0.84	96,0 ± 1.49	0.803
BMI (Kg/m^2)	27.6 ± 0.25	27.1 ± 0.39	27.9 ± 0.34	0.098
SBP (mmHg)	130.6 ± 0.9	131.2 ± 1.3	130.1 ± 1.2	0.523
DBP (mmHg)	79.8 ± 0.5	80.5 ± 0.8	79.2 ± 0.69	0.220
HR (bpm)	72.2 ± 0.6	72.1 ± 0.8	72.28 ± 0.82	0.877
Fasting Glucose (mg/dl)	84.4 ± 1.2	91.28 ± 1.7	79.41 ± 1.5	0.001
Serum Insulin (µU/dl)	17.7 ± 0.97	21.4 ± 1.7	14.9 ± 1.1	0.001
Creatinine (mg/dl)	0.85 ± 0.02	0.88 ± 0.05	0.82 ± 0.01	0.19
Current Smokers (%)	32.0	30.0	34.0	0.427
Cholesterol (Total, mg/dl)	201.4 ± 1.9	201.36 ± 3.2	201.48 ± 2.5	0.977
Cholesterol (HDL, mg/dl)	59.3 ± 0.7	59.03 ± 1.2	59.56 ± 1.0	0.737
Cholesterol (LDL, mg/dl)	124.6 ± 2.1	127.02 ± 3.9	123.43 ± 2.4	0.418
TG (mg/dl)	121.7 ± 3.6	136.14 ± 5.9	110.95 ± 4.3	0.001
Metabolic Syndrome (%)	24.81	31.46	19.65	0.007
Trichopoulous Score	4.98 ± 0.08	4.86 ± 0.13	5.08 ± 0.10	0.180

Frequencies are reported as %, continuous variables as mean ± SE; DBP: Diastolic/systolic blood pressure; HR: Heart rate; HDL/LDL: High-density/low-density lipoproteins; LSC/SSC: Long/short supply chain; TG: Triglycerides; Trichopoulous Score: Score of the adherence to a Mediterranean-style diet (9 = max, 0 = min; p value was calculated applying the t test or χ^2, as appropriate).

Our data indicate that SSCs are associated with lower levels of triglycerides and glucose, and therefore have a marked impact on the occurrence of MetS: indeed, MetS is less frequent among populations that consume SSC food. Interestingly, adherence to the Mediterranean diet, assessed using a validated questionnaire, was similar between the two populations, indicating a homogenous high adherence between the consumers of SSC and LSC foods.

3.3. Effects of SSCs on Insulin Sensitivity

Given the notion that MetS is a hallmark of insulin resistance, we assayed insulin resistance by means of the HOMA index. As shown in Figure 1, the HOMA index was lower in the SSC than in the LSC group (2.67 ± 0.20 vs. 4.66 ± 0.44, respectively; p = 0.0002).

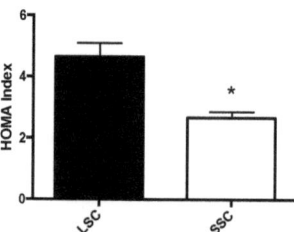

Figure 1. Impact of SSCs and the LSC on insulin resistance. LSC: Long supply chain; SSC: Short supply chain; * p = 0.0002.

4. Discussion

Our results indicate that the Mediterranean diet with food from a SSC significantly reduces the prevalence of MetS. These results are consistent with recent observations suggesting that local food environments might affect health outcomes [27]. Our data are corroborated by the evidence that insulin resistance is significantly more common among LSC subjects compared with SSC individuals. With our data, we are among the first investigators to introduce the concept that freshness of food is a key determinant of health outcomes.

Prevalence of MetS in Southern Italy is reported to be ~25% in young adults [23] and ~65% in older women after menopause [28]; of note, the area of assessment might slightly impact the occurrence of MetS [29]. Our population showed overall a prevalence of 35%, and we consider this number to be fairly representative, given the large age range (from 30 to 80 years) of our population.

Substantial evidence indicates that local food environments might affect health outcomes [27,30–36]. It is therefore possible to speculate that length of a food supply chain might affect cardiovascular risk. To verify this hypothesis, it is crucial to compare populations that present similar dietary patterns that derive from different sources (i.e., retail market vs. locally grown food). In this sense, Southern Italy features examples of urbanization, where retail food is the most important source of food, which is the opposite to rural areas, where consuming locally grown, seasonal vegetables, as well as meat of courtyard animals is a fairly regular habit [28,29,37]. These contrasting local food environments, somehow superimposed on the Mediterranean diet, represent a unique setting to test the impact on health phenotypes, such as intermediate metabolism and cardiovascular risk [4,38,39].

Our findings are particularly relevant because they provide for the first time an actual evaluation of how critical the food supply chain is in the context of the Mediterranean diet. Indeed, it is well established that the Mediterranean diet can ameliorate cardiovascular risk [40]. Therefore, to verify the existence of a further improvement in health outcomes from SSCs versus the LSC, it is imperative to compare groups that consume the same diet, with no difference in macro- and micronutrients. Based on our data on insulin resistance, we can speculate that insulin sensitivity is better preserved among subjects adhering to the Mediterranean diet who eat SSC foods. Using a previously published questionnaire [18], we were indeed able to verify the high adherence of Southern Italians to the Mediterranean diet, and no differences were observed when we divided our population according to LSC and SSC groups. Therefore, we can conclude that the difference observed in terms of MetS prevalence cannot be attributable to a different attitude towards the Mediterranean diet.

Our findings should be interpreted in light of several limitations. First and foremost, the cross-sectional design of the study prevents a determination of causality. Another major issue that was not addressed by our questionnaires is the lifestyle that accompanies the provision of SSC food, nor did our questionnaire did not measure the time spent in the production of such food, such as the time spent looking after crops and/or courtyard animals, which would imply a more active lifestyle. Likewise, the use of food from the LSC is more distinctive of urban centers, where alternative healthy lifestyles are also more common (practicing sports, attending the gym). This aspect was also testified by our observation of no significant differences in body weight or waist between the two populations, with a tendency of heavier weights detected in the SSC group. Therefore, while we cannot completely rule out an effect of physical activity on MetS in our study, the evidence that SSC is associated with a lower prevalence of MetS is suggestive of a fundamental impact of fresh food on metabolic parameters.

If confirmed in larger prospective studies, these results could promote public interventions to improve lifestyle, preferring, whenever possible, SSCs to the LSC. Therefore, an assessment of cardiovascular risk should include dietary habits of the studied population.

5. Conclusions

Taken together, our findings indicate for the first time that the length of food supply chain is crucial in determining the risk of developing MetS as well as in the assessment of cardiovascular risk in a population adhering to the Mediterranean diet.

Supplementary Materials: The following are available online at http://www.mdpi.com/2077-0383/8/12/2061/s1, Figure S1: Determination of the optimal cut off value in our questionnaire.

Author Contributions: Methodology, G.S., M.C., and G.I.; validation, G.S., C.M., M.I., G.I., and E.C.; formal analysis, G.S. and G.I.; investigation, V.P., R.F., V.V., R.G., A.M., and M.C.; data curation, G.S., G.I., and E.C.; writing, G.S. and G.I.

Funding: G.S. is supported by the National Institutes of Health (NIH: R01 DK123259, R00 DK107895, R01 HL146691, R01 DK033823). G.I. holds grants from the Italian Ministry of Research (PRIN 2017 and PON Campania Bioscience PON03PE0006008), POR MOVIE from Regione Campania, and the Italian Society of Hypertension (SIIA). M.C. holds funds from University of Salerno's Funds for Basic Research.

Conflicts of Interest: None of the authors have any financial associations that might pose a conflict of interest in connection with the submitted article.

References

1. Salas-Salvado, J.; Guasch-Ferre, M.; Lee, C.H.; Estruch, R.; Clish, C.B.; Ros, E. Protective effects of the Mediterranean diet on Type 2 Diabetes and metabolic syndrome. *J. Nutr.* **2016**, *146*, 920S–927S. [CrossRef]
2. Grosso, G.; Mistretta, A.; Marventano, S.; Purrello, A.; Vitaglione, P.; Calabrese, G.; Drago, F.; Galvano, F. Beneficial effects of the Mediterranean diet on metabolic syndrome. *Curr. Pharm. Des.* **2014**, *20*, 5039–5044. [CrossRef] [PubMed]
3. Estruch, R.; Ros, E.; Salas-Salvadó, J.; Covas, M.I.; Corella, D.; Arós, F.; Gómez-Gracia, E.; Ruiz-Gutiérrez, V.; Fiol, M.; Lapetra, J.; et al. Primary prevention of cardiovascular disease with a Mediterranean diet. *N. Engl. J. Med.* **2013**, *368*, 12. [CrossRef] [PubMed]
4. Franquesa, M.; Pujol-Busquets, G.; Garcia-Fernandez, E.; Rico, L.; Shamirian-Pulido, L.; Aguilar-Martinez, A.; Medina, F.X.; Serra-Majem, L.; Bach-Faig, A. Mediterranean diet and cardiodiabesity: A systematic review through evidence-based answers to key clinical questions. *Nutrients* **2019**, *11*, 655. [CrossRef] [PubMed]
5. Santulli, G. Dietary components and metabolic dysfunction: Translating preclinical studies into clinical practice. *Nutrients.* **2016**, *8*, 632. [CrossRef] [PubMed]
6. Smith, G.I.; Mittendorfer, B.; Klein, S. Metabolically healthy obesity: Facts and fantasies. *J. Clin. Investig.* **2019**, *129*, 3978–3989. [CrossRef] [PubMed]
7. Alberti, K.G.; Eckel, R.H.; Grundy, S.M.; Zimmet, P.Z.; Cleeman, J.I.; Donato, K.A.; Fruchart, J.C.; James, W.P.; Loria, C.M.; Smith, S.C., Jr.; et al. Harmonizing the metabolic syndrome: A joint interim statement of the International Diabetes Federation Task Force on Epidemiology and Prevention; National Heart, Lung, and Blood Institute; American Heart Association; World Heart Federation; International Atherosclerosis Society; and International Association for the Study of Obesity. *Circulation* **2009**, *120*, 1640–1645. [PubMed]
8. Hernandez-Rubio, J.; Perez-Mesa, J.C.; Piedra-Munoz, L.; Galdeano-Gomez, E. Determinants of Food Safety Level in Fruit and Vegetable Wholesalers' Supply Chain: Evidence from Spain and France. *Int. J. Environ. Res. Public Health* **2018**, *15*, 2246. [CrossRef]
9. Pettinger, C.; Holdsworth, M.; Gerber, M. 'All under one roof?' differences in food availability and shopping patterns in Southern France and Central England. *Eur. J. Public Health* **2008**, *18*, 109–114. [CrossRef]
10. Wible, B.; Mervis, J.; Wigginton, N.S. The global supply chain. Rethinking the global supply chain. Introduction. *Science* **2014**, *344*, 1100–1103. [CrossRef]
11. Gregorio, M.J.; Rodrigues, A.M.; Graca, P.; de Sousa, R.D.; Dias, S.S.; Branco, J.C.; Canhao, H. Food insecurity is associated with low adherence to the Mediterranean diet and adverse health conditions in Portuguese adults. *Front. Public Health* **2018**, *6*, 38. [CrossRef] [PubMed]
12. Bonaccio, M.; Di Castelnuovo, A.; Bonanni, A.; Costanzo, S.; De Lucia, F.; Persichillo, M.; Zito, F.; Donati, M.B.; de Gaetano, G.; Iacoviello, L. Decline of the Mediterranean diet at a time of economic crisis. Results from the Moli-sani study. *Nutr. Metab. Cardiovasc. Dis.* **2014**, *24*, 853–860. [CrossRef] [PubMed]
13. Agnoli, C.; Sieri, S.; Ricceri, F.; Giraudo, M.T.; Masala, G.; Assedi, M.; Panico, S.; Mattiello, A.; Tumino, R.; Giurdanella, M.C.; et al. Adherence to a Mediterranean diet and long-term changes in weight and waist circumference in the EPIC-Italy cohort. *Nutr. Diabetes* **2018**, *8*, 22. [CrossRef] [PubMed]
14. Theodoridis, X.; Grammatikopoulou, M.G.; Gkiouras, K.; Papadopoulou, S.E.; Agorastou, T.; Gkika, I.; Maraki, M.I.; Dardavessis, T.; Chourdakis, M. Food insecurity and Mediterranean diet adherence among Greek university students. *Nutr. Metab. Cardiovasc. Dis.* **2018**, *28*, 477–485. [CrossRef] [PubMed]

15. Pascale, A.V.; Finelli, R.; Giannotti, R.; Visco, V.; Fabbricatore, D.; Matula, I.; Mazzeo, P.; Ragosa, N.; Massari, A.; Izzo, R.; et al. Vitamin D, parathyroid hormone and cardiovascular risk: The good, the bad and the ugly. *J. Cardiovasc. Med. (Hagerstown)* **2018**, *19*, 62–66. [CrossRef] [PubMed]
16. Williams, B.; Mancia, G.; Spiering, W.; Agabiti Rosei, E.; Azizi, M.; Burnier, M.; Clement, D.L.; Coca, A.; de Simone, G.; Dominiczak, A.; et al. 2018 ESC/ESH Guidelines for the management of arterial hypertension. *Eur. Heart J.* **2018**, *39*, 3021–3104. [CrossRef]
17. Gambardella, J.; Sardu, C.; Sacra, C.; Del Giudice, C.; Santulli, G. Quit smoking to outsmart atherogenesis: Molecular mechanisms underlying clinical evidence. *Atherosclerosis* **2017**, *257*, 242–245. [CrossRef]
18. Trichopoulou, A.; Costacou, T.; Bamia, C.; Trichopoulos, D. Adherence to a Mediterranean diet and survival in a Greek population. *N. Engl. J. Med.* **2003**, *348*, 2599–2608. [CrossRef]
19. Hajian-Tilaki, K. The choice of methods in determining the optimal cut-off value for quantitative diagnostic test evaluation. *Stat. Methods Med. Res.* **2018**, *27*, 2374–2383. [CrossRef]
20. Youden, W.J. Index for rating diagnostic tests. *Cancer* **1950**, *3*, 32–35. [CrossRef]
21. Alberti, K.G.; Zimmet, P.; Shaw, J. Metabolic syndrome—A new world-wide definition. A Consensus Statement from the International Diabetes Federation. *Diabet. Med.* **2006**, *23*, 469–480. [CrossRef] [PubMed]
22. Haffner, S.M.; Kennedy, E.; Gonzalez, C.; Stern, M.P.; Miettinen, H. A prospective analysis of the HOMA model. The Mexico City Diabetes Study. *Diabetes Care* **1996**, *19*, 1138–1141. [CrossRef] [PubMed]
23. Caserta, C.A.; Mele, A.; Surace, P.; Ferrigno, L.; Amante, A.; Messineo, A.; Vacalebre, C.; Amato, F.; Baldassarre, D.; Amato, M.; et al. Association of non-alcoholic fatty liver disease and cardiometabolic risk factors with early atherosclerosis in an adult population in Southern Italy. *Ann. Ist. Super Sanita* **2017**, *53*, 77–81. [PubMed]
24. Ruggiero, E.; Di Castelnuovo, A.; Costanzo, S.; Persichillo, M.; Bracone, F.; Cerletti, C.; Donati, M.B.; de Gaetano, G.; Iacoviello, L.; Bonaccio, M.; et al. Socioeconomic and psychosocial determinants of adherence to the Mediterranean diet in a general adult Italian population. *Eur. J. Public Health* **2019**, *29*, 328–335. [CrossRef] [PubMed]
25. Knoops, K.T.; de Groot, L.C.; Kromhout, D.; Perrin, A.E.; Moreiras-Varela, O.; Menotti, A.; van Staveren, W.A. Mediterranean diet, lifestyle factors, and 10-year mortality in elderly European men and women: The HALE project. *JAMA* **2004**, *292*, 1433–1439. [CrossRef]
26. Cruz, J.A. Dietary habits and nutritional status in adolescents over Europe—Southern Europe. *Eur. J. Clin. Nutr.* **2000**, *54* (Suppl. 1), S29–S35. [CrossRef]
27. Story, M.; Kaphingst, K.M.; Robinson-O'Brien, R.; Glanz, K. Creating Healthy Food and Eating Environments: Policy and Environmental Approaches. *Annu. Rev. Public Health* **2008**, *29*, 253–272. [CrossRef]
28. Maiello, M.; Zito, A.; Ciccone, M.M.; Palmiero, P. Metabolic syndrome and its components in postmenopausal women living in Southern Italy, Apulia region. *Diabetes Metab. Syndr.* **2017**, *11*, 43–46. [CrossRef]
29. Martino, F.; Puddu, P.E.; Pannarale, G.; Colantoni, C.; Zanoni, C.; Martino, E.; Barilla, F. Metabolic syndrome among children and adolescents from Southern Italy: Contribution from the Calabrian Sierras Community Study (CSCS). *Int. J. Cardiol.* **2014**, *177*, 455–460. [CrossRef]
30. Morland, K.B.; Evenson, K.R. Obesity prevalence and the local food environment. *Health Place* **2009**, *15*, 491–495. [CrossRef]
31. Cobb, L.K.; Appel, L.J.; Franco, M.; Jones-Smith, J.C.; Nur, A.; Anderson, C.A. The relationship of the local food environment with obesity: A systematic review of methods, study quality, and results. *Obesity* **2015**, *23*, 1331–1344. [CrossRef] [PubMed]
32. Lamb, K.E.; Thornton, L.E.; Olstad, D.L.; Cerin, E.; Ball, K. Associations between major chain fast-food outlet availability and change in body mass index: A longitudinal observational study of women from Victoria, Australia. *BMJ Open* **2017**, *7*, e016594. [CrossRef] [PubMed]
33. Stark, J.H.; Neckerman, K.; Lovasi, G.S.; Konty, K.; Quinn, J.; Arno, P.; Viola, D.; Harris, T.G.; Weiss, C.C.; Bader, M.D.; et al. Neighbourhood food environments and body mass index among New York City adults. *J. Epidemiol. Community Health* **2013**, *67*, 736–742. [CrossRef] [PubMed]
34. Pitt, E.; Gallegos, D.; Comans, T.; Cameron, C.; Thornton, L. Exploring the influence of local food environments on food behaviours: A systematic review of qualitative literature. *Public Health Nutr.* **2017**, *20*, 2393–2405. [CrossRef] [PubMed]

35. Biboloni, M.D.M.; Bouzas, C.; Abbate, M.; Martinez-Gonzalez, M.A.; Corella, D.; Salas-Salvado, J.; Zomeno, M.D.; Vioque, J.; Romaguera, D.; Martinez, J.A.; et al. Nutrient adequacy and diet quality in a Mediterranean population with metabolic syndrome: A cross-sectional study. *Clin. Nutr.* **2019**. [CrossRef] [PubMed]
36. Julibert, A.; Biboloni, M.D.M.; Bouzas, C.; Martinez-Gonzalez, M.A.; Salas-Salvado, J.; Corella, D.; Zomeno, M.D.; Romaguera, D.; Vioque, J.; Alonso-Gomez, A.M.; et al. Total and Subtypes of Dietary Fat Intake and Its Association with Components of the Metabolic Syndrome in a Mediterranean Population at High Cardiovascular Risk. *Nutrients* **2019**, *11*, 1493. [CrossRef] [PubMed]
37. Scuteri, A.; Laurent, S.; Cucca, F.; Cockcroft, J.; Cunha, P.G.; Manas, L.R.; Mattace Raso, F.U.; Muiesan, M.L.; Ryliskyte, L.; Rietzschel, E.; et al. Metabolic syndrome across Europe: Different clusters of risk factors. *Eur. J. Prev. Cardiol.* **2015**, *22*, 486–491. [CrossRef]
38. Lacatusu, C.M.; Grigorescu, E.D.; Floria, M.; Onofriescu, A.; Mihai, B.M. The Mediterranean Diet: From an Environment-Driven Food Culture to an Emerging Medical Prescription. *Int. J. Environ. Res. Public Health* **2019**, *16*, 942. [CrossRef]
39. Salas-Salvado, J.; Diaz-Lopez, A.; Ruiz-Canela, M.; Basora, J.; Fito, M.; Corella, D.; Serra-Majem, L.; Warnberg, J.; Romaguera, D.; Estruch, R.; et al. Effect of a Lifestyle Intervention Program With Energy-Restricted Mediterranean Diet and Exercise on Weight Loss and Cardiovascular Risk Factors: One-Year Results of the PREDIMED-Plus Trial. *Diabetes Care* **2019**, *42*, 777–788. [CrossRef]
40. Kastorini, C.M.; Milionis, H.J.; Esposito, K.; Giugliano, D.; Goudevenos, J.A.; Panagiotakos, D.B. The effect of Mediterranean diet on metabolic syndrome and its components: A meta-analysis of 50 studies and 534,906 individuals. *J. Am. Coll. Cardiol.* **2011**, *57*, 1299–1313. [CrossRef]

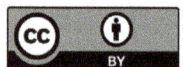

© 2019 by the authors. Licensee MDPI, Basel, Switzerland. This article is an open access article distributed under the terms and conditions of the Creative Commons Attribution (CC BY) license (http://creativecommons.org/licenses/by/4.0/).

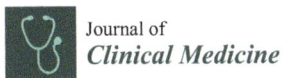

Article

Neopterin is Associated with Disease Severity and Outcome in Patients with Non-Ischaemic Heart Failure

Lukas Lanser [1], Gerhard Pölzl [2], Dietmar Fuchs [3], Günter Weiss [1] and Katharina Kurz [1,*]

1. Department of Internal Medicine II, Medical University of Innsbruck, 6020 Innsbruck, Austria; lukas.lanser@i-med.ac.at (L.L.); guenter.weiss@i-med.ac.at (G.W.)
2. Department of Internal Medicine III, Medical University of Innsbruck, 6020 Innsbruck, Austria; gerhard.poelzl@tirol-kliniken.at
3. Division of Biological Chemistry, Biocenter, Medical University of Innsbruck, 6020 Innsbruck, Austria; dietmar.fuchs@i-med.ac.at
* Correspondence: katharina.kurz@tirol-kliniken.at; Tel.: +43-512-504-23260

Received: 22 October 2019; Accepted: 13 December 2019; Published: 17 December 2019

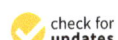

Abstract: Inflammation and immune activation play an important role in the pathogenesis of cardiac remodelling in patients with heart failure. The aim of this study was to assess whether biomarkers of inflammation and immune activation are linked to disease severity and the prognosis of heart failure patients. In 149 patients (65.8% men, median age 49.7 years) with heart failure from nonischaemic cardiomyopathy, the biomarkers neopterin and C-reactive protein were tested at the time of diagnosis. Patients were followed-up for a median of 58 months. During follow-up, nineteen patients died, five had a heart transplantation, two needed a ventricular assistance device, and twenty-one patients had to be hospitalised because of heart failure decompensation. Neopterin concentrations correlated with N-terminal prohormone of brain natriuretic peptide (NT-proBNP) concentrations (rs = 0.399, $p < 0.001$) and rose with higher New York Heart Association (NYHA) class (I: 5.60 nmol/L, II: 6.90 nmol/L, III/IV: 7.80 nmol/L, $p = 0.033$). Higher neopterin levels were predictive for an adverse outcome (death or hospitalisation due to HF decompensation), independently of age and sex and of established predictors in heart failure such as NYHA class, NT-proBNP, estimated glomerular filtration rate (eGFR), and left ventricular ejection fraction (LV-EF) (HR 2.770; 95% CI 1.419–5.407; $p = 0.003$). Patients with a neopterin/eGFR ratio ≥ 0.133 (as a combined marker for immune activation and kidney function) had a more than eightfold increased risk of reaching an endpoint compared to patients with a neopterin/eGFR ratio ≤0.065 (HR 8.380; 95% CI 2.889–24.308; $p < 0.001$). Neopterin is associated with disease severity and is an independent predictor of prognosis in patients with heart failure.

Keywords: Neopterin; inflammation; heart failure; adverse outcome

1. Introduction

Activation and down-regulation of the immune response are important mechanisms to control tissue damage, initiate the healing process, and to remove dead cells and debris after a harmful stimulus [1]. However, prolonged immune activation promotes local and systemic inflammatory processes, thereby contributing to tissue damage and organ failure over time. This has also been shown in patients with chronic heart failure (CHF) [2], where increased concentrations of circulating cytokines and biomarkers of inflammation were associated with a poor outcome [3–5]. Therefore, the balance of physiological and pathological immune activation contributes to heart failure (HF) progression and determines the outcomes of these patients [2]. Immune activation in CHF is driven by several factors:

pro-inflammatory cells are found in the failing myocardium itself [3] but systemic immune activation also plays a role [6]. In fact, low-grade immune activation has been established to greatly contribute to atherogenesis [7]. Additionally, circulating endotoxins, which translocate from the intestinal tract into the systemic circulation [8], as well as the hypoxia of body tissues [9–11] and central inhibition of the parasympathetic nervous system appear to be involved [6].

Elevated parameters of inflammation have been shown to predict an unfavourable clinical course of patients with cardiovascular diseases [12–14]. Several studies have demonstrated that the pteridine neopterin is a good prognostic marker for an adverse outcome in patients with clinically inapparent atherosclerosis [12,15], chronic stable angina pectoris [16–18], and acute coronary syndrome [19].

Neopterin is produced by activated monocytes, macrophages and dendritic cells (DCs) upon stimulation with interferon gamma (IFN-γ). Therefore, neopterin levels reflect the extent of T-helper cell type 1 (Th1) immune activation. Monocytes stimulated by IFN-γ also produce reactive oxygen species (ROS) [20] concomitantly with neopterin, thus inducing oxidative stress, which also plays a key role in the progress of HF [21–23]. Neopterin was demonstrated to correlate with cardiac dysfunction following cardiac surgery [24] and cardiac remodelling in patients with CHF [25]. In addition, neopterin concentrations correlated with the severity of heart failure in patients with preserved ejection fraction (HFpEF) and the probability of future cardiovascular events [26].

The aim of this study was to assess the relationship between the inflammatory biomarkers, C-reactive protein (CRP), neopterin, and disease severity, as well as to evaluate the predictive value of these parameters for the outcome of HF patients with nonischaemic cardiomyopathy (CMP).

2. Experimental Section

2.1. Study Population

We retrospectively analysed the data of 475 caucasian patients with HF caused by nonischaemic CMP. Patients with more than mild-to-moderate valve disease as well as ischaemic cardiomyopathy were not included in the study, since there are studies describing significant differences in immune activation between patients with ischemic and non-ischemic cardiomyopathy [27]. At our department, specific investigations such as echocardiography, coronary angiography (CAG), right heart catheterization, and endomyocardial biopsy (EMB) were performed in patients with nonischaemic CAG. These investigations took place between 2009 and 2014 over the course of an elective hospitalisation, and only patients with compensated HF were investigated. All patients were diagnosed and treated according to prevailing guidelines at the cardiology department at Innsbruck University Hospital. Data of all HF patients with available neopterin and C-reactive protein concentrations (n = 149) were analysed. The final study population consisted of 98 men and 51 women. The study conformed to the ethical principles outlined in the Declaration of Helsinki and was approved by the ethics committee of the Innsbruck Medical University (ID of the ethical votum: UN4280, session number 298/4.11). All patients gave written informed consent to participate in this study.

2.2. Follow-Up Analysis

Patients were followed up until May 2017. For the outcome analysis, we defined the event-free survival as time between invasive diagnosis and laboratory testing, and the occurrence of the combined endpoint. Components of the combined event were death or hospitalisation for cardiac decompensation, whatever came first. Information about patients' events was obtained from the clinical information system (KIS), the local mortality registry, from the patients' relatives or from the patients themselves.

2.3. Measurements

Blood samples were taken from all patients at their first hospitalisation and stored at −80°C. Concentrations of all laboratory variables were measured at the central laboratory of the Innsbruck University Hospital, which undergoes regular internal and external quality control and evaluation.

Neopterin was measured by an enzyme-linked immunosorbent assay (IBL International GmbH, Hamburg, Germany). C-reactive protein (CRP) was detected with an immunoturbidimetry test (Roche, Mannheim, Germany). In order to estimate the glomerular filtration rate (eGFR), we used the IDMS-traceable MDRD study equation (eGFR(mL/min/1.73 m2) = 175 × (serum creatinine) − 1.154 × age − 0.203 (×0.742 if female)).

Hemodynamic parameters were measured in the course of a right and left heart catheterisation, while the left ventricular ejection fraction (LV-EF) was measured during an echocardiography.

2.4. Statistical Analysis

Quantitative variables are presented as medians (25th, 75th percentile) because there was no Gaussian distribution given. Categorical variables are presented as prevalence and percentage. The Kolmogorov-Smirnov test was used to evaluate the normal distribution of the measured data. To test for differences between two or more groups, Mann-Whitney-U test (two unpaired groups), Kruskal-Wallis test (more than two unpaired groups) and Pearson chi-square test were used. Spearman rank correlation was used to assess cross-sectional relations between neopterin, HF severity and kidney function. We used proportional hazard regression analysis to analyse the potential risk factors for an adverse outcome and logarithmised parameters that showed a skewed distribution. All tests used were two-tailed and p-values < 0.05 were considered as statistically significant. The statistical analysis was performed with SPSS Statistics Version 24.0 for Macintosh (IBM Corporation, Armonk, NY, USA).

3. Results

Demographic and clinical characteristics, laboratory measurements, and haemodynamic parameters of the whole population and separately for patients with and without an event within five years are depicted in Table 1.

Table 1. Patient characteristics.

Variable	Total	No Event *	Event *	Significance
	n = 149	n = 115	n = 34	p-Value
	Median (IQR)	Median	Median	
Demographic and clinical characteristics				
Age (years)	49.7 (38.5–61.7)	48.9	51.4	0.074
BMI (kg/m^2)	24.81 (22.00–27.74)	25.25	23.55	0.025
Heart rate (bpm)	70 (60–82)	70	73	0.220
Diast. BP (mmHg)	80 (70–85)	80	77	0.751
Syst. BP (mmHg)	120 (110–132)	120	115	0.193
Hypertension	45.2%	45.5%	44.1%	0.884
Atrial fibrillation	9.7%	9.7%	9.4%	0.952
NYHA class, overall	-	-	-	0.072
NYHA class I	22.4%	26.3%	9.1%	-
NYHA class II	44.2%	43.9%	45.5%	-
NYHA class III/IV	33.3%	29.8%	45.5%	-
Laboratory measurements				
Neopterin (nmol/L)	6.90 (5.00–9.70)	6.50	10.00	<0.001
CRP (mg/L)	0.20 (0.10–0.63)	0.20	0.20	0.966
eGFR (mL/min/1.73m^2)	74.11 (58.39–90.47)	78.29	65.57	0.001
Neopterin/eGFR ratio	0.097 (0.057–0.148)	0.082	0.162	<0.001
NT-proBNP (ng/L)	1340 (501–3266)	1025	3835	<0.001
Hemodynamics				
LV-EF (%)	37.0 (25.7–49.7)	36.0	46.0	0.052
Cardiac index (L/min/m^2)	1.93 (1.68–2.45)	2.01	1.78	0.003
mean PAP (mmHg)	26.0 (19.0–33.0)	24.0	32.5	0.001
PCWP (mmHg)	17 (11–25)	15	24	<0.001
RAP (mmHg)	9 (6–12)	8	11	0.003

Table 1. *Cont.*

Variable	Total n = 149 Median (IQR)	No Event * n = 115 Median	Event * n = 34 Median	Significance *p*-Value
Medication and Treatment				
ACE inhibitor/ARB	77.7%	79.8%	70.6%	0.256
Beta-blocker	74.8%	78.8%	61.8%	0.045
MRA	34.5%	33.3%	38.2%	0.598
Diuretics	57.8%	52.6%	75.8%	0.018
Cardiac glycosides	2.0%	1.8%	2.9%	0.666
Pacemaker	3.4%	3.5%	2.9%	0.872

Data from 149 patients are presented as medians (interquartile range). (*) Event within five years. Parameters that differed significantly are printed in italic letters. IQR = interquartile range; BMI = body mass index; BP = blood pressure; NYHA = New York Heart Association; CRP = C-reactive protein; eGFR = estimated glomerular filtration rate; NT-proBNP = N-terminal prohormone of brain natriuretic peptide; RAP = right atrial pressure; mean PAP = mean pulmonary artery pressure; PCWP = pulmonary capillary wedge pressure; LV-EF = left ventricular ejection fraction; ACE = angiotensin converting enzyme; ARB = angiotensin II receptor blocker; MRA = mineralocorticoid receptor antagonist.

The percentage of patients with reduced LV-EF <40% was 63.4% (66.3% of men, 58.0% of women, $p = 0.323$). Reduced kidney function (eGFR $\leq$ 60 mL/min/1.73m^2) was found in 40 patients (26.8%) but only seven of them (4.7%) were presented with advanced renal insufficiency (eGFR $\leq$ 45 mL/min/1.73m^2).

3.1. Inflammation Correlates With HF Severity and Cardiac Function

Inflammatory parameters (CRP and/or neopterin) were elevated in 72 patients (48.3%). Out of these, 25 patients (16.8%) showed elevated CRP concentrations (>0.5 mg/L), 27 patients (18.1%) elevated neopterin concentrations (>8.7 nmol/L), and 20 patients (13.4%) showed both elevated CRP and neopterin concentrations.

Neopterin concentrations were positively correlated with CRP concentrations (rs = 0.343, $p < 0.001$; Figure 1A). Additionally, significant correlations were found between neopterin concentrations and NT-proBNP concentrations (rs = 0.399, $p < 0.001$, Figure 1B), cardiac index (rs = −0.287, $p = 0.001$), right atrial pressure (RAP, rs = 0.170, $p = 0.043$), pulmonary artery mean pressure (mean PAP, rs = 0.227, $p = 0.007$) and pulmonary capillary wedge pressure (PCWP, rs = 0.244, $p = 0.004$) were found. Neopterin progressively increased with higher NYHA class (I: 5.60 nmol/L, II: 6.90 nmol/L, III/IV: 7.80 nmol/L, $p = 0.033$, Figure 1C).

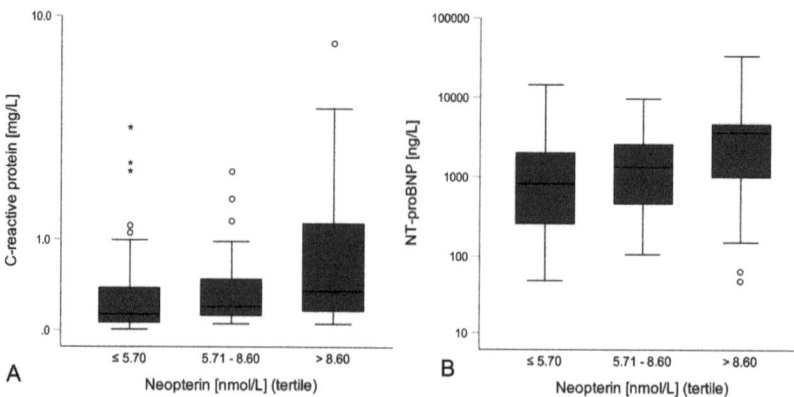

Figure 1. *Cont.*

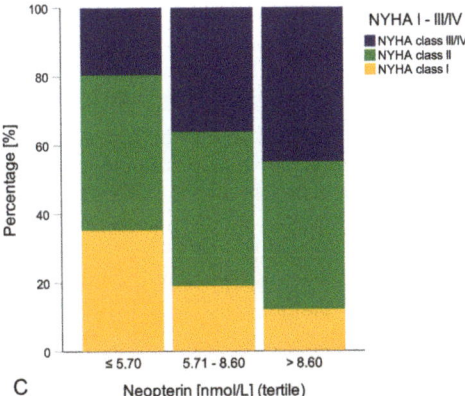

Figure 1. Inflammation and HF severity: Higher neopterin concentrations were associated with higher CRP (**A**) and NT-proBNP concentrations (**B**). Patients with higher neopterin concentrations also had higher NYHA classes (**C**).

CRP concentrations also correlated significantly with NT-proBNP concentrations (rs = 0.232, $p = 0.006$) and showed a positive dose-response relationship with increasing NYHA class (l: 0.16 mg/L, ll: 0.17 mg/L, lll/lV: 0.25 mg/L, $p = 0.030$).

3.2. Neopterin/eGFR Ratio and HF Severity

As patients with reduced eGFR (≤60 mL/min/1.73m^2) had significantly higher neopterin concentrations than patients with preserved kidney function (8.90 nmol/L vs. 6.00 nmol/L, $p < 0.001$), we adjusted neopterin concentrations for the kidney function and calculated a neopterin/eGFR ratio. Correlation analysis showed a highly significant correlation of the neopterin/eGFR ratio with NT-proBNP concentrations (rs = 0.438, $p < 0.001$), cardiac index (rs = −0.383, $p < 0.001$), right atrial pressure (RAP, rs = 0.172, $p = 0.041$), pulmonary artery mean pressure (mean PAP, rs = 0.281, $p = 0.001$) and pulmonary capillary wedge pressure (PCWP, rs = 0.302, $p < 0.001$). Patients with a higher NYHA class showed a significant higher neopterin/eGFR ratio (l: 0.060, ll: 0.098, lll/lV: 0.131, $p = 0.003$).

3.3. Neopterin/eGFR Ratio and Left Ventricular Ejection Fraction

The LV-EF was reduced (<40%) in 49.7% of our patients (Heart Failure with reduced Ejection Fraction—HFrEF), while 22.1% had a preserved LV-EF ≥ 50% (Heart Failure with preserved Ejection Fraction—HFpEF) and 21.5% a LV-EF between 40%–49.9% (Heart Failure with mid-range Ejection Fraction—HFmrEF). Patients with HFmrEF had the lowest neopterin concentrations (5.35 nmol/L, $p = 0.021$) and the highest eGFR (84.28 mL/min/1.73m2, $p = 0.003$) compared to patients with HFrEF and HFpEF (Appendix A, Table A1). Interestingly enough, neopterin concentrations did not differ significantly between patients with HFrEF and HFpEF (7.00 nmol/L vs. 7.40 nmol/L, $p = 0.235$), while patients with HFpEF had a significantly lower eGFR compared to patients with HFrEF (66.15 mL/min/1.73m2 vs. 76.48 mL/min/1.73m2, $p = 0.026$).

3.4. Laboratory Parameters and Event-Free Survival

The median follow-up of patients in this study was 58 months (0–98). A total of 40 patients reached the combined endpoint: 19 patients (12.8%) died and 21 patients (14.1%) were hospitalised for cardiac decompensation.

Patients with an event within five years had significantly higher neopterin and NT-proBNP concentrations, as well as a higher RAP and were found to have a higher NYHA class, while the cardiac index and eGFR were significantly lower compared to patients without an event. Interestingly enough,

CRP concentrations, LV-EF, or age did not differ between patients with or without an event, while patients with an event showed a higher BMI compared to patients with no event (Table 1).

3.5. Neopterin is a Predictor for an Adverse Outcome in Patients with HF

Patients with neopterin concentrations >8.60 nmol/L (highest tertile) had a fourfold higher risk of reaching an endpoint compared to patients with neopterin concentrations ≤5.70 nmol/L (lowest tertile) in Cox regression analysis sex-stratified and adjusted for age (HR 4.118; 95% CI 1.727–9.820; p = 0.001; Figure 2A). The cumulative five-year event rates for the neopterin tertiles were 8.4% (≤5.70 nmol/L), 20.0% (5.71–8.60 nmol/L) and 46.6% (≥8.61 nmol/L). This was even independent of kidney function since a higher neopterin/eGFR ratio (logarithmised) was also predictive for future adverse events in Cox regression analysis sex-stratified and adjusted for age (Table 2). Patients with a neopterin/eGFR ratio ≥ 0.133 had a more than eightfold increased risk of reaching an endpoint compared to patients with a neopterin/eGFR ratio ≤ 0.065 (HR 8.380; 95% CI 2.889–24.308; p < 0.001, Figure 2B).

Table 2. Cox regression analysis.

Variable	Univariate Model			Multivariate Model		
	HR	95% CI	p-Value	HR	95% CI	p-Value
Neopterin (nmol/L) _Ln *	2.874	1.663–4.966	<0.001	2.770	1.419–5.407	0.003
eGFR (mL/min/1.73m^2) _Ln	0.321	0.174–0.593	<0.001	2.723	0.936–7.926	0.066
NT-proBNP (ng/L) _Ln	1.665	1.253–2.214	<0.001	1.368	0.972–1.926	0.072
NYHA class II vs. I	2.542	0.852–7.578	0.094	3.200	0.830–12.329	0.091
NYHA class III/IV vs. I	3.245	1.070–9.840	0.038	3.126	0.751–13.006	0.117
LV-EF (%) _Ln	2.245	0.989–5.096	0.053	2.884	1.096–7.589	0.032
Neopterin/eGFR ratio _Ln	1.748	1.420–2.152	<0.001			
Cardiac index (L/min/m^2) _Ln	0.250	0.062–1.008	0.051			
mean PAP (mmHg) _Ln	2.979	1.168–7.599	0.022			
PCWP (mmHg) _Ln	2.453	1.203–5.002	0.014			
RAP (mmHg) _Ln	3.536	1.584–7.894	0.002			
BMI (kg/m^2) _Ln	0.188	0.032–1.114	0.066			

Univariate and multivariate Cox regression analyses models are adjusted for age and stratified for sex. * Neopterin levels were also adjusted for the eGFR in the univariate model. Variables showing a skewed distribution were logarithmised with the natural logarithm and marked with "_Ln". HR = hazard ratio; CI = confidence interval; eGFR = estimated glomerular filtration rate; NT-proBNP = N-terminal prohormone of brain natriuretic peptide; NYHA = New York Heart Association; LV-EF = left ventricular ejection fraction; mean PAP = pulmonary artery mean pressure; PCWP = pulmonary capillary wedge pressure; RAP = right atrial pressure; BMI = body mass index.

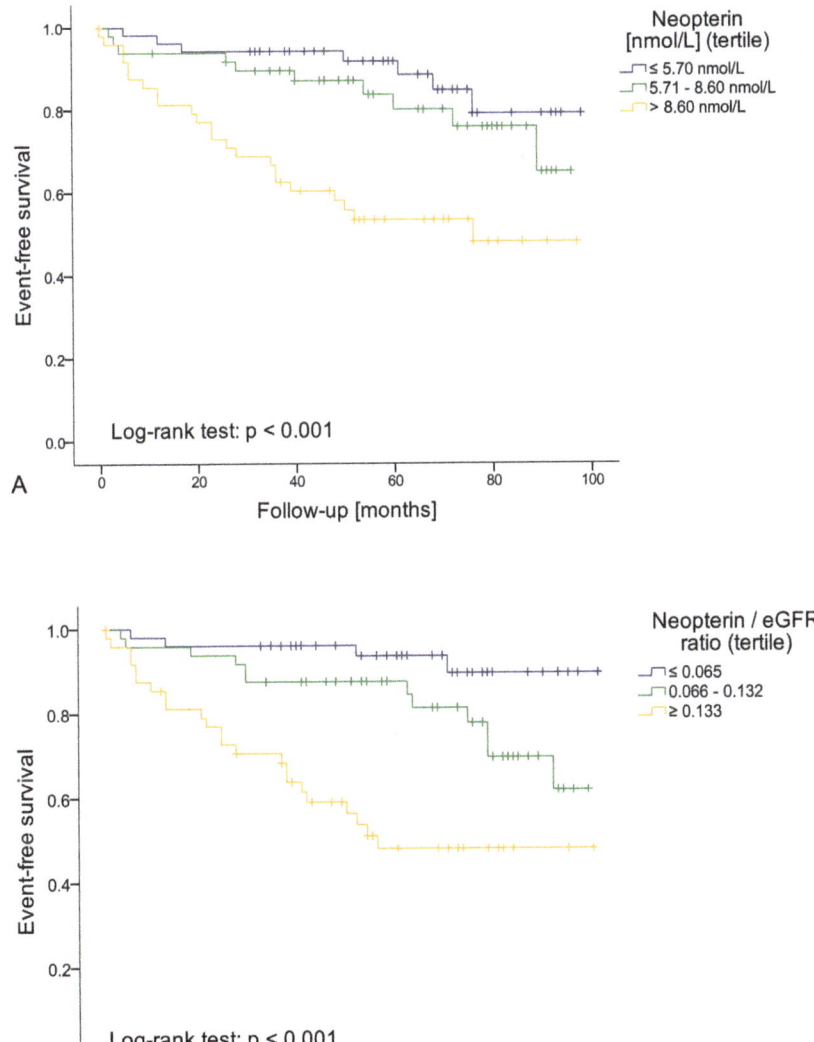

Figure 2. (**A**) Patients with higher neopterin levels (Neopterin > 8.60 nmol/L) had a fourfold higher risk of reaching an endpoint compared to patients within neopterin levels ≤5.70 nmol/L in Cox regression analysis sex-stratified and adjusted for age ($p = 0.001$); (**B**) The same was also true for patients with a higher neopterin/eGFR ratio: Patients with a neopterin/eGFR ratio ≥ 0.133 had a more than eight-fold increased risk of reaching an endpoint compared to patients with a neopterin/eGFR ratio ≤ 0.065 ($p < 0.001$).

A multivariate regression model stratified for sex was calculated with neopterin, age, eGFR, NT-proBNP, NYHA functional class, and LV-EF as co-variates that were considered clinically meaningful. Multivariate Cox regression analysis showed that baseline neopterin levels were associated with the combined endpoint, independently of established and widely available predictors of HF such as eGFR,

NT-proBNP, NYHA class and LV-EF (Table 2). Neopterin was also an independent predictor for an unfavourable outcome when correcting for co-medications (ACE inhibitor/ARB, beta-blocker, MRA, diuretics or cardiac glycosides) in Cox regression analysis. Patients with diuretics had significantly higher neopterin concentrations than those without (7.50 nmol/L vs. 5.80 nmol/L, $p = 0.001$).

4. Discussion

This study demonstrates that serum neopterin concentrations are linked to disease severity and can predict a worse outcome in patients with HF caused by non-ischaemic CMP. We also show that calculation of the neopterin/eGFR ratio is very useful to predict a worse outcome of patients and might be well suited as a "combined" marker for immune activation and decreased kidney function.

Recent studies have proposed a key role of inflammation in the determination of cardiovascular risk [28]. Levels of inflammatory cytokines are elevated in HF patients and related to an adverse outcome [29]. Activation of the immune system following cardiac injury is, per se, a protective (i.e., physiological) mechanism. Several studies have demonstrated that a short-term low-grade expression of stress-activated proinflammatory cytokines within the failing heart has beneficial consequences [30–32]. These cytokines induce the upregulation of so-called protective proteins in the heart that are part of the myocardial stress response such as cardiac hypertrophy, cardiac remodeling, and cardiac repair. However, the sustained or excessive expression of proinflammatory cytokines can cause tissue injury, consequently leading to progressive LV dysfunction and adverse LV remodeling [1,5,30]. Accordingly, patients with chronic inflammatory disease including rheumatoid arthritis [33], systemic lupus erythematosus [34] or atopic dermatitis [35] were shown to have an increased cardiovascular risk.

Our data show that higher neopterin concentrations, which originate from activated monocytes and macrophages upon stimulation with the proinflammatory cytokine IFN-γ, are associated with an impaired cardiac function: Elevated neopterin concentrations were found in patients with higher NYHA class, lower cardiac index, and increased NT-proBNP concentrations.

The association of neopterin concentrations with the combined endpoint was independent of age or sex and established predictors in HF such as NT-proBNP, NYHA class, eGFR, and LV-EF. Interestingly enough, CRP concentrations were not associated with the outcome in our population, although CRP is regarded as a powerful predictor of adverse outcome in cardiovascular disease (CVD) and HF [36]. While CRP is an acute phase protein and synthesised by the liver mainly upon IL-6 [37], neopterin is a more specific marker reflecting the interaction of T-cells (IFN-γ signalling) and monocytes/macrophages within Th1 immune activation. While CRP was shown earlier to be elevated in patients with acute cardiac events (unstable angina pectoris, non-ST-elevation myocardial infarction, or ST-elevation myocardial infarction), neopterin did not differ between these patients, but was predictive for a higher risk of an adverse long-term outcome in patients with coronary artery disease compared to high CRP concentrations [12].

There are only few studies in which CRP and neopterin levels were tested in parallel in large populations: In all these trials, neopterin was predictive for an increased cardiovascular mortality, but also for the overall mortality, independent of other established risk factors [12,14,19], and also independent of the acute phase marker CRP. Hazard ratios for adverse outcomes were higher for elevated neopterin concentrations as compared with high CRP concentrations in the LURIC study (patients with different kinds of cardiovascular diseases) [12,38], and neopterin was also predictive of an adverse outcome after adjusting for NT-ProBNP values, while CRP was not. Contrarily, in the HUSK study (population-based study in West Norway) CRP seemed slightly better for the prediction of CVD mortality, while IFN-γ-mediated inflammatory markers (neopterin and tryptophan degradation) better predicted non-CVD mortality [14]. Unfortunately, testing for neopterin is not performed in most routine labs, while the measurement of CRP is easily available everywhere.

Previous studies have also shown that neopterin, but not CRP, is associated with LV dysfunction [16] and predicts an increased cardiovascular risk [18] in patients with stable angina pectoris. On the other hand, elevated CRP levels are an established cardiovascular risk factor [39], which has also been used recently in the CANTOS trial, which assessed the effect of anti-inflammatory treatment with the monoclonal antibody Canakinumab (targeting interleukin-1β) in patients with prior myocardial infarction and elevated CRP [40]. Canakinumab was very effective in preventing adverse cardiac events and decreasing CRP concentrations in patients, indicating that the downregulation of chronic inflammatory processes is able to improve patient outcomes.

Considering this possible role of immune activation in the pathogenesis of cardiovascular disease, the determination of other inflammatory markers like neopterin appears to be a promising strategy to assess the actual risk of HF patients for a cardiovascular event. In particular, it may also serve as decision-making tool for anti-inflammatory therapy to decide if immune activation is over-whelming or within the normal range. In our population, the neopterin/eGFR ratio was also correlated with all relevant risk markers as well as with HF severity and it was predictive for a worse outcome. Calculation of the neopterin/eGFR ratio might in fact allow an even better risk stratification of patients with HF, as it combines the information from two risk factors (inflammation and decreased renal function). Thus, it would certainly be interesting to investigate the predictive power of this combined marker in future HF trials with a higher number of patients.

Still, it has to be emphasised that there are also other very important factors that contribute importantly to the development of inflammation. Moreover, the interaction between genetic and environmental factors might play a prominent role and significantly modulates inflammatory processes [41]. In patients with HF other mechanisms such as transthyretin amyloidosis or HF with preserved ejection fraction should also be investigated in more detail [42]. Further studies examining the effects of an impaired cholesterol efflux, which is linked to an increased CV risk, might provide interesting new data [43]. Last but not least, the role of diet should be evaluated in more detail in patients with CVD and HF. A very interesting recent study reviewed the impact of diet on inflammation, and in fact, the change of diet might represent a relatively easy and reasonable strategy to reduce the risk of CVD [41].

Strengths and Limitations

This study shows the clinical potential of neopterin and neopterin/eGFR ratio for the prediction of the course of CHF. Unfortunately, neopterin and CRP were not available in all patients who were initially included in the study, which resulted in a smaller sample size. This must be taken into account when interpreting the results of multivariate Cox regression analysis. The fact that the study was carried out with patients with non-ischemic CMP does not allow for a sweeping generalisation about all HF patients. The collection of event data, including patients questioning themselves and relative driven information, also represents a certain bias.

5. Conclusions

This study indicates that Th_1 immune activation, reflected by neopterin concentrations, plays a crucial role in the pathogenesis of HF caused by nonischaemic CMP. Neopterin concentrations as well as the neopterin/eGFR ratio are linked to disease severity and are associated with disease progression and an adverse outcome for patients with HF. Further longitudinal studies with a higher number of patients are needed to prove the role of neopterin in HF.

Author Contributions: Conceptualization, G.W. and G.P.; methodology, G.W. and G.P.; software, L.L. and K.K.; validation, L.L., G.P., D.F., G.W., and K.K.; formal analysis, L.L. and K.K.; investigation, L.L. and K.K.; data curation, L.L. and K.K.; writing—original draft preparation, L.L. and K.K.; writing—review and editing, G.W., G.P. and D.F.; visualization, L.L.

Funding: This research received no external funding.

Conflicts of Interest: The authors declare no conflict of interest.

Appendix A

Table A1. Heart failure classification, demographic and clinical characteristics and laboratory measurements.

Variable	HFrEF, LV-EF < 40% n = 74 Median (IQR)	HFmrEF, LV-EF 40–49.9% n = 32 Median (IQR)	HFpEF, LV-EF ≥ 50% n = 33 Median (IQR)	Sig. p-Value
Demographic and clinical characteristics				
Age (years)	46.3 (36.2–55.8)	46.3 (35.3–55.8)	55.6 (48.2–69.2)	0.005
BMI (kg/m^2)	24.00 (21.60–27.30)	24.76 (22.35–28.05)	24.40 (22.00–28.90)	0.516
Heart rate (bpm)	72 (63–85)	69 (60–79)	70 (60–81)	0.385
Syst. BP (mmHg)	115 (110 – 140)	126 (110–140)	126 (120–150)	0.003
Laboratory measurements				
Neopterin (nmol/L)	7.00 (5.20–9.20)	5.35 (3.95–8.10)	7.40 (5.90–11.50)	0.021
CRP (mg/L)	0.24 (0.13–0.63)	0.25 (0.07–0.63)	0.15 (0.10–0.25)	0.120
eGFR (mL/min/1.73m^2)	76.48 (58.09–94.34)	84.28 (71.12–101.40)	66.15 (54.16–74.23)	0.003
Neopterin/eGFR ratio	0.104 (0.059–0.144)	0.061 (0.046–0.103)	0.126 (0.082–0.190)	0.005
NT-proBNP (ng/L)	2072 (949–3681)	198 (96–745)	1989 (703–4644)	<0.001

Data from 149 patients are presented as medians (interquartile range). Parameters that differed significantly are printed in italic letters. HFrEF = Heart failure with reduced Ejection Fraction; HFmrEF = Heart failure with mid-range Ejection Fraction; HFpEF = Heart Failure with preserved Ejection Fraction; IQR = interquartile range; BMI = body mass index; Syst. BP = systolic blood pressure; CRP = C-reactive protein; eGFR = estimated glomerular filtration rate; NT-proBNP = N-terminal prohormone of brain natriuretic peptide; RAP = right atrial pressure; mean PAP = mean pulmonary artery pressure.

References

1. Medzhitov, R. Inflammation 2010: New adventures of an old flame. *Cell* **2010**, *140*, 771–776. [CrossRef]
2. Dick, S.A.; Epelman, S. Chronic heart failure and inflammation: What do we really know? *Circ. Res.* **2016**, *119*, 159–176. [CrossRef] [PubMed]
3. Torre-Amione, G.; Kapadia, S.; Lee, J.; Durand, J.B.; Bies, R.D.; Young, J.B.; Mann, D.L. Tumor necrosis factor-alpha and tumor necrosis factor receptors in the failing human heart. *Circulation* **1996**, *93*, 704–711. [CrossRef] [PubMed]
4. Vasan, R.S.; Sullivan, L.M.; Roubenoff, R.; Dinarello, C.A.; Harris, T.; Benjamin, E.J.; Sawyer, D.B.; Levy, D.; Wilson, P.W.; D'Agostino, R.B.; et al. Inflammatory markers and risk of heart failure in elderly subjects without prior myocardial infarction: The Framingham Heart Study. *Circulation* **2003**, *107*, 1486–1491. [CrossRef]
5. Mann, D.L. Innate immunity and the failing heart: The cytokine hypothesis revisited. *Circ. Res.* **2015**, *116*, 1254–1268. [CrossRef] [PubMed]
6. Jankowska, E.A.; Ponikowski, P.; Piepoli, M.F.; Banasiak, W.; Anker, S.D.; Poole-Wilson, P.A. Autonomic imbalance and immune activation in chronic heart failure—pathophysiological links. *Cardiovasc. Res.* **2006**, *70*, 434–445. [CrossRef]
7. Libby, P.; Lichtman, A.H.; Hansson, G.K. Immune effector mechanisms implicated in atherosclerosis: From mice to humans. *Immunity* **2013**, *38*, 1092–1104. [CrossRef]
8. Niebauer, J.; Volk, H.D.; Kemp, M.; Dominguez, M.; Schumann, R.R.; Rauchhaus, M.; Poole-Wilson, P.A.; Coats, A.J.; Anker, S.D. Endotoxin and immune activation in chronic heart failure: A prospective cohort study. *Lancet* **1999**, *353*, 1838–1842. [CrossRef]
9. Hasper, D.; Hummel, M.; Kleber, F.X.; Reindl, I.; Volk, H.D. Systemic inflammation in patients with heart failure. *Eur. Heart J.* **1998**, *19*, 761–765. [CrossRef]
10. Suzuki, K.; Nakaji, S.; Yamada, M.; Totsuka, M.; Sato, K.; Sugawara, K. Systemic inflammatory response to exhaustive exercise. Cytokine kinetics. *Exerc. Immunol. Rev.* **2002**, *8*, 6–48.
11. Shephard, R.J. Sepsis and mechanisms of inflammatory response: Is exercise a good model? *Br. J. Sports Med.* **2001**, *35*, 223–230. [CrossRef] [PubMed]
12. Grammer, T.B.; Fuchs, D.; Boehm, B.O.; Winkelmann, B.R.; Maerz, W. Neopterin as a predictor of total and cardiovascular mortality in individuals undergoing angiography in the Ludwigshafen Risk and Cardiovascular Health study. *Clin. Chem.* **2009**, *55*, 1135–1146. [CrossRef] [PubMed]

13. Fuchs, D.; Avanzas, P.; Arroyo-Espliguero, R.; Jenny, M.; Consuegra-Sanchez, L.; Kaski, J.C. The role of neopterin in atherogenesis and cardiovascular risk assessment. *Curr. Med. Chem.* **2009**, *16*, 4644–4653. [CrossRef] [PubMed]
14. Zuo, H.; Ueland, P.M.; Ulvik, A.; Eussen, S.J.; Vollset, S.E.; Nygård, O.; Midttun, Ø.; Theofylaktopoulou, D.; Meyer, K.; Tell, G.S. Plasma biomarkers of inflammation, the kynurenine pathway, and risks of all-cause, cancer, and cardiovascular disease mortality: The Hordaland health study. *Am. J. Epidemiol.* **2016**, *183*, 249–258. [CrossRef] [PubMed]
15. Weiss, G.; Willeit, J.; Kiechl, S.; Fuchs, D.; Jarosch, E.; Oberhollenzer, F.; Reibnegger, G.; Tilz, G.P.; Gerstenbrand, F.; Wachter, H. Increased concentrations of neopterin in carotid atherosclerosis. *Atherosclerosis* **1994**, *106*, 263–271. [CrossRef]
16. Estévez-Loureiro, R.; Recio-Mayoral, A.; Sieira-Rodríguez-Moret, J.A.; Trallero-Araguás, E.; Kaski, J.C. Neopterin levels and left ventricular dysfunction in patients with chronic stable angina pectoris. *Atherosclerosis* **2009**, *207*, 514–518. [CrossRef]
17. Avanzas, P.; Arroyo-Espliguero, R.; Quiles, J.; Roy, D.; Kaski, J.C. Elevated serum neopterin predicts future adverse cardiac events in patients with chronic stable angina pectoris. *Eur. Heart J.* **2005**, *26*, 457–463. [CrossRef]
18. Bjørnestad, E.; Borsholm, R.A.; Svingen, G.F.T.; Pedersen, E.R.; Seifert, R.; Midttun, Ø.; Ueland, P.M.; Tell, G.S.; Bønaa, K.H.; Nygård, O. Neopterin as an effect modifier of the cardiovascular risk predicted by total homocysteine: A prospective 2-cohort study. *J. Am. Heart Assoc.* **2017**, *6*, e006500. [CrossRef]
19. Ray, K.K.; Morrow, D.A.; Sabatine, M.S.; Shui, A.; Rifai, N.; Cannon, C.P.; Braunwald, E. Long-term prognostic value of neopterin: A novel marker of monocyte activation in patients with acute coronary syndrome. *Circulation* **2007**, *115*, 3071–3078. [CrossRef]
20. Nathan, C.F.; Murray, H.W.; Wiebe, M.E.; Rubin, B.Y. Identification of interferon-gamma as the lymphokine that activates human macrophage oxidative metabolism and antimicrobial activity. *J. Exp. Med.* **1983**, *158*, 670–689. [CrossRef]
21. Eisenhut, M. Neopterin in diagnosis and monitoring of infectious diseases. *J. Biomark.* **2013**, *2013*, 196432. [CrossRef] [PubMed]
22. Wirleitner, B.; Reider, D.; Ebner, S.; Böck, G.; Widner, B.; Jaeger, M.; Schennach, H.; Romani, N.; Fuchs, D. Monocyte-derived dendritic cells release neopterin. *J. Leukoc. Biol.* **2002**, *72*, 1148–1153. [PubMed]
23. Gostner, J.M.; Becker, K.; Fuchs, D.; Sucher, R. Redox regulation of the immune response. *Redox. Rep.* **2013**, *18*, 88–94. [CrossRef] [PubMed]
24. Berg, K.S.; Stenseth, R.; Pleym, H.; Wahba, A.; Videm, V. Neopterin predicts cardiac dysfunction following cardiac surgery. *Interact. Cardiovasc. Thorac. Surg.* **2015**, *21*, 598–603. [CrossRef] [PubMed]
25. Caruso, R.; De Chiara, B.; Campolo, J.; Verde, A.; Musca, F.; Belli, O.; Parolini, M.; Cozzi, L.; Moreo, A.; Frigerio, M.; et al. Neopterin levels are independently associated with cardiac remodeling in patients with chronic heart failure. *Clin. Biochem.* **2013**, *46*, 94–98. [CrossRef] [PubMed]
26. Yamamoto, E.; Hirata, Y.; Tokitsu, T.; Kusaka, H.; Tabata, N.; Tsujita, K.; Yamamuro, M.; Kaikita, K.; Watanabe, H.; Hokimoto, S.; et al. The clinical significance of plasma neopterin in heart failure with preserved left ventricular ejection fraction. *ESC Heart Fail.* **2016**, *3*, 53–59. [CrossRef]
27. Karabacak, M.; Doğan, A.; Varol, E.; Uysal, B.A.; Yıldız, İ. Comparison of Inflammatory Markers in Patients with Ischemic and Non-ischemic Heart Failure. *J. Am. Coll. Cardiol.* **2013**, *62*, C137–C138. [CrossRef]
28. Sorriento, D.; Iaccarino, G. Inflammation and cardiovascular diseases: The most recent findings. *Int. J. Mol. Sci.* **2019**, *20*, 3879. [CrossRef]
29. Fiordelisi, A.; Iaccarino, G.; Morisco, C.; Coscioni, E.; Sorriento, D. NFkappaB is a key player in the crosstalk between inflammation and cardiovascular diseases. *Int. J. Mol. Sci.* **2019**, *20*, 1599. [CrossRef]
30. Mann, D.L. Stress-activated cytokines and the heart: From adaptation to maladaptation. *Annu. Rev. Physiol.* **2003**, *65*, 81–101. [CrossRef]
31. Samsonov, M.; Fuchs, D.; Reibnegger, G.; Belenkov, J.N.; Nassonov, E.L.; Wachter, H. Patterns of serological markers for cellular immune activation in patients with dilated cardiomyopathy and chronic myocarditis. *Clin. Chem.* **1992**, *38*, 678–680. [PubMed]
32. Rudzite, V.; Skards, J.I.; Fuchs, D.; Reibnegger, G.; Wachter, H. Serum kynurenine and neopterin concentrations in patients with cardiomyopathy. *Immunol. Lett.* **1992**, *32*, 125–129. [CrossRef]

33. England, B.R.; Thiele, G.M.; Anderson, D.R.; Mikuls, T.R. Increased cardiovascular risk in rheumatoid arthritis: Mechanisms and implications. *BMJ* **2018**, *361*, k1036. [CrossRef] [PubMed]
34. Sinicato, N.A.; da Silva Cardoso, P.A.; Appenzeller, S. Risk factors in cardiovascular disease in systemic lupus erythematosus. *Curr. Cardiol. Rev.* **2013**, *9*, 15–19. [CrossRef] [PubMed]
35. Silverwood, R.J.; Forbes, H.J.; Abuabara, K.; Ascott, A.; Schmidt, M.; Schmidt, S.A.J.; Smeeth, L.; Langan, S.M. Severe and predominantly active atopic eczema in adulthood and long term risk of cardiovascular disease: Population based cohort study. *BMJ* **2018**, *361*, k1786. [CrossRef] [PubMed]
36. Araújo, J.P.; Lourenço, P.; Azevedo, A.; Friões, F.; Rocha-Gonçalves, F.; Ferreira, A.; Bettencourt, P. Prognostic value of high-sensitivity C-reactive protein in heart failure: A systematic review. *J. Card. Fail.* **2009**, *15*, 256–266. [CrossRef] [PubMed]
37. Abrams, J. C-reactive protein, inflammation, and coronary risk: An update. *Cardiol. Clin.* **2003**, *21*, 327–331. [CrossRef]
38. Avanzas, P.; Arroyo-Espliguero, R.; Kaski, J.C. Neopterin—marker of coronary artery disease activity or extension in patients with chronic stable angina? *Int. J. Cardiol.* **2010**, *144*, 74–75. [CrossRef]
39. Fonseca, F.A.; Izar, M.C. High-sensitivity C-reactive protein and cardiovascular disease across countries and ethnicities. *Clinics* **2016**, *71*, 235–242. [CrossRef]
40. Ridker, P.M.; Everett, B.M.; Thuren, T.; MacFadyen, J.G.; Chang, W.H.; Ballantyne, C.; Fonseca, F.; Nicolau, J.; Koenig, W.; Anker, S.D.; et al. Antiinflammatory therapy with canakinumab for atherosclerotic disease. *N. Engl. J. Med.* **2017**, *377*, 1119–1131. [CrossRef]
41. Gambardella, J.; Santulli, G. Integrating diet and inflammation to calculate cardiovascular risk. *Atherosclerosis* **2016**, *253*, 258–261. [CrossRef] [PubMed]
42. Michels da Silva, D.; Langer, H.; Graf, T. Inflammatory and molecular pathways in heart failure-ischemia, HFpEF and transthyretin cardiac amyloidosis. *Int. J. Mol. Sci.* **2019**, *20*, 2322. [CrossRef] [PubMed]
43. Riggs, K.A.; Joshi, P.H.; Khera, A.; Singh, K.; Akinmolayemi, O.; Ayers, C.R.; Rohatgi, A. Impaired HDL metabolism links GlycA, A novel inflammatory marker, with incident cardiovascular events. *J. Clin. Med.* **2019**, *8*, 2137. [CrossRef] [PubMed]

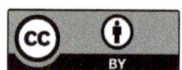

© 2019 by the authors. Licensee MDPI, Basel, Switzerland. This article is an open access article distributed under the terms and conditions of the Creative Commons Attribution (CC BY) license (http://creativecommons.org/licenses/by/4.0/).

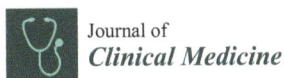

Review

Inositol 1,4,5-Trisphosphate Receptors in Human Disease: A Comprehensive Update

Jessica Gambardella [1,2,3], **Angela Lombardi** [1,4], **Marco Bruno Morelli** [1,5], **John Ferrara** [1] and **Gaetano Santulli** [1,2,3,5,*]

1. Department of Medicine, Einstein-Mount Sinai Diabetes Research Center (ES-DRC), Fleischer Institute for Diabetes and Metabolism, Albert Einstein College of Medicine, New York, NY 10461, USA; jessica.gambardella@einsteinmed.org (J.G.); angela.lombardi@einsteinmed.org (A.L.); marco.morelli@einstein.yu.edu (M.B.M.); j.ferraraeastchester@gmail.com (J.F.)
2. International Translational Research and Medical Education Consortium (ITME), 80100 Naples, Italy
3. Department of Advanced Biomedical Sciences, "Federico II" University, 80131 Naples, Italy
4. Department of Microbiology and Immunology, Albert Einstein College of Medicine, New York, NY 10461, USA
5. Department of Molecular Pharmacology, Wilf Family Cardiovascular Research Institute, Albert Einstein College of Medicine, New York, NY 10461, USA
* Correspondence: gsantulli001@gmail.com

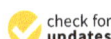

Received: 9 March 2020; Accepted: 10 April 2020; Published: 12 April 2020

Abstract: Inositol 1,4,5-trisphosphate receptors (ITPRs) are intracellular calcium release channels located on the endoplasmic reticulum of virtually every cell. Herein, we are reporting an updated systematic summary of the current knowledge on the functional role of ITPRs in human disorders. Specifically, we are describing the involvement of its loss-of-function and gain-of-function mutations in the pathogenesis of neurological, immunological, cardiovascular, and neoplastic human disease. Recent results from genome-wide association studies are also discussed.

Keywords: Alzheimer; ataxia; autoimmune disease; cancer; cardiovascular disease; diabetes; GWAS; IP3 Receptors; ITPRs; mutations

---

1. Introduction

Since their discovery in the 1970s, several studies have provided substantial evidence that inositol 1,4,5-trisphosphate receptors (ITPRs) play a pleiotropic role in the regulation of cellular functions. Indeed, their ability to regulate calcium handling poses ITPRs at the heart of molecular networks underlying cellular homeostasis: From proliferation, apoptosis, and differentiation to metabolism and neurotransmission.

ITPR was identified for the first time as a large membrane protein called P400 [1,2] that was able to regulate intracellular calcium spikes [1–3]. After protein purification and cDNA isolation, it became clear that P400 was a channel releasing calcium from the endoplasmic reticulum (ER) [4–6]. Later, ITPR was shown to be a rather peculiar channel, as two-second messengers are needed for its activation: IP3 and calcium [7–12].

Three isoforms of ITPR have been identified (ITPR13) in mammals, which, albeit produced by different genes, show 70% of homology in the primary protein sequence [13]. The similarity in amino acid sequence also reflects the resemblance in protein conformation and spatial organization. All three isoforms consist of five domains: Suppressor domain (SD), IP3 binding core domain (IBC), regulatory domain, transmembrane domain (TD), and C-terminus domain (CTD) [14–17]. These domains are organized in a complex tetrameric "mushroom-like" structure (Figure 1), with the stalk inserted in the ER membrane and the cap exposed to the cytosol [18]. The stalk is mainly represented by the transmembrane TM domain, with its six-helices forming the ion-conducting pore [16]. All the other domains are in the "cap", exposed to the cytosol. This organization makes the IBC domain available to IP3 binding, and the regulatory domain to the many interactions and post-transcriptional modifications that regulate the receptor activity, including phosphorylation and oxidation [16].

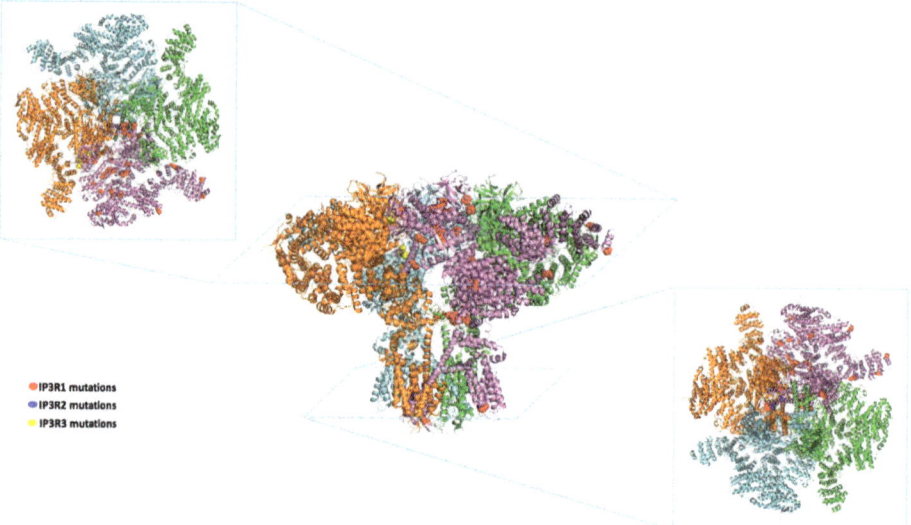

Figure 1. Representative structure of inositol 1,4,5-trisphosphate receptors (ITPRs) (1-3) showing disease-related mutations. In the middle, representative "mushroom-like structure" of ITPRs. For clarity, only the crystal of human isoform 3 is shown. Top left corner: View from the top; bottom right corner: View from the bottom. The residues in red, blue, and yellow indicate the mutations in ITPR1, 2, and 3, respectively, that have been hitherto reported in humans.

Nevertheless, the information on the ITPR molecular organization is still not sufficient for a complete mechanistic definition of its structure–function relationship [10,19]. If the central calcium conducting pore is similar to other ion channels, as suggested by the 4.7 Å structure of ITPR [16], the spatial arrangement of the cytosolic C-terminus is quite unique for ITPR; in particular, these carboxyl tails have the ability to interact with the N-terminal domains of the near subunits, suggesting a mechanism of allosteric regulation dictated by intracellular signals [16]. The feature of ITPR of being prone to modulation by nearby signals gives an idea of the complexity of the ITPR-interactome. In other words, ITPRs have the structural complexity to participate in and regulate a dense network of cellular processes. ITPRs are differently expressed in human tissues, as reported in Table 1, obtained with data retrieved from the Human Protein Atlas [20]. The effects of ITPRs have been extensively studied in preclinical models [21–29]. Here, we offer an overview of the human pathologies where ITPR alterations have a clear causative role. Moreover, we summarize the information derived from innovative studies of the disease-genome profile association, which also suggests the potential, under-investigated role of ITPR in several human pathologies.

Table 1. Protein expression levels of IP3Rs in different human tissues and organs.

Tissue	IP3R1	IP3R2	IP3R3
Cerebral cortex	XX	XX	X
Cerebellum	XX	X	XXX
Hippocampus	XX		
Caudate	XX		
Thyroid gland		X	X
Parathyroid gland		XXX	
Adrenal gland		XX	X
Nasopharynx		X	XX
Bronchus		XX	XX
Lung	X	X	XX
Oral mucosa		X	XX
Salivary gland		XX	
Esophagus		X	XX
Stomach	X	XX	XX
Duodenum		XX	XX
Small intestine		XX	XXX
Colon		XX	XX
Rectum		XX	XX
Liver		XX	XX
Gallbladder		XX	X
Pancreas		XX	X
Kidney	X	XXX	X
Urinary bladder		X	XX
Testis	X	XX	XXX
Epididymis	X	XX	X
Seminal vesicle	X	X	X
Prostate	X		X
Vagina			XX
Ovary		X	
Fallopian tube		XX	X
Endometrium		XX	XXX
Cervix, uterine		X	XX
Placenta		X	X
Breast	X	XXX	XX
Heart	X	XX	
Smooth muscle		XX	
Skeletal muscle		XX	
Soft tissue			
Adipose tissue		XX	
Skin		XX	XX
Appendix		XX	XX
Spleen	X		
Lymph node	X		X
Tonsil	X	X	XXX
Bone marrow		X	

X: Low, XX: Medium, XXX: High protein expression level.

2. ITPRs and Neurological Disorders

The function of ITPR has been historically assessed in the neurological field. Indeed, the first identification of P400 protein occurred in Purkinje cells and the neurological signs were the first to be studied in mice [30]. The highest number of ITPR human mutations has been identified in neurological disorders, in particular affecting the isoform 1. Indeed, ITPR1 is the most abundant isoform in the brain, regulating important functions including memory and motor coordination [31].

2.1. Spinocerebellar Ataxia

Spinocerebellar ataxia (SCA) is a term referring to a group of hereditary ataxias characterized by degenerative alterations in the part of the brain related to the movement control (cerebellum) and sometimes in the spinal cord. Van de Leemput was the first to identify the deletion of a 5′ portion of ITPR1 in British and Australian families with type 15 SCA [32]. Thereafter, the deletion of exons 1-48 of ITPR1 was identified in other populations, demonstrating that the haploinsufficiency of ITPR1 is involved in SCA15-16 [33,34]. Missense mutations in the ITPR1 gene have been later associated with SCA15: P1059L and P1074L in a Japanese family, and V494I in an Australian family [35,36].

Another form of SCA, SCA29, characterized by an early-onset motor delay, hypotonia, and gait ataxia, is one of the forms more frequently associated with ITPR1 mutations [37]. The missense mutations V1553M and N602D, identified by Huang et al. [38], are among the first mutations observed; G2547A was identified as a de novo mutation but only in one case [39]. In a cohort study on a population of 21 patients with SCA29, Zambonin et al. identified six novel mutations in the ITPR1 gene [40]: Three mutations in the IP3 binding domain (R269G, K279E, K418ins), two mutations in the transmembrane domain (G2506R, I2550T), and one in the regulatory domain (T1386M); no specific genotype–phenotype correlations were observed, but the recurrence in affected subjects suggested the pathogenic role of these mutations.

SCA has been generally associated with a loss of function of ITPR1, however, Casey et al. recently identified a gain-of-function pathogenic mutation [41], detecting a R36C missense variant in three SCA29 affected members of the same family. The resultant ITPR1 mutant displayed a higher IP3 binding affinity than the wild type counterpart, converting the pattern of intracellular calcium release from transient to sigmoidal. This evidence supports the idea that the enhancement of calcium release can contribute to SCA29 pathogenesis. In addition to missense mutations of the ITPR1 gene, a splicing variant was also associated with SCA29: The c.1207-2A-T transition was identified in exon 14 of ITPR1 in four SCA29 patients and was not found in unaffected members of the same family [42].

Notably, all the mutations described above are autosomal dominant variants; however, a missense mutation in the ITPR1 gene was similarly associated with autosomal recessive SCA: In a family with congenital SCA history, the homozygous missense mutation L1787P was identified in all affected individuals, while the heterozygous carriers were asymptomatic [43]. The ability of this mutation to alter the receptor function is only predictive, but the concerned residue is highly conserved and the transition of leucine to proline can affect the protein stability with a high probability. Moreover, missense mutations (T267M, T594I, S277I, T267R) were observed in sporadic infantile-onset SCA [44,45], in congenital ataxias (R269W, R241K, A280D, E512K) [46], and in another subtype of ataxia, ataxic cerebral palsy (S1493D) [47]; other mutations have been reported [48–51] in molecularly unassigned SCA forms (V2541A, T2490M) and in rare forms of cerebellar hypoplasia (T2552P, I2550N).

Intriguingly, there are SCA variants not directly associated with ITPR1 gene mutations, but involving genes functionally close to ITPR1 and its signaling. A good example comes from SCA2 and SCA3, where the causative mutations are alterations in ataxin-2 and -3, respectively. In both cases, the mutant forms of ATXs are able to bind ITPR1 increasing the sensitivity of the channel for IP3 and enhancing channel gating [52,53]. Of interest, ITPR1-functional alterations by ATXs seem to have a pathogenic role, as they increase the apoptosis of Purkinje cells in animal models of ataxia [54]. This evidence supports the key role of calcium homeostasis regulation by ITPR1 in these neurological disorders even if the channel function is not directly altered.

2.2. Huntington's Disease and Alzheimer's Disease

To date, genetic mutations in the ITPR1 gene with a pathological relevance in human Huntington's Disease (HD) and Alzheimer's Disease (AD) have not been detected. However, both disorders are major examples of indirect involvement of ITPR1.

In HD, the causative mutation is the poliQ expansion of Huntingtin (Htt), although the cellular and molecular mechanisms of GABAergic neurons loss are not clearly understood [55]. Of note, the polyQ-Htt can bind ITPR1 with high affinity, sensitizing the receptor activity by IP3 [56,57]. Blocking the Htt–ITPR1 interaction in vivo was shown to regulate the abnormal calcium signaling in response to glutamate, protecting the neurons from death, and improving motor coordination [58], posing ITPR1 in a key position in HD pathophysiology and supporting the use of ITPR1-based therapies.

In AD, the pathogenic hypothesis of the beta-amyloid plaque has been extensively and historically investigated. However, in the last years, new and additional potential mechanisms have been suggested, including the dysregulation of calcium handling. In particular, ITPRs seem to have a key role in modulating calcium signals in AD [59]. Alterations in the ITPR function have been detected in cells derived from patients with AD already in 1994 [60,61]. Later, Ferreiro et al. demonstrated that antibody-aggregates are able to induce calcium release by ITPR in cortical neurons, leading to apoptosis, which was prevented by the ITPR inhibitor Xestopongin C [62].

2.3. Gillespie Syndrome

The Gillespie syndrome (GS) is a rare form of aniridia, cerebellar ataxia, and mental deficiency, described in 1965 by the American ophthalmologist Fredrick Gillespie [63]. Until 2016, its causative gene and mutations were unknown. Using a whole-exome sequencing approach, Gerber et al. identified several ITPR1 mutations in five GS-affected families [64]. In particular, the Authors detected truncating mutations in homozygous (Q1558*, R728*) or in composed heterozygous (G2102Valfs5/A2221Valfs23); the resultant truncated mutants were unable to generate a functional channel in a heterologous cell system. In the other two families, the Authors found one missense mutation (F2553L) and one deletion (K2563del) in the transmembrane domain. The latter, in addition to producing a dysfunctional channel, was able to exert a negative effect on the product derived from the wild type allele, with a dominant-negative action.

Later, next-generation sequencing approaches were used to study other GS families. The results evidenced novel missense mutations in the region of the calcium pore (N2543I), and in the regulatory domain (E2061G, E2061Q), further extending the ITPR1 mutations spectrum associated to GS [65,66].

2.4. Autism Spectrum Disorder

The Autism spectrum disorder (ASD) is a complex heterogeneous disorder with a poorly defined etiology and diagnosis criteria. Its high heritability, however, suggests a strong genetic component [67] and several genetic studies suggest that calcium homeostasis is a key determinant in its pathophysiology [68]. Recent studies demonstrate that IP_3-mediated calcium signals are significantly depressed in fibroblasts isolated from patients with ASD, identifying ITPR as a functional target in this disease [69]. These data are consistent with another study done in patients with autism in which a genetic variant of the oxytocin receptor (implicated in the etiology of ASD), causes a decline in the IP3/calcium signaling pathway in vitro [70].

2.5. Amyotrophic Lateral Sclerosis

Amyotrophic lateral sclerosis (ALS) is a condition characterized by a progressive degeneration of motor neurons in the brain and spinal cord. ITPR1 and ITPR2 are the main isoforms expressed in motor neurons [71]. ITPR2 mRNA levels are elevated in peripheral blood samples of patients with ALS [72] and studies done in human cells suggest that the pharmacological inhibition of ITPR1 is a potential strategy to prevent motor neuron deterioration in ALS [73].

3. ITPRs in Autoimmune Disorders

ITPRs are important for exocrine fluid secretion including saliva, pancreatic juice, and tear secretion [74]. Interestingly, anti-ITPR antibodies have been detected in sera from patients with Sjogren's syndrome (SS) [75], a chronic autoimmune disease involving lymphocytic infiltration and loss of secretory function in salivary and lacrimal glands [76]. A recent study demonstrates that the expression of ITPR2 and ITPR3 is significantly reduced in the salivary gland of SS patients, suggesting that deficits in ITPRs may underlie the secretory defect in SS [77].

Antibodies against ITPRs were also found in patients with rheumatoid arthritis and systemic lupus erythematosus, although the locations of the antigenic epitopes were different among the disease conditions [75].

4. ITPRs and Anhidrosis

Anhidrosis is the inability to sweat, which is responsible for heat tolerance; it is a rare disorder occurring even in the presence of morphologically normal eccrine glands, which are the main glands that respond to thermal stress with a high secretion rate. The whole-genome analysis of a family with anhidrosis and normal eccrine glands unveiled a novel missense mutation (G2498S) in ITPR type 2 [78]. This mutation occurs in the calcium pore-forming region. This association was corroborated by the observation of anhidrosis and hyperhidrosis in human pathologies linked to ITPR dysfunction; also, there was a marked reduction of sweat secretion in ITPR2$^{-/-}$ animals. Interestingly, ITPR2 inhibitors have the potential to reduce sweat production in hyperhidrosis, suggesting that ITPR2 is a potential pharmacological target in the treatment of sweat secretion conditions [78].

5. ITPRs and Cancer

Calcium has a key role in proliferation, differentiation, and migration; therefore, it is not surprising that ITPR, one of the main regulators of calcium handling, is involved in neoplastic transformation and progression [79]. Neck squamous cell carcinoma (HNSCC) was one of the first diseases connected to ITPR [80]; a whole-exome sequencing analysis of HNSCC patients revealed missense mutations affecting the ITPR3 gene, R64H, and R149L, both in the regulatory domain of the receptor [80]. Importantly, ITPR3 gene mutations were detectable only in metastatic or in recurrent tumors, but not in the respective primary tumors. This finding strongly suggests a role for ITPR3 in the metastatic process and malignant transformation, very significant if we take into account that the major problem related to HNSCC is given by recurrent metastases, which occur in more than half of the patients.

An increased expression of ITPR3 was detected in clear renal cell carcinoma compared to the unaffected part of the kidney [81]; ITPR3 silencing affected tumor growth, in vitro as well as in vivo, providing a direct proof of the involvement of this receptor in the carcinogenesis. An increased expression of ITPR3 has been also observed in cholangiocarcinoma [82] and in colorectal cancer [83]; in both cases the expression of ITPR3 correlated with the degree of neoplasia severity [82,83].

Alterations of ITPR1 and ITPR2 have been associated with the Sézary syndrome, a T-cell lymphoma with an aggressive clinical course. The analysis of gene mutations in 15 patients with the neoplastic syndrome unveiled somatic point mutations in ITPR1 including A95T in the regulatory domain and S2454F in the trans-membrane domain, and mutation in ITPR2, such as S2508L, in the trans-membrane domain [84]. These discoveries have important implications in considering ITPRs as new therapeutic targets in cancer.

6. Potential Role of ITPRs in Human Disease: Evidence from GWAS

While an evident role of ITPRs has been recognized for several human pathologies by identifying specific mutations, a potential role of this channel in other human conditions has been suggested by genome whole association studies (GWASs). Eleftherohorinou et al. have shown that a defective second messenger signaling could be involved in the predisposition to rheumatoid arthritis [85]. Specifically, alterations in ITPRs were proposed to be responsible for calcium signaling deregulations in this disease [85]. As revealed by another GWAS, the involvement of ITPR3 in the release of the macrophage migration inhibitory factor (MIF) confirmed the role of this receptor in rheumatoid arthritis [86]. In the same study, ITPR was also associated with type 1 diabetes mellitus [86], reflecting the similarity of genetic perturbations and the comparable immunological dysfunctions underlying these diseases, further corroborated by genetic analyses identifying ITPR3 as an independent risk locus in

Graves' disease [87] and allergic disorders including asthma, allergic rhinitis, atopic dermatitis [88,89], and airflow obstruction [90]. The involvement of ITPR3 in diabetes has been also confirmed by the significant recurrence of single nucleotides polymorphisms (SNPs) in the ITPR3 gene in diabetic American women [91], as well as in a Swedish nationwide study [92]. The latter study reported that a variation at rs2296336 (a SNP within ITPR3) might influence the risk of developing diabetes through an effect on alternative splicing. Moreover, rs3748079, a SNP located in the promoter region of ITPR3, has been associated with several autoimmune diseases including systemic lupus erythematosus, rheumatoid arthritis, and Graves' disease in a Japanese population [93], and the variant rs999943 of ITPR3 has been linked to obesity [94]. Equally important, ITPR1 has been associated in different GWASs with diabetic kidney disease [95] and obesity-related traits [96]. Of note, a recent GWAS in a Chinese population identified *ITPR2* as a susceptibility gene for the Kashin-Beck disease, a chronic osteochondropathy characterized by cartilage degeneration [97]; in this study, a significant association between the disease and nine SNPs of *ITPR2* was described. Interestingly, the regulatory role of ITPR2 in apoptosis is a possible contributor to the Kashin-Beck disease, since excessive chondrocyte apoptosis was found to be related to cartilage lesions in affected patients [98]. Moreover, a GWAS has revealed that the ITPR signaling pathway is genetically associated with epilepsy [99], and the anti-epileptic drug levetiracetum is known to act inhibiting the release of calcium by ITPRs, highlighting the relevance of enhanced ITPRs action in epilepsy [100].

Other association studies have underlined the role of ITPRs in the cardiovascular field. The association between gene expression and dilated cardiomyopathy (DCM) has been studied by assessing the presence of CpG sites in the proximity of gene-promoters, as an index of promoter methylation and consequent downregulation of transcription [101]; using this strategy, the CpG site "cg26395694" close to the ITPR1 locus (ENSG00000150995) has been shown to be significantly associated to DCM (p-value: 2.57E-02). More in general, ITPR3-mediated pathways have been also linked to ischemic heart disease [86] and coronary artery disease [102]. ITPR3 has been associated with the risk of developing coronary artery aneurism in Taiwanese children with Kawasaki disease [103], a multisystemic vasculitis that can result in coronary artery lesions and that had been linked to aberrant calcium signaling [104]. In a case-control study involving 93 Kawasaki disease patients and 680 healthy controls, the frequency of the rs2229634 T/T genotype was significantly higher in Kawasaki disease patients with coronary artery aneurism than in patients without coronary artery aneurism [103]. The key importance of ITPRs in cardiovascular medicine is confirmed by the crucial role of ITPRs in cardiogenesis [105–107]; ergo, it may be difficult to detect mutations causing severe heart defects by using genetic analyses of patient samples postnatally, especially if considering that ITPRs have been shown to be essential in very early embryogenesis and some mutations might cause lethality in utero [108,109].

An international GWAS identified ITPR1 between the novel loci associated with blood pressure in children and adolescents [110]. Finally, in the Hispanic population, ITPR1 was associated to the pathophysiology of childhood obesity [96], while ITPR3 was linked to body mass index variants conferring a high risk of extreme obesity [94].

The GWAS demonstrated an association of ITPR1–2 with different forms of cancer, especially breast cancer [111–113]. Other studies associated the expression level of ITPR3 with the aggressiveness of different types of tumors, including colorectal carcinoma, gastric cancers [114], and head and neck squamous cell carcinoma [80]. *ITPR3* variants were also found to be implied in cervical squamous cell carcinoma [115]. Interestingly, ITPR3 appears also to actively participate in cell death in several tissues and its increased activity was demonstrated to induce apoptosis in T lymphocytes [116,117]. These findings indicate that compounds aimed at controlling the ITPR activity may be useful as a therapeutic approach for modulating immune responses in cancer.

7. Conclusions

In this systematic review, we illustrated the association of ITPRs mutations with human disorders. The mutations of ITPRs reported in humans are summarized in Table 2 and represented in Figure 1. Throughout the analysis of current literature, the involvement of ITPRs in human disease appears to be under-investigated.

Table 2. Spectrum of IP3Rs mutations identified in humans.

Mutation	IP3R Isoform	Effect on Protein	Disease	Reference
5′ deletion	IP3R1	Downregulation	SCA15	[32]
1-48 exons deletion	IP3R1	Downregulation	SCA15-16	[33,34]
P1059L	IP3R1	Missense (ND)	SCA15	[35]
P1074L	IP3R1	Missense (ND)	SCA15	[35]
V494I	IP3R1	Missense (ND)	SCA15	[36]
V1553M	IP3R1	Missense (ND)	SCA29	[38]
N602D	IP3R1	Missense (ND)	SCA29	[38]
G2547A	IP3R1	Missense (ND)	SCA29	[39]
R269G	IP3R1	Missense (ND)	SCA29	[40]
K279E	IP3R1	Missense (ND)	SCA29	[40]
G2506R	IP3R1	Missense (ND)	SCA29	[40]
I2550T	IP3R1	Missense (ND)	SCA29	[40]
T1386M	IP3R1	Missense (ND)	SCA29	[40]
R36C	IP3R1	Gain-of-function Increase of IP3 binding affinity	SCA29	[41]
c.1207-2A-T	IP3R1	Splicing variant	SCA29	[42]
L1787P	IP3R1	Protein-instability*	Autosomal-recessive SCA	[43]
T267M	IP3R1	Missense (ND)	Sporadic infantile-onset-SCA	[44,45]
T594I	IP3R1	Missense (ND)	Sporadic infantile-onset-SCA	[44,45]
S277I	IP3R1	Missense (ND)	Sporadic infantile-onset-SCA	[44,45]
T267R	IP3R1	Missense (ND)	Sporadic infantile-onset-SCA	[44,45]
R269W	IP3R1	Missense (ND)	Congenital-ataxias	[46]
R241K	IP3R1	Missense (ND)	Congenital-ataxias	[46]
A280D	IP3R1	Missense (ND)	Congenital-ataxias	[46]
E512K	IP3R1	Missense (ND)	Congenital-ataxias	[46]
S1493D	IP3R1	Missense (ND)	Ataxic-cerebral-palsy	[47]
V2541A	IP3R1	Missense (ND)	Molecular-unassigned SCA	[48]
T2490M	IP3R1	Missense (ND)	Molecular-unassigned SCA	[48]
T2552P	IP3R1	Missense (ND)	Cerebellar-hypoplasia	[50]
I2550N	IP3R1	Missense (ND)	Cerebellar-hypoplasia	[51]
Q1558	IP3R1	Truncating-protein, no functional channel	Gillespie syndrome	[64]
R728	IP3R1	Truncating-protein, no functional channel	Gillespie syndrome	[64]
F2553L	IP3R1	Missense (ND)	Gillespie syndrome	[64]
K2563 deletion	IP3R1	Dysfunctional channel with dominant negative action	Gillespie syndrome	[64]
N2543I	IP3R1	Missense (ND)	Gillespie syndrome	[65]
E2061G	IP3R1	Missense (ND)	Gillespie syndrome	[66]
E2061Q	IP3R1	Missense (ND)	Gillespie syndrome	[66]
A95T	IP3R1	Missense (ND)	Sézary syndrome	[84]
S2454F	IP3R1	Missense (ND)	Sézary syndrome	[84]
S2508L	IP3R1	Missense (ND)	Sézary syndrome	[84]
G2498S	IP3R2	Missense: dysfunctional channel *	Anhidrosis	[78]
R64H	IP3R3	Missense (ND)	HNSCC	[80]
R149L	IP3R3	Missense (ND)	HNSCC	[80]

HNSCC: Head and neck squamous cell carcinoma; ND: Not determined; SCA: Spinocerebellar ataxia; * predicted effect on protein.

The currently known contribution of the receptor to the pathogenesis of human disease is only the top of the iceberg. The information about causative genetic alterations affecting ITPRs mainly come from the neurology-related fields, cancer fields, or rare disease field, where the genetic analysis is a more common approach included in diagnostic procedures. However, in several studies of large-scale genome analysis, ITPRs recurrently emerge as a susceptibility gene for several pathological conditions. This evidence confirms that only little is known about this channel, particularly in cardiac and vascular homeostasis or metabolism. The recent findings of the physical link between ER and mitochondria, mediated by a protein complex including ITPR, suggest a potential role of the receptor in the regulation of calcium-dependent mitochondrial metabolism [118–130]. The ability of ITPR to indirectly regulate mitochondrial energetic metabolism could have a significant impact on the health and homeostasis of the tissues strongly dependent on mitochondrial energetic production, such as cardiac and skeletal muscle. However, this aspect needs to be further explored.

The underestimated pathophysiological role of ITPR might also depend on the fact that the cellular context strongly affects the impact of ITPR alterations on calcium handling and the relative cell fate. A good example comes from a study in neuronal cells about the P1059L affecting the regulatory domain of ITPR1; this mutation increases the affinity of ITPR1 to IP3, altering the functional output of Purkinje cells, however, no differences were detected in calcium signaling between the wild type and the same mutant in B-cells [131]. The regulatory domain of ITPR is the target of several molecular partners whose expression and activity profile are different among the different cellular contexts. Therefore, the regulation around the P1059 residue of ITPR could be different—and/or of different impact—in Purkinje cells compared to other cells, such as B-cells. Nevertheless, the experiments performed in stable cell lines can alter the impact of ITPR alterations, as several adaptive pathways could affect the expression of ITPR regulatory proteins minimizing the effects of mutations. These observations encourage future studies on ITPR in the appropriate native cellular context, both in physiological and pathological conditions.

Author Contributions: Conceptualization, G.S.; data curation, M.B.M. and J.F.; writing—original draft preparation, J.G., A.L. and M.B.M.; writing—review and editing, J.F. and G.S. All authors have read and agreed to the published version of the manuscript.

Funding: The Santulli's lab is supported in part by the NIH (R01-HL146691, R01-DK123259, R01-DK033823, P30-DK020541, and R00-DK107895, to G.S.) and by the American Heart Association (AHA-20POST35211151 to J.G.).

Conflicts of Interest: The authors declare no conflict of interest.

References

1. Mikoshiba, K.; Changeux, J.P. Morphological and biochemical studies on isolated molecular and granular layers from bovine cerebellum. *Brain Res.* **1978**, *142*, 487–504. [CrossRef]
2. Mikoshiba, K.; Huchet, M.; Changeux, J.P. Biochemical and immunological studies on the P400 protein, a protein characteristic of the Purkinje cell from mouse and rat cerebellum. *Dev. Neurosci.* **1979**, *2*, 254–275. [CrossRef] [PubMed]
3. Crepel, F.; Dupont, J.L.; Gardette, R. Selective absence of calcium spikes in Purkinje cells of staggerer mutant mice in cerebellar slices maintained in vitro. *J. Physiol.* **1984**, *346*, 111–125. [CrossRef] [PubMed]
4. Maeda, N.; Niinobe, M.; Nakahira, K.; Mikoshiba, K. Purification and characterization of P400 protein, a glycoprotein characteristic of Purkinje cell, from mouse cerebellum. *J. Neurochem.* **1988**, *51*, 1724–1730. [CrossRef]
5. Furuichi, T.; Yoshikawa, S.; Miyawaki, A.; Wada, K.; Maeda, N.; Mikoshiba, K. Primary structure and functional expression of the inositol 1,4,5-trisphosphate-binding protein P400. *Nature* **1989**, *342*, 32–38. [CrossRef]
6. Furuichi, T.; Yoshikawa, S.; Mikoshiba, K. Nucleotide sequence of cDNA encoding P400 protein in the mouse cerebellum. *Nucleic Acids Res.* **1989**, *17*, 5385–5386. [CrossRef]
7. Iino, M. Biphasic Ca2+ dependence of inositol 1,4,5-trisphosphate-induced Ca release in smooth muscle cells of the guinea pig taenia caeci. *J. Gen. Physiol* **1990**, *95*, 1103–1122. [CrossRef]
8. Finch, E.A.; Turner, T.J.; Goldin, S.M. Calcium as a coagonist of inositol 1,4,5-trisphosphate-induced calcium release. *Science* **1991**, *252*, 443–446. [CrossRef]
9. Santulli, G.; Nakashima, R.; Yuan, Q.; Marks, A.R. Intracellular calcium release channels: An update. *J. Physiol.* **2017**, *595*, 3041–3051. [CrossRef]
10. Paknejad, N.; Hite, R.K. Structural basis for the regulation of inositol trisphosphate receptors by Ca(2+) and IP3. *Nat. Struct. Mol. Biol.* **2018**, *25*, 660–668. [CrossRef]
11. Belkacemi, A.; Hui, X.; Wardas, B.; Laschke, M.W.; Wissenbach, U.; Menger, M.D.; Lipp, P.; Beck, A.; Flockerzi, V. IP3 Receptor-Dependent Cytoplasmic Ca(2+) Signals Are Tightly Controlled by Cavbeta3. *Cell Rep.* **2018**, *22*, 1339–1349. [CrossRef] [PubMed]

12. Rong, Y.P.; Bultynck, G.; Aromolaran, A.S.; Zhong, F.; Parys, J.B.; De Smedt, H.; Mignery, G.A.; Roderick, HL.; Bootman, M.D.; Distelhorst, C.W. The BH4 domain of Bcl-2 inhibits ER calcium release and apoptosis by binding the regulatory and coupling domain of the IP3 receptor. *Proc. Natl. Acad. Sci. USA* **2009**, *106*, 14397–14402. [CrossRef] [PubMed]
13. Prole, D.L.; Taylor, C.W. Structure and Function of IP3 Receptors. *Cold Spring Harb Perspect Biol* **2019**, *11*. [CrossRef] [PubMed]
14. Lin, C.C.; Baek, K.; Lu, Z. Apo and InsP(3)-bound crystal structures of the ligand-binding domain of an InsP(3) receptor. *Nat. Struct Mol. Biol.* **2011**, *18*, 1172–1174. [CrossRef] [PubMed]
15. Seo, M.D.; Velamakanni, S.; Ishiyama, N.; Stathopulos, P.B.; Rossi, A.M.; Khan, S.A.; Dale, P.; Li, C.; Ames, J.B.; Ikura, M.; et al. Structural and functional conservation of key domains in InsP3 and ryanodine receptors. *Nature* **2012**, *483*, 108–112. [CrossRef]
16. Fan, G.; Baker, M.L.; Wang, Z.; Baker, M.R.; Sinyagovskiy, P.A.; Chiu, W.; Ludtke, S.J.; Serysheva, I.I. Gating machinery of InsP3R channels revealed by electron cryomicroscopy. *Nature* **2015**, *527*, 336–341. [CrossRef]
17. Chandran, A.; Chee, X.; Prole, D.L.; Rahman, T. Exploration of inositol 1,4,5-trisphosphate (IP3) regulated dynamics of N-terminal domain of IP3 receptor reveals early phase molecular events during receptor activation. *Sci. Rep.* **2019**, *9*, 2454. [CrossRef]
18. Hamada, K.; Miyatake, H.; Terauchi, A.; Mikoshiba, K. IP3-mediated gating mechanism of the IP3 receptor revealed by mutagenesis and X-ray crystallography. *Proc. Natl. Acad. Sci. USA* **2017**, *114*, 4661–4666. [CrossRef]
19. Lock, J.T.; Alzayady, K.J.; Yule, D.I.; Parker, I. All three IP3 receptor isoforms generate Ca(2+) puffs that display similar characteristics. *Sci. Signal.* **2018**, *11*, eaau0344. [CrossRef]
20. Thul, P.J.; Akesson, L.; Wiking, M.; Mahdessian, D.; Geladaki, A.; Ait Blal, H.; Alm, T.; Asplund, A.; Bjork, L.; Breckels, L.M.; et al. A subcellular map of the human proteome. *Science* **2017**, *356*, eaal3321. [CrossRef]
21. Chan, C.; Ooashi, N.; Akiyama, H.; Fukuda, T.; Inoue, M.; Matsu-Ura, T.; Shimogori, T.; Mikoshiba, K.; Kamiguchi, H. Inositol 1,4,5-Trisphosphate Receptor Type 3 Regulates Neuronal Growth Cone Sensitivity to Guidance Signals. *iScience* **2020**, *23*, 100963. [CrossRef] [PubMed]
22. Yuan, Q.; Yang, J.; Santulli, G.; Reiken, S.R.; Wronska, A.; Kim, M.M.; Osborne, B.W.; Lacampagne, A.; Yin, Y.; Marks, A.R. Maintenance of normal blood pressure is dependent on IP3R1-mediated regulation of eNOS. *Proc. Natl. Acad. Sci. USA* **2016**, *113*, 8532–8537. [CrossRef] [PubMed]
23. Perry, R.J.; Zhang, D.; Guerra, M.T.; Brill, A.L.; Goedeke, L.; Nasiri, A.R.; Rabin-Court, A.; Wang, Y.; Peng, L.; Dufour, S.; et al. Glucagon stimulates gluconeogenesis by INSP3R1-mediated hepatic lipolysis. *Nature* **2020**, *579*, 279–283. [CrossRef] [PubMed]
24. Santulli, G.; Xie, W.; Reiken, S.R.; Marks, A.R. Mitochondrial calcium overload is a key determinant in heart failure. *Proc. Natl. Acad. Sci. USA* **2015**, *112*, 11389–11394. [CrossRef]
25. Wang, Y.; Li, G.; Goode, J.; Paz, J.C.; Ouyang, K.; Screaton, R.; Fischer, W.H.; Chen, J.; Tabas, I.; Montminy, M. Inositol-1,4,5-trisphosphate receptor regulates hepatic gluconeogenesis in fasting and diabetes. *Nature* **2012**, *485*, 128–132. [CrossRef]
26. Kuchay, S.; Giorgi, C.; Simoneschi, D.; Pagan, J.; Missiroli, S.; Saraf, A.; Florens, L.; Washburn, M.P.; Collazo-Lorduy, A.; Castillo-Martin, M.; et al. PTEN counteracts FBXL2 to promote IP3R3- and Ca(2+)-mediated apoptosis limiting tumour growth. *Nature* **2017**, *546*, 554–558. [CrossRef]
27. Cheung, K.H.; Mei, L.; Mak, D.O.; Hayashi, I.; Iwatsubo, T.; Kang, D.E.; Foskett, J.K. Gain-of-function enhancement of IP3 receptor modal gating by familial Alzheimer's disease-linked presenilin mutants in human cells and mouse neurons. *Sci. Signal.* **2010**, *3*, ra22. [CrossRef]
28. Gambardella, J.; Trimarco, B.; Iaccarino, G.; Santulli, G. New Insights in Cardiac Calcium Handling and Excitation-Contraction Coupling. *Adv. Exp. Med. Biol* **2018**, *1067*, 373–385.
29. Huang, W.; Cane, M.C.; Mukherjee, R.; Szatmary, P.; Zhang, X.; Elliott, V.; Ouyang, Y.; Chvanov, M.; Latawiec, D.; Wen, L.; et al. Caffeine protects against experimental acute pancreatitis by inhibition of inositol 1,4,5-trisphosphate receptor-mediated Ca2+ release. *Gut* **2017**, *66*, 301–313. [CrossRef]
30. Maeda, N.; Niinobe, M.; Mikoshiba, K. A cerebellar Purkinje cell marker P400 protein is an inositol 1,4,5-trisphosphate (InsP3) receptor protein. Purification and characterization of InsP3 receptor complex. *EMBO J.* **1990**, *9*, 61–67. [CrossRef]

31. Hisatsune, C.; Mikoshiba, K. IP3 receptor mutations and brain diseases in human and rodents. *J. Neurochem.* **2017**, *141*, 790–807. [CrossRef] [PubMed]
32. van de Leemput, J.; Chandran, J.; Knight, M.A.; Holtzclaw, L.A.; Scholz, S.; Cookson, M.R.; Houlden, H.; Gwinn-Hardy, K.; Fung, H.C.; Lin, X.; et al. Deletion at ITPR1 underlies ataxia in mice and spinocerebellar ataxia 15 in humans. *PLoS Genet.* **2007**, *3*, e108. [CrossRef] [PubMed]
33. Marelli, C.; van de Leemput, J.; Johnson, J.O.; Tison, F.; Thauvin-Robinet, C.; Picard, F.; Tranchant, C.; Hernandez, D.G.; Huttin, B.; Boulliat, J.; et al. SCA15 due to large ITPR1 deletions in a cohort of 333 white families with dominant ataxia. *Arch. Neurol.* **2011**, *68*, 637–643. [CrossRef] [PubMed]
34. Novak, M.J.; Sweeney, M.G.; Li, A.; Treacy, C.; Chandrashekar, H.S.; Giunti, P.; Goold, R.G.; Davis, M.B.; Houlden, H.; Tabrizi, S.J. An ITPR1 gene deletion causes spinocerebellar ataxia 15/16: A genetic, clinical and radiological description. *Mov. Disord.* **2010**, *25*, 2176–2182. [CrossRef]
35. Hara, K.; Shiga, A.; Nozaki, H.; Mitsui, J.; Takahashi, Y.; Ishiguro, H.; Yomono, H.; Kurisaki, H.; Goto, J.; Ikeuchi, T.; et al. Total deletion and a missense mutation of ITPR1 in Japanese SCA15 families. *Neurology* **2008**, *71*, 547–551. [CrossRef]
36. Ganesamoorthy, D.; Bruno, D.L.; Schoumans, J.; Storey, E.; Delatycki, M.B.; Zhu, D.; Wei, M.K.; Nicholson, G.A.; McKinlay Gardner, R.J.; Slater, H.R. Development of a multiplex ligation-dependent probe amplification assay for diagnosis and estimation of the frequency of spinocerebellar ataxia type 15. *Clin. Chem.* **2009**, *55*, 1415–1418. [CrossRef]
37. Ando, H.; Hirose, M.; Mikoshiba, K. Aberrant IP3 receptor activities revealed by comprehensive analysis of pathological mutations causing spinocerebellar ataxia 29. *Proc. Natl. Acad. Sci. USA* **2018**, *115*, 12259–12264. [CrossRef]
38. Huang, L.; Chardon, J.W.; Carter, M.T.; Friend, K.L.; Dudding, T.E.; Schwartzentruber, J.; Zou, R.; Schofield, P.W.; Douglas, S.; Bulman, D.E.; et al. Missense mutations in ITPR1 cause autosomal dominant congenital nonprogressive spinocerebellar ataxia. *Orphanet. J. Rare Dis.* **2012**, *7*, 67. [CrossRef]
39. Gonzaga-Jauregui, C.; Harel, T.; Gambin, T.; Kousi, M.; Griffin, L.B.; Francescatto, L.; Ozes, B.; Karaca, E.; Jhangiani, S.N.; Bainbridge, M.N.; et al. Exome Sequence Analysis Suggests that Genetic Burden Contributes to Phenotypic Variability and Complex Neuropathy. *Cell Rep.* **2015**, *12*, 1169–1183. [CrossRef]
40. Zambonin, J.L.; Bellomo, A.; Ben-Pazi, H.; Everman, D.B.; Frazer, L.M.; Geraghty, M.T.; Harper, A.D.; Jones, J.R.; Kamien, B.; Kernohan, K.; et al. Spinocerebellar ataxia type 29 due to mutations in ITPR1: A case series and review of this emerging congenital ataxia. *Orphanet J. Rare. Dis.* **2017**, *12*, 121. [CrossRef]
41. Casey, J.P.; Hirouchi, T.; Hisatsune, C.; Lynch, B.; Murphy, R.; Dunne, A.M.; Miyamoto, A.; Ennis, S.; van der Spek, N.; O'Hici, B.; et al. A novel gain-of-function mutation in the ITPR1 suppressor domain causes spinocerebellar ataxia with altered Ca(2+) signal patterns. *J. Neurol.* **2017**, *264*, 1444–1453. [CrossRef] [PubMed]
42. Wang, L.; Hao, Y.; Yu, P.; Cao, Z.; Zhang, J.; Zhang, X.; Chen, Y.; Zhang, H.; Gu, W. Identification of a Splicing Mutation in ITPR1 via WES in a Chinese Early-Onset Spinocerebellar Ataxia Family. *Cerebellum* **2018**, *17*, 294–299. [CrossRef] [PubMed]
43. Klar, J.; Ali, Z.; Farooq, M.; Khan, K.; Wikstrom, J.; Iqbal, M.; Zulfiqar, S.; Faryal, S.; Baig, S.M.; Dahl, N. A missense variant in ITPR1 provides evidence for autosomal recessive SCA29 with asymptomatic cerebellar hypoplasia in carriers. *Eur J. Hum. Genet.* **2017**, *25*, 848–853. [CrossRef] [PubMed]
44. Sasaki, M.; Ohba, C.; Iai, M.; Hirabayashi, S.; Osaka, H.; Hiraide, T.; Saitsu, H.; Matsumoto, N. Sporadic infantile-onset spinocerebellar ataxia caused by missense mutations of the inositol 1,4,5-triphosphate receptor type 1 gene. *J. Neurol* **2015**, *262*, 1278–1284. [CrossRef]
45. Fogel, B.L.; Lee, H.; Deignan, J.L.; Strom, S.P.; Kantarci, S.; Wang, X.; Quintero-Rivera, F.; Vilain, E.; Grody, W.W.; Perlman, S.; et al. Exome sequencing in the clinical diagnosis of sporadic or familial cerebellar ataxia. *JAMA Neurol.* **2014**, *71*, 1237–1246. [CrossRef] [PubMed]
46. Barresi, S.; Niceta, M.; Alfieri, P.; Brankovic, V.; Piccini, G.; Bruselles, A.; Barone, M.R.; Cusmai, R.; Tartaglia, M.; Bertini, E.; et al. Mutations in the IRBIT domain of ITPR1 are a frequent cause of autosomal dominant nonprogressive congenital ataxia. *Clin. Genet.* **2017**, *91*, 86–91. [CrossRef]
47. Parolin Schnekenberg, R.; Perkins, E.M.; Miller, J.W.; Davies, W.I.; D'Adamo, M.C.; Pessia, M.; Fawcett, K.A.; Sims, D.; Gillard, E.; Hudspith, K.; et al. De novo point mutations in patients diagnosed with ataxic cerebral palsy. *Brain* **2015**, *138*, 1817–1832. [CrossRef]

48. Valencia, C.A.; Husami, A.; Holle, J.; Johnson, J.A.; Qian, Y.; Mathur, A.; Wei, C.; Indugula, S.R.; Zou, F.; Meng, H.; et al. Clinical Impact and Cost-Effectiveness of Whole Exome Sequencing as a Diagnostic Tool: A Pediatric Center's Experience. *Front. Pediatr.* **2015**, *3*, 67. [CrossRef]
49. Hsiao, C.T.; Liu, Y.T.; Liao, Y.C.; Hsu, T.Y.; Lee, Y.C.; Soong, B.W. Mutational analysis of ITPR1 in a Taiwanese cohort with cerebellar ataxias. *PLoS ONE* **2017**, *12*, e0187503. [CrossRef]
50. Hayashi, S.; Uehara, D.T.; Tanimoto, K.; Mizuno, S.; Chinen, Y.; Fukumura, S.; Takanashi, J.I.; Osaka, H.; Okamoto, N.; Inazawa, J. Comprehensive investigation of CASK mutations and other genetic etiologies in 41 patients with intellectual disability and microcephaly with pontine and cerebellar hypoplasia (MICPCH). *PLoS ONE* **2017**, *12*, e0181791. [CrossRef]
51. van Dijk, T.; Barth, P.; Reneman, L.; Appelhof, B.; Baas, F.; Poll-The, B.T. A de novo missense mutation in the inositol 1,4,5-triphosphate receptor type 1 gene causing severe pontine and cerebellar hypoplasia: Expanding the phenotype of ITPR1-related spinocerebellar ataxia's. *Am. J. Med. Genet. A* **2017**, *173*, 207–212. [CrossRef] [PubMed]
52. Chen, X.; Tang, T.S.; Tu, H.; Nelson, O.; Pook, M.; Hammer, R.; Nukina, N.; Bezprozvanny, I. Deranged calcium signaling and neurodegeneration in spinocerebellar ataxia type 3. *J. Neurosci.* **2008**, *28*, 12713–12724. [CrossRef] [PubMed]
53. Liu, J.; Tang, T.S.; Tu, H.; Nelson, O.; Herndon, E.; Huynh, D.P.; Pulst, S.M.; Bezprozvanny, I. Deranged calcium signaling and neurodegeneration in spinocerebellar ataxia type 2. *J. Neurosci.* **2009**, *29*, 9148–9162. [CrossRef] [PubMed]
54. Kasumu, A.W.; Hougaard, C.; Rode, F.; Jacobsen, T.A.; Sabatier, J.M.; Eriksen, B.L.; Strobaek, D.; Liang, X.; Egorova, P.; Vorontsova, D.; et al. Selective positive modulator of calcium-activated potassium channels exerts beneficial effects in a mouse model of spinocerebellar ataxia type 2. *Chem. Biol.* **2012**, *19*, 1340–1353. [CrossRef]
55. Vonsattel, J.P.; Myers, R.H.; Stevens, T.J.; Ferrante, R.J.; Bird, E.D.; Richardson, E.P. Jr. Neuropathological classification of Huntington's disease. *J. Neuropathol. Exp. Neurol.* **1985**, *44*, 559–577. [CrossRef]
56. Tang, T.S.; Tu, H.; Chan, E.Y.; Maximov, A.; Wang, Z.; Wellington, C.L.; Hayden, M.R.; Bezprozvanny, I. Huntingtin and huntingtin-associated protein 1 influence neuronal calcium signaling mediated by inositol-(1,4,5) triphosphate receptor type 1. *Neuron* **2003**, *39*, 227–239. [CrossRef]
57. Tang, T.S.; Tu, H.; Orban, P.C.; Chan, E.Y.; Hayden, M.R.; Bezprozvanny, I. HAP1 facilitates effects of mutant huntingtin on inositol 1,4,5-trisphosphate-induced Ca release in primary culture of striatal medium spiny neurons. *Eur. J. Neurosci.* **2004**, *20*, 1779–1787. [CrossRef]
58. Tang, T.S.; Guo, C.; Wang, H.; Chen, X.; Bezprozvanny, I. Neuroprotective effects of inositol 1,4,5-trisphosphate receptor C-terminal fragment in a Huntington's disease mouse model. *J. Neurosci.* **2009**, *29*, 1257–1266. [CrossRef]
59. Green, K.N.; Demuro, A.; Akbari, Y.; Hitt, B.D.; Smith, I.F.; Parker, I.; LaFerla, F.M. SERCA pump activity is physiologically regulated by presenilin and regulates amyloid beta production. *J. Cell Biol.* **2008**, *181*, 1107–1116. [CrossRef]
60. Ito, E.; Oka, K.; Etcheberrigaray, R.; Nelson, T.J.; McPhie, D.L.; Tofel-Grehl, B.; Gibson, G.E.; Alkon, D.L. Internal Ca2+ mobilization is altered in fibroblasts from patients with Alzheimer disease. *Proc. Natl. Acad. Sci. USA* **1994**, *91*, 534–538. [CrossRef]
61. Hirashima, N.; Etcheberrigaray, R.; Bergamaschi, S.; Racchi, M.; Battaini, F.; Binetti, G.; Govoni, S.; Alkon, D.L. Calcium responses in human fibroblasts: A diagnostic molecular profile for Alzheimer's disease. *Neurobiol. Aging* **1996**, *17*, 549–555. [CrossRef]
62. Ferreiro, E.; Oliveira, C.R.; Pereira, C. Involvement of endoplasmic reticulum Ca2+ release through ryanodine and inositol 1,4,5-triphosphate receptors in the neurotoxic effects induced by the amyloid-beta peptide. *J. Neurosci. Res.* **2004**, *76*, 872–880. [CrossRef] [PubMed]
63. Gillespie, F.D. Aniridia, Cerebellar Ataxia, and Oligophrenia in Siblings. *Arch. Ophthalmol.* **1965**, *73*, 338–341. [CrossRef] [PubMed]
64. Gerber, S.; Alzayady, K.J.; Burglen, L.; Bremond-Gignac, D.; Marchesin, V.; Roche, O.; Rio, M.; Funalot, B.; Calmon, R.; Durr, A.; et al. Recessive and Dominant De Novo ITPR1 Mutations Cause Gillespie Syndrome. *Am. J. Hum. Genet.* **2016**, *98*, 971–980. [CrossRef]

65. Dentici, M.L.; Barresi, S.; Nardella, M.; Bellacchio, E.; Alfieri, P.; Bruselles, A.; Pantaleoni, F.; Danieli, A.; Iarossi, G.; Cappa, M.; et al. Identification of novel and hotspot mutations in the channel domain of ITPR1 in two patients with Gillespie syndrome. *Gene* **2017**, *628*, 141–145. [CrossRef]
66. McEntagart, M.; Williamson, K.A.; Rainger, J.K.; Wheeler, A.; Seawright, A.; De Baere, E.; Verdin, H.; Bergendahl, L.T.; Quigley, A.; Rainger, J.; et al. A Restricted Repertoire of De Novo Mutations in ITPR1 Cause Gillespie Syndrome with Evidence for Dominant-Negative Effect. *Am. J. Hum. Genet.* **2016**, *98*, 981–992. [CrossRef]
67. Schmunk, G.; Gargus, J.J. Channelopathy pathogenesis in autism spectrum disorders. *Front. Genet.* **2013**, *4*, 222. [CrossRef]
68. Cross-Disorder Group of the Psychiatric Genomics, C. Identification of risk loci with shared effects on five major psychiatric disorders: A genome-wide analysis. *Lancet* **2013**, *381*, 1371–1379.
69. Schmunk, G.; Boubion, B.J.; Smith, I.F.; Parker, I.; Gargus, J.J. Shared functional defect in IP(3)R-mediated calcium signaling in diverse monogenic autism syndromes. *Transl. Psychiatry* **2015**, *5*, e643. [CrossRef]
70. Ma, W.J.; Hashii, M.; Munesue, T.; Hayashi, K.; Yagi, K.; Yamagishi, M.; Higashida, H.; Yokoyama, S. Non-synonymous single-nucleotide variations of the human oxytocin receptor gene and autism spectrum disorders: A case-control study in a Japanese population and functional analysis. *Mol. Autism* **2013**, *4*, 22. [CrossRef]
71. Van Den Bosch, L.; Verhoeven, K.; De Smedt, H.; Wuytack, F.; Missiaen, L.; Robberecht, W. Calcium handling proteins in isolated spinal motoneurons. *Life Sci.* **1999**, *65*, 1597–1606. [CrossRef]
72. van Es, M.A.; Van Vught, P.W.; Blauw, H.M.; Franke, L.; Saris, C.G.; Andersen, P.M.; Van Den Bosch, L.; de Jong, S.W.; van 't Slot, R.; Birve, A.; et al. ITPR2 as a susceptibility gene in sporadic amyotrophic lateral sclerosis: A genome-wide association study. *Lancet Neurol.* **2007**, *6*, 869–877. [CrossRef]
73. Kim, S.H.; Zhan, L.; Hanson, K.A.; Tibbetts, R.S. High-content RNAi screening identifies the Type 1 inositol triphosphate receptor as a modifier of TDP-43 localization and neurotoxicity. *Hum. Mol. Genet.* **2012**, *21*, 4845–4856. [CrossRef] [PubMed]
74. Futatsugi, A.; Nakamura, T.; Yamada, M.K.; Ebisui, E.; Nakamura, K.; Uchida, K.; Kitaguchi, T.; Takahashi-Iwanaga, H.; Noda, T.; Aruga, J.; et al. IP3 receptor types 2 and 3 mediate exocrine secretion underlying energy metabolism. *Science* **2005**, *309*, 2232–2234. [CrossRef]
75. Miyachi, K.; Iwai, M.; Asada, K.; Saito, I.; Hankins, R.; Mikoshiba, K. Inositol 1,4,5-trisphosphate receptors are autoantibody target antigens in patients with Sjogren's syndrome and other systemic rheumatic diseases. *Mod. Rheumatol.* **2007**, *17*, 137–143. [CrossRef]
76. Vivino, F.B. Sjogren's syndrome: Clinical aspects. *Clin. Immunol.* **2017**, *182*, 48–54. [CrossRef]
77. Teos, L.Y.; Zhang, Y.; Cotrim, A.P.; Swaim, W.; Won, J.H.; Ambrus, J.; Shen, L.; Bebris, L.; Grisius, M.; Jang, S.I.; et al. IP3R deficit underlies loss of salivary fluid secretion in Sjogren's Syndrome. *Sci. Rep.* **2015**, *5*, 13953. [CrossRef]
78. Klar, J.; Hisatsune, C.; Baig, S.M.; Tariq, M.; Johansson, A.C.; Rasool, M.; Malik, N.A.; Ameur, A.; Sugiura, K.; Feuk, L.; et al. Abolished InsP3R2 function inhibits sweat secretion in both humans and mice. *J. Clin. Invest.* **2014**, *124*, 4773–4780. [CrossRef]
79. Sneyers, F.; Rosa, N.; Bultynck, G. Type 3 IP3 receptors driving oncogenesis. *Cell Calcium* **2020**, *86*, 102141. [CrossRef]
80. Hedberg, M.L.; Goh, G.; Chiosea, S.I.; Bauman, J.E.; Freilino, M.L.; Zeng, Y.; Wang, L.; Diergaarde, B.B.; Gooding, W.E.; Lui, V.W.; et al. Genetic landscape of metastatic and recurrent head and neck squamous cell carcinoma. *J. Clin. Invest.* **2016**, *126*, 169–180. [CrossRef]
81. Rezuchova, I.; Hudecova, S.; Soltysova, A.; Matuskova, M.; Durinikova, E.; Chovancova, B.; Zuzcak, M.; Cihova, M.; Burikova, M.; Penesova, A.; et al. Type 3 inositol 1,4,5-trisphosphate receptor has antiapoptotic and proliferative role in cancer cells. *Cell Death Dis.* **2019**, *10*, 186. [CrossRef] [PubMed]
82. Ueasilamongkol, P.; Khamphaya, T.; Guerra, M.T.; Rodrigues, M.A.; Gomes, D.A.; Kong, Y.; Wei, W.; Jain, D.; Trampert, D.C.; Ananthanarayanan, M.; et al. Weerachayaphorn, J. Type 3 Inositol 1,4,5-Trisphosphate Receptor Is Increased and Enhances Malignant Properties in Cholangiocarcinoma. *Hepatology* **2020**, *71*, 583–599. [CrossRef] [PubMed]
83. Shibao, K.; Fiedler, M.J.; Nagata, J.; Minagawa, N.; Hirata, K.; Nakayama, Y.; Iwakiri, Y.; Nathanson, M.H.; Yamaguchi, K. The type III inositol 1,4,5-trisphosphate receptor is associated with aggressiveness of colorectal carcinoma. *Cell Calcium* **2010**, *48*, 315–323. [CrossRef] [PubMed]

84. Prasad, A.; Rabionet, R.; Espinet, B.; Zapata, L.; Puiggros, A.; Melero, C.; Puig, A.; Sarria-Trujillo, Y.; Ossowski, S.; Garcia-Muret, M.P.; et al. Identification of Gene Mutations and Fusion Genes in Patients with Sezary Syndrome. *J. Invest. Derm.* **2016**, *136*, 1490–1499. [CrossRef] [PubMed]
85. Eleftherohorinou, H.; Hoggart, C.J.; Wright, V.J.; Levin, M.; Coin, L.J. Pathway-driven gene stability selection of two rheumatoid arthritis GWAS identifies and validates new susceptibility genes in receptor mediated signalling pathways. *Hum. Mol. Genet.* **2011**, *20*, 3494–3506. [CrossRef] [PubMed]
86. Torkamani, A.; Topol, E.J.; Schork, N.J. Pathway analysis of seven common diseases assessed by genome-wide association. *Genomics* **2008**, *92*, 265–272. [CrossRef]
87. Nakabayashi, K.; Tajima, A.; Yamamoto, K.; Takahashi, A.; Hata, K.; Takashima, Y.; Koyanagi, M.; Nakaoka, H.; Akamizu, T.; Ishikawa, N.; et al. Identification of independent risk loci for Graves' disease within the MHC in the Japanese population. *J. Hum. Genet.* **2011**, *56*, 772–778. [CrossRef]
88. Ferreira, M.A.; Vonk, J.M.; Baurecht, H.; Marenholz, I.; Tian, C.; Hoffman, J.D.; Helmer, Q.; Tillander, A.; Ullemar, V.; van Dongen, J.; et al. Shared genetic origin of asthma, hay fever and eczema elucidates allergic disease biology. *Nat. Genet.* **2017**, *49*, 1752–1757. [CrossRef]
89. Kichaev, G.; Bhatia, G.; Loh, P.R.; Gazal, S.; Burch, K.; Freund, M.K.; Schoech, A.; Pasaniuc, B.; Price, A.L. Leveraging Polygenic Functional Enrichment to Improve GWAS Power. *Am. J. Hum. Genet.* **2019**, *104*, 65–75. [CrossRef]
90. Wilk, J.B.; Shrine, N.R.; Loehr, L.R.; Zhao, J.H.; Manichaikul, A.; Lopez, L.M.; Smith, A.V.; Heckbert, S.R.; Smolonska, J.; Tang, W.; et al. Genome-wide association studies identify CHRNA5/3 and HTR4 in the development of airflow obstruction. *Am. J. Respir. Crit. Care Med.* **2012**, *186*, 622–632. [CrossRef]
91. Reddy, M.V.; Wang, H.; Liu, S.; Bode, B.; Reed, J.C.; Steed, R.D.; Anderson, S.W.; Steed, L.; Hopkins, D.; She, J.X. Association between type 1 diabetes and GWAS SNPs in the southeast US Caucasian population. *Genes Immun.* **2011**, *12*, 208–212. [CrossRef] [PubMed]
92. Roach, J.C.; Deutsch, K.; Li, S.; Siegel, A.F.; Bekris, L.M.; Einhaus, D.C.; Sheridan, C.M.; Glusman, G.; Hood, L.; Lernmark, A.; et al. Swedish Childhood Diabetes Study, G.; Diabetes Incidence in Sweden Study, G. Genetic mapping at 3-kilobase resolution reveals inositol 1,4,5-triphosphate receptor 3 as a risk factor for type 1 diabetes in Sweden. *Am. J. Hum. Genet.* **2006**, *79*, 614–627. [CrossRef] [PubMed]
93. Oishi, T.; Iida, A.; Otsubo, S.; Kamatani, Y.; Usami, M.; Takei, T.; Uchida, K.; Tsuchiya, K.; Saito, S.; Ohnisi, Y.; et al. A functional SNP in the NKX2.5-binding site of ITPR3 promoter is associated with susceptibility to systemic lupus erythematosus in Japanese population. *J. Hum. Genet.* **2008**, *53*, 151–162. [CrossRef]
94. Cotsapas, C.; Speliotes, E.K.; Hatoum, I.J.; Greenawalt, D.M.; Dobrin, R.; Lum, P.Y.; Suver, C.; Chudin, E.; Kemp, D.; Reitman, M.; et al. Consortium, G. Common body mass index-associated variants confer risk of extreme obesity. *Hum. Mol. Genet.* **2009**, *18*, 3502–3507. [CrossRef] [PubMed]
95. Iyengar, S.K.; Sedor, J.R.; Freedman, B.I.; Kao, W.H.; Kretzler, M.; Keller, B.J.; Abboud, H.E.; Adler, S.G.; Best, L.G.; Bowden, D.W.; et al. Diabetes, Genome-Wide Association and Trans-ethnic Meta-Analysis for Advanced Diabetic Kidney Disease: Family Investigation of Nephropathy and Diabetes (FIND). *PLoS Genet.* **2015**, *11*, e1005352. [CrossRef] [PubMed]
96. Comuzzie, A.G.; Cole, S.A.; Laston, S.L.; Voruganti, V.S.; Haack, K.; Gibbs, R.A.; Butte, N.F. Novel genetic loci identified for the pathophysiology of childhood obesity in the Hispanic population. *PLoS ONE* **2012**, *7*, e51954. [CrossRef] [PubMed]
97. Zhang, F.; Wen, Y.; Guo, X.; Zhang, Y.; Wang, X.; Yang, T.; Shen, H.; Chen, X.; Tian, Q.; Deng, H.W. Genome-wide association study identifies ITPR2 as a susceptibility gene for Kashin-Beck disease in Han Chinese. *Arthritis Rheumatol.* **2015**, *67*, 176–181. [CrossRef]
98. Wang, S.J.; Guo, X.; Zuo, H.; Zhang, Y.G.; Xu, P.; Ping, Z.G.; Zhang, Z.; Geng, D. Chondrocyte apoptosis and expression of Bcl-2, Bax, Fas, and iNOS in articular cartilage in patients with Kashin-Beck disease. *J. Rheumatol.* **2006**, *33*, 615–619.
99. Mirza, N.; Appleton, R.; Burn, S.; Carr, D.; Crooks, D.; du Plessis, D.; Duncan, R.; Farah, J.O.; Josan, V.; Miyajima, F.; et al. Identifying the biological pathways underlying human focal epilepsy: From complexity to coherence to centrality. *Hum. Mol. Genet.* **2015**, *24*, 4306–4316. [CrossRef]
100. Nagarkatti, N.; Deshpande, L.S.; DeLorenzo, R.J. Levetiracetam inhibits both ryanodine and IP3 receptor activated calcium induced calcium release in hippocampal neurons in culture. *Neurosci. Lett.* **2008**, *436*, 289–293. [CrossRef]

101. Meder, B.; Haas, J.; Sedaghat-Hamedani, F.; Kayvanpour, E.; Frese, K.; Lai, A.; Nietsch, R.; Scheiner, C.; Mester, S.; Bordalo, D.M.; et al. Epigenome-Wide Association Study Identifies Cardiac Gene Patterning and a Novel Class of Biomarkers for Heart Failure. *Circulation* **2017**, *136*, 1528–1544. [CrossRef] [PubMed]
102. Consortium, C.A.D.; Deloukas, P.; Kanoni, S.; Willenborg, C.; Farrall, M.; Assimes, T.L.; Thompson, J.R.; Ingelsson, E.; Saleheen, D.; Erdmann, J.; et al. Large-scale association analysis identifies new risk loci for coronary artery disease. *Nat. Genet.* **2013**, *45*, 25–33.
103. Huang, Y.C.; Lin, Y.J.; Chang, J.S.; Chen, S.Y.; Wan, L.; Sheu, J.J.; Lai, C.H.; Lin, C.W.; Liu, S.P.; Chen, C.P.; et al. Single nucleotide polymorphism rs2229634 in the ITPR3 gene is associated with the risk of developing coronary artery aneurysm in children with Kawasaki disease. *Int J. Immunogenet.* **2010**, *37*, 439–443. [CrossRef] [PubMed]
104. Bijnens, J.; Missiaen, L.; Bultynck, G.; Parys, J.B. A critical appraisal of the role of intracellular Ca(2+)-signaling pathways in Kawasaki disease. *Cell Calcium* **2018**, *71*, 95–103. [CrossRef]
105. Nakazawa, M.; Uchida, K.; Aramaki, M.; Kodo, K.; Yamagishi, C.; Takahashi, T.; Mikoshiba, K.; Yamagishi, H. Inositol 1,4,5-trisphosphate receptors are essential for the development of the second heart field. *J. Mol. Cell Cardiol.* **2011**, *51*, 58–66. [CrossRef]
106. Uchida, K.; Aramaki, M.; Nakazawa, M.; Yamagishi, C.; Makino, S.; Fukuda, K.; Nakamura, T.; Takahashi, T.; Mikoshiba, K.; Yamagishi, H. Gene knock-outs of inositol 1,4,5-trisphosphate receptors types 1 and 2 result in perturbation of cardiogenesis. *PLoS ONE* **2010**, *5*, e12500. [CrossRef]
107. Uchida, K.; Nakazawa, M.; Yamagishi, C.; Mikoshiba, K.; Yamagishi, H. Type 1 and 3 inositol trisphosphate receptors are required for extra-embryonic vascular development. *Dev. Biol* **2016**, *418*, 89–97. [CrossRef]
108. Miyazaki, S.; Yuzaki, M.; Nakada, K.; Shirakawa, H.; Nakanishi, S.; Nakade, S.; Mikoshiba, K. Block of Ca2+ wave and Ca2+ oscillation by antibody to the inositol 1,4,5-trisphosphate receptor in fertilized hamster eggs. *Science* **1992**, *257*, 251–255. [CrossRef]
109. Saneyoshi, T.; Kume, S.; Amasaki, Y.; Mikoshiba, K. The Wnt/calcium pathway activates NF-AT and promotes ventral cell fate in Xenopus embryos. *Nature* **2002**, *417*, 295–299. [CrossRef]
110. Parmar, P.G.; Taal, H.R.; Timpson, N.J.; Thiering, E.; Lehtimaki, T.; Marinelli, M.; Lind, P.A.; Howe, L.D.; Verwoert, G.; Aalto, V.; et al. International Genome-Wide Association Study Consortium Identifies Novel Loci Associated With Blood Pressure in Children and Adolescents. *Circ. Cardiovasc. Genet.* **2016**, *9*, 266–278. [CrossRef]
111. Michailidou, K.; Beesley, J.; Lindstrom, S.; Canisius, S.; Dennis, J.; Lush, M.J.; Maranian, M.J.; Bolla, M.K.; Wang, Q.; Shah, M.; et al. Genome-wide association analysis of more than 120,000 individuals identifies 15 new susceptibility loci for breast cancer. *Nat. Genet.* **2015**, *47*, 373–380. [CrossRef] [PubMed]
112. Michailidou, K.; Lindstrom, S.; Dennis, J.; Beesley, J.; Hui, S.; Kar, S.; Lemacon, A.; Soucy, P.; Glubb, D.; Rostamianfar, A.; et al. Association analysis identifies 65 new breast cancer risk loci. *Nature* **2017**, *551*, 92–94. [CrossRef] [PubMed]
113. Lee, J.Y.; Kim, J.; Kim, S.W.; Park, S.K.; Ahn, S.H.; Lee, M.H.; Suh, Y.J.; Noh, D.Y.; Son, B.H.; Cho, Y.U.; et al. BRCA1/2-negative, high-risk breast cancers (BRCAX) for Asian women: Genetic susceptibility loci and their potential impacts. *Sci Rep.* **2018**, *8*, 15263. [CrossRef] [PubMed]
114. Sakakura, C.; Hagiwara, A.; Fukuda, K.; Shimomura, K.; Takagi, T.; Kin, S.; Nakase, Y.; Fujiyama, J.; Mikoshiba, K.; Okazaki, Y.; et al. Possible involvement of inositol 1,4,5-trisphosphate receptor type 3 (IP3R3) in the peritoneal dissemination of gastric cancers. *Anticancer Res.* **2003**, *23*, 3691–3697. [PubMed]
115. Yang, Y.C.; Chang, T.Y.; Chen, T.C.; Lin, W.S.; Chang, S.C.; Lee, Y.J. ITPR3 gene haplotype is associated with cervical squamous cell carcinoma risk in Taiwanese women. *Oncotarget* **2017**, *8*, 10085–10090. [CrossRef] [PubMed]
116. Blackshaw, S.; Sawa, A.; Sharp, A.H.; Ross, C.A.; Snyder, S.H.; Khan, A.A. Type 3 inositol 1,4,5-trisphosphate receptor modulates cell death. *FASEB J.* **2000**, *14*, 1375–1379.
117. Mendes, C.C.; Gomes, D.A.; Thompson, M.; Souto, N.C.; Goes, T.S.; Goes, A.M.; Rodrigues, M.A.; Gomez, M.V.; Nathanson, M.H.; Leite, M.F. The type III inositol 1,4,5-trisphosphate receptor preferentially transmits apoptotic Ca2+ signals into mitochondria. *J. Biol. Chem.* **2005**, *280*, 40892–40900. [CrossRef]
118. Bartok, A.; Weaver, D.; Golenar, T.; Nichtova, Z.; Katona, M.; Bansaghi, S.; Alzayady, K.J.; Thomas, V.K.; Ando, H.; Mikoshiba, K.; et al. IP3 receptor isoforms differently regulate ER-mitochondrial contacts and local calcium transfer. *Nat. Commun.* **2019**, *10*, 3726. [CrossRef]

119. Diaz-Vegas, A.R.; Cordova, A.; Valladares, D.; Llanos, P.; Hidalgo, C.; Gherardi, G.; De Stefani, D.; Mammucari, C.; Rizzuto, R.; Contreras-Ferrat, A.; et al. Mitochondrial Calcium Increase Induced by RyR1 and IP3R Channel Activation After Membrane Depolarization Regulates Skeletal Muscle Metabolism. *Front. Physiol.* **2018**, *9*, 791. [CrossRef]
120. Carreras-Sureda, A.; Jana, F.; Urra, H.; Durand, S.; Mortenson, D.E.; Sagredo, A.; Bustos, G.; Hazari, Y.; Ramos-Fernandez, E.; Sassano, M.L.; et al. Non-canonical function of IRE1alpha determines mitochondria-associated endoplasmic reticulum composition to control calcium transfer and bioenergetics. *Nature cell biology* **2019**, *21*, 755–767. [CrossRef]
121. Cardenas, C.; Muller, M.; McNeal, A.; Lovy, A.; Jana, F.; Bustos, G.; Urra, F.; Smith, N.; Molgo, J.; Diehl, J.A.; et al. Selective Vulnerability of Cancer Cells by Inhibition of Ca(2+) Transfer from Endoplasmic Reticulum to Mitochondria. *Cell Rep.* **2016**, *14*, 2313–2324. [CrossRef] [PubMed]
122. Arruda, A.P.; Pers, B.M.; Parlakgul, G.; Guney, E.; Inouye, K.; Hotamisligil, G.S. Chronic enrichment of hepatic endoplasmic reticulum-mitochondria contact leads to mitochondrial dysfunction in obesity. *Nat. Med.* **2014**, *20*, 1427–1435. [CrossRef] [PubMed]
123. Straub, S.V.; Giovannucci, D.R.; Yule, D.I. Calcium wave propagation in pancreatic acinar cells: Functional interaction of inositol 1,4,5-trisphosphate receptors, ryanodine receptors, and mitochondria. *J. Gen. Physiol.* **2000**, *116*, 547–560. [CrossRef] [PubMed]
124. Wiel, C.; Lallet-Daher, H.; Gitenay, D.; Gras, B.; Le Calve, B.; Augert, A.; Ferrand, M.; Prevarskaya, N.; Simonnet, H.; Vindrieux, D.; et al. Endoplasmic reticulum calcium release through ITPR2 channels leads to mitochondrial calcium accumulation and senescence. *Nat. Commun.* **2014**, *5*, 3792. [CrossRef]
125. Bononi, A.; Giorgi, C.; Patergnani, S.; Larson, D.; Verbruggen, K.; Tanji, M.; Pellegrini, L.; Signorato, V.; Olivetto, F.; Pastorino, S.; et al. BAP1 regulates IP3R3-mediated Ca(2+) flux to mitochondria suppressing cell transformation. *Nature* **2017**, *546*, 549–553. [CrossRef]
126. D'Eletto, M.; Rossin, F.; Occhigrossi, L.; Farrace, M.G.; Faccenda, D.; Desai, R.; Marchi, S.; Refolo, G.; Falasca, L.; Antonioli, M.; et al. Transglutaminase Type 2 Regulates ER-Mitochondria Contact Sites by Interacting with GRP75. *Cell Rep.* **2018**, *25*, 3573–3581. [CrossRef]
127. De Stefani, D.; Bononi, A.; Romagnoli, A.; Messina, A.; De Pinto, V.; Pinton, P.; Rizzuto, R. VDAC1 selectively transfers apoptotic Ca2+ signals to mitochondria. *Cell Death Differ.* **2012**, *19*, 267–273. [CrossRef]
128. Marchi, S.; Marinello, M.; Bononi, A.; Bonora, M.; Giorgi, C.; Rimessi, A.; Pinton, P. Selective modulation of subtype III IP(3)R by Akt regulates ER Ca(2)(+) release and apoptosis. *Cell Death Dis.* **2012**, *3*, e304. [CrossRef]
129. Suman, M.; Sharpe, J.A.; Bentham, R.B.; Kotiadis, V.N.; Menegollo, M.; Pignataro, V.; Molgo, J.; Muntoni, F.; Duchen, M.R.; Pegoraro, E.; et al. Inositol trisphosphate receptor-mediated Ca2+ signalling stimulates mitochondrial function and gene expression in core myopathy patients. *Hum. Mol. Genet.* **2018**, *27*, 2367–2382. [CrossRef]
130. Hohendanner, F.; Maxwell, J.T.; Blatter, L.A. Cytosolic and nuclear calcium signaling in atrial myocytes: IP3-mediated calcium release and the role of mitochondria. *Channels (Austin)* **2015**, *9*, 129–138. [CrossRef]
131. Yamazaki, H.; Nozaki, H.; Onodera, O.; Michikawa, T.; Nishizawa, M.; Mikoshiba, K. Functional characterization of the P1059L mutation in the inositol 1,4,5-trisphosphate receptor type 1 identified in a Japanese SCA15 family. *Biochem. Biophys. Res. Commun.* **2011**, *410*, 754–758. [CrossRef] [PubMed]

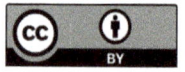

© 2020 by the authors. Licensee MDPI, Basel, Switzerland. This article is an open access article distributed under the terms and conditions of the Creative Commons Attribution (CC BY) license (http://creativecommons.org/licenses/by/4.0/).

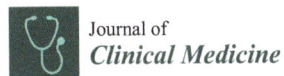

Article

The Circulating GRP78/BiP Is a Marker of Metabolic Diseases and Atherosclerosis: Bringing Endoplasmic Reticulum Stress into the Clinical Scenario

Josefa Girona [1,2], Cèlia Rodríguez-Borjabad [1,2], Daiana Ibarretxe [1,2], Joan-Carles Vallvé [1,2], Raimon Ferré [1,2], Mercedes Heras [1,2], Ricardo Rodríguez-Calvo [1,2], Sandra Guaita-Esteruelas [1], Neus Martínez-Micaelo [1,2], Núria Plana [1,2] and Lluís Masana [1,2,*]

[1] Vascular Medicine and Metabolism Unit, Research Unit on Lipids and Atherosclerosis, Sant Joan University Hospital, Universitat Rovira i Virgili, IISPV, 43201 Reus, Spain; josefa.girona@urv.cat (J.G.); celia.nutricio@gmail.com (C.R.-B.); daiana.ibarretxe@urv.cat (D.I.); jc.vallve@urv.cat (J.-C.V.); rferre@grupsagessa.cat (R.F.); mercedes.heras@urv.cat (M.H.); ricardo.rodriguez@ciberdem.com (R.R.-C.); sandra.guaita@urv.cat (S.G.-E.); neus.martinez@urv.cat (N.M.-M.); nplana@grupsagessa.cat (N.P.)
[2] Spanish Biomedical Research Centre in Diabetes and Associated Metabolic Disorders (CIBERDEM), 28029 Madrid, Spain
* Correspondence: luis.masana@urv.cat; Tel.: +34-977759366; Fax: +34-977759322

Received: 3 October 2019; Accepted: 24 October 2019; Published: 26 October 2019

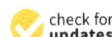

Abstract: Background: Glucose-regulated protein 78/Binding immunoglobulin protein (GRP78/BiP) is a protein associated with endoplasmic reticulum stress and is upregulated by metabolic alterations at the tissue-level, such as hypoxia or glucose deprivation, and it is hyper-expressed in fat tissue of obese individuals. Objective: To investigate the role of the GRP78/BiP level as a metabolic and vascular disease biomarker in patients with type 2 diabetes (DM), obesity and metabolic syndrome (MS). Methods: Four hundred and five patients were recruited, of whom 52.5% were obese, 72.8% had DM, and 78.6% had MS. The intimae media thickness (cIMT) was assessed by ultrasonography. The plasma GRP78/BiP concentration was determined, and its association with metabolic and vascular parameters was assessed. Circulating GRP78/BiP was also prospectively measured in 30 DM patients before and after fenofibrate/niacin treatment and 30 healthy controls. Results: In the cross-sectional study, the GRP78/BiP level was significantly higher in the patients with obesity, DM, and MS. Age-, gender- and BMI-adjusted GRP78/BiP was directly associated with LDL-cholesterol, non-HDL-cholesterol, triglycerides, apoB, and cIMT. GRP78/BiP was positively associated to carotid plaque presence in the adjusted model, irrespective of obesity, DM and MS. In the prospective study, nicotinic acid treatment produced a significant reduction in the GRP78/BiP levels that was not observed with fenofibrate. Conclusions: GRP78/BiP plasma concentrations are increased in patients with both metabolic derangements and subclinical atherosclerosis. GRP78/BiP could be a useful marker of metabolic and cardiovascular risk.

Keywords: GRP78/BiP; endoplasmic reticulum stress; atherosclerosis; carotid intima–media thickness; obesity; type 2 diabetes; metabolic syndrome; cardiovascular risk; fenofibrate/niacin treatment

1. Introduction

Glucose-regulated protein 78/Binding immunoglobulin protein (GRP78/BiP) is an endoplasmic reticulum stress (ERS) protein that belongs to the Hsp70 multigene family and is located in the inner membrane of the endoplasmic reticulum. Its main function is associated with the unfolded protein response (UPR) in ERS situations. GRP78/BiP chaperons newly synthesized proteins until full maturation. In ERS situations, the proteins are titrated away, which frees ERS proteins that function to reduce protein synthesis and increase misfolded protein degradation and the protein-folding capacity [1]. GRP78/BiP is overexpressed in several tissues under ERS. The GRP78/BiP mRNA levels are elevated in the livers of obese mice, and high glucose levels result in reduced GRP78/BiP expression [2]. Additionally, the GRP78/BiP levels are increased in the adipose tissue of patients with diabetes and obesity [3,4]. Hypoxia and glucose deprivation account for the induction of GRP78/BiP [5,6]. Interestingly, this protein has also been detected in cell membranes, where it acts as a multireceptor and signal receptor transducer and mediates other functions [7,8]. These aspects are particularly relevant in some neoplastic tissues [9]. GRP78/BiP is released into culture medium from challenged cells to induce ERS. A soluble part of the protein can be detected in circulation, probably due to active secretion rather than simply a result of cell necrosis or apoptosis [10–12].

Alterations in ER homeostasis have been observed in obese and diabetic subjects [13]. The pathophysiological role of the UPR in obesity, insulin resistance and diabetes has been demonstrated in several studies in animal models [14] and humans [15,16]. One of the main findings was the demonstration that both genetically and diet-induced obese mice exhibited chronic activation of the UPR [2]. Consistent with these findings, treatment of obese and diabetic mice with chemical chaperones alleviated ERS and restored glucose homeostasis in the liver, muscle, and adipose tissues [17]. Furthermore, mice heterozygous for Grp78/BiP ($Grp78^{+/-}$) were protected from the metabolic disorders linked to a high-fat diet [18]. A decrease in the BMI resulting from bariatric surgery reduced ERS in insulin-resistant, obese, human patients [19]. In this regard, physical exercise alleviates ERS in obese individuals through reduction of GRP78/BiP expression and release [4].

Atherosclerosis is the major cause of cardiovascular disease, and UPR activation occurs at all stages of atherosclerotic lesion development. GRP78/BiP has been found to be highly expressed in macrophages, smooth muscle cells, and endothelial cells of atherosclerotic lesions [20]. Increased ERS occurs in unstable plaques, suggesting that ERS-induced apoptosis of smooth muscle cells and macrophages may contribute to plaque vulnerability. Moreover, unstable atherosclerotic plaques present abnormal numbers of apoptotic cells, which is related to ERS [21] mainly via robust CHOP expression. ERS markers, such as GRP78/BiP, are strongly associated with atherosclerotic plaques in human coronary artery lesions [22]. Hemodynamic shear stress in atherosclerotic regions regulates GRP78/BiP expression in vivo and in vitro, and GRP78/BiP upregulation in the endothelium has been hypothesized to provide a protective compensatory effect in response to ERS within early or developing atherosclerotic lesions [23].

ERS is a pathophysiological process that is involved in many metabolic derangements. Therefore, an ERS biomarker should be highly informative at the clinical level.

To the best of our knowledge, no studies have addressed the relationship between GRP78/BiP, diabetes, metabolic alterations, and subclinical atherosclerosis. In the present study, we have studied the associations between GRP78/BiP and metabolic indexes and atherosclerosis in patients with obesity, type 2 diabetes mellitus (DM), and/or metabolic syndrome (MS). We have also investigated the effect of lipid-modifying drugs on GRP78/BiP in patients with DM.

2. Research Design and Methods

2.1. Design and Study Subjects

Cross-Sectional Study: For the cross-sectional study, we recruited 405 consecutive individuals attending the vascular medicine and metabolism unit of our university hospital due to lipid metabolism disturbances and associated disorders (obesity, DM, and MS) who were willing to participate. DM, MS, and obesity were diagnosed according to standard clinical criteria. Prediabetes was diagnosed according to the fasting glucose level (>100 mg/dL and <126 mg/dL). Subjects with chronic lung, renal, or liver disease, cancer, or any other serious disease were excluded. Patients on lipid-lowering drugs underwent a 6-week wash-out period (8 weeks if they were on fibrates). Anamnesis, anthropometric, and physical examination data were recorded.

Prospective Study: GRP78/BiP was analyzed in deep-frozen stored sera from 29 patients with DM and 30 gender- and age-matched, apparently healthy, individuals (control group) who participated in an open randomized control trial to evaluate the impact of fenofibrate and niacin on HDL quality in DM patients. The details of this study including the flow chart scheme have been published [24] (ClinicalTrials.gov Identifier: NCT02153879). Briefly, after a 6-week lipid-lowering drug wash-out period, the patients with DM were randomly distributed into two groups. One group received 20 mg of simvastatin plus 145 mg of fenofibrate, and the other group received 20 mg of simvastatin plus 2 g of niacin plus laropiprant for a 12-week period. After a new 6-week lipid-lowering drug wash-out period, they were shifted to the other lipid-lowering drug in a crossover design for a 12-week period.

The Hospital Ethics Committee approved the study, and all patients provided their written consent to participate in the study.

2.2. Clinical and Laboratory Determinations

A blood sample was obtained from each patient in the study cohort after overnight fasting. Aliquots were prepared for immediate storage at −80 °C in the BioBanc at our center prior to use. Biochemical parameters, lipids, and apolipoproteins were measured using colorimetric, enzymatic and immunoturbidimetric assays, respectively (Spinreact, SA, Spain; Wako Chemicals GmbH, Germany; and Polymedco, New York, NY, USA; CV < 4%), which were adapted to the Cobas Mira Plus Autoanalyser (Roche Diagnostics, Spain). The lipid profile was analyzed according to the Spintrol "H" CAL (Spinreact, SA, Spain) GC–MS reference methods. Spintrol "H" Normal was used as a quality control. The circulating PCSK9 levels were measured by an enzyme-linked immunosorbent assay (ELISA) kit (R&D Systems, Minneapolis, MN, USA). The FABP5, FABP4 and HMW-adiponectin levels were assessed using commercial ELISA kits (BioVendor Laboratory Medicine Inc., Brno, Czech Republic; RayBiotech, Inc., Georgia, GA, USA; CV, 5%). The serum GRP78/BiP levels were measured with an ELISA kit (Enzo Life Sciences, Inc., New York, NY, USA) following the reagent manufacturer's instructions. The optical density (OD) of the well was measured at a wavelength of 450 nm ± 2 nm (Synergy, BioTek Instruments, Inc., Winooski, VT, USA). Each sample was analyzed in duplicate. The serum GRP78/BiP levels were measured using a standard curve constructed with the kit's standards. The homeostasis model assessment–insulin resistance (HOMA–IR) index was calculated from the fasting glucose and insulin concentrations, as previously reported [25].

2.3. Carotid Ultrasound Imaging

A total of 316 subjects from the entire cohort underwent a vascular study with the Mylab 50 X-Vision ultrasound (Esaote, Italy). A 7.5 MHz linear array and semiautomated software were used to measure the carotid intima–media thickness (cIMT) in the far wall of both common carotid arteries. The cIMT mean was the average of 2 territories. Bifurcations and internal carotids were also measured using a manual method. A plaque was defined as a focal structure that either encroached into the arterial lumen by at least 0.5 mm or 50% of the surrounding cIMT value or demonstrated a thickness >1.5 mm, as measured from the media–adventitia interface to the intima-lumen interface, according to the Mannheim carotid intima–media thickness consensus [26].

2.4. Statistical Analyses

Data are presented as medians and 25th and 75th percentiles or percentages, unless otherwise indicated. The normality of continuous variables was determined by the Kolmogorov–Smirnov test. GRP78/BiP was log-transformed to reduce skewness. Unadjusted associations between GRP78/BiP and continuous variables were assessed by Spearman's correlation test. Differences in GRP78/BiP between patients with obesity, DM, and MS were analyzed by the Mann–Whitney test, and differences between MS components were analyzed using the Kruskal–Wallis test. Group differences between treatments in the validation cohort were analyzed with the paired Wilcoxon test. Adjusted differences were investigated using analysis of covariance (ANCOVA). Multivariate linear regression models were constructed to search for independent relationships between GRP78/BiP (dependent variable) and clinical and biochemical variables in the whole study group and in the obese, type 2 diabetic, and MS subjects. Logistic binary regression models were also performed for dichotomous variables to assess the risk of obesity, DM, MS, or atherosclerotic plaques based on the serum GRP78/BiP levels. All statistical analyses were conducted with SPSS 25 (IBM, Armonk, NY, USA). A p value < 0.05 was considered statistically significant.

3. Results

3.1. Subjects' Characterisctics

The clinical, anthropometric, and biochemical characteristics of the patients participating in the cross-sectional study are shown in Table 1. The median (25th percentile–75th percentile) age of the study subjects was 60 (50–67) years, and 50.9% were women. Obesity was present in 52.5%, DM in 72.8%, and MS in 78.6% of the patients. Carotid atherosclerotic plaques were present in 33.2% of the patients. The median GRP/BiP level was 7.43 (4.42–13.49) μg/mL. Analysis of our full cohort revealed no differences in GRP78/BiP between genders, and the level was unrelated to age.

Table 1. Clinical and biochemical characteristics of the study subjects.

	N = 405
Women (%)	50.9
Age (years)	60 (50–67)
BMI (kg/m^2)	27.53 (27.33–34.75)
Waist circumference (cm)	103.0 (95.0–112.0)
Systolic BP (mmHg)	133 (124–146)
Diastolic BP (mmHg)	80 (71–85)
Glucose (mg/dL)	126.7 (101.0–163.0)
Insulin (%) *	10.43 (6.95–16.48)
HbA1c (%) †	6.40 (5.70–7.50)
HOMA-IR *	3.13 (1.75–6.19)
Lipids and Apolipoproteins	
Total cholesterol (mmol/L)	5.20 (4.50–6.19)
LDL-C (mmol/L)	3.18 (2.55–3.97)
HDL-C (mmol/L)	1.38 (1.19–1.59)
Non-HDL-C (mmol/L)	3.80 (3.14–4.73)
Total triglycerides (mmol/L)	1.65 (1.04–2.58)
ApoB100 (mg/dL)	103 (85–120)
ApoA1 (mg/dL)	136 (128–146)
Lp(a) (mg/dL)	8.10 (2.70–22.00)
Protein Biomarkers	
GRP78/BiP (μg/mL)	7.43 (4.42–13.49)
PCSK9 (ng/mL)	320.2 (254.4–404.7)
hsCRP (mg/L)	2.09 (1.12–3.75)
FABP4 (ng/mL)	26.06 (16.84–37.24)
FABP5 (ng/mL)	7.74 (6.13–9.92)
HMW-Adiponectin (μg/mL)	5.44 (2.96–8.98)
Disease	
Obesity (%)	52.5
Type 2 diabetes (%)	72.8
Metabolic syndrome (%)	78.6
Subclinical Atherosclerosis	
cIMT (mm) ‡	0.685 (0.619–0.776)
Carotid atherosclerotic plaque (%) §	33.2

Data are shown as n (percentage) or median (25th percentile–75th percentile). BMI = body mass index; BP = blood pressure; LDL-C = LDL cholesterol; HDL-C = HDL cholesterol; Non-HDL-C = non-HDL cholesterol; ApoB100 = apolipoprotein B100; ApoA1 = apolipoprotein A1, Lp(a) = lipoprotein a; GRP78/BiP = 78 kDa glucose-regulated protein/binding immunoglobulin protein; PCSK9 = proprotein convertase subtilisin/kexin type 9; hsCRP = high-sensitivity C-reactive protein; FABP4 = fatty acid binding protein 4; FABP5 = fatty acid binding protein 5; HMW-adiponectin = high-molecular-weight adiponectin; cIMT = carotid intima–media thickness. Measurements were available in a subpopulation of: * n = 168; † n = 314; ‡ n = 312; § n = 316.

3.2. Association of GRP78/BiP with the Metabolic Status

The GRP78/BiP serum concentrations were higher in patients with obesity, DM, and MS compared with patients without metabolic disturbances (5.67 (3.74–11.62) µg/mL vs. 9.15 (5.74–16.38) µg/mL, $p < 0.001$; 4.72 (3.63–9.94) µg/mL vs. 8.57 (5.27–16.73) µg/mL, $p < 0.001$ and 4.15 (2.91–5.76) µg/mL vs. 9.15 (5.85–16.73) µg/mL, $p < 0.001$, respectively) (Figure 1A,B,C). A direct and positive association was found with the number of MS components ($p < 0.001$) (Figure 1D). The differences were independent of covariates ($p < 0.001$ for obesity, DM, and MS) (Figure 1).

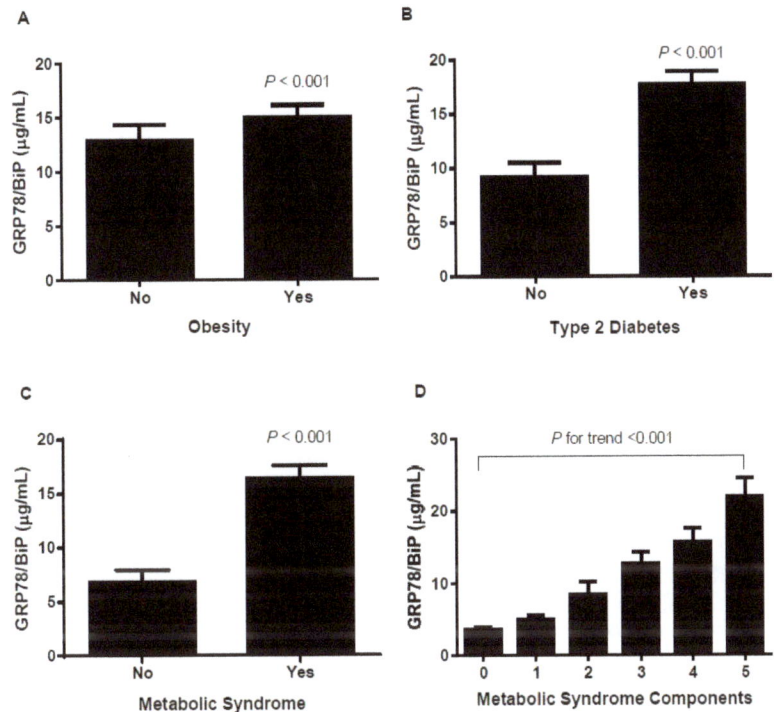

Figure 1. Circulating 78 kDa glucose-regulated protein/binding immunoglobulin protein (GRP78/BiP) levels according to obesity (**A**), type 2 diabetes (**B**), metabolic syndrome (**C**) and metabolic syndrome components (**D**). The results are expressed as the mean ± SEM. p values for group comparisons are reported for the age- and gender-adjusted ANCOVA test.

A logistic regression analysis revealed that the serum GRP78/BiP levels were associated with the presence of obesity, DM, and MS in the crude and in the gender- and age-adjusted model (model 1). After adjusting for other risk factors (model 2), GRP78/BiP levels remained directly associated with DM and MS (Supplemental Table S1).

3.3. Associations of GRP78/BiP with the Clinical, Biochemical and Vascular Imaging Data

The associations among GRP78/BiP and the clinical, anthropometric, and standard biochemical data and the adipokine and vascular values are shown in Table 2. Notably, GRP78/BiP was directly related to all adiposity indexes, including the BMI, standard lipids, lipoprotein levels, glucose concentrations, inflammation and adipokines, and was inversely related to apo A1 and HMW-adiponectin. The mean GRP78/BiP was also directly related to cIMT.

Table 2. Relationships between log-GRP78/BiP and continuous variables.

	Log GRP78/BiP	p Value	Log GRP78/BiP *	p Value *
Age	0.034	0.499	-	-
BMI	0.307	<0.001	-	-
Waist Circumference	0.269	<0.001	0.125	0.121
Systolic BP	0.394	<0.001	0.154	0.055
Diastolic BP	0.153	<0.001	0.122	0.129
Glucose	0.296	<0.001	−0.045	0.576
Total cholesterol	0.429	<0.001	0.156	0.052
LDL-C	0.351	<0.001	0.099	0.217
HDL-C	−0.011	0.830	0.038	0.637
Non-HDL-C	0.472	<0.001	0.176	0.028
Total triglycerides	0.392	<0.001	0.243	0.002
ApoB100	0.420	<0.001	0.169	0.035
ApoA1	−0.165	0.001	−0.137	0.088
Lp(a)	0.065	0.190	0.039	0.626
PCSK9	0.191	<0.001	0.077	0.340
hsCRP	0.256	<0.001	0.084	0.297
FABP4	0.141	0.005	0.104	0.195
FABP5	0.274	<0.001	0.095	0.236
HMW-Adiponectin	−0.176	0.001	−0.055	0.493
cIMT	0.165	0.003	0.244	0.002

GRP78/BiP = 78 kDa glucose-regulated protein/binding immunoglobulin protein; BMI = body mass index; BP = blood pressure; LDL-C = LDL cholesterol; HDL-C = HDL cholesterol; Non-HDL-C = non-HDL cholesterol; ApoB100 = apolipoprotein B100; ApoA1 = apolipoprotein A1, Lp(a) = lipoprotein a; PCSK9 = proprotein convertase subtilisin/kexin type 9; hsCRP = high-sensitivity C-reactive protein; FABP4 = fatty acid binding protein 4; FABP5 = fatty acid binding protein 5; HMW-adiponectin = high-molecular-weight adiponectin; cIMT = carotid intima–media thickness. p values for Spearman's correlations are reported. * p values corrected by age, gender and BMI.

After adjusting for age, gender, and BMI, the relationships that remained statistically significant with GRP78/BiP were cholesterol, non-HDL-C, triglycerides, apoB100 and cIMT ($p < 0.05$ for all comparisons) (Table 2).

Thereafter, a multivariate stepwise regression analysis was used to identify factors influencing circulating GRP78/BiP across obesity, DM, and MS. In the entire study population, gender, systolic blood pressure, triglycerides, and cIMT were the determinants of circulating GRP78/BiP, accounting for 32.7% of the observed variance (Supplemental Table S2). Further analysis of obese individuals revealed that gender accounted for 15.4% of the variance observed in the circulating GRP78/BiP levels. In diabetic individuals, gender, BMI, triglycerides, and cIMT accounted for 25.3% of the variance. For MS, the determinants of circulating GRP78/BiP were gender, triglycerides, and cIMT, which accounted for 20.3% of the variance.

3.4. Associations Between GRP68/BiP and the Carotid Plaque Burden

Age- and gender-adjusted GRP78/BiP was higher in patients with carotid plaques (7.13 (4.56–12.63) µg/mL vs 11.8 (7.91–24.99) µg/mL, $p < 0.001$, $n = 316$, respectively) (Figure 2). GRP78/BiP was directly related to the carotid plaque presence (odds ratio OR, 95% confidence interval [CI] = 7.077 (3.357–14.922), $p < 0.001$) in the age- and gender-adjusted model. The direct association of GRP78/BiP with the presence of a plaque was significant in the patients with obesity (OR [CI] = 5.053 (1.716–14.876), $p = 0.003$), DM (OR [CI] = 6.296 (2.521–15.724), $p < 0.001$), and MS (OR [CI] = 5.109 (2.216–11.778), $p < 0.001$) (Supplemental Table S3).

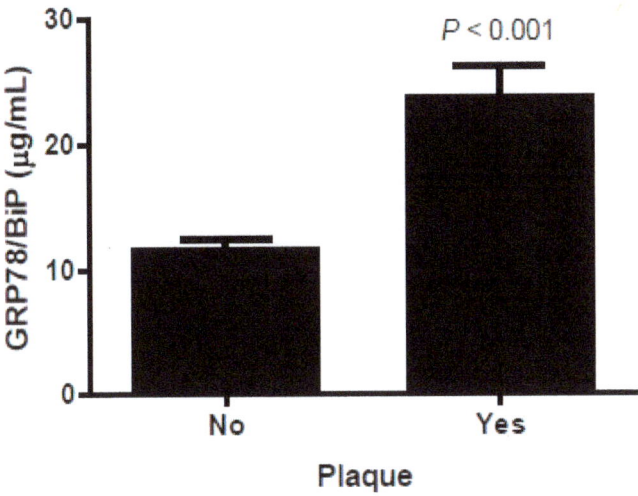

Figure 2. Circulating 78 kDa glucose-regulated protein/binding immunoglobulin protein (GRP78/BiP) levels according to the presence of atherosclerotic plaques. The results are expressed as the mean ± SEM. p values for group comparison are reported for the age- and gender-adjusted ANCOVA test.

3.5. GRP68/BiP and Prediabetes

GRP78/BiP was increased in the subjects with prediabetes compared with the levels in the subjects with neither prediabetes nor diabetes (4.46 (3.22–8.66) µg/mL vs. 7.23 (4.54–13.96) µg/mL, $p < 0.001$, respectively). Additionally, a positive association was detected with the HOMA-IR ($r = 0.407$; $p < 0.001$, $n = 168$) that persisted after age and gender adjustment ($r = 0.231$; $p = 0.003$). In the patients with triglycerides < 2.26 mmol/L, GRP78/BiP was significantly higher in those with prediabetes and diabetes than in the controls, whereas the levels in the patients with high triglycerides (>2.26 mmol/L) were equally altered (Supplemental Figure S1).

3.6. Effect of Treatment on Circulating GRP78/BiP in DM Patients

The clinical characteristics of the patients participating in the intervention trial were previously published [24]. The median (25th percentile–75th percentiles) age was 58 (53–65) years, and 36.7% were women. Similar to the main study cohort, the age- and gender-matched GRP78/BiP levels were higher in the DM patients than in the control group ($p < 0.001$). Similar to those of the main study cohort, GRP78/BiP showed a direct association with triglycerides ($r = 0.581$; $p < 0.001$) and the cIMT ($r = 0.509$; $p = 0.016$, $n = 22$). Interestingly, in the DM patients, treatment with nicotinic acid for a 12-week period ($n = 26$) significantly reduced GRP78/BiP by 11% ($p = 0.038$) (Figure 3). This reduction was accompanied by the expected reduction in triglycerides (39%, $p = 0.003$). Treatment with fenofibrate ($n = 29$) also accounted for a significant reduction of triglycerides (32%, $p = 0.002$) but resulted in a non-significant reduction of GRP78/BiP ($p = 0.705$).

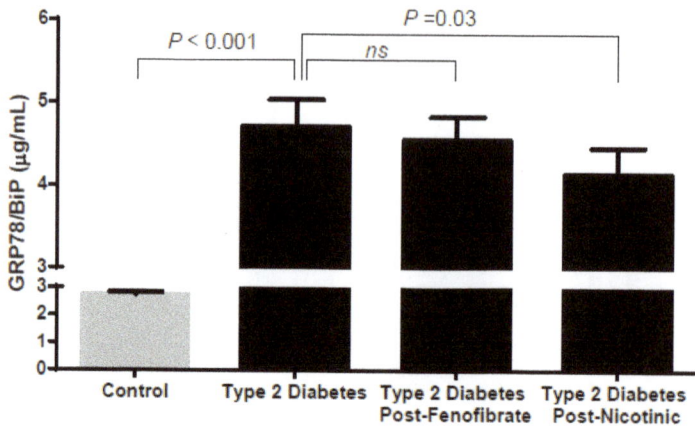

Figure 3. Circulating 78 kDa glucose-regulated protein/binding immunoglobulin protein (GRP78/BiP) in the control group and the type 2 diabetes patients before and after fenofibrate and nicotinic treatment in a validation cohort. The results are expressed as the mean ± SEM. p values for the group comparisons are reported for the age- and gender-adjusted ANCOVA test or paired Wilcoxon test.

4. Discussion

We communicate that the circulating GRP78/BiP levels are significantly increased in obese, DM, and MS patients. Higher GRP78/BiP concentrations are also associated with subclinical atherosclerosis. The data are robust enough to support the use of GRP78/BiP serum concentrations as a biomarker of metabolic and vascular derangements. The endoplasmic reticulum is a crucial subcellular organelle that is responsible for protein, lipid, glucose, and calcium metabolism. Conditions in which its physiological capacity is overwhelmed are referred to as ERS, in which a complex molecular reaction is activated and proteins are not properly processed due to the UPR [27]. GRP78/BiP is a cornerstone protein of this process [1]. It is physiologically located in the inner layer of the ER and maintains the localization of several proteins associated with the ERS response. In ERS situations, GRP78/BiP frees these proteins to counterbalance the UPR by reducing protein synthesis, increasing misfolded protein removal and improving the protein folding capacity. Increased extracellular delivery of GRP78/BiP occurs because of this process. According to the results of our and other studies [4], this increased secretion leads to higher circulating GRP78/BiP concentrations in humans. Thus, a high serum GRP78/BiP level should be interpreted as an ERS marker. Triglycerides and cholesterol esters are assembled in the ER. ER homeostasis is altered in the presence of a high amount of lipids, leading to ERS [28–30]. Therefore, our data showing an increased amount of a circulating protein associated with ERS in subjects with important alterations in intermediate metabolism are logical. According to our data, GRP78/BiP can be detected in the sera at very low levels, which increase in the presence of obesity, DM, and MS. Interestingly, a robust direct association exists between GRP78/BiP and cholesterol and triglycerides, suggesting that alterations in lipid metabolism are involved in ERS and the increase in circulating GRP78/BiP. This finding could be of interest, given that GRP78/BiP expression in vitro is associated with an increase in expression of the very low-density lipoprotein receptor [6], which is important in tissues with active fatty acid metabolism. In other words, the high fat pools in tissues involved in lipid metabolism, such as the liver and adipose tissue, would be at least partially responsible for ERS. This possibility is of interest in patients with normal triglyceride levels but signs of prediabetes or resistance to insulin; we observed that GRP78/BiP was already high in these patients, suggesting that other metabolic alterations might play a role in GRP78/BiP secretion.

On the other hand, inflammation is also associated with ERS [31]. This fact could also explain ERS in diabetes and obesity because they are associated to chronic subclinical inflammation. In our hands, GRP78/BiP was also correlated with the hsCRP concentration.

Interestingly, triglyceride-lowering drugs have different impacts on the GRP78/BiP plasma concentration, although, as expected, both drugs produced a significant triglyceride-lowering effect. Niacin but not fenofibrate induced a significant reduction of GRP78/BiP. The lipid-lowering effect of niacin is not completely understood but seems to be mediated by a decrease in adipose tissue lipolysis, which reduces the substrate for triglyceride synthesis in the liver, whereas fenofibrate acts mainly during the catabolic phase [32,33]. The decrease in the intracellular lipid burden mediated by niacin can most likely explain the observed differences.

An interesting observation of our study is the significant association between GRP78/BiP and the presence of subclinical atherosclerosis, particularly in those with carotid plaques. We have no elements to link a direct impact of GRP78/BiP with atherosclerotic pathogenesis, although the protein is expressed in macrophages, smooth muscle cells, and endothelial cells of atherosclerotic lesions in animal models [20]. We cannot exclude the possibility that high circulating GRP78/BiP levels are signaling individuals with more severe metabolic alterations, although the correlation between GRP78/BiP and carotid plaques is maintained after multiple adjustments.

Our work has some limitations. The cross-sectional design precludes obtaining causal relationships between GRP78/BiP and metabolic and vascular alterations. The prospective, randomized and controlled validation study was open, the sample size was small, and the study was not designed for this objective. However, the data obtained are in concordance with the results from the main part of the study and provide additional information on the reversibility of ERS.

In conclusion, the circulating GRP78/BiP levels are significantly increased in people with DM, obesity, and its associated metabolic alterations. The associated hyperlipidemia probably plays a role in ERS in these patients. GRP78/BiP was also associated with subclinical atherosclerosis. Taking all of these results together, our work supports the use of the circulating GRP78/BiP level as a marker of vascular and metabolic risk. Our data provide elements to bring derangement of a crucial cellular mechanism to the clinical setting.

Supplementary Materials: The following are available online at http://www.mdpi.com/2077-0383/8/11/1793/s1.

Author Contributions: Conceptualization, J.G., N.P. and L.M.; Data curation, J.G., D.I., R.F., N.P. and L.M.; Formal analysis, J.G., J.-C.V. and L.M.; Funding acquisition, J.G. and L.M.; Investigation, J.G., C.R.-B., R.F., N.P. and L.M.; Methodology, J.G., C.R.-B., D.I., J.-C.V., M.H., R.R.-C., S.G.-E. and N.M.-M.; Supervision, J.G., C.R.-B., D.I. and L.M.; Writing—original draft, J.G., J.-C.V. and L.M.; Writing—review & editing, J.G., C.R.-B., D.I., J.-C.V. and L.M.

Funding: This study was funded by grants from Instituto de Salud Carlos III (ISCIII), Madrid, Spain (PI15/00627; PI18/00515). This work was jointly supported by national funding from the Spanish Biomedical Research Centre in Diabetes and Associated Metabolic Disorders (CIBERDEM). This work was co-funded by the European Regional Development Fund (ERDF).

Acknowledgments: The authors thank the UVASMET in Sant Joan University Hospital for assistance and all patients who gave time to this study. The authors acknowledge the IISPV-BIOBANC for sample handling.

Conflicts of Interest: The authors declare no conflict of interest.

References

1. Pobre, K.F.R.; Poet, G.J.; Hendershot, L.M. The endoplasmic reticulum (ER) chaperone BiP is a master regulator of ER functions: Getting by with a little help from ERdj friends. *J. Biol. Chem.* **2019**, *294*, 2098–2108. [CrossRef] [PubMed]
2. Ozcan, U.; Cao, Q.; Yilmaz, E.; Lee, A.-H.; Iwakoshi, N.N.; Ozdelen, E.; Tuncman, G.; Görgün, C.; Glimcher, L.H.; Hotamisligil, G.S. Endoplasmic reticulum stress links obesity, insulin action, and type 2 diabetes. *Science* **2004**, *306*, 457–461. [CrossRef] [PubMed]

3. Fang, L.; Kojima, K.; Zhou, L.; Crossman, D.K.; Mobley, J.A.; Grams, J. Analysis of the Human Proteome in Subcutaneous and Visceral Fat Depots in Diabetic and Non-Diabetic Patients with Morbid Obesity. *J. Proteom. Bioinform.* **2015**, *8*, 133–141.
4. Khadir, A.; Kavalakatt, S.; Abubaker, J.; Cherian, P.; Madhu, D.; Al-Khairi, I.; Abu-Farha, M.; Warsame, S.; Elkum, N.; Dehbi, M.; et al. Physical exercise alleviates ER stress in obese humans through reduction in the expression and release of GRP78 chaperone. *Metabolism* **2016**, *65*, 1409–1420. [CrossRef] [PubMed]
5. Shiu, R.P.; Pouyssegur, J.; Pastan, I. Glucose depletion accounts for the induction of two transformation-sensitive membrane proteinsin Rous sarcoma virus-transformed chick embryo fibroblasts. *Proc. Natl. Acad. Sci. USA* **1977**, *74*, 3840–3844. [CrossRef]
6. Yang, D.; Gao, L.; Wang, T.; Qiao, Z.; Liang, Y.; Zhang, P. Hypoxia triggers endothelial endoplasmic reticulum stress and apoptosis via induction of VLDL receptor. *FEBS Lett.* **2014**, *588*, 4448–4456. [CrossRef]
7. Tsai, Y.-L.; Zhang, Y.; Tseng, C.-C.; Stanciauskas, R.; Pinaud, F.; Lee, A.S. Characterization and Mechanism of Stress-induced Translocation of 78-Kilodalton Glucose-regulated Protein (GRP78) to the Cell Surface. *J. Biol. Chem.* **2015**, *290*, 8049–8064. [CrossRef]
8. Mazaki, Y.; Higashi, T.; Onodera, Y.; Nam, J.-M.; Hashimoto, A.; Hashimoto, S.; Horinouchi, T.; Miwa, S. Endothelin type B receptor interacts with the 78-kDa glucose-regulated protein. *FEBS Lett.* **2019**, *593*, 644–651. [CrossRef]
9. Li, Z.; Zhuang, M.; Zhang, L.; Zheng, X.; Yang, P.; Li, Z. Acetylation modification regulates GRP78 secretion in colon cancer cells. *Sci. Rep.* **2016**, *6*, 30406. [CrossRef]
10. Li, R.; Yanjiao, G.; Wubin, H.; Yue, W.; Jianhua, H.; Huachuan, Z.; Rongjian, S.; Zhidong, L. Secreted GRP78 activates EGFR-SRC-STAT3 signaling and confers the resistance to sorafeinib in HCC cells. *Oncotarget* **2017**, *8*, 19354–19364.
11. Ma, X.; Guo, W.; Yang, S.; Zhu, X.; Xiang, J.; Li, H. Serum GRP78 as a Tumor Marker and Its Prognostic Significance in Non-Small Cell Lung Cancers: A Retrospective Study. *Dis. Markers* **2015**, *2015*, 814670. [CrossRef] [PubMed]
12. Aksoy, M.O.; Kim, V.; Cornwell, W.D.; Rogers, T.J.; Kosmider, B.; Bahmed, K.; Barrero, C.; Merali, S.; Shetty, N.; Kelsen, S.G. Secretion of the endoplasmic reticulum stress protein, GRP78, into the BALF is increased in cigarette smokers. *Respir. Res.* **2017**, *18*, 78. [CrossRef] [PubMed]
13. Back, S.H.; Kaufman, R.J. Endoplasmic reticulum stress and type 2 diabetes. *Annu. Rev. Biochem.* **2012**, *81*, 767–793. [CrossRef] [PubMed]
14. Nakatani, Y.; Kaneto, H.; Kawamori, D.; Yoshiuchi, K.; Hatazaki, M.; Matsuoka, T.; Ozawa, K.; Ogawa, S.; Hori, M.; Yamasaki, Y.; et al. Involvement of Endoplasmic Reticulum Stress in Insulin Resistance and Diabetes. *J. Biol. Chem.* **2005**, *280*, 847–851. [CrossRef]
15. Sharma, N.K.; Das, S.K.; Mondal, A.K.; Hackney, O.G.; Chu, W.S.; Kern, P.A.; Rasouli, N.; Spencer, H.J.; Yao-Borengasser, A.; Elbein, S.C. Endoplasmic reticulum stress markers are associated with obesity in nondiabetic subjects. *J. Clin. Endocrinol. Metab.* **2008**, *93*, 4532–4541. [CrossRef]
16. Boden, G.; Duan, X.; Homko, C.; Molina, E.J.; Song, W.; Perez, O.; Cheung, P.; Merali, S. Increase in Endoplasmic Reticulum Stress-Related Proteins and Genes in Adipose Tissue of Obese, Insulin-Resistant Individuals. *Diabetes* **2008**, *57*, 2438–2444. [CrossRef]
17. Ozcan, U.; Yilmaz, E.; Ozcan, L.; Furuhashi, M.; Vaillancourt, E.; Smith, R.O.; Görgün, C.Z.; Hotamisligil, G.S. Chemical chaperones reduce ER stress and restore glucose homeostasis in a mouse model of type 2 diabetes. *Science* **2006**, *313*, 1137–1140. [CrossRef]
18. Ye, R.; Jung, D.Y.; Jun, J.Y.; Li, J.; Luo, S.; Ko, H.J.; Kim, J.K.; Lee, A.S. Grp78 heterozygosity promotes adaptive unfolded protein response and attenuates diet-induced obesity and insulin resistance. *Diabetes* **2010**, *59*, 6–16. [CrossRef]
19. Gregor, M.F.; Yang, L.; Fabbrini, E.; Mohammed, B.S.; Eagon, J.C.; Hotamisligil, G.S.; Klein, S. Endoplasmic reticulum stress is reduced in tissues of obese subjects after weight loss. *Diabetes* **2009**, *58*, 693–700. [CrossRef]
20. Zhou, J.; Lhoták, S.; Hilditch, B.A.; Austin, R.C. Activation of the unfolded protein response occurs at all stages of atherosclerotic lesion development in apolipoprotein E-deficient mice. *Circulation* **2005**, *111*, 1814–1821. [CrossRef]

21. Cominacini, L.; Garbin, U.; Mozzini, C.; Stranieri, C.; Pasini, A.; Solani, E.; Tinelli, I.A.; Pasini, A.F. The atherosclerotic plaque vulnerability: Focus on the oxidative and endoplasmic reticulum stress in orchestrating the macrophage apoptosis in the formation of the necrotic core. *Curr. Med. Chem.* **2015**, *22*, 1565–1572. [CrossRef] [PubMed]
22. Myoishi, M.; Hao, H.; Minamino, T.; Watanabe, K.; Nishihira, K.; Hatakeyama, K.; Asada, Y.; Okada, K.; Ishibashi-Ueda, H.; Gabbiani, G.; et al. Increased Endoplasmic Reticulum Stress in Atherosclerotic Plaques Associated with Acute Coronary Syndrome. *Circulation* **2007**, *116*, 1226–1233. [CrossRef] [PubMed]
23. Feaver, R.E.; Hastings, N.E.; Pryor, A.; Blackman, B.R. GRP78 upregulation by atheroprone shear stress via p38-, alpha2beta1-dependent mechanism in endothelial cells. *Arterioscler. Thromb. Vasc. Biol.* **2008**, *28*, 1534–1541. [CrossRef] [PubMed]
24. Masana, L.; Cabré, A.; Heras, M.; Amigó, N.; Correig, X.; Martínez-Hervás, S.; Real, J.T.; Ascaso, J.F.; Quesada, H.; Julve, J.; et al. Remarkable quantitative and qualitative differences in HDL after niacin or fenofibrate therapy in type 2 diabetic patients. *Atherosclerosis* **2015**, *238*, 213–219. [CrossRef] [PubMed]
25. Levy, J.C.; Matthews, D.R.; Hermans, M.P. Correct homeostasis model assessment (HOMA) evaluation uses the computer program. *Diabetes Care* **1998**, *21*, 2191–2192. [CrossRef]
26. Touboul, P.-J.; Hennerici, M.G.; Meairs, S.; Adams, H.; Amarenco, P.; Bornstein, N.; Csiba, L.; Desvarieux, M.; Ebrahim, S.; Hernandez Hernandez, R.; et al. Mannheim Carotid Intima-Media Thickness and Plaque Consensus (2004–2006–2011). *Cerebrovasc. Dis.* **2012**, *34*, 290–296. [CrossRef]
27. Todd, D.J.; Lee, A.-H.; Glimcher, L.H. The endoplasmic reticulum stress response in immunity and autoimmunity. *Nat. Rev. Immunol.* **2008**, *8*, 663–674. [CrossRef]
28. Sozen, E.; Ozer, N.K. Impact of high cholesterol and endoplasmic reticulum stress on metabolic diseases: An updated mini-review. *Redox Biol.* **2017**, *12*, 456–461. [CrossRef]
29. Han, J.; Kaufman, R.J. The role of ER stress in lipid metabolism and lipotoxicity. *J. Lipid Res.* **2016**, *57*, 1329–1338. [CrossRef]
30. Balasus, D.; Way, M.; Fusilli, C.; Mazza, T.; Morgan, M.Y.; Cervello, M.; Giannitrapani, L.; Soresi, M.; Agliastro, R.; Vinciguerra, M.; et al. The association of variants in PNPLA3 and GRP78 and the risk of developing hepatocellular carcinoma in an Italian population. *Oncotarget* **2016**, *7*, 86791–86802. [CrossRef]
31. McGrath, K.C.Y.; Heather, A.K. Endoplasmic Reticulum Stress in Inflammatory Disease. *Endocrinology* **2012**, *153*, 2949–2952. [CrossRef] [PubMed]
32. Ali, A.H.; Mundi, M.; Koutsari, C.; Bernlohr, D.A.; Jensen, M.D. Adipose Tissue Free Fatty Acid Storage In Vivo: Effects of Insulin Versus Niacin as a Control for Suppression of Lipolysis. *Diabetes* **2015**, *64*, 2828–2835. [CrossRef] [PubMed]
33. Forcheron, F.; Cachefo, A.; Thevenon, S.; Pinteur, C.; Beylot, M. Mechanisms of the triglyceride- and cholesterol-lowering effect of fenofibrate in hyperlipidemic type 2 diabetic patients. *Diabetes* **2002**, *51*, 3486–3491. [CrossRef] [PubMed]

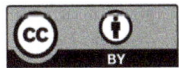

© 2019 by the authors. Licensee MDPI, Basel, Switzerland. This article is an open access article distributed under the terms and conditions of the Creative Commons Attribution (CC BY) license (http://creativecommons.org/licenses/by/4.0/).

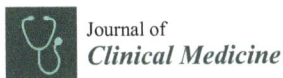

Article

Association of Trimethylamine, Trimethylamine N-oxide, and Dimethylamine with Cardiovascular Risk in Children with Chronic Kidney Disease

Chien-Ning Hsu [1,2], Guo-Ping Chang-Chien [3,4], Sufan Lin [3,4], Chih-Yao Hou [5], Pei-Chen Lu [6] and You-Lin Tain [6,7,*]

1. Department of Pharmacy, Kaohsiung Chang Gung Memorial Hospital, Kaohsiung 833, Taiwan; chien_ning_hsu@hotmail.com
2. School of Pharmacy, Kaohsiung Medical University, Kaohsiung 807, Taiwan
3. Center for Environmental Toxin and Emerging-Contaminant Research, Cheng Shiu University, Kaohsiung 833, Taiwan; guoping@csu.edu.tw (G.-P.C.-C.); linsufan2003@gmail.com (S.L.)
4. Super Micro Mass Research and Technology Center, Cheng Shiu University, Kaohsiung 833, Taiwan
5. Department of Seafood Science, National Kaohsiung University of Science and Technology, Kaohsiung 811, Taiwan; chihyaohou@gmail.com
6. Department of Pediatrics, Kaohsiung Chang Gung Memorial Hospital and College of Medicine, Chang Gung University, Kaohsiung 833, Taiwan; alexiellu@gmail.com
7. Institute for Translational Research in Biomedicine, Kaohsiung Chang Gung Memorial Hospital and Chang Gung University, College of Medicine, Kaohsiung 833, Taiwan
* Correspondence: tainyl@cgmh.org.tw; Tel.: +886-975-056-995; Fax: +886-7733-8009

Received: 2 January 2020; Accepted: 22 January 2020; Published: 25 January 2020

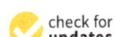

Abstract: Chronic kidney disease (CKD) is associated with high risk for cardiovascular disease (CVD). Gut microbiota-dependent metabolites trimethylamine (TMA), trimethylamine N-oxide (TMAO), and dimethylamine (DMA) have been linked to CKD and CVD. We examined whether these methylamines are correlated with cardiovascular risk in CKD children. A total of 115 children and adolescents with CKD stage G1–G4 were enrolled in this cross-sectional study. Children with CKD stage G2–G4 had higher plasma levels of DMA, TMA, and TMAO, but lower urinary levels of DMA and TMAO than those with CKD stage G1. Up to 53% of CKD children and adolescents had blood pressure (BP) abnormalities on 24-h ambulatory BP monitoring (ABPM). Plasma TMA and DMA levels inversely associated with high BP load as well as estimated glomerular filtration rate (eGFR). Additionally, CKD children with an abnormal ABPM profile had decreased abundance of phylum *Cyanobacteria*, genera *Subdoligranulum*, *Faecalibacterium*, *Ruminococcus*, and *Akkermansia*. TMA and DMA are superior to TMAO when related to high BP load and other CV risk factors in children and adolescents with early-stage CKD. Our findings highlight that gut microbiota-dependent methylamines are related to BP abnormalities and CV risk in pediatric CKD. Further studies should determine whether these microbial markers can identify children at risk for CKD progression.

Keywords: ambulatory blood pressure monitoring; cardiovascular disease; children; chronic kidney disease; dimethylamine; gut microbiota; hypertension; trimethylamine; trimethylamine N-oxide

1. Introduction

Chronic kidney disease (CKD) is associated with high risk for cardiovascular disease (CVD), not just for adults but also for children [1,2]. Even though overt CVD barely presents in children, the process of atherosclerosis can originate in early life. Therefore, heightened efforts are needed to identify CKD children at higher risk for CVD during their lifetimes to develop effective interventions for preemption [3]. Several noninvasive procedures, such as 24-h ambulatory blood pressure monitoring (ABPM) [4], ambulatory arterial stiffness index (AASI) [5], and left ventricular mass [6], are available to evaluate risk for CVD in children with CKD.

Gut microbiome has been identified as a source of pathogenic mediators in CKD [7]. Certain gut microbiota-derived metabolites have been shown to correlate with CVD in patients with CKD [8,9]. Among them, trimethylamine N-oxide (TMAO) has attracted increasing notoriety recently as a causative factor in various CVD. Emerging evidence has linked higher blood levels of TMAO with a higher risk of CVD [10].

TMAO production is a two-step process. The first step involves the liberation of trimethylamine (TMA) from dietary precursors (e.g., choline and carnitine) by gut microbes. In the second step, TMA is oxidized to TMAO by hepatic flavin-containing monooxygenases (FMOs). Both TMAO and TMA can be subsequently converted to dimethylamine (DMA). Thus, the plasma TMAO-to-TMA ratio may reflect FMO activity, while DMA-to-TMAO ratio is related to TMAO-metabolizing activity.

Although plasma levels of TMAO, TMA, and DMA are all increased in uremic patients [11], little attention has been paid to understand the role of their levels and combined ratios in the development of CVD in children with early-stage CKD. Because TMAO, TMA, and DMA are all tightly linked to each other and because all these methylamines are excreted into urine [12], we assume that simultaneous analysis of their combined ratios in the plasma and urine may provide more information to reflect the TMA–TMAO metabolic pathway. Thus, we assessed the association between CVD assessments, microbial markers, and TMA–TMAO metabolic pathway in early pediatric CKD.

2. Materials and Methods

2.1. Study Population

This is a cross-sectional study of 115 children and adolescents with CKD who were enrolled in the Kaohsiung Chang Gung Memorial Hospital from January 2019 to December 2019. Human subjects review board approval was obtained from the Institution Review Board and Ethics Committee of Chang Gung Medical Foundation, Taoyuan, Taiwan (Permit number: 201701735A3C501). Our study protocol was conducted in accordance with the 1964 Helsinki Declaration and its later amendments. Written informed consent was obtained from all participants. CKD is defined as abnormal kidney structure or function lasting more than three months [13]. We calculated estimated glomerular filtration rate (eGFR) with the Schwartz formula according to body height and blood creatinine (Cr) level [14]. Kidney damage included proteinuria, urine sediment abnormalities, or structural abnormalities and was detected by histology or imaging. Participants were categorized according to eGFR (mL/min/1.73 m^2): G1 ≥90, G2 60–89, G3 30–59, or G4 15–29. The causes of kidney diseases were divided to two categories: Congenital anomalies of the kidney and urinary tract (CAKUT) or non-CAKUT. CAKUT structural anomalies ranged from renal agenesis, kidney hypo-/dysplasia, horseshoe kidney, duplex collecting system, multi-cystic kidney dysplasia, posterior urethral valves, and ureter abnormalities [15]. Patients were excluded from the study if they (1) had a history of congenital heart disease; (2) were already documented as being pregnant; (3) had eGFR <15 mL/min/1.73 m^2 or were on dialysis maintenance, or had ever received renal transplantation; (4) were unable to cooperate with CV assessment.

2.2. Biochemical Analysis

Fasting plasma and spot urine samples were stored at −80 °C until analysis. We directed the family to have their children avoid excessive intake of foods rich in choline and carnitine (e.g., eggs, fish, or red meat) for 1 week before blood and urine sampling. Blood urea nitrogen (BUN), creatinine, total cholesterol, low-density lipoprotein (LDL), triglyceride, sodium, potassium, calcium, phosphate, uric acid, glucose, hemoglobin, hematocrit, and urine total protein-to-creatinine ratio were measured by the hospital central laboratory as described previously [16].

2.3. Liquid Chromatography–Mass Spectrometry (LC–MS/MS) Analysis

We analyzed plasma and urinary concentrations of DMA, TMA, and TMAO by LC–MS/MS analysis using an Agilent 6410 Series Triple Quadrupole mass spectrometer (Agilent Technologies, Wilmington, DE, USA) equipped with an electrospray ionization source [16]. The multiple-reaction-monitoring mode was set up using characteristic precursor-product ion transitions to detect m/z 46.1→30, m/z 60.1→44.1, and m/z 76.1→58.1, for DMA, TMA, and TMAO, respectively. Separation was performed in the Agilent Technologies 1200 HPLC system consisting of an autosampler and a binary pump. Chromatographic separation was performed on a SeQuant ZIC-HILIC column (150 × 2.1 mm, 5 µm; Merck KGaA, Darmstadt, Germany) protected by an Ascentis C18 column (2 cm × 4 mm, 5 µm; Merck KGaA, Darmstadt, Germany). Diethylamine was added to samples as an internal standard. The mobile phase containing methanol with 15mmol/L ammonium formate (phase A) and acetonitrile (phase B) was used at a ratio of 20:80 (phase A: phase B), with the flow rate set as 0.3–1 mL/min. The urinary concentration of each methylamine was corrected for urine Cr concentration, which was represented in ng/mg Cr.

2.4. Blood Pressure Measurement and Echocardiography

Participants were instructed to measure office blood pressure (BP) at the clinic visit after a 5 min rest with at least 1 min between recordings. The mean value was used for calculations. The 24-h ABPM data were collected for subjects aged 6–18 years, handled by an experienced specialist nurse as described previously [16]. We used the Oscar II monitoring device (SunTech Medical, Morrisville, NC) to measure BP and pulse rate at 20-min intervals over 24 h. The participants and their parents were requested to complete a diary of sleeping and waking times, as well as activities that may influence BP measurements. An abnormal ABPM profile was defined as (1) awake, asleep, systolic, or diastolic BP loads ≥95th percentile based on gender and height using ABPM reference data [17]; (2) awake, asleep, systolic or diastolic BP load ≥25%; and (3) asleep decrease of BP load <10% compared with average awake BP load. Next, the ambulatory arterial stiffness index (AASI) is an index derived from 24-h ABPM for the evaluation of arterial stiffness [5]. The AASI was defined as 1 minus the regression slope of diastolic BP (DBP) on systolic BP (SBP) [18]. Echocardiographic examination was performed with commercially available machines (Philips IE33 system, Philips, Bothell, WA, USA). The left ventricular (LV) mass was calculated using images obtained in the parasternal long-axis or short-axis view of the left ventricle by M-mode echocardiography. The LV mass index (LVMI) was obtained by indexing LV mass to height$^{2.7}$ [19].

2.5. Analysis of Gut Microbiota Composition

Metagenomic DNA was extracted from frozen fecal samples. Simple centrifugation processing was carried out to remove impurity, proteins, and other organic compounds. As described previously [16], all polymerase chain-reaction amplicons were mixed together with the Biotools Co., Ltd. (Taipei, Taiwan) for sequencing using an Illumina Miseq platform (Illumina, CA, USA). Amplicons were prepared according to the 16S Metagenomics Sequencing Library Preparation protocol (Illumina, CA, USA), and sequenced using the variable V3–V4 regions of the 16S rRNA gene with the Illumina MiSeq platform (Illumina, CA, USA) in paired-end mode with 600-cycle sequencing reagent. The sequences were analyzed using QIIME version 1.9.1. A median of 116,776 raw sequencing reads and 79,067 effective tag sequences per sample was obtained, respectively. Sequences with a distance-based similarity of 97% or greater were grouped into operational taxonomic units (OTUs) using the USEARCH algorithm. The phylogenetic relationships were determined based on a representative sequence alignment using Fast-Tree. Shannon's index accounting for both abundance and evenness of the taxa present was analyzed by QIIME version 1.9.1. We evaluated the β-diversity changes in gut microbiota across groups by the Partial Least Squares Discriminant Analysis (PLS-DA) and the weighted or unweighted UniFrac distances. To determine the significantly differential taxa, we applied linear discriminant analysis effect size (LEfSe) to compare samples between groups. The LEfSe uses linear discriminant analysis (LDA) to estimate the effect size of each differentially abundant feature. The threshold of the linear discriminant was set to 3.

2.6. Statistical Analysis

Continuous variables were expressed with the median (25th–75th percentile), and categorical variables were indicated by number (%). The Mann–Whitney U test or Chi-square test was used to test the differences in variables between children with normal and abnormal ABPM. The associations between variables were examined using Spearman's correlation coefficient. A linear regression model was performed, followed by the stepwise multivariable analyses integrating relevant parameters to explain BP load, AASI, and LV mass. A value of $p < 0.05$ was considered statistically significant. Analyses were performed using the Statistical Package for the Social Sciences (SPSS) software 14.0 (Chicago, IL, USA).

3. Results

Characteristics of the study subjects are shown in Table 1. A total of 115 children and adolescents with CKD were enrolled in this study, including 79 G1 subjects (68.7%), 27 G2 subjects (23.5%), seven G3 subjects (6.1%), and two G4 subjects (1.7%). The median age was 11.3 years. Our study population had a slight preponderance of males (M:F = 1.4:1). The median eGFR was 100.7 mL/min/1.73 m^2, demonstrating most participants were in the early stage of CKD. The major cause of CKD was due to CAKUT (66.1%). Among them, 49 cases (42.6%) had office BP exceeding the 95th percentile for age, gender, and height. As illustrated in Table 1, in terms of biochemical parameters, most patients were well controlled for common complications of CKD. Thirty-one patients (27%) displayed proteinuria. There was a trend toward moderate hyperlipidemia: 23 (20%) and 10 (9%) patients were above the upper normal limit of 200 and 130 mg/dL for total cholesterol and triglyceride, respectively. Moreover, 20 patients (17%) had hyperuricemia. Neither severe anemia nor hyperkalemia was observed.

Table 1. Descriptive statistics for clinical, anthropometric, and biomedical characteristics of 115 study participants.

Characteristics	
Age, years	11.3 (7.2–15.5)
Male	67 (58.3%)
CKD staging	
Stage G1	79 (68.7%)
Stage G2	27 (23.5%)
Stage G3	7 (6.1%)
Stage G4	2 (1.7%)
CAKUT	76 (66.1%)
Hypertension (by office BP)	49 (42.6%)
Body height, percentile	50 (25–75)
Body weight, percentile	50 (15–85)
Systolic blood pressure, mmHg	112 (101–122)
Diastolic blood pressure, mmHg	71 (66–80)
Body mass index, kg·m^{-2}	17.9 (15.2–21.5)
Blood urea nitrogen, mg/dL	13 (10–15)
Creatinine, mg/dL	0.58 (0.46–0.77)
eGFR, mL/min/1.73 m^2	100.7 (82.3–113.4)
Urine total protein-to-creatinine ratio, mg/g	62.7 (33.9–176.9)
Hemoglobin, g/dL	13.3 (12.7–14.1)
Hematocrit, %	40.5 (38.5–43)
Total cholesterol, mg/dL	169 (144–197)
Low-density lipoprotein, mg/dL	93 (74–118)
Triglyceride, mg/dL	70 (51–92)
Uric acid, mg/dL	5.2 (4.3–6.7)
Sodium, mEq/L	140 (139–141)
Potassium, mEq/L	4.3 (4.2–4.6)
Calcium, mg/dL	9.8 (9.6–10.1)
Phosphate, mg/dL	4.6 (4.2–5)

Data are medians (25th, 75th percentile) or n (%). CAKUT = Congenital anomalies of the kidney and urinary tract.

Table 2 summarizes the results of cardiovascular assessments in children and adolescents with CKD: 75 patients (65%) aged 6–18 years had undergone 24-h ABPM. In total, 53% (40/75) of them had at least one BP load abnormality. Among them, seven (9%), seven (9%), and eight patients (11%) had SBP or DBP load ≥95th percentile at 24-h, awake, and asleep stages, respectively. Additionally, there were 23 patients (31%) with BP load ≥25% and 31 patients (41%) with a non-dipping nocturnal BP profile. CKD children with stage G2–G4 had a higher awake SBP load than that in CKD stage 1. Moreover, the cases with asleep BP ≥95th percentile and BP load ≥25% were greater in CKD stage G2–G4 vs. stage G1 group. The AASI and LV mass were higher in children with CKD stage G2–G4 than those with stage G1. However, LVMI was not different between the two groups.

Table 2. Cardiovascular assessments in children and adolescents with chronic kidney disease (CKD) stage G1–G4.

CKD Stage	G1	G2–G4
24-h ABPM	N = 48	N = 27
Awake SBP load (%)	6.5 (0–13)	15 (1–36) *
Asleep SBP load (%)	8.5 (0–25.3)	21 (6–69)
Awake DBP load (%)	2 (0–6)	3 (0–10)
Asleep DBP load (%)	9 (0–18.8)	7 (0–41)
Abnormal ABPM profile (with any of the following abnormalities)	23 (48%)	17 (63%)
Average 24-h BP >95th percentile	2 (4%)	5 (19%)
Average awake BP >95th percentile	2 (4%)	5 (19%)
Average asleep BP >95th percentile	2 (4%)	6 (22%) *
BP load ≥25%	10 (21%)	13 (48%) *
Nocturnal decrease of BP <10%	18 (38%)	13 (48%)
AASI	0.33 (0.21–0.45)	0.41 (0.33–0.57) *
Left ventricular mass (g)	74.6 (54.6–102)	96 (51.8–141.3) *
LVMI (g/m$^{2.7}$)	30.8 (25.2–37.1)	32.7 (28.4–36.3)

Data are medians (25th, 75th percentile) or n (%). * $p < 0.05$ by the Chi-square test or the Mann–Whitney U-test. ABPM = 24-h ambulatory blood pressure monitoring. AASI = ambulatory arterial stiffness index. LVMI = left ventricular mass index.

We next analyzed methylamines in the plasma and urine. Children with CKD stage G2–G4 had higher plasma levels of DMA, TMA, and TMAO compared to those with CKD stage 1 (Table 3). Conversely, urinary levels of DMA and TMAO were lower in patients with CKD stage G2–G4 vs. stage G1. However, both TMAO-to-TMA and DMA-to-TMAO ratios in the plasma and urine did not differ between the two groups. Additionally, fractional excretion of DMA, TMA, and TMAO was comparable between CKD children with stage G1 and stage G2–G4.

Using data pooled from all subjects, correlations between plasma and urinary methylamine levels and CV risk factors were analyzed (Table 4). We observed that urinary DMA level was negatively correlated with awake SBP load ($r = -0.235$, $p = 0.043$), asleep SBP load ($r = -0.289$, $p = 0.012$), awake DBP load ($r = -0.288$, $p = 0.012$), and LV mass ($r = -0.554$, $p < 0.001$). Additionally, LV mass exhibited negative correlations with urinary TMA ($r = -0.226$, $p = 0.016$) and TMAO levels ($r = -0.324$, $p < 0.001$). In CKD children and adolescents, there were significantly inverse correlations between eGFR and plasma DMA ($r = -0.718$, $p < 0.001$), TMA ($r = -0.371$, $p < 0.001$), and TMAO ($r = -0.283$, $p = 0.002$) (Figure 1).

Table 3. Plasma and urinary levels of dimethylamine (DMA), trimethylamine (TMA), and trimethylamine N-oxide (TMAO) in children and adolescents with CKD stage G1–G4.

CKD Stage	G1	G2–G4
	N = 73	N = 36
Plasma level, ng/ml		
DMA	91 (81.7–104.8)	124.4 (107.7–147.4) *
TMA	100.8 (83.9–123.1)	112.6 (105.2–138.6) *
TMAO	170.5 (112.9–232.7)	245.7 (129.6–477.1) *
TMAO-to-TMA ratio	1.56 (1.05–2.33)	2.11 (1.17–4.33)
DMA-to-TMAO ratio	0.57 (0.4–0.86)	0.45 (0.34–1)
Urine level, ng/mg Cr		
DMA	222.2 (164.7–281.3)	196.8 (123.8–243.2) *
TMA	3.18 (2.46–5.75)	2.96 (1.44–6.62)
TMAO	271.1 (167.3–417.8)	183.8 (107.5–291.6) *
TMAO-to-TMA ratio	87.5 (55.8–113.7)	68.7 (38.2–112.9)
DMA-to-TMAO ratio	0.84 (0.55–1.15)	0.89 (0.51–1.48)
Fractional excretion of DMA	44.2 (30.2–61.2)	48.8 (36.9–69.6)
Fractional excretion of TMA	1.6 (1.13–2.84)	1.87 (1.13–4.99)
Fractional excretion of TMAO	82.3 67.9–96.8)	81.3 (61–92.1)

Data are medians (25th, 75th percentile). * $p < 0.05$ by the Mann–Whitney U-test. DMA = dimethylamine; TMA = trimethylamine; TMAO = trimethylamine N-oxide.

Table 4. Correlation between plasma and urinary methylamines and cardiovascular risk factors in children with CKD stage G1–G4.

CV Risk Factors	Awake SBP Load		Asleep SBP Load		Awake DBP Load		Asleep DBP Load		LV Mass	
	r	p	r	p	r	p	r	p	r	p
Plasma										
DMA	0.144	0.221	0.141	0.232	0.117	0.32	0.039	0.74	0.059	0.534
TMA	0.115	0.329	0.133	0.26	−0.029	0.807	0.137	0.244	0.093	0.326
TMAO	0.113	0.339	−0.018	0.879	0.088	0.457	−0.08	0.945	0.024	0.797
Urine										
DMA	−0.235	0.043 *	−0.289	0.012 *	−0.288	0.012 *	−0.022	0.854	−0.554	<0.001 *
TMA	0.212	0.067	0.07	0.548	0.105	0.368	0.131	0.261	−0.226	0.016 *
TMAO	0.043	0.716	−0.223	0.055	0.013	0.91	0.003	0.980	−0.324	<0.001 *

* $p < 0.05$ by Spearman's correlation coefficient. DMA = dimethylamine; TMA = trimethylamine; TMAO = trimethylamine N-oxide.

As illustrated in Table 5, associations between methylamines and CV risk were further examined in a multivariate linear regression model. To specify the exact role of each methylamine biomarker in CV risk, a multivariate linear regression model using the stepwise selection was applied for age, sex, eGFR, and other methylamines. In the best predictive model ($r = 0.479$, $p < 0.001$), office DBP was associated with urinary TMA ($p = 0.009$) as well as plasma TMA level ($p = 0.02$), controlling for age. Urine DMA-to-TMAO ratio was inversely associated with office DBP controlling for age ($r = 0.441$, $p < 0.001$). A positive association between plasma TMA level and awake DBP was found in the adjusted regression model ($r = 0.283$, $p = 0.015$). Additionally, plasma TMA level was associated with asleep DBP (p = 0.036), controlling for age. We also found that urine DMA-to-TMAO ratio had a negative association with LV mass controlling for age and sex ($r = 0.771$, $p < 0.001$). Furthermore, an inverse association between plasma DMA-to-TMAO ratio and LVMI was found in the adjusted regression model controlling for eGFR and sex ($r = 0.465$, $p < 0.001$).

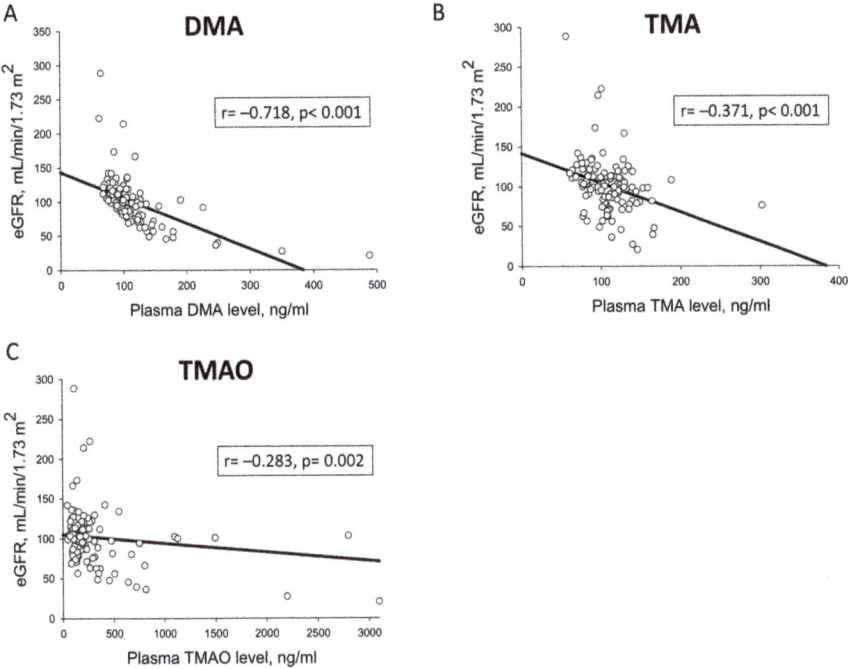

Figure 1. Correlation of plasma (**A**) DMA, (**B**) TMA, and (**C**) TMAO levels (ng/mL) with estimated glomerular filtration rate (eGFR) (ml/min/1.73m^2) by Spearman's correlation coefficient. DMA = dimethylamine; TMA = trimethylamine; TMAO = trimethylamine N-oxide.

Table 5. Adjusted regression model estimates of the association between plasma and urinary methylamines and cardiovascular risk factors in children with CKD stage G1–G4.

Dependent Variable	Explanatory Variable	Adjusted [a]		Model	
		Beta	p Value	r	p Value
Office DBP	Urine TMA	−0.227	0.009	0.479	<0.001
	Plasma TMA	0.202	0.02		
	Urine DMA-to-TMAO ratio	−0.221	0.012	0.441	<0.001
Awake DBP	Plasma TMA	0.283	0.015	0.283	0.015
Asleep DBP	Plasma TMA	0.232	0.036	0.423	0.001
LV mass	Urine DMA-to-TMAO ratio	−0.148	0.018	0.771	<0.001
LVMI	Plasma DMA-to-TMAO ratio	−0.218	0.012	0.465	<0.001

DMA = dimethylamine; TMA = trimethylamine; TMAO = trimethylamine N-oxide. LVMI = left ventricular mass index. [a] Adjusted for age, sex, eGFR, and other methylamines.

We further analyzed the composition of the gut microbiota. We determined α-diversity as the mean species richness, quantified by the Shannon index, and found that there was no significant difference between CKD children with normal vs. abnormal ABPM (Figure 2A; $p = 0.723$). The β-diversity was measured by calculating the unweighted UniFrac distances between each pair of samples, and the unweighted UniFrac distance matrix was measured and visualized using a partial least squares discriminant analysis (PLS-DA) analysis. The score plots of PLS-DA analysis showed that two groups were well separated (Figure 2B). The unweighted UniFrac results differed from the normal, and the abnormal ABPM group reached significance ($p = 0.005$). At the phylum level, we observed that the main phyla were *Firmicutes*, *Actinobacteria*, *Proteobacteria*, *Bacteroidetes*, and *Verrucomicrobia*

(Figure 2C). Although several phyla showed lower abundance in the abnormal vs. normal ABPM group (Figure 2D), only phylum *Cyanobacteria* reached the significance ($p < 0.05$; Figure 2E). Moreover, the *Firmicutes* to *Bacteroidetes* ratio was comparable between two groups.

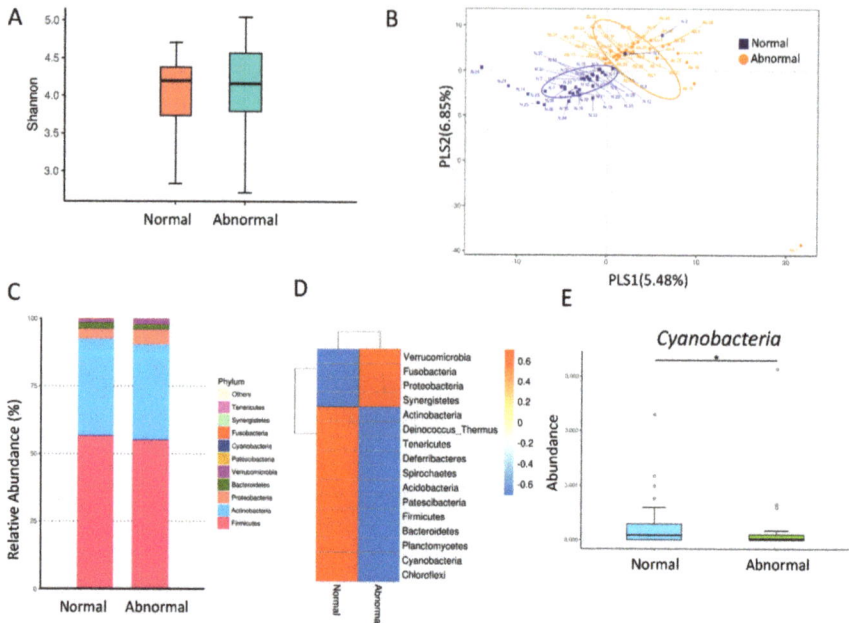

Figure 2. (**A**) Fecal bacterial α-diversity in CKD children with normal and abnormal ABPM represented by the Shannon's diversity indexes. (**B**) β-diversity changes in gut microbiota between CKD children with normal and abnormal ABPM by the partial least squares discriminant analysis (PLS-DA). (**C**) Relative abundance of top 10 phyla of the gut microbiota between the normal and abnormal ABPM group. (**D**) Heat map of 16S rRNA gene sequencing analysis of gut microbiome at the phylum level. (**E**) The abundance of phylum *Cyanobacteria* in CKD children with normal vs. abnormal ABPM. The asterisk indicates $p < 0.05$.

At the genus level (Figure 3A), the abundances of most top 10 genera were not different between the normal and abnormal ABPM group, except genera *Subdoligranulum* ($p = 0.034$) and *Ruminococcus* ($p = 0.033$). Finally, we ran the LEfSe algorithm to identify metagenomic biomarkers (Figure 3B). Our results identified that genera *Subdoligranulum*, *Holdemanella*, and *Actinomyces* are detected by LEfSe with a high LDA score (more than three orders of magnitude), reflecting marked higher abundance in the normal ABPM group. In contrast, the abnormal ABPM group had decreased abundance of genera *Faecalibacterium* and *Akkermansia*. Additionally, the abnormal ABPM group showed a decreased abundance of genera *Providencia* (Figure 3C), *Gemella* (Figure 3D), and *Peptosreptoccocus* (Figure 3E) (all $p < 0.05$).

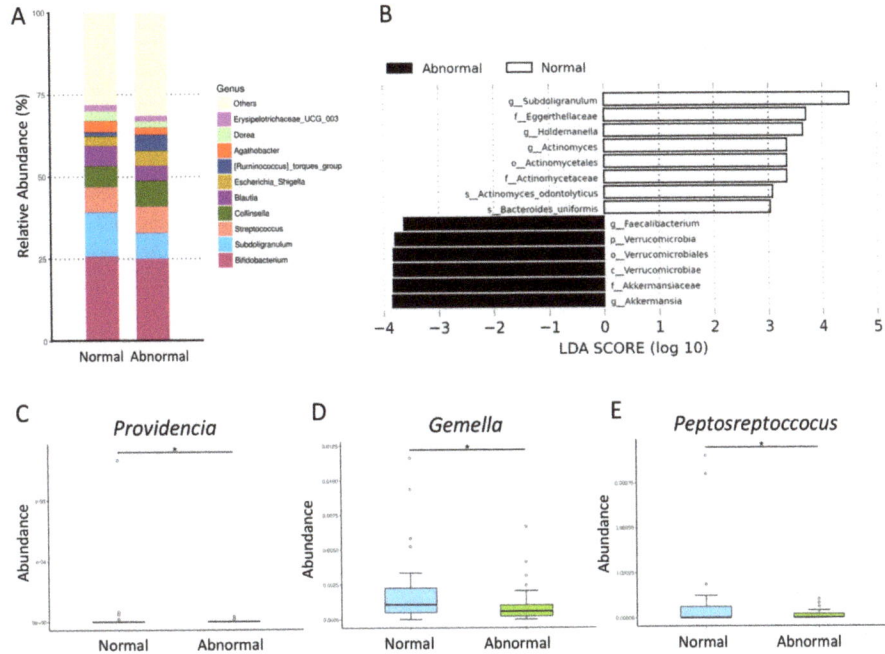

Figure 3. (**A**) Relative abundance of top 10 genera of the gut microbiota in CKD children with normal and abnormal ABPM group. (**B**) Linear discriminant analysis effect size (LEfSe) to identify the taxa that were significantly different between normal vs. abnormal ABPM group. The threshold of the linear discriminant was set to 3. (**C**) The abundance of genus *Providencia*, (**D**) *Gemella*, and (**E**) *Peptosreptoccocus* in CKD children with normal vs. abnormal ABPM. The asterisk indicates $p < 0.05$.

4. Discussion

To the best of our knowledge, this study is the first to evaluate the association between gut microbiota-dependent methylamines and CV risk in early-stage pediatric CKD. The key findings are (1) children with CKD stage G2–G4 had higher plasma levels of DMA, TMA, and TMAO, but lower urinary levels of DMA and TMAO compared to those with CKD stage G1; (2) plasma TMA and DMA levels were not only inversely associated with high BP load, but also eGFR; (3) CKD children with abnormal and normal ABPM associated into two distinct enterotypes; (4) CKD children with an abnormal ABPM profile had decreased abundance of phylum *Cyanobacteria*, genera *Subdoligranulum*, *Faecalibacterium*, *Ruminococcus*, and *Akkermansia*; and (5) TMA and DMA are superior to TMAO related to CV risk in early-stage CKD children.

In the current study, more than half of CKD children exhibited BP abnormalities on ABPM. Our data showed the cases with nocturnal hypertension and increased BP load were greater in children with CKD stage G2–G4 than those with stage G1. Of note is that up to 48% of children with CKD stage G1 had BP abnormalities on ABPM. Our findings are consistent with previous reports wherein hypertension is extremely prevalent in CKD children, even in an early stage [20–23]. The present study supported the notion that ABPM is superior to office BP in identifying children with BP abnormalities [24]. As expected, the severity of CKD is associated with certain markers of CV risk, like AASI and LV mass in the current study. AASI, an index of arterial stiffness, has been proposed as a surrogate marker to predict CV morbidity and mortality [18]. Our previous report demonstrated that high AASI is related to BP abnormalities in CKD children, even in an early stage [23]. The present results showed AASI was higher in children with CKD stage G2–G4 than those with stage G1, which ties well with the previous study in that high AASI worsens GFR decline in adult CKD patients [25]. Left ventricular hypertrophy is an index of target organ damage as well as a risk factor for CVD in adult CKD patients [26]. In keeping with previous studies showing that LV mass is greater in CKD children on dialysis and ABPM correlates with LV hypertrophy in CKD children [6,27,28], we observed children with advanced CKD displayed higher degree of LV mass and BP abnormalities.

Gut microbiota-derived metabolites TMAO, TMA, and DMA from dietary methylamines have recently gained much attention due to their high association with CV risk [8–10,29,30]. In the present study, our results are consistent with previous reported data in CKD adults [31,32], showing that TMAO is increased in CKD with a weak inverse correlation ($r = -0.283$) between plasma TMAO level and eGFR. Our results are also in agreement with a previous report in CKD adults showing urinary excretion is a dominant route for TMAO elimination with a steady fractional excretion of TMAO, regardless of the CKD stages [32]. However, we observed lower urinary TMAO levels in children with CKD stage G2–G4 than those with stage G1. Either increased or decreased urinary TMAO levels have been reported in adult CKD patients [32,33]. Conflicting results are likewise seen in this study showing that decreased urinary but increased plasma TMAO levels in children with advanced-stage CKD may represent reduced renal excretion of circulating TMAO or increased local renal TMAO metabolism. Although observational and experimental studies suggest a positive correlation between high plasma TMAO levels and increased CV risk [10], data are contradictory and the underlying mechanism is not yet validated [34]. Therefore, it is debated whether TMAO is harmful or beneficial for CV health. Our data showed no significant association between TMAO and most CV surrogate markers, except that urinary TMAO level had a negative correlation with LV mass. Therefore, whether plasma and urinary TMAO may aid in predicting CVD in early-stage pediatric CKD awaits further elucidation.

Strikingly, less attention has been paid to the TMAO precursor TMA in CV risk. TMA is generated by the metabolism of gut microbes using dietary precursors such as choline or carnitine [34]. Like TMAO, TMA is considered as a uremic toxin [29]. Results from this study identified plasma TMA level is increased in CKD children, which is in accordance with data from CKD adults [29,35]. Children with stage G2–G4 had higher plasma TMA levels than those with stage G1. There was also a trend towards a higher plasma TMAO-to-TMA ratio, an index of FMO activity, in this group. Taking into account that plasma TMA and TMAO levels both are simultaneously elevated in children with advanced CKD, our data suggest their increases could be due to increased gut bacterial production and TMA-to-TMAO conversion. Of note, eGFR exhibited a stronger correlation with the TMA than with TMAO. Additionally, TMAO and BP abnormalities were unrelated, whereas plasma TMA level was positively correlated with awake DBP, asleep DBP, and office DBP. Our findings suggest the superiority for the TMA over TMAO as a cardiovascular risk index in children with early-stage CKD.

Another important result of this study is the description of an inverse association between plasma DMA level and cardiovascular risk. Since we found a strong inverse association between plasma DMA level and eGFR, high plasma level but low urinary level of DMA in advanced CKD is possible due to decreased renal excretion. On the other hand, both TMAO and TMA can be metabolized to DMA. It is presumably that an increased plasma DMA level in children with advanced CKD is due to, at least in part, increased gut microbiota-derived TMA and TMAO production. Our previous study showed that urine DMA level was negatively associated with asleep BP load in CKD children [36]. In the present study, we further confirm that urinary DMA level is inversely associated with awake SBP load, asleep SBP load, awake DBP load, and LV mass. These findings suggest that DMA is superior to TMAO in predicting CV risk in early-stage pediatric CKD. On the other hand, our data demonstrated that DMA-to-TMAO ratio, but not TMAO, in the plasma and urine related to several CV risk markers. Given that phases of TMAO synthesis and metabolism happens simultaneously and that DMA-to-TMAO is considered as an index of TMAO-metabolizing activity, data from this study suggest that measures of the combined ratio instead of individual methylamine (i.e., DMA, TMA, and TMAO) may provide us a better understanding of TMA-TMAO metabolic pathway on CVD in CKD children. On the other hand, a previous study demonstrated that the presence of gut microbes might not be essential for DMA production as its excretion is the same in germ-free and control animals [37]. Therefore, DMA might be produced from other endogenous pathways. Indeed, DMA is also a derivative of nitric oxide (NO) metabolism [38]. Asymmetric dimethylarginine (ADMA), an endogenous inhibitor of NO synthase, can be metabolized by dimethylarginine dimethylaminohydrolase to generate DMA and citrulline [38]. Noteworthily, DMA can come from the TMA–TMAO pathway as well the ADMA–NO pathway, and TMAO and ADMA both are uremic toxins related to cardiovascular risk [34,39]. Whether DMA links two pathways together to play a role in the development of hypertension in CKD awaits further elucidation.

In the current study, CKD children with abnormal and normal ABPM associated into two distinct enterotypes, represented by β-diversity changes. Our data support the notion that gut microbiota is linked to the development of hypertension [40,41]. At the phylum level, the abundance of *Cyanobacteria* was lower in the abnormal vs. normal ABPM group. This finding is in line with an animal study showing that minocycline-treated Dahl salt-sensitive rats developed hypertension related to a decrease in *Cyanobacteria* [42]. Although the *Firmicutes*-to-*Bacteroidetes* ratio has been linked to hypertension [41], we did not find the difference of this ratio between CKD children with normal and abnormal ABPM profile. The reason is possibly because we analyzed gut microbiota in CKD children preceding hypertension onset but not in the stage of established hypertension. According to our data, CKD children with abnormal ABPM group had decreased abundance of genera *Subdoligranulum*, *Faecalibacterium*, *Ruminococcus*, and *Akkermansia*. Low abundance of genera *Subdoligranulum* and *Faecalibacterium* has been identified as a microbial marker in adult hypertensive patients [40,43]. *Ruminococcus* abundance was shown to be deficient in hypertension mice [40]. *Akkermansia* is known as a beneficial gut microbe [44]. Overall, these observations suggest that these certain bacteria populations might have beneficial cardiovascular properties in CKD children to halt the development of hypertension. Moreover, CKD children with abnormal ABPM had decreased abundance of genera *Providencia*, *Gemella*, and *Peptosreptoccocus*. Interestingly, these genera of bacteria have been reported to be involved in TMA production [45]. Thus, whether these microbes play a crucial role on the development of hypertension via mediating the TMA–TMAO metabolic pathway in children with early-stage CKD deserves further clarification. Of note is that a key factor in determining gut microbiota composition is the type of diet in patients with CKD [46]. Since the Mediterranean diet that is rich in fiber has been proven to reduce cardiovascular risk [47], it can be speculated that high-fiber dietary intervention might be an efficient way to control microbiota to further prevent CVD in CKD children [48,49].

This study has several limitations that should be acknowledged. First, a low number of CKD children from one hospital would not be representative of an entire population. Multicenter studies of large numbers of patients may be required to elucidate the true relationship. Second, we presented the associations between certain microbes and BP abnormalities but we do not reveal the pathophysiological mechanism by which those specific microbes contribute to the TMA–TMAO pathway and hypertension. Third, our data might not be applicable to other populations for ethnic reasons. Lastly, there remains a lack of reference for AASI and LVMI to define a cut-off value to indicate normal versus abnormal in a pediatric population. We also did not recruit non-CKD controls because children with CKD stage G1 were served as the controls to compare the differences of BP abnormalities and methylamines levels between two different levels of renal function (i.e., CKD stage G1 vs. stage G2–G4). Although age was different between the two groups, we adjusted the age factor in the multivariate linear regression model.

5. Conclusions

Our study in early-stage CKD children demonstrates the associations between gut microbiota-dependent methylamines and BP abnormalities assessed by ABPM. Our results cast a new light on the link between the TMA–TMAO metabolic pathway, gut microbiota, and cardiovascular risk in CKD children. As hypertension and CKD both can originate from early life, early identification of microbial markers related to cardiovascular risk may aid in developing the ideal intervention to improve cardiovascular outcomes in pediatric CKD.

Author Contributions: C.-N.H.: contributed to concept generation, data interpretation, drafting of the manuscript, critical revision of the manuscript and approval of the article; G.-P.C.-C.: contributed to methodology and approval of the article; S.L.: contributed to methodology and approval of the article; C.-Y.H.: contributed to methodology and approval of the article; P.-C.L.: contributed to data interpretation, critical revision of the manuscript and approval of the article; Y.-L.T.: contributed to concept generation, data interpretation, drafting of the manuscript, critical revision of the manuscript and approval of the article. All authors have read and agreed to the published version of the manuscript.

Funding: This work was supported by grant CMRPG8I0101 from the Kaohsiung Chang Gung Memorial Hospital, Taiwan.

Acknowledgments: We would like to thank the Super Micro Mass Research and Technology Center and the Center for Environmental Toxin and Emerging-Contaminant Research, Cheng Shiu University, Kaohsiung for technical support.

Conflicts of Interest: The authors declare no conflict of interest.

References

1. Go, A.S.; Chertow, G.M.; Fan, D.; McCulloch, C.E.; Hsu, C.Y. Chronic kidney disease and the risks of death, cardiovascular events, and hospitalization. *N. Engl. J. Med.* **2004**, *351*, 1296–1305. [CrossRef]
2. Weaver, D.J.; Mitsnefes, M. Cardiovascular Disease in Children and Adolescents with Chronic Kidney Disease. *Semin. Nephrol.* **2018**, *38*, 559–569. [CrossRef] [PubMed]
3. Ingelfinger, J.R.; Kalantar-Zadeh, K.; Schaefer, F.; World Kidney Day Steering Committee. World Kidney Day 2016: Averting the legacy of kidney disease-focus on childhood. *Pediatr. Nephrol.* **2016**, *31*, 343–348. [CrossRef] [PubMed]
4. Urbina, E.M.; Williams, R.V.; Alpert, B.S.; Collins, R.T.; Daniels, S.R.; Hayman, L.; Jacobson, M.; Mahoney, L.; Mietus-Snyder, M.; Rocchini, A.; et al. Noninvasive assessment of subclinical atherosclerosis in children and adolescents: Recommendations for standard assessment for clinical research: A scientific statement from the American Heart Association. *Hypertension* **2009**, *54*, 919–950. [PubMed]
5. Taal, M.W. Arterial stiffness in chronic kidney disease: An update. *Curr. Opin. Nephrol. Hypertens.* **2014**, *23*, 169–173. [CrossRef] [PubMed]
6. Kupferman, J.C.; Aronson Friedman, L.; Cox, C.; Flynn, J.; Furth, S.; Warady, B.; Mitsnefes, M. CKiD Study Group. BP control and left ventricular hypertrophy regression in children with CKD. *J. Am. Soc. Nephrol.* **2014**, *25*, 167–174. [CrossRef]
7. Ramezani, A.; Raj, D.S. The gut microbiome, kidney disease, and targeted interventions. *J. Am. Soc. Nephrol.* **2014**, *25*, 657–670. [CrossRef]
8. Meijers, B.; Jouret, F.; Evenepoel, P. Linking gut microbiota to cardiovascular disease and hypertension: Lessons from chronic kidney disease. *Pharmacol. Res.* **2018**, *133*, 101–107. [CrossRef]
9. Jovanovich, A.; Isakova, T.; Stubbs, J. Microbiome and Cardiovascular Disease in CKD. *Clin. J. Am. Soc. Nephrol.* **2018**, *13*, 1598–1604. [CrossRef]
10. Schiattarella, G.G.; Sannino, A.; Toscano, E.; Giugliano, G.; Gargiulo, G.; Franzone, A.; Trimarco, B.; Esposito, G.; Perrino, C. Gut microbe-generated metabolite trimethylamine-N-oxide as cardiovascular risk biomarker: A systematic review and dose-response meta-analysis. *Eur. Heart J.* **2017**, *38*, 2948–2956. [CrossRef]
11. Duranton, F.; Cohen, G.; De Smet, R.; Rodriguez, M.; Jankowski, J.; Vanholder, R.; Argiles, A.; European Uremic Toxin Work Group. Normal and pathologic concentrations of uremic toxins. *J. Am. Soc. Nephrol.* **2012**, *23*, 1258–1270. [CrossRef] [PubMed]
12. Smith, J.L.; Wishnok, J.S.; Deen, W.M. Metabolism and excretion of methylamines in rats. *Toxicol. Appl. Pharmacol.* **1994**, *125*, 296–308. [CrossRef] [PubMed]
13. Kidney Disease: Improving Global Outcomes (KDIGO) CKD Work Group. KDIGO 2012 clinical practice guideline for the evaluation and management of chronic kidney disease. *Kidney Int. Suppl.* **2013**, *3*, 1–150.
14. Schwartz, G.J.; Muñoz, A.; Schneider, M.F.; Mak, R.H.; Kaskel, F.; Warady, B.A.; Furth, S.L. New equations to estimate GFR in children with CKD. *J. Am. Soc. Nephrol.* **2009**, *20*, 629–637. [CrossRef] [PubMed]
15. Renkema, K.Y.; Winyard, P.J.; Skovorodkin, I.N.; Levtchenko, E.; Hindryckx, A.; Jeanpierre, C.; Weber, S.; Salomon, R.; Antignac, C.; Vainio, S.; et al. Novel perspectives for investigating congenital anomalies of the kidney and urinary tract (CAKUT). *Nephrol. Dial. Transplant.* **2011**, *26*, 3843–3851. [CrossRef]

16. Hsu, C.N.; Lu, P.C.; Lo, M.H.; Lin, I.C.; Chang-Chien, G.P.; Lin, S.; Tain, Y.L. Gut Microbiota-Dependent Trimethylamine N-Oxide Pathway Associated with Cardiovascular Risk in Children with Early-Stage Chronic Kidney Disease. *Int. J. Mol. Sci.* **2018**, *19*, 3699. [CrossRef]
17. Kollias, A.; Stergiou, W.E.; Witte, K.; Soergelm, M.; Mehls, O.; Schaefer, F. German Working Group on Pediatric Hypertension. Distribution of 24-h ambulatory blood pressure in children: Normalized reference values and role of body dimensions. *J. Hypertens.* **2002**, *20*, 1995–2007.
18. Kollias, A.; Stergiou, G.S.; Dolan, E.; O'Brien, E. Ambulatory arterial stiffness index: A systematic review and meta-analysis. *Atherosclerosis* **2012**, *224*, 291–301. [CrossRef]
19. Daniels, S.R.; Kimball, T.R.; Morrison, J.A.; Khoury, P.; Meyer, R.A. Indexing left ventricular mass to account for differences in body size in children and adolescents without cardiovascular disease. *Am. J. Cardiol.* **1995**, *76*, 699–701. [CrossRef]
20. Flynn, J.T.; Mitsnefes, M.; Pierce, C.; Cole, S.R.; Parekh, R.S.; Furth, S.L.; Warady, B.A. Chronic Kidney Disease in Children Study Group: Blood pressure in children with chronic kidney disease: A report from the Chronic Kidney Disease in Children study. *Hypertension* **2008**, *52*, 631–637. [CrossRef]
21. Wühl, E.; Trivelli, A.; Picca, S.; Litwin, M.; Peco-Antic, A.; Zurowska, A.; Testa, S.; Jankauskiene, A.; Emre, S.; Caldas-Afonso, A.; et al. ESCAPE Trial Group: Strict blood-pressure control and progression of renal failure in children. *N. Engl. J. Med.* **2009**, *361*, 1639–1650.
22. Chou, H.H.; Lin, C.Y.; Chiou, Y.H.; Tain, Y.L.; Wang, Y.F.; Wang, H.H.; Chiou, Y.Y. Clinical characteristics and prevalence of complications of chronic kidney disease in children: The Taiwan Pediatric Renal Collaborative study. *Pediatr. Nephrol.* **2016**, *31*, 1113–1120. [CrossRef] [PubMed]
23. Hsu, C.N.; Lu, P.C.; Lo, M.H.; Lin, I.C.; Tain, Y.L. The association between nitric oxide pathway, blood pressure abnormalities, and cardiovascular risk profile in pediatric chronic kidney disease. *Int. J. Mol. Sci.* **2019**, *20*, 5301. [CrossRef] [PubMed]
24. Graves, J.W.; Althaf, M.M. Utility of ambulatory blood pressure monitoring in children and adolescents. *Pediatr. Nephrol.* **2006**, *21*, 1640–1652. [CrossRef]
25. Eriksen, B.O.; Stefansson, V.T.N.; Jenssen, T.G.; Mathisen, U.D.; Schei, J.; Solbu, M.D.; Wilsgaard, T.; Melsom, T. High Ambulatory Arterial Stiffness Index Is an Independent Risk Factor for Rapid Age-Related Glomerular Filtration Rate Decline in the General Middle-Aged Population. *Hypertension* **2017**, *69*, 651–659. [CrossRef] [PubMed]
26. K/DOQI Workgroup. K/DOQI clinical practice guidelines for cardiovascular disease in dialysis patients. *Am. J. Kidney Dis.* **2005**, *45*, S1–S153.
27. Robinson, R.F.; Nahata, M.C.; Sparks, E.; Daniels, C.; Batisky, D.L.; Hayes, J.R.; Mahan, J.D. Abnormal left ventricular mass and aortic distensibility in pediatric dialysis patients. *Pediatr. Nephrol.* **2005**, *20*, 64–68. [CrossRef]
28. Mitsnefes, M.; Flynn, J.; Cohn, S.; Samuels, J.; Blydt-Hansen, T.; Saland, J.; Kimball, T.; Furth, S.; Warady, B.; CKiD Study Group. Masked hypertension associates with left ventricular hypertrophy in children with CKD. *J. Am. Soc. Nephrol.* **2010**, *21*, 137–144. [CrossRef]
29. Jaworska, K.; Hering, D.; Mosieniak, G.; Bielak-Zmijewska, A.; Pilz, M.; Konwerski, M.; Gasecka, A.; Kapłon-Cieślicka, A.; Filipiak, K.; Sikora, E.; et al. TMA, A Forgotten Uremic Toxin, but Not TMAO, Is Involved in Cardiovascular Pathology. *Toxins* **2019**, *11*, 490. [CrossRef]
30. Kuo, H.C.; Hsu, C.N.; Huang, C.F.; Lo, M.H.; Chien, S.J.; Tain, Y.L. Urinary arginine methylation index associated with ambulatory blood pressure abnormalities in children with chronic kidney disease. *J. Am. Soc. Hypertens.* **2012**, *6*, 385–392. [CrossRef] [PubMed]
31. Stubbs, J.R.; House, J.A.; Ocque, A.J.; Zhang, S.; Johnson, C.; Kimber, C.; Schmidt, K.; Gupta, A.; Wetmore, J.B.; Nolin, T.D.; et al. Serum Trimethylamine-N-Oxide is Elevated in CKD and Correlates with Coronary Atherosclerosis Burden. *J. Am. Soc. Nephrol.* **2016**, *27*, 305–313. [CrossRef] [PubMed]
32. Pelletier, C.C.; Croyal, M.; Ene, L.; Aguesse, A.; Billon-Crossouard, S.; Krempf, M.; Lemoine, S.; Guebre-Egziabher, F.; Juillard, L.; Soulage, C.O. Elevation of Trimethylamine-N-Oxide in Chronic Kidney Disease: Contribution of Decreased Glomerular Filtration Rate. *Toxins* **2019**, *11*, 635. [CrossRef] [PubMed]
33. Posada-Ayala, M.; Zubiri, I.; Martin-Lorenzo, M.; Sanz-Maroto, A.; Molero, D.; Gonzalez-Calero, L.; Fernandez-Fernandez, B.; de la Cuesta, F.; Laborde, C.M.; Barderas, M.G.; et al. Identification of a urine metabolomics signature in patients with advanced-stage chronic kidney disease. *Kidney Int.* **2014**, *85*, 103–111. [CrossRef] [PubMed]

34. Velasquez, M.T.; Ramezani, A.; Manal, A.; Raj, D.S. Trimethylamine N-Oxide: The Good, the Bad and the Unknown. *Toxins* **2016**, *8*, 326. [CrossRef] [PubMed]
35. Storino, G.; Moraes, C.; Saldanha, J.; Mafra, D. Cardiovascular mortality in chronic kidney patients: The role of uremic toxins. *Int. J. Cardiovasc. Sci.* **2015**, *28*, 327–334. [CrossRef]
36. Zeisel, S.H.; DaCosta, K.A.; Fox, J.G. Endogenous formation of dimethylamine. *Biochem. J.* **1985**, *232*, 403–408. [CrossRef]
37. Lin, I.C.; Hsu, C.N.; Lo, M.H.; Chien, S.J.; Tain, Y.L. Low urinary citrulline/arginine ratio associated with blood pressure abnormalities and arterial stiffness in childhood chronic kidney disease. *J. Am. Soc. Hypertens.* **2016**, *10*, 115–123. [CrossRef]
38. Tain, Y.L.; Hsu, C.N. Toxic dimethylarginines: Asymmetric dimethylarginine (ADMA) and symmetric dimethylarginine (SDMA). *Toxins* **2017**, *9*, 92. [CrossRef]
39. Hsu, C.N.; Tain, Y.L. Regulation of Nitric Oxide Production in the Developmental Programming of Hypertension and Kidney Disease. *Int. J. Mol. Sci.* **2018**, *20*, 681. [CrossRef]
40. Li, J.; Zhao, F.; Wang, Y.; Chen, J.; Tao, J.; Tian, G.; Wu, S.; Liu, W.; Cui, Q.; Geng, B.; et al. Gut microbiota dysbiosis contributes to the development of hypertension. *Microbiome* **2017**, *5*, 14. [CrossRef]
41. Galla, S.; Chakraborty, S.; Cheng, X.; Yeo, J.; Mell, B.; Zhang, H.; Mathew, A.V.; Vijay-Kumar, M.; Joe, B. Disparate effects of antibiotics on hypertension. *Physiol. Genomics* **2018**, *50*, 837–845. [CrossRef]
42. Yang, T.; Santisteban, M.M.; Rodriguez, V.; Li, E.; Ahmari, N.; Carvajal, J.M.; Zadeh, M.; Gong, M.; Qi, Y.; Zubcevic, J.; et al. Gut dysbiosis is linked to hypertension. *Hypertension* **2015**, *65*, 1331–1340. [CrossRef] [PubMed]
43. Kim, S.; Goel, R.; Kumar, A.; Qi, Y.; Lobaton, G.; Hosaka, K.; Mohammed, M.; Handberg, E.M.; Richards, E.M.; Pepine, C.J.; et al. Imbalance of gut microbiome and intestinal epithelial barrier dysfunction in patients with high blood pressure. *Clin. Sci. (Lond.)* **2018**, *132*, 701–718. [CrossRef] [PubMed]
44. Cani, P.D.; de Vos, W.M. Next-Generation Beneficial Microbes: The Case of Akkermansia muciniphila. *Front. Microbiol.* **2017**, *8*, 1765. [CrossRef] [PubMed]
45. Nelson, T.M.; Borgogna, J.L.; Brotman, R.M.; Ravel, J.; Walk, S.T.; Yeoman, C.J. Vaginal biogenic amines: Biomarkers of bacterial vaginosis or precursors to vaginal dysbiosis? *Front. Physiol.* **2015**, *6*, 253. [CrossRef] [PubMed]
46. Koppe, L.; Fouque, D.; Soulage, C.O. The Role of Gut Microbiota and Diet on Uremic Retention Solutes Production in the Context of Chronic Kidney Disease. *Toxins* **2018**, *10*, 155. [CrossRef] [PubMed]
47. Estruch, R.; Ros, E.; Salas-Salvado, J.; Covas, M.I.; Corella, D.; Aros, F.; Gómez-Gracia, E.; Ruiz-Gutiérrez, V.; Fiol, M.; Lapetra, J.; et al. Primary prevention of cardiovascular disease with a Mediterranean diet. *N. Engl. J. Med.* **2013**, *368*, 1279–1290. [CrossRef]
48. Sonnenburg, J.L.; Bäckhed, F. Diet-microbiota interactions as moderators of human metabolism. *Nature* **2016**, *535*, 56–64. [CrossRef]
49. Zhang, C.; Yin, A.; Li, H.; Wang, R.; Wu, G.; Shen, J.; Zhang, M.; Wang, L.; Hou, Y.; Ouyang, H.; et al. Dietary Modulation of Gut Microbiota Contributes to Alleviation of Both Genetic and Simple Obesity in Children. *EBioMedicine* **2015**, *2*, 968–984. [CrossRef]

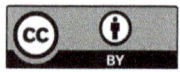

© 2020 by the authors. Licensee MDPI, Basel, Switzerland. This article is an open access article distributed under the terms and conditions of the Creative Commons Attribution (CC BY) license (http://creativecommons.org/licenses/by/4.0/).

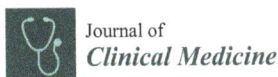

Review

Natriuretic Peptides, Cognitive Impairment and Dementia: An Intriguing Pathogenic Link with Implications in Hypertension

Giovanna Gallo [1], Franca Bianchi [2], Maria Cotugno [2], Massimo Volpe [1,2] and Speranza Rubattu [1,2,*]

1. Department of Clinical and Molecular Medicine, School of Medicine and Psychology, Sapienza University of Rome, 00189 Rome, Italy; giovanna.gallo@uniroma1.it (G.G.); massimo.volpe@uniroma1.it (M.V.)
2. IRCCS Neuromed, 86077 Pozzilli (Isernia), Italy; franca.bianchi@neuromed.it (F.B.); maria.cotugno@neuromed.it (M.C.)
* Correspondence: rubattu.speranza@neuromed.it

Received: 5 June 2020; Accepted: 15 July 2020; Published: 16 July 2020

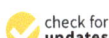

Abstract: The natriuretic peptides (NPs) belong to a family of cardiac hormones that exert relevant protective functions within the cardiovascular system. An increase of both brain and atrial natriuretic peptide levels, particularly of the amino-terminal peptides (NT-proBNP and NT-proANP), represents a marker of cardiovascular damage. A link between increased NP levels and cognitive decline and dementia has been reported in several human studies performed both in general populations and in cohorts of patients affected by cardiovascular diseases (CVDs). In particular, it was reported that the elevation of NP levels in dementia can be both dependent and independent from CVD risk factors. In the first case, it may be expected that, by counteracting early on the cardiovascular risk factor load and the pathological processes leading to increased aminoterminal natriuretic peptide (NT-proNP) level, the risk of dementia could be significantly reduced. In case of a link independent from CVD risk factors, an increased NP level should be considered as a direct marker of neuronal damage. In the context of hypertension, elevated NT-proBNP and mid-regional (MR)-proANP levels behave as markers of brain microcirculatory damage and dysfunction. The available evidence suggests that they could help in identifying those subjects who would benefit most from a timely antihypertensive therapy.

Keywords: natriuretic peptides; brain; cognitive decline; dementia; cardiovascular diseases; stroke; hypertension

---

1. Introduction

Natriuretic peptides (NPs) are a family of cardiovascular hormones mainly secreted by the heart (atrial (ANP) and brain (BNP) natriuretic peptides) and by the endothelium (C-type natriuretic peptide (CNP)) that play important protective functions within the cardiovascular system [1,2]. Apart from their relevant implications in pathophysiology, diagnosis, prognosis and therapeutics of cardiovascular diseases (CVD) [3], a role of BNP and ANP has been convincingly documented in cardiovascular prevention in several population studies, both in apparently healthy individuals and in CVD affected patients [4]. In all circumstances, higher levels of the amino-terminal natriuretic peptides (NT-proBNP and NT-proANP), the more stable forms, predict future cardiovascular events [4]. Whereas the prognostic impact of NPs in patients with CVD can be easily explained as a reflection of the underlying cardiovascular dysfunction and damage, the predictive role of increased NP levels toward future cardiovascular events in apparently healthy individuals is a very intriguing and still unexplained issue. Based on current knowledge on the functional role of the system, it may be supposed that an elevated level of the amino-terminal-NPs in apparently healthy subjects is an index of a subtle initial cardiac and vascular damage that becomes later an overt CVD condition. Therefore, NPs appear able to detect the cardiovascular damage earlier before it could be clinically diagnosed and, while serving as useful markers, they play an important role in the activation of a timely defensive reaction. However, despite these important observations, no clinical guidelines include the use of NT-proBNP level for CVD risk prediction.

Interestingly, the evidence regarding the link between NP level and cardiovascular risk prediction in both healthy subjects and patients with a known history of CVD appears tightly connected to another relevant issue in the context of disease prevention, which is the emerging relationship of NP circulating levels with cognitive decline, vascular dementia and any type of dementia. This important aspect of the pathophysiological implications of NPs has been highlighted over the last recent years, and it certainly deserves to be further characterized. Moreover, its underlying pathophysiological mechanisms need to be better understood.

This article discusses the available evidence on the intriguing relationship between NPs and cognitive decline/dementia, the most plausible explanations and the clinical implications, particularly focusing on hypertension-mediated organ damage.

2. Populations-Based Evidence

In the last few years, an increasing body of literature has reported a significant association between NP level and the development of dementia. One of the first investigation on this matter showed that NT-proBNP level predicted accelerated cognitive and functional decline as well as cardiovascular morbidity and mortality in a prospective cohort study of individuals aged 85 years with a 5-year follow-up [5]. In a Japanese population, NT-proBNP was revealed as a biomarker for the future development of dementia [6]. Moreover, some population studies conducted in the general population reported that serum NT-proBNP level was associated with cognitive impairment and microstructural changes detected by neuroimaging. In particular, Zonnefeld et al. [7] detected an association between NT-proBNP level and reduction of total brain volume, of grey matter volume and of microstructural organization of normal white matter, with a consequent increase of white matter volume. In a community-based middle-aged cohort, higher levels of NT-proBNP were significantly associated with a smaller total grey matter volume, although this association was attenuated after adjusting for cardiovascular risk factors and cardiac output [8]. Thus, based on these observations and on the well-recognized heart–brain link [9], NT-proBNP level can be interpreted as a marker of subclinical cardiac dysfunction, underlying subclinical brain damage and ultimately dementia. If this hypothesis holds true, it is expected that, by disrupting early the pathological processes leading to a rise of NT-proBNP level, we can prevent dementia in older people.

A recent study underscored for the first time the relevance of incremental changes of NT-proBNP level over time by reporting that they were able to predict future dementia in a Caucasian population [10]. In this study, the baseline NT-proBNP level was associated with the future development of impaired cognitive function. Most importantly, a 3-year increase of NT-proBNP level over time was associated with an increased risk of future dementia whereas a decrease of NT-proBNP level was associated with reduced risk of dementia. The NT-proBNP level increase was correlated to the presence of cardiovascular risk factors and concomitant comorbidities, such as impaired renal function, hypertension, diabetes mellitus, smoking habit and coronary artery calcification, which represent potential targets in order to prevent dementia [11,12]. In fact, this study suggested that early treatment of these risk conditions and adequate cardiovascular prevention could avoid dementia development in the elderly. Notably, a higher circulating BNP level appears as a suitable marker for adequate interventional strategies toward these risk conditions and for a successful prevention of progressive cognitive impairment and dementia.

In line with this evidence, a study by Hilal et al. showed that a significant association of NT-proBNP and cognitive impairment exists only in the presence of cerebrovascular disease. Herein, NT-proBNP should be considered as a marker of ischemic brain damage [13,14]. These studies supported the role of circulating markers of cardiac dysfunction reflecting silent brain injury or systemic vascular damage.

On the other hand, few studies have shown that the elevation of NPs in dementia can also occur independently from CVD risk factors and that an increased NT-proBNP level is an independent risk marker for dementia particularly among men [15]. Thus, based on this evidence, it has been proposed that BNP may be a direct marker of neuronal damage and of a pathogenic process located within the brain. In accordance with this hypothesis, the plasma level of BNP was found associated with levels of amyloid-β in the cerebrospinal fluid [16]. The association of NT-proBNP level with dementia in a CVD-free population, as reported by Tynkkynen et al. [15], indicates that the neurodegenerative changes start very early in the course of CVD, as reflected by early changes of the NT-proBNP level. The data obtained by Ferguson et al. in a middle-aged population also support, at least in part, a direct link between BNP and brain damage [8]. Accordingly, in a study by Sabayan et al. [17], a higher NT-proBNP level was associated with alterations of brain structure and function, independently of cardiovascular risk factors and of cardiac output, suggesting that NT-proBNP may be directly related to age-dependent structural and functional brain changes, including decline in brain tissue volume, cognitive impairment, and increased depressive symptoms. Thus, BNP level can be considered as a potential marker for timely preventive and treatment strategies in order to avoid development of dementia later in life [18].

With regard to the relation with age, it is evident that the majority of the studies showing an association between elevated BNP level and mild cognitive impairment (MCI), including conversion from MCI to Alzheimer's disease (AD), and with AD and vascular dementia are confounded by the fact that, often, the patient population is older than the controls. However, few studies have shown that the increase of BNP may be also independent from age. In particular, a study by Hiltunen et al. demonstrated that its prognostic capacity may be only valid among subjects below 79 years of age [19]. With regard to sex, women are disproportionately affected by AD and other types of dementia compared to men, have a greater risk of developing cognitive decline in the presence of risk factors and experience a faster progression of hippocampal atrophy [20,21]. However, although NP levels are higher in women [22], no evidence exists about its influence in the different evolutions of dementia according to sex.

Another important component of the NP family was explored for its ability to predict and possibly associate with dementia. In fact, it was demonstrated that the mid-regional (MR)-proANP level behaved as a marker of microvascular dysfunction and neurodegenerative process in the transition from MCI to AD. Interestingly, MR-proANP played its predictive role independently from blood pressure (BP) level [23]. More recently, an elevated level of MR-proANP was reported to be independently associated with a higher risk of incident all-cause and vascular dementia in a population-based prospective study [24]. Thus, these studies highlighted a CVD-independent role of ANP in dementia and supported some of the findings previously obtained with regard to a direct role of BNP in the brain [15,18].

3. Mechanistic Insights on the Link between NPs and Cognitive Decline/Dementia

3.1. CVD-Dependent Pathogenic Mechanisms

As discussed above, a high NT-proBNP level associates closely with white matter microstructural damage and brain atrophy in subjects with prior onset of CVD and diabetes and in subjects without cardio- and cerebrovascular diseases. Due to the fact that the link between NPs and risk of dementia can be both dependent and independent from CVD and cardiovascular risk factors, the exact pathophysiological mechanisms underlying this association are complex and they are still in part unclear. It may be supposed that subjects with subclinical vascular disease, reflected by an increased NT-proBNP level, first manifest CVD and then dementia. Since BNP is protective and not neurotoxic, its increase should be mainly considered as a marker reflecting mechanisms of cerebral hypoperfusion and neurodegeneration, microemboli and cardioembolic stroke, as the consequence of the cardiovascular risk factors load [25]. In fact, the latter may contribute to the development of atherosclerotic disease responsible for ischemia, endothelial dysfunction, abnormalities in microcirculation, hypoxia, increased inflammation and oxidative stress, interstitial fibrosis, breakdown of blood–brain barrier (BBB) function and damage of the neurovascular unit. The establishment of cerebral microinfarcts might explain the consequent development of clinical dementia. For instance, heart failure leads, as a consequence of reduced cardiac function, to cerebral hypoperfusion, oxidative stress and neuronal dysfunction via deposition of amyloid-β or neurovascular damage [26]. In hypertension, the loss of cerebral vascular autoregulation, resulting in hypoxia and regional cerebral atrophy, mediates the reduction of cognitive function. Thus, an increased NT-proBNP level reflects subclinical disease, particularly poor cardiac function and volume overload in the presence of CVD. In this view, the BNP level increase may reflect a combination of cardiac, neurovascular and neurodegenerative aetiologies. It is also possible that common systemic vascular processes drive both cardiac and brain pathologies. Importantly, given that a higher NT-proBNP level is detected in subjects with higher loads of vascular damage, it should be assessed if timely treatment of CVDs and of cardiovascular risk factors would influence the link between NT-proBNP and brain structural and functional impairments, ultimately preventing the development of cognitive impairment and dementia.

3.2. CVD-Independent Pathogenic Mechanisms

As mentioned before, a second potential mechanism linking NPs and cognitive impairment/dementia is a direct relationship between NT-proBNP and brain structure explained by the presence of BNP [27] and of its receptor in neuronal tissue [28,29]. Several animal and human studies showed an abundant extensive distribution of all NPs in the central nervous system [27]. Their receptors may affect cerebral function through the regulation of BBB integrity, synaptic transmission, and modulation of both systemic and central nervous system stress responses. In fact, it is known that NPs are involved in neural development, in neurotransmitter release, in synaptic transmission, in regulation of inflammatory processes at the level of microglia and in neuroprotection [27–30]. Consistently, ANP has been shown as a neuroprotective agent via upregulation of the Wnt/β-catenin pathway in an in vitro model of Parkinson disease [31]. An increase of ANP upon neprilysin inhibition therapy protected from stroke occurrence in a high-salt-fed stroke-prone spontaneously hypertensive rat model [32]. Furthermore, an increase of circulating ANP levels predicted stroke in apparently healthy individuals [33]. Based on this knowledge, it may be expected that increased levels of NP can indicate the presence of initial brain and vascular damage that will become later on a conclamant disease condition. In this context, as pointed out in the introduction of this article, the NP increase could be considered both as a marker and as a defensive endogenous reaction toward brain damage. Moreover, due to the role that NPs play in regulating several functions that are involved in the course of cognitive impairment, we cannot definitively rule out the possibility that abnormalities of NP regulation and function, as expressed by high levels, may themselves be involved in the development of cognitive impairment/dementia. In all cases, the measurement of NT-proNP levels may represent a useful tool to identify individuals at high risk of developing abnormal brain aging.

It is interesting to note that the protective role of NPs in the brain is strongly supported by the positive results obtained in the past with the use of nesiritide (a human recombinant form of BNP). In fact, its infusion led to an improvement of cerebral blood flow and of brain injury, with a better functional outcome [34]. Moreover, infusion of BNP in ischemic animal models showed a significant infarct volume reduction and a better sensorimotor recovery [35]. The same study reported that patients affected by cardioembolic stroke carrying higher circulating BNP levels presented a better outcome at a 3-month follow-up. Moreover, available evidence shows that low concentrations of NPs in the brain along with elevated systemic concentration are linked to structural and functional cerebral alterations. On the other hand, higher levels of NPs in the brain are crucial for the maintenance of brain homeostasis [27]. This evidence supports the hypothesis that BNP exerts direct protective effects in the brain through its own receptor, its increase may truly be a marker of an ongoing pathological process within the brain and, finally, elevation of BNP level may be a suitable target for therapeutic purposes.

It is likely that both direct and indirect mechanisms underlie the pathogenic relationship between NPs and cognitive decline/dementia. We also need to point out that the intriguing relationship does not necessarily mean causation but that it may rather indicate a correlation/association between NPs and cognitive deficit/dementia.

4. NPs, Cognitive Impairment and Dementia: Implications in Hypertension

Hypertension represents one of the most commonly known risk factors for cognitive impairment and dementia, also including low levels of education, smoking, high total cholesterol, obesity, diabetes, atherosclerosis, arteriolosclerosis, hypertensive vascular damage, impaired vascular autoregulation, heart failure and anaemia. Previous studies showed that high-to-normal BP levels correlated with lower grey matter volume in several brain regions in young adults. Thus, BP-associated grey matter alterations start early in adulthood and emerge continuously across the range of BP [36]. High BP in mid-life has been involved in the development of dementia [37] and even with AD-type pathophysiology, later in life [38]. Interestingly, BP level is increased from 5 to 15 years before the onset of dementia, and it declines within the years before overt development of dementia [39].

The relationship between BP and cognitive decline is known to be age dependent. In particular, low BP level has been constantly associated with poor cognitive function especially in older subjects. It is known that autoregulation of cerebral vasculature increases the blood flow to the brain during reduced cardiac function and in the presence of low BP levels. However, this compensatory mechanism is compromised when systemic blood flow reduction is chronic or subclinical, particularly in the elderly. On the other hand, since low BP levels associate with impaired cognitive function in the elderly, it is likely that elevated BP in the same range of age is an indicator of good cardiac pump function required for adequate perfusion of the brain.

Interestingly, it was observed that the harmful effect of hypertension on the risk of dementia is higher in females than in males [40]. Also, blacks are more likely than whites to develop hypertension and the related cognitive decline [41].

At the tissue level, hypertension induces alterations in neurovascular function that, together with reduced cerebral perfusion, alterations in BBB permeability and deficiency of vascular growth factors, alter neuronal function in regions involved in cognitive function (hippocampus, entorhinal cortex and prefrontal cortex) [42]. At the molecular level, the processes of inflammation and of oxidative stress within the brain tissue may contribute to the link between subclinical CVD and neurodegenerative changes in hypertension (Figure 1), particularly in the presence of other vascular risk factors such as diabetes. In fact, endothelial dysfunction may also play a role. In this context, biomarkers for the microvascular contribution to cognitive impairment and dementia in hypertension are needed.

The relevance of the NP system in this regard is supported by evidence linking BNP to arterial stiffness and BP variability. Arterial stiffness is known to predict cognitive decline in hypertension [43-45]. Of interest, a recent study found a significant association between higher NT-proBNP level and increased arterial stiffness modulated by BP variability [46]. This finding provides a major strength to the pathophysiological implications of BNP, as a marker of arterial stiffness, in the prediction of cognitive decline/dementia in hypertension.

It has been reported that NT-proBNP level reflects poor cardiac function and volume overload in hypertension [47]. An increased NT-proBNP level was independently associated with the presence of subclinical MRI signs of brain small vessel disease in a cohort of hypertensive patients free of stroke and dementia [48]. Thus, NT-proBNP level may provide a useful inexpensive tool to identify subclinical CVD causing subclinical neurodegenerative changes and the need for a timely intervention strategy. In this regard, a few limitations need to be taken into account when using NPs as markers. For instance, it is still uncertain the role that NPs may play in the higher predisposition of both female sex and black subjects to develop cognitive decline and dementia in the presence of hypertension. Of note, females have higher NP levels [22] and blacks have lower NP levels [49]. Apart from sex and race, NP levels are known to be influenced by age, renal function, body mass index and comorbidities so that the assessed plasma NP level has to be considered once adjusted for the above parameters [4].

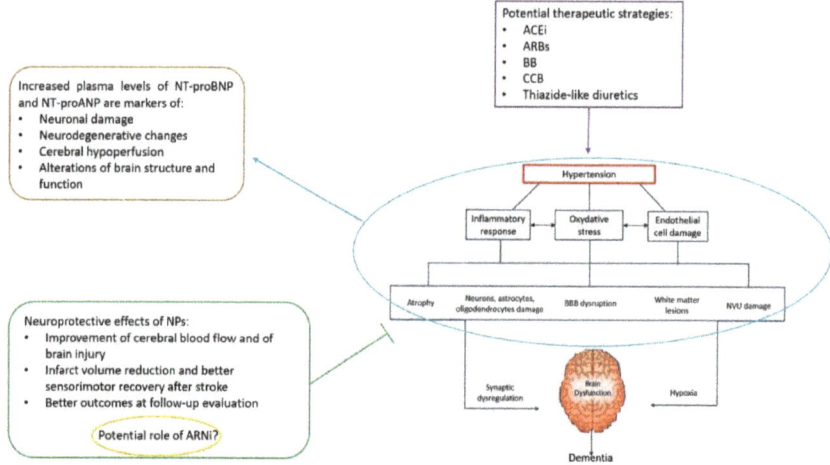

Figure 1. Schematic representation of the pathophysiological mechanisms underlying the development of dementia in hypertension: The role of aminoterminal natriuretic peptides (NT-proNPs) as both markers of brain damage and neuroprotective agents is highlighted. An appropriate antihypertensive treatment can be started on time by taking advantage of the NT-proNP levels in order to counteract the evolution to dementia in older patients.

A study by Kerola et al. [50] reported a trend toward low diastolic BP and new onset of dementia. In this study, the diagnosis of hypertension was associated with lower incidence of dementia in the follow-up, independent of known risk factors for dementia, and it was a likely consequence of the appropriate antihypertensive medications used. Notably, this study, while demonstrating an independent predictive role of BNP towards dementia in the elderly, indicated that cardiovascular morbidity and stress significantly affected cognitive decline in older subjects. Therefore, early initiation of antihypertensive therapy appears of crucial relevance for the prevention of dementia development. In this regard, a few trials have also shown that treatment of hypertension lowered the incidence of cognitive decline in the elderly [51–53]. Thus, it is worthwhile considering the impact of antihypertensive medications on cognitive decline in this group of subjects based on the level of BNP, and, particularly, considering the opportunity to start early the treatment in those patients with elevated BNP levels.

Of note, antihypertensive therapy was shown to reduce the rate of conversion from MCI to AD also in subjects with high MR-proANP [54]. Based on these findings, elevated MR-proANP, as a marker of microcirculatory function in the brain, could help to identify those subjects who would most benefit from antihypertensive therapy.

However, contrasting data also exist. Some studies have demonstrated that treatment of hypertension decreased the risk of vascular and all-cause dementia but it did not decrease the risk for AD, cognitive impairment and cognitive decline. Of note, there are also data regarding the effect of specific antihypertensive treatments. Observational studies reported potential preventive effects toward cognitive decline and dementia with the use of calcium channel blockers and of renin-angiotensin system blockers [55]. Another study [56] has reported that the use of angiotensin converting enzyme inhibitors (ACEI) might associate with a better outcome in terms of cognitive decline. This is probably secondary to the decrease in cardiac workload with a consequent reduction of BNP level rather than to a direct effect of ACEI on local BNP in the brain. The beneficial effects of ACEI toward cognitive impairment were more recently confirmed [57]. In the Perindopril protection against recurrent stroke study (PROGRESS), use of perindopril or indapamide led to a benefit in dementia reduction among individuals with recurrent stroke [58]. In a recent study, telmisartan (an AT1R blocker) synergistically interacted with low-dose rosuvastatin to reduce white matter hypertensive progression and cognitive function decline [59]. Contrasting findings are available with the new pharmacological approach based on neprilysin inhibition in association with an AT1R blocker (ARNi) [60]. Since neprilysin normally degrades amyloid-β, its inhibition was initially seen with particular concern due to the possible risk of increased occurrence of dementia and AD [61]. Other studies, however, have denied a relationship between neprilysin inhibition and AD. It has been supposed that the increased NPs level, as a consequence of ARNi treatment, may counterbalance the detrimental effects of cerebral deposition of amyloid-β [62–64].

It is clear that the optimal antihypertensive regimen able to prevent future cognitive decline or dementia is difficult to assess for each individual, considering that comorbidities, socioeconomic and demographic characteristics may impact on the effect of the therapy.

Based on all abovementioned evidence, it is recommended to diagnose early high BP and to start an appropriate treatment with the aim to avoid cognitive decline and dementia in elderly subjects [65,66]. In this regard, higher NT-proBNP and MR-proANP levels may adequately identify subgroups of patients with marked endothelial dysfunction and microvascular pathology as the most suitable inexpensive markers to indicate a timely and efficacious therapeutic intervention to prevent dementia in hypertensive patients. Finally, based on current knowledge on the neurological functions of NPs, these hormones and their receptors might be a suitable therapeutic target to treat cognitive impairment and dementia (Figure 1).

Author Contributions: Conceptualization, S.R.; methodology, F.B., M.C. and S.R.; investigation, G.G. and S.R.; data curation, G.G. and S.R.; writing—original draft preparation, G.G. and S.R.; writing—review and editing, S.R. and M.V.; funding acquisition, S.R. and M.V. All authors have read and agreed to the published version of the manuscript.

Funding: This research was funded by a grant from the Italian Ministry of Health, and the APC will be funded by a grant from the Italian Ministry of Health.

Conflicts of Interest: The authors declare no conflicts of interest. The funders had no role in the design of the study; in the collection, analyses or interpretation of data; in the writing of the manuscript; or in the decision to publish the results.

Abbreviations

ARNi = angiotensin receptor neprilysin inhibitor; ACEi = angiotensin converting enzyme inhibitor; ARB = angiotensin receptor blocker; BB = beta blocker; CCB = calcium channel blocker; CVD = cardiovascular disease; BBB = blood–brain barrier; NVU = neurovascular unit; NPs = natriuretic peptides; NTproANP= aminoterminal atrial natriuretic peptide; NTproBNP = aminoterminal brain natriuretic peptide.

References

1. Levin, E.R.; Gardner, D.G.; Samson, W.K. Natriuretic peptides. *N. Engl. J. Med.* **1998**, *339*, 321–328. [CrossRef] [PubMed]
2. Rubattu, S.; Sciarretta, S.; Valenti, V.; Stanzione, R.; Volpe, M. Natriuretic peptides: An update on bioactivity, potential therapeutic use, and implication in cardiovascular diseases. *Am. J. Hypertens.* **2008**, *21*, 733–741. [CrossRef] [PubMed]
3. Nakagawa, Y.; Nishikimi, T.; Kuwahara, K. Atrial and brain natriuretic peptides: Hormones secreted from the heart. *Peptides* **2019**, *111*, 18–25. [CrossRef]
4. Volpe, M.; Rubattu, S.; Burnett, J., Jr. Natriuretic peptides in cardiovascular diseases: Current use and perspectives. *Eur. Heart J.* **2014**, *35*, 419–425. [CrossRef]
5. van Peet, P.G.; de Craen, A.J.; Gussekloo, J.; de Ruijter, W. Plasma NT-proBNP as predictor of change in functional status, cardiovascular morbidity and mortality in the oldest old: The Leiden 85-plus study. *Age (Dordr)* **2014**, *36*, 9660. [CrossRef] [PubMed]

6. Nagata, T.; Ohara, T.; Hata, J.; Sakata, S.; Furuta, Y.; Yoshida, D.; Honda, T.; Hirakawa, Y.; Ide, T.; Kanba, S.; et al. NT-proBNP and Risk of Dementia in a General Japanese Elderly Population: The Hisayama Study. *J. Am. Heart Assoc.* **2019**, *8*, e011652. [CrossRef]
7. Zonneveld, H.I.; Arfan Ikram, M.; Hofman, A.; Niessen, W.J.; van der Lugt, A.; Krestin, G.P.; Franco, O.H.; Vernooij, M.W. N-Terminal Pro-B-Type Natriuretic Peptide and Subclinical Brain Damage in the General Population. *Radiology* **2017**, *283*, 205–214. [CrossRef] [PubMed]
8. Ferguson, I.T.; Elbejjani, M.; Sabayan, B.; Jacobs, D.R., Jr.; Meirelles, O.; Sanchez, O.A.; Tracy, R.; Bryan, N.; Launer, L.J. N-Terminal pro-Brain Natriuretic Peptide and Associations With Brain Magnetic Resonance Imaging (MRI) Features in Middle Age: The CARDIA Brain MRI Study. *Front. Neurol.* **2018**, *9*, 307. [CrossRef]
9. Riching, A.S.; Major, J.L.; Londono, P.; Bagchi, R.A. The Brain-Heart Axis: Alzheimer's, Diabetes, and Hypertension. *ACS Pharmacol. Transl. Sci.* **2019**, *3*, 21–28. [CrossRef]
10. Ostovaneh, M.R.; Moazzami, K.; Yoneyama, K.; Venkatesh, B.A.; Heckbert, S.R.; Wu, C.O.; Shea, S.; Post, W.S.; Fitzpatrick, A.L.; Burke, G.L.; et al. Change in NT-proBNP (N-Terminal Pro-B-Type Natriuretic Peptide) Level and Risk of Dementia in Multi-Ethnic Study of Atherosclerosis (MESA). *Hypertension* **2020**, *75*, 316–323. [CrossRef]
11. Di Daniele, N.; Celotto, R.; Alunni Fegatelli, D.; Gabriele, M.; Rovella, V.; Scuteri, A. Common Carotid Artery Calcification Impacts on Cognitive Function in Older Patients. *High Blood Press. Cardiovasc. Prev.* **2019**, *26*, 127–134. [CrossRef] [PubMed]
12. Rizzoni, D.; Rizzoni, M.; Nardin, M.; Chiarini, G.; Agabiti-Rosei, C.; Aggiusti, C.; Paini, A.; Salvetti, M.; Muiesan, M.L. Vascular Aging and Disease of the Small Vessels. *High Blood Press. Cardiovasc. Prev.* **2019**, *26*, 183–189. [CrossRef]
13. Hilal, S.; Chai, Y.L.; Ikram, M.K.; Elangovan, S.; Yeow, T.B.; Xin, X.; Chong, J.Y.; Venketasubramanian, N.; Richards, A.M.; Chong, J.P.C.; et al. Markers of Cardiac Dysfunction in Cognitive Impairment and Dementia. *Medicine (Baltimore)* **2015**, *94*, e297. [CrossRef] [PubMed]
14. Hilal, S.; Chai, Y.L.; van Veluw, S.; Shaik, M.A.; Ikram, M.K.; Venketasubramanian, N.; Richards, A.M.; Biessels, G.J.; Chen, C. Association Between Subclinical Cardiac Biomarkers and Clinically Manifest Cardiac Diseases With Cortical Cerebral Microinfarcts. *JAMA Neurol.* **2017**, *74*, 403–410. [CrossRef] [PubMed]
15. Tynkkynen, J.; Hernesniemi, J.A.; Laatikainen, T.; Havulinna, A.S.; Salo, P.; Blankenberg, S.; Zeller, T.; Salomaa, V. High-sensitivity cardiac troponin I and NT-proBNP as predictors of incident dementia and Alzheimer's disease: The FINRISK Study. *J. Neurol.* **2017**, *264*, 503–511. [CrossRef] [PubMed]
16. Hu, W.T.; Holtzman, D.M.; Fagan, A.M.; Shaw, L.M.; Perrin, R.; Arnold, S.E.; Grossman, M.; Xiong, C.; Craig-Schapiro, R.; Clark, C.M.; et al. Alzheimer's Disease Neuroimaging Initiative. Plasma multianalyte profiling in mild cognitive impairment and Alzheimer disease [published correction appears in Neurology. 2012 Oct 30;79(18):1935]. *Neurology* **2012**, *79*, 897–905. [CrossRef]
17. Sabayan, B.; van Buchem, M.A.; Sigurdsson, S.; Zhang, Q.; Harris, T.B.; Gudnason, V.; Arai, A.E.; Launer, L.J. Cardiac hemodynamics are linked with structural and functional features of brain aging: The age, gene/environment susceptibility (AGES)-Reykjavik Study. *J. Am. Heart Assoc.* **2015**, *4*, e001294. [CrossRef]
18. Mirza, S.S.; de Bruijn, R.F.; Koudstaal, P.J.; van den Meiracker, A.H.; Franco, O.H.; Hofman, A.; Tiemeier, H.; Ikram, M.A. The N-terminal pro B-type natriuretic peptide, and risk of dementia and cognitive decline: A 10-year follow-up study in the general population. *J. Neurol. Neurosurg. Psychiatry* **2016**, *87*, 356–362. [CrossRef]
19. Hiltunen, M.; Kerola, T.; Kettunen, R.; Hartikainen, S.; Sulkava, R.; Vuolteenaho, O.; Nieminen, T. The prognostic capacity of B-type natriuretic peptide on cognitive disorder varies by age. *Ann. Med.* **2013**, *45*, 74–78. [CrossRef]
20. Mazure, C.M.; Swendsen, J. Sex differences in Alzheimer's disease and other dementias. *Lancet Neurol.* **2016**, *15*, 451–452. [CrossRef]
21. Rocca, W.A.; Mielke, M.M.; Vemuri, P.; Miller, V.M. Sex and gender differences in the causes of dementia: A narrative review. *Maturitas* **2014**, *79*, 196–201. [CrossRef] [PubMed]
22. Lam, C.S.; Cheng, S.; Choong, K.; Larson, M.G.; Murabito, J.M.; Newton-Cheh, C.; Bhasin, S.; McCabe, E.L.; Miller, K.K.; Redfield, M.M.; et al. Influence of sex and hormone status on circulating natriuretic peptides. *J. Am. Coll. Cardiol.* **2011**, *58*, 618–626. [CrossRef] [PubMed]

23. Buerger, K.; Uspenskaya, O.; Hartmann, O.; Hansson, O.; Minthon, L.; Blennow, K.; Moeller, H.J.; Teipel, S.J.; Ernst, A.; Bergmann, A.; et al. Prediction of Alzheimer's disease using midregional proadrenomedullin and midregional proatrial natriuretic peptide: A retrospective analysis of 134 patients with mild cognitive impairment. *J. Clin. Psychiatry* **2011**, *72*, 556–563. [CrossRef] [PubMed]
24. Holm, H.; Nägga, K.; Nilsson, E.D.; Ricci, F.; Melander, O.; Hansson, O.; Bachus, E.; Magnusson, M.; Fedorowski, A. Biomarkers of microvascular endothelial dysfunction predict incident dementia: A population-based prospective study. *J. Intern. Med.* **2017**, *282*, 94–101. [CrossRef] [PubMed]
25. Abete, P.; Della-Morte, D.; Gargiulo, G.; Basile, C.; Langellotto, A.; Galizia, G.; Testa, G.; Canonico, V.; Bonaduce, D.; Cacciatore, F. Cognitive impairment and cardiovascular diseases in the elderly. A heart-brain continuum hypothesis. *Ageing Res. Rev.* **2014**, *18*, 41–52. [CrossRef]
26. Mueller, K.; Thiel, F.; Beutner, F.; Teren, A.; Frisch, S.; Ballarini, T.; Möller, H.E.; Ihle, K.; Thiery, J.; Schuler, G.; et al. Brain Damage With Heart Failure: Cardiac Biomarker Alterations and Gray Matter Decline. *Circ. Res.* **2020**, *126*, 750–764. [CrossRef]
27. Mahinrad, S.; de Craen, A.J.M.; Yasar, S.; van Heemst, D.; Sabayan, B. Natriuretic peptides in the central nervous system: Novel targets for cognitive impairment. *Neurosci. Biobehav. Rev.* **2016**, *68*, 148–156. [CrossRef]
28. Cao, L.H.; Yang, X.L. Natriuretic peptides and their receptors in the central nervous system. *Prog. Neurobiol.* **2008**, *84*, 234–248. [CrossRef]
29. Prado, J.; Baltrons, M.A.; Pifarré, P.; García, A. Glial cells as sources and targets of natriuretic peptides. *Neurochem. Int.* **2010**, *57*, 367–374. [CrossRef]
30. Quirion, R. Receptor sites for atrial natriuretic factors in brain and associated structures: An overview. *Cell. Mol. Neurobiol.* **1989**, *9*, 45–55. [CrossRef]
31. Colini Baldeschi, A.; Pittaluga, E.; Andreola, F.; Rossi, S.; Cozzolino, M.; Nicotera, G.; Sferrazza, G.; Pierimarchi, P.; Serafino, A. Atrial Natriuretic Peptide Acts as a Neuroprotective Agent in in Vitro Models of Parkinson's Disease via Up-regulation of the Wnt/β-Catenin Pathway. *Front. Aging Neurosci.* **2018**, *10*, 20. [CrossRef] [PubMed]
32. Rubattu, S.; Cotugno, M.; Forte, M.; Stanzione, R.; Bianchi, F.; Madonna, M.; Marchitti, S.; Volpe, M. Effects of dual angiotensin type 1 receptor/neprilysin inhibition vs. angiotensin type 1 receptor inhibition on target organ injury in the stroke-prone spontaneously hypertensive rat. *J. Hypertens.* **2018**, *36*, 1902–1914. [CrossRef]
33. Wang, T.J.; Larson, M.G.; Levy, D.; Benjamin, E.J.; Leip, E.P.; Omland, T.; Wolf, P.A.; Vasan, R.S. Plasma natriuretic peptide levels and the risk of cardiovascular events and death. *N. Engl. J. Med.* **2004**, *350*, 655–663. [CrossRef]
34. James, M.L.; Wang, H.; Venkatraman, T.; Song, P.; Lascola, C.D.; Laskowitz, D.T. Brain natriuretic peptide improves long-term functional recovery after acute CNS injury in mice. *J. Neurotrauma* **2010**, *27*, 217–228. [CrossRef] [PubMed]
35. Fernández-Susavila, H.; Rodríguez-Yáñez, M.; Dopico-López, A.; Arias, S.; Santamaría, M.; Ávila-Gómez, P.; Doval-García, J.M.; Sobrino, T.; Iglesias-Rey, R.; Castillo, J.; et al. Heads and Tails of Natriuretic Peptides: Neuroprotective Role of Brain Natriuretic Peptide. *J. Am. Heart Assoc.* **2017**, *6*, e007329. [CrossRef]
36. Schaare, H.L.; Kharabian Masouleh, S.; Beyer, F.; Kumral, D.; Uhlig, M.; Reinelt, J.D.; Reiter, A.M.F.; Lampe, L.; Babayan, A.; Erbey, M.; et al. Association of peripheral blood pressure with gray matter volume in 19-to 40-year-old adults [published correction appears in Neurology. 2019 Mar 5;92(10):495]. *Neurology* **2019**, *92*, e758–e773. [CrossRef] [PubMed]
37. Launer, L.J.; Ross, G.W.; Petrovitch, H.; Masaki, K.; Foley, D.; White, L.R.; Havlik, R.J. Midlife blood pressure and dementia: The Honolulu-Asia aging study. *Neurobiol. Aging* **2000**, *21*, 49–55. [CrossRef]
38. Iadecola, C.; Yaffe, K.; Biller, J.; Bratzke, L.C.; Faraci, F.M.; Gorelick, P.B.; Gulati, M.; Kamel, H.; Knopman, D.S.; Launer, L.J.; et al. Impact of Hypertension on Cognitive Function: A Scientific Statement From the American Heart Association. *Hypertension* **2016**, *68*, e67–e94. [CrossRef] [PubMed]
39. Pandav, R.; Dodge, H.H.; DeKosky, S.T.; Ganguli, M. Blood pressure and cognitive impairment in India and the United States: A cross-national epidemiological study. *Arch. Neurol.* **2003**, *60*, 1123–1128. [CrossRef] [PubMed]
40. Gilsanz, P.; Mayeda, E.R.; Glymour, M.M.; Quesenberry, C.P.; Mungas, D.M.; DeCarli, C.; Dean, A.; Whitmer, R.A. Female sex, early-onset hypertension, and risk of dementia. *Neurology* **2017**, *89*, 1886–1893. [CrossRef] [PubMed]

41. Levine, D.A.; Galecki, A.T.; Langa, K.M.; Unverzagt, F.W.; Kabeto, M.U.; Giordani, B.; Cushman, M.; McClure, L.A.; Safford, M.M.; Wadley, V.G. Blood Pressure and Cognitive Decline Over 8 Years in Middle-Aged and Older Black and White Americans. *Hypertension* **2019**, *73*, 310–318. [CrossRef] [PubMed]
42. Iadecola, C.; Gottesman, R.F. Neurovascular and Cognitive Dysfunction in Hypertension. *Circ. Res.* **2019**, *124*, 1025–1044. [CrossRef] [PubMed]
43. Scuteri, A.; Brancati, A.M.; Gianni, W.; Assisi, A.; Volpe, M. Arterial stiffness is an independent risk factor for cognitive impairment in the elderly: A pilot study. *J. Hypertens.* **2005**, *23*, 1211–1216. [CrossRef]
44. Rouch, L.; Cestac, P.; Sallerin, B.; Andrieu, S.; Bailly, H.; Beunardeau, M.; Cohen, A.; Dubail, D.; Hernandorena, I.; Seux, M.L.; et al. Pulse Wave Velocity Is Associated With Greater Risk of Dementia in Mild Cognitive Impairment Patients. *Hypertension* **2018**, *72*, 1109–1116. [CrossRef] [PubMed]
45. Neves, M.F.; Cunha, A.R.; Cunha, M.R.; Gismondi, R.A.; Oigman, W. The Role of Renin-Angiotensin-Aldosterone System and Its New Components in Arterial Stiffness and Vascular Aging. *High Blood Press. Cardiovasc. Prev.* **2018**, *25*, 137–145. [CrossRef] [PubMed]
46. Ishiyama, Y.; Hoshide, S.; Kanegae, H.; Kario, K. Increased Arterial Stiffness Amplifies the Association Between Home Blood Pressure Variability and Cardiac Overload: The J-HOP Study. *Hypertension* **2020**, *75*, 1600–1606. [CrossRef] [PubMed]
47. McDonagh, T.A.; Robb, S.D.; Murdoch, D.R.; Morton, J.J.; Ford, I.; Morrison, C.E.; Tunstall-Pedoe, H.; McMurray, J.J.; Dargie, H.J. Biochemical detection of left-ventricular systolic dysfunction. *Lancet* **1998**, *351*, 9–13. [CrossRef]
48. Vilar-Bergua, A.; Riba-Llena, I.; Penalba, A.; Cruz, L.M.; Jiménez-Balado, J.; Montaner, J.; Delgado, P. N-terminal pro-brain natriuretic peptide and subclinical brain small vessel disease. *Neurology* **2016**, *87*, 2533–2539. [CrossRef]
49. Rubattu, S.; Stanzione, R.; Cotugno, M.; Bianchi, F.; Marchitti, S.; Forte, M. Epigenetic control of natriuretic peptides: Implications for health and disease. *Cell. Mol. Life Sci.* **2020**, in press. [CrossRef]
50. Kerola, T.; Nieminen, T.; Hartikainen, S.; Sulkava, R.; Vuolteenaho, O.; Kettunen, R. B-type natriuretic peptide as a predictor of declining cognitive function and dementia—A cohort study of an elderly general population with a 5-year follow-up. *Ann. Med.* **2010**, *42*, 207–215. [CrossRef]
51. Staessen, J.A.; Fagard, R.; Thijs, L.; Celis, H.; Arabidze, G.G.; Birkenhäger, W.H.; Bulpitt, C.J.; de Leeuw, P.W.; Dollery, C.T.; Fletcher, A.E.; et al. Randomised double-blind comparison of placebo and active treatment for older patients with isolated systolic hypertension. The Systolic Hypertension in Europe (Syst-Eur) Trial Investigators. *Lancet* **1997**, *350*, 757–764. [CrossRef]
52. Hanon, O.; Forette, F. Prevention of dementia: Lessons from SYST-EUR and PROGRESS. *J. Neurol. Sci.* **2004**, *226*, 71–74. [CrossRef]
53. Ikram, M.A.; Brusselle, G.G.O.; Murad, S.D.; van Duijn, C.M.; Franco, O.H.; Goedegebure, A.; Klaver, C.C.W.; Nijsten, T.E.C.; Peeters, R.P.; Stricker, B.H.; et al. The Rotterdam Study: 2018 update on objectives, design and main results. *Eur. J. Epidemiol.* **2017**, *32*, 807–850. [CrossRef] [PubMed]
54. Schneider, P.; Buerger, K.; Teipel, S.; Uspenskaya, O.; Hartmann, O.; Hansson, O.; Minthon, L.; Rujescu, D.; Moeller, H.J.; Zetterberg, H.; et al. Antihypertensive therapy is associated with reduced rate of conversion to Alzheimer's disease in midregional proatrial natriuretic peptide stratified subjects with mild cognitive impairment. *Biol. Psychiatry* **2011**, *70*, 145–151. [CrossRef] [PubMed]
55. Hernandorena, I.; Duron, E.; Vidal, J.S.; Hanon, O. Treatment options and considerations for hypertensive patients to prevent dementia. *Expert Opin. Pharmacother.* **2017**, *18*, 989–1000. [CrossRef] [PubMed]
56. Sink, K.M.; Leng, X.; Williamson, J.; Kritchevsky, S.B.; Yaffe, K.; Kuller, L.; Yasar, S.; Atkinson, H.; Robbins, M.; Psaty, B.; et al. Angiotensin-converting enzyme inhibitors and cognitive decline in older adults with hypertension: Results from the Cardiovascular Health Study. *Arch. Intern. Med.* **2009**, *169*, 1195–1202. [CrossRef]
57. Csikai, E.; Andrejkovics, M.; Balajthy-Hidegh, B.; Hofgárt, G.; Kardos, L.; Diószegi, Á.; Rostás, R.; Czuriga-Kovács, K.R.; Csongrádi, É.; Csiba, L. Influence of angiotensin-converting enzyme inhibition on reversibility of alterations in arterial wall and cognitive performance associated with early hypertension: A follow-up study. *Medicine (Baltimore)* **2019**, *98*, e16945. [CrossRef]

58. Tzourio, C.; Anderson, C.; Chapman, N.; Woodward, M.; Neal, B.; MacMahon, S.; Chalmers, J.; PROGRESS Collaborative Group. Effects of blood pressure lowering with perindopril and indapamide therapy on dementia and cognitive decline in patients with cerebrovascular disease. *Arch. Intern. Med.* **2003**, *163*, 1069–1075. [CrossRef] [PubMed]
59. Zhang, H.; Cui, Y.; Zhao, Y.; Dong, Y.; Duan, D.; Wang, J.; Sheng, L.; Ji, T.; Zhou, T.; Hu, W.; et al. Effects of sartans and low-dose statins on cerebral white matter hyperintensities and cognitive function in older patients with hypertension: A randomized, double-blind and placebo-controlled clinical trial. *Hypertens. Res.* **2019**, *42*, 717–729. [CrossRef]
60. Bavishi, C.; Messerli, F.H.; Kadosh, B.; Ruilope, L.M.; Kario, K. Role of neprilysin inhibitor combinations in hypertension: Insights from hypertension and heart failure trials. *Eur. Heart J.* **2015**, *36*, 1967–1973. [CrossRef]
61. McMurray, J.J.; Packer, M.; Desai, A.S.; Gong, J.; Lefkowitz, M.P.; Rizkala, A.R.; Rouleau, J.L.; Shi, V.C.; Solomon, S.D.; Swedberg, K.; et al. Angiotensin-neprilysin inhibition versus enalapril in heart failure. *N. Engl. J. Med.* **2014**, *371*, 993–1004. [CrossRef]
62. Cannon, J.A.; Shen, L.; Jhund, P.S.; Kristensen, S.L.; Køber, L.; Chen, F.; Gong, J.; Lefkowitz, M.P.; Rouleau, J.L.; Shi, V.C.; et al. Dementia-related adverse events in PARADIGM-HF and other trials in heart failure with reduced ejection fraction. *Eur. J. Heart Fail.* **2017**, *19*, 129–137. [CrossRef] [PubMed]
63. Packer, M. Kicking the tyres of a heart failure trial: Physician response to the approval of sacubitril/valsartan in the USA. *Eur. J. Heart Fail.* **2016**, *18*, 1211–1219. [CrossRef] [PubMed]
64. Langenickel, T.H.; Tsubouchi, C.; Ayalasomayajula, S.; Pal, P.; Valentin, M.A.; Hinder, M.; Jhee, S.; Gevorkyan, H.; Rajman, I. The effect of LCZ696 (sacubitril/valsartan) on amyloid-β concentrations in cerebrospinal fluid in healthy subjects. *Br. J. Clin. Pharmacol.* **2016**, *81*, 878–890. [CrossRef] [PubMed]
65. Lowy, A.; Munk, V.C.; Ong, S.H.; Burnier, M.; Vrijens, B.; Tousset, E.P.; Urquhart, J. Effects on blood pressure and cardiovascular risk of variations in patients' adherence to prescribed antihypertensive drugs: Role of duration of drug action. *Int. J. Clin. Pract.* **2011**, *65*, 41–53. [CrossRef] [PubMed]
66. Peters, R.; Yasar, S.; Anderson, C.S.; Andrews, S.; Antikainen, R.; Arima, H.; Beckett, N.; Beer, J.C.; Bertens, A.S.; Booth, A. Investigation of antihypertensive class, dementia, and cognitive decline: A meta-analysis. *Neurology* **2020**, *94*, e267–e281. [CrossRef]

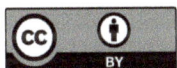

© 2020 by the authors. Licensee MDPI, Basel, Switzerland. This article is an open access article distributed under the terms and conditions of the Creative Commons Attribution (CC BY) license (http://creativecommons.org/licenses/by/4.0/).

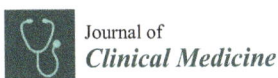

Article

Risk Stratification in Hypertrophic Cardiomyopathy. Insights from Genetic Analysis and Cardiopulmonary Exercise Testing

Damiano Magrì [1,*,†], Vittoria Mastromarino [1,2], Giovanna Gallo [1], Elisabetta Zachara [3], Federica Re [3], Piergiuseppe Agostoni [4,5], Dario Giordano [1], Speranza Rubattu [1,6,*], Maurizio Forte [6], Maria Cotugno [6], Maria Rosaria Torrisi [1,7], Simona Petrucci [1,7], Aldo Germani [1,7], Camilla Savio [7], Antonello Maruotti [8,9,10], Massimo Volpe [1,6], Camillo Autore [1], Maria Piane [1,7,†] and Beatrice Musumeci [1]

1. Department of Clinical and Molecular Medicine, Sapienza University, 00100 Rome, Italy; vittoriamastromarino@libero.it (V.M.); giovanna.gallo@uniroma1.it (G.G.); dariogiordano@outlook.com (D.G.); mara.torrisi@uniroma1.it (M.R.T.); simona.petrucci@uniroma1.it (S.P.); aldo.germani@uniroma1.it (A.G.); massimo.volpe@uniroma1.it (M.V.); camillo.autore@uniroma1.it (C.A.); maria.piane@uniroma1.it (M.P.); beatrice.musumeci@uniroma1.it (B.M.)
2. Unit of Pediatric Cardiology and Cardiac Surgery, Sant'Orsola Hospital, 40100 Bologna, Italy
3. Cardiac Arrhythmia Center and Cardiomyopathies Unit, San Camillo—Forlanini Hospital, 00100 Rome, Italy; elisabettazachara@gmail.com (E.Z.); re.federica77@gmail.com (F.R.)
4. Centro Cardiologico Monzino, IRCCS, 20100 Milan, Italy; piergiuseppe.agostoni@unimi.it
5. Department of Clinical Sciences and Community Health, University of Milan, 20100 Milan, Italy
6. IRCCS Neuromed, 86077 Pozzilli (IS), Italy; maurizio.forte@neuromed.it (M.F.); maria.cotugno@neuromed.it (M.C.)
7. UOC Medical Genetics and Advanced Cell Diagnostics, S. Andrea University Hospital, 00100 Rome, Italy; camilla.savio@ospedalesantandrea.it
8. Department of Scienze Economiche, Politiche e delle Lingue Moderne—Libera Università SS Maria Assunta, 00100 Rome, Italy; a.maruotti@lumsa.it
9. Department of Mathematics, University of Bergen, 5052 Bergen, Norway
10. School of Computing, University of Portsmouth, Portsmouth PO1, UK
* Correspondence: damiano.magri@uniroma1.it (D.M.); rubattu.speranza@neuromed.it (S.R.)
† These authors contributed equally.

Received: 4 May 2020; Accepted: 26 May 2020; Published: 28 May 2020

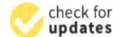

Abstract: The role of genetic testing over the clinical and functional variables, including data from the cardiopulmonary exercise test (CPET), in the hypertrophic cardiomyopathy (HCM) risk stratification remains unclear. A retrospective genotype–phenotype correlation was performed to analyze possible differences between patients with and without likely pathogenic/pathogenic (LP/P) variants. A total of 371 HCM patients were screened at least for the main sarcomeric genes *MYBPC3* (myosin binding protein C), *MYH7* (β-myosin heavy chain), *TNNI3* (cardiac troponin I) and *TNNT2* (cardiac troponin T): 203 patients had at least an LP/P variant, 23 patients had a unique variant of uncertain significance (VUS) and 145 did not show any LP/P variant or VUS. During a median 5.4 years follow-up, 51 and 14 patients developed heart failure (HF) and sudden cardiac death (SCD) or SCD-equivalents events, respectively. The LP/P variant was associated with a more aggressive HCM phenotype. However, left atrial diameter (LAd), circulatory power (peak oxygen uptake*peak systolic blood pressure, CP%) and ventilatory efficiency (C-index = 0.839) were the only independent predictors of HF whereas only LAd and CP% were predictors of the SCD end-point (C-index = 0.738). The present study reaffirms the pivotal role of the clinical variables and, particularly of those CPET-derived, in the HCM risk stratification.

Keywords: hypertrophic cardiomyopathy; cardiopulmonary exercise test; genetic testing

1. Introduction

Hypertrophic cardiomyopathy (HCM), the most common genetic heart disease, inherited with an autosomal dominant pattern, incomplete penetrance and variable expressivity, is characterized by markedly different instrumental and clinical spectra [1–3]. Accordingly, there is always great interest in investigating approaches potentially able to identify early those HCM patients at high risk of cardiovascular events both in terms of sudden cardiac death (SCD) and heart failure (HF). Indeed, albeit the SCD is a devastating but relatively rare event, HF development and its related complications still represent an incoming concern in HCM patients [4–6].

In such a context, due to its genetic nature, many researchers attempted not only an HCM genotype–phenotype correlation but also a possible genotype-based risk stratification. Indeed, HCM is predominantly a sarcomeric disease and variants in *MYH7* and *MYBPC3* genes, encoding for the cardiac thick myofilament proteins β-myosin heavy chain and myosin binding protein C, respectively, together account about 50% of the HCM families. Conversely, likely pathogenic/pathogenic (LP/P) variants in thin filament protein genes, such as *TNNT2*, *TNNI3* and *TPM1* encoding for cardiac troponin T, troponin I and alpha-tropomyosin, account for less than 10% [6–9]. Several studies have demonstrated that being carriers of sarcomeric variants might exert a negative prognostic impact on outcome, as well as multiple simultaneous variants, such as the so-called "gene dosage effect" [8–13]. What remains unclear, up to now, is whether the genetic profile of the single HCM patient might provide a real significant incremental risk prediction beyond the clinical risk factors, including those derived from a maximal cardiopulmonary exercise test (CPET) [2,3]. Indeed, growing evidence suggests that a CPET assessment, combined with other clinical and instrumental variables, represents a useful tool in stratifying both the SCD and the HF-related events' risk in HCM patients [14–18].

Therefore, the current multicenter retrospective study investigates a possible adjunctive role of genetic testing analysis in the HCM patients' management over the main clinical and functional parameters. Particularly, a genotype–phenotype correlation was performed to analyze possible differences between HCM patients with and without LP/P variants with respect to their main clinical and functional features and, mainly, their SCD and HF-related events' rate.

2. Methods

2.1. Study Sample

Data from a total of 665 consecutive outpatients with HCM were analyzed. All patients were part of a cohort recruited and prospectively followed in three HCM Italian centers between September 2007 and December 2019: Azienda Ospedaliera Universitaria Sant'Andrea, "Sapienza" University, Rome (n = 437); Azienda Ospedaliera San Camillo Forlanini, Rome (n = 189); Centro Cardiologico Monzino, University of Milan, Milan (n = 39). The diagnosis of HCM was based on maximal wall thickness (MWT) ≥ 15 mm unexplained by abnormal loading conditions or in accordance with published criteria for the diagnosis of disease in relatives of patients with unequivocal disease [2,3]. Patients with known metabolic diseases or syndromic causes of HCM were excluded from the present study.

The study complied with the ethical standards of the Declaration of Helsinki and was reviewed and approved by the institutional ethics committees. Written informed consent was obtained from all participants. The authors from each participating center guarantee the integrity of data from their institution and have agreed to the article as written.

2.2. Patients Clinical and Functional Assessment

Data were independently collected at each participating center using a uniform methodology. Each HCM patient underwent a clinical assessment, including history with pedigree analysis and the New York Heart Association (NYHA) classification, 24 h ECG Holter monitoring, transthoracic Doppler echocardiography and maximal CPET. The usual five SCD risk factors were also collected [2,3]: (a) FH-SCD (history of HCM-related SCD in at least one first-degree or other relatives younger than 50 years old); (b) massive left ventricular (LV) hypertrophy (maximal wall thickness, MWT, ≥30 mm); (c) at least one run of nonsustained ventricular tachycardia (NSVT, ≥3 consecutive ventricular beats at a rate of ≥120 beats per minute and <30 s in duration on 24 h ECG Holter monitoring); (d) unexplained syncope judged inconsistent with neurocardiogenic origin; (e) abnormal blood pressure response to exercise (ABPRE, failure to increase systolic blood pressure, SBP, by at least 20 mmHg from rest to peak exercise or a fall of ≥20 mmHg from SBP).

The following echocardiographic measurements, obtained according to the international guidelines [19], were considered: LV end-diastolic diameter (LVEDd, parasternal long axis), the greatest LV thickness (MWT, measured at any LV site), left atrial diameter (LAd, parasternal long axis), the highest maximal LV outflow tract gradient among those measured at rest, in orthostatic position and after Valsalva maneuver (LVOTGmax, apical four-chamber view) [20] and LV ejection fraction with Simpson's biplane methods (LVEF, apical four-chamber view).

All CPETs were performed using an electronically braked cycle ergometer. A personalized ramp exercise protocol was performed, aiming at a test duration of 10 ± 2 min [21]. The exercise was preceded by a few minutes of resting breath-by-breath gas exchange monitoring and by an unloaded warm-up. In the absence of clinical events, CPET was interrupted when patients stated that they had reached maximal effort. A 12-lead ECG, diastolic and systolic blood pressure were recorded during CPET, in order to obtain the following parameters: rest heart rate (HR), peak HR, %pHR ((peak HR/(220 − age)) × 100), and ΔSBP (peak SBP − rest SBP) [22]. A breath-by-breath analysis of expiratory gases and ventilation (VE) has been performed, and peak values were obtained in the last 20 s of exercise. The predicted peak VO_2 was determined by using the gender-, age- and weight-adjusted formula. Circulatory power (CP = peak VO_2 × SBP) was obtained considering peak VO_2 value as a percentage of predicted (CP%) [19,23]. Anaerobic threshold (AT) was measured by V-slope analysis of VO_2 and VCO_2, and it was confirmed by ventilator equivalents and end-tidal pressures of CO_2 and O_2 [24]. The end of the isocapnic buffering period was identified when VE/VCO_2 increased and the end-tidal pressure of CO_2 decreased. VE/VCO_2 slope was calculated as the slope of the linear relationship between VE and VCO_2 from the 1st minute after the beginning of the loaded exercise and the end of the isocapnic buffering period [24].

2.3. Genetic Testing

All patients included in the study received genetic counseling and underwent genetic testing for HCM, performed by Sanger sequencing (from 2007 to 2010) or NGS (next-generation sequencing, from 2011 to 2019). The genes analyzed in the participating laboratories from the HCM centers had changed and/or added over time. In this retrospective study, we report the genotype–phenotype correlation analysis only for those patients screened at least for the sarcomeric genes *MYBPC3* (myosin binding protein C, cardiac) *MYH7* (β-myosin heavy chain, cardiac), *TNNI3* (troponin I, cardiac) and *TNNT2* (troponin T type 2, cardiac). All coding regions and boundaries of flanking introns ±25 were analyzed for all genes considered in this study. In addition, all variants reported in this paper, identified by NGS technology, were validated by Sanger sequencing. Patients with variants located in nonsarcomeric genes were also excluded.

All the identified variants were re-evaluated based on new evidence from the scientific literature and classified according to the criteria of the American College of Medical Genetics and Genomics (ACMG) [25,26]. Only the genetic variants predicted to alter the protein and with a minor allele frequency (MAF) ≤0.2% (considering the prevalence of HCM disease in the general population), were considered. For this evaluation, we used MAF data derived from GnomAD (Genome Aggregation Database https://gnomad.broadinstitute.org/). The clinical classification of variants was carried out according to the 5-class system: benign (B), likely benign (LB), likely pathogenic (LP), pathogenic (P) and variants of uncertain significance (VUS). Genetic results were considered informative for LP or P variants, noninformative for B, LB or VUS variants. Variants are reported using the Human Genome Variation Society nomenclature guidelines (https://varnomen.hgvs.org/).

2.4. Clinical Outcomes

All patients had planned clinical reviews every 6–12 months or earlier according to the clinical status. Follow-up duration was defined as the time interval between the clinical examination and either the first event or the last visit/telephone interview in case of no events.

The HF end-point was represented by the following events: death due to HF, cardiac transplantation, progression to a stable NYHA class III–IV due to an end-stage phase with or without LVEF < 50% (hypokinetic dilated phase or restrictive phenotype evolution), severe functional deterioration leading to hospitalization for septal reduction, hospitalization due to HF symptoms or signs development. The SCD end-point was also tested, which included SCD or an equivalent event. SCD was defined as witnessing sudden death with or without documented ventricular fibrillation or death within 1 h of new symptoms or nocturnal deaths with no antecedent history of worsening symptoms. Aborted SCD during follow-up and appropriate ICD therapies (defined as intervention triggered by ventricular fibrillation or rapid ventricular tachycardia at >180 bpm) were considered equivalent to SCD in accordance with previous studies [17,18,27,28].

The causes of death, as well as the other events, were ascertained by experienced cardiologists at each center using hospital and primary health care records, death certificates, post-mortem reports, and interviews with relatives and/or physicians. To avoid a composite cardiovascular end-point including also cerebrovascular events, due to the small number of such events and in accordance with other studies by our research group [17,18,22], death due to ischemic or hemorrhagic stroke (n. 2 events) and nonfatal cerebrovascular (n. 5 events), as well as death due to noncardiovascular causes (n. 2 events), were excluded from the survival analysis.

2.5. Statistical Analysis

All data are expressed as mean ± standard deviation or as absolute number (percentage). Preliminarily, an extension of the Shapiro–Wilk test of normality was performed. Categorical variables were compared with a difference between proportion tests whereas a two-sample *t*-test was used to compare the continuous data between the two study groups (no variants and VUS Versus LP/P variants). In comparing the two populations, the variance was estimated separately for both groups and the Welch–Satterthwaite modification to the degrees of freedom was used.

We, therefore, focused on the distribution of survival times by adopting the Cox proportional hazards regression model. We performed a backward selection of the predictors to be included in the model. A 5% significance level was used in the backward elimination procedure to select covariates for the final multivariate model for the combined as well as the HF end-point while, due to the low events' number, a 15% significance level was adopted for the SCD one. To avoid the inclusion of collinear variables in the multivariate Cox analysis, we built several models in which VO_2-derived variables, known to be collinear, were added to the prognostic model one at a time. We retain the model with the best trade-off between model complexity and model fit judged by the log-likelihood. We also performed a calibration analysis. We computed the average calibration error for both approaches and tested the observed versus average predicted probabilities for each class of risk. The Brier quadratic error score and a χ^2 test of goodness of fit based on the Brier score were also checked. We did not find any clear indication of overfitting from the post hoc analysis and, consequently, in the present paper we simply reported results based on the backward elimination procedure only. Discrimination of variables included in the final multivariate model specification was performed by Harrell's C-index.

Therefore, we investigated the proportional hazards assumption by tests and graphical diagnostics based on scaled Schoenfeld residuals. Test of proportional hazards assumption for each covariate was obtained by correlating the corresponding set of scaled Schoenfeld residuals with the Kaplan–Meier estimate of the survival distribution. To check for the presence of influential observations, we produced a matrix of estimated changes in the regression coefficients upon deleting each observation in turn and comparing the magnitudes of the largest values to the regression coefficients.

Statistical analysis was performed using R (R Development Core Team, 2014). A *p*-value lower than or equal to 0.05 was generally considered as statistically significant.

3. Results

From an initial study sample of 665 consecutive HCM outpatients, a total of 294 patients (44%) were excluded because they did not undergo genetic testing ($n = 197$), because they were lost at follow-up ($n = 39$), because of the presence of nonsarcomeric variants ($n = 22$) or, eventually, because the genetic analysis was not performed according to the previously described inclusion criteria ($n = 36$). Thus, a total of 371 HCM patients were effectively enrolled and analyzed in the present study. The diagram displayed in Figure 1 resumes the step-by-step classification of the study population.

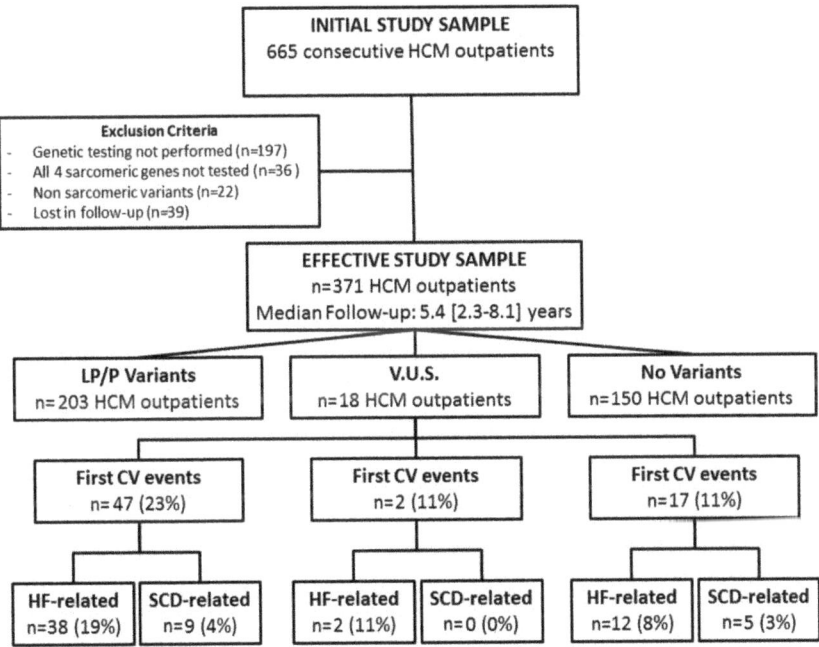

Figure 1. Diagram showing the step-by-step classification of the hypertrophic cardiomyopathy (HCM) population considered in our study. LP/P: likely pathogenic/pathogenic sarcomeric variants; V.U.S.: variant of uncertain significance; CV: cardiac events; HF: heart failure; SCD: sudden cardiac death.

3.1. Genetic Results

Two hundred and three (55%) genetic tests were informative as they detected at least an LP/P variant, whereas the percentage of patients with VUS was 6% ($n = 23$ patients); 39% ($n = 145$ patients) did not show any P/LP variant or VUS (Figure 2). Excluding the B/LB variants, 124 unique variants were identified and detailed extensively in the Supplementary files (Tables S1 and S2). These variants included 91 (73%) missense, 2 (2%) intronic, 10 (8%) frameshift, 8 (6%) splicing, 11 (9%) nonsense, 1 (1%) inframe variants (Figure S1). According to ACMG criteria, 94 variants were classified as LP/P and 30 of them as VUS. *MYBPC3* and *MYH7* resulted in the most mutated genes with 88 LP/P variants (75%, Figure 2). Twenty-four patients resulted to be carriers of multiple variants, considering those with at least one P/LP variant and other P/LP or VUS variants (Table S3). Among these, 14 patients were double heterozygous with one variant in two different genes while the remaining 10 had multiple variants in the same gene. It was not possible to determinate the phase of these variants, since segregation studies among relatives could not be performed.

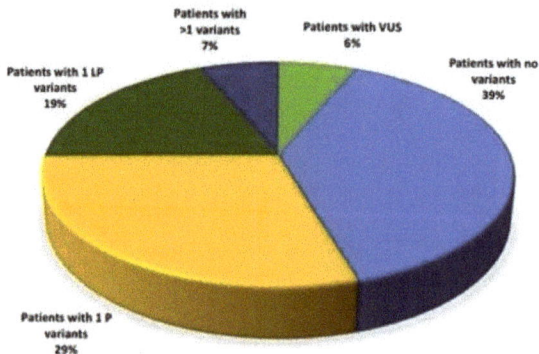

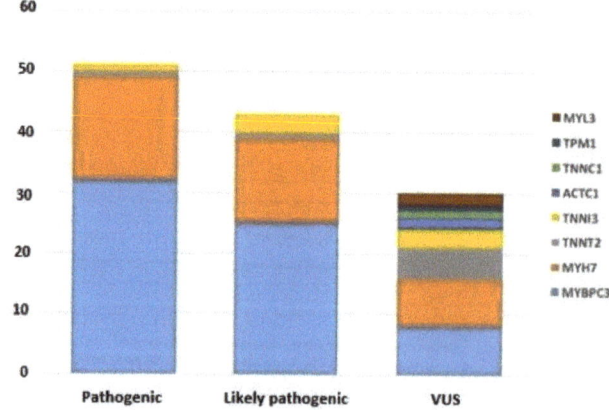

Figure 2. (**Top panel**): results of genetic testing analysis in the overall study sample. (**Bottom panel**): type and distribution of likely pathogenic/pathogenic (LP/P) variants and variants of uncertain significance (VUS). *MYL3*: myosin light chain 3; *TPM1*: tropomyosin 1; *TNNC1*: troponin C1; *ACTC1*: actin alpha cardiac muscle 1; *TNNI3*: cardiac troponin I; *TNNT2*: cardiac troponin T; *MYH7*: β-myosin heavy chain; *MYBPC3*: myosin binding protein C.

3.2. Clinical and Functional Characteristics

The demographic and clinical data of the entire cohort are reported in Table 1. The population mainly consisted of middle-aged predominantly male (64%) patients with a quite preserved NYHA class (NYHA I–II 94%). At the study run-in, echocardiographic evidence of the end-stage phase was present in 4%, atrial fibrillation in 3% and a septal myectomy had been performed in 11% patients.

Documented cardiovascular comorbidities included systemic hypertension (27%), diabetes (6%) and coronary artery disease (4%).

Table 1. Main clinical variables of the entire study sample at the study run-in (n = 371 patients).

General Data	
Age, years	49 ± 16
Male, n (%)	238 (64)
Age at diagnosis, years	40 ± 19
NYHA III–IV, n (%)	24 (6)
ICD, n (%)	43 (12)
Previous myectomy, n (%)	20 (5)
SCD risk factors	
NSVT, n (%)	121 (32)
FH-SCD, n (%)	48 (13)
MWT > 30 mm, n (%)	26 (7)
Unexplained syncope, n (%)	56 (15)
ABPRE, n (%)	45 (16)
Echocardiographic data	
LVEDd, mm	45 ± 5
LAd, mm	43 ± 7
MWT, mm	20 ± 5
LVOT obstruction, n (%)	125 (33)
LVOTG$_{max}$, mmHg	11 (6–39)
LVEF, %	62 ± 7
CPET data	
Peak HR, % of predicted	79 ± 13
Peak VO$_2$, mL/kg/min	23 ± 7
Peak VO$_2$, % of predicted	77 ± 18
Peak SBP, mmHg	164 ± 27
CP%, % of predicted * mmHg	12,937 ± 4300
VE/VCO$_2$ slope	28.4 ± 5.5
Medical treatment	
β-blocker, n (%)	228 (61)
Nondihydropyridine CCB, n (%)	31 (8)
ACE-I/ARB, n (%)	107 (29)
Diuretics, n (%)	78 (21)
Amiodaron, n (%)	33 (9)

Data are expressed as mean ± SD, as an absolute number of patients (% on total sample) or as median (25th–75th percentile). VUS: variant of uncertain significance; LP: likely pathogenic; P: pathogenic; NYHA: New York Heart Association; ICD: implantable cardioverter defibrillator; SCD: sudden cardiac death; NSVT: nonsustained ventricular tachycardia; FH: family history; ABPRE: abnormal blood pressure response at exercise; LVEDd: left ventricular end-diastolic diameter; LAd: left atrial diameter; MWT: maximum wall thickness; LVOTG$_{max}$: maximal LV outflow tract gradient; LVEF: LV ejection fraction; SBP: peak systolic blood pressure; HR: heart rate; VO$_2$: oxygen uptake; CP: circulatory power; VE/VCO$_2$ slope: relation between ventilation versus carbon dioxide production; CCB: calcium channel blocker; ACE-I/ARB: angiotensin-converting enzyme inhibitors/angiotensin receptor blocker.

Table 2 shows the comparison of clinical features between patients with and without LP/P variants. The LP/P variants group showed a younger age, a slightly higher prevalence of FH-SCD and ABPRE and a worse functional capacity in terms of pVO$_2$, CP% and VE/VCO$_2$ slope. With respect to the other clinical features, at the study run-in, the LP/P variants group had a greater prevalence of patients with end-stage phase (6% vs. 2%, p = 0.011) and atrial fibrillation (3% vs. 1%, p = 0.032), whereas no difference in the prevalence of previous myectomy was found (5% for both groups). Concerning the documented cardiovascular comorbidities, no difference was found in coronary artery disease (3% vs. 5%), whereas the LP/P variants group showed a lower prevalence of systemic hypertension (15% vs. 31%, p < 0.001) and diabetes (3% vs. 8%, p = 0.007).

Table 2. Main clinical variables of the study sample at the study run-in according to genetic testing results.

General Data	No Variants and VUS (n = 168)	LP/P Variants (n = 203)	p-Values
Age, years	53 ± 18	45 ± 16	<0.001
Male, n (%)	112 (67)	124 (61)	NS
Age at diagnosis, years	47 ± 20	35 ± 17	<0.001
NYHA III-IV, n (%)	10 (6)	14 (7)	NS
ICD, n (%)	11 (6)	32 (16)	0.019
Previous myectomy, n (%)	9 (5)	11 (5)	NS
SCD risk factors			
NSVT, n (%)	48 (28)	73 (36)	NS
FH-SCD, n (%)	16 (9)	32 (16)	0.049
MWT > 30 mm, n (%)	10 (6)	16 (8)	NS
Unexplained syncope, n (%)	29 (17)	26 (13)	NS
ABPRE, n (%)	11 (7)	34 (17)	0.003
Echocardiographic data			
LVEDd, mm	46 ± 4	45 ± 6	NS
LAd, mm	43 ± 7	43 ± 7	NS
MWT, mm	20 ± 5	20 ± 5	NS
LVOT obstruction, n (%)	79 (47)	45 (22)	<0.001
$LVOTG_{max}$, mmHg	16 (9–39)	10 (5–33)	0.023
LVEF, %	63 ± 4	61 ± 6	<0.001
CPET data			
Peak HR, % of predicted	78 ± 12	79 ± 13	NS
Peak VO_2, mL/kg/min	23 ± 7	23 ± 7	NS
Peak VO_2, % of predicted	79 ± 18	75 ± 18	0.032
Peak SBP, mmHg	175 ± 26	157 ± 26	<0.001
CP%, % of predicted * mmHg	14,070 ± 4269	12,015 ± 4020	<0.001
VE/VCO_2 slope	27.5 ± 4.9	29.1 ± 6.0	0.019
Medical treatment			
β-blocker, n (%)	105 (62)	122 (60)	NS
Non dihydropyridine CCB, n (%)	11 (7)	20 (10)	NS
ACE-I/ARB, n (%)	58 (34)	48 (24)	0.014
Diuretics, n (%)	37 (22)	41 (21)	NS
Amiodaron, n (%)	16 (9)	17 (8)	NS

Data are expressed as mean ± SD, as the absolute number of patients (% on total sample) or as median (25th–75th percentile). NS: not significant. See Table 1 for other abbreviations.

3.3. End-Point Analysis

Median follow-up was 5.4 years (25th–75th centile: 2.3 to 8.1 years) with a total of 2271 patients-year. During the entire follow-up, a total of 129 (35%) patients experienced at least one of the pre-specified events. In patients who developed multiple events, time to the first was used as an event time cutoff and, accordingly, SCD or HF-related events at five-years' cumulative hazard equal to 0.369 was estimated. Patients who completed the follow-up period before the tenth year were censored at the time of the last clinical evaluation.

A total of 14 SCD or SCD-equivalents were analyzed. Specifically, SCD occurred in three patients; four patients experienced a resuscitated SCD and seven patients had an appropriate ICD intervention. A total of 52 HF-related events were analyzed. Specifically, HF-related death occurred in two patients, seven patients underwent cardiac transplantation, 20 patients were hospitalized due to HF signs/symptoms, 12 patients were hospitalized for septal reduction procedure due to significant HF signs/symptoms development and 11 patients evolved to end-stage or restrictive phenotype evolution. Table 3 reports the detailed Cox proportional univariate survival analysis for both the study end-points. Most of the single variables were significantly associated with the HF end-point whereas few of them to the SCD end-point. Particularly, besides a number of clinical variables, the LP/P variant presence was significantly associated with the HF but not to the SCD end-point (Figure 3). Instead, at multivariate analysis, covariates showing significant effects for the primary HF-related end-point were the following: LAd, CP% and VE/VCO$_2$ slope (C-index 0.839, $p < 0.001$) while LAd and the CP% remained independently associated with the SCD end-point (C-index 0.738, Table 4).

Table 3. Main significant univariate Cox proportional survival analysis according to the clinical variables for the two main study end-points.

	HF Endpoint (n = 52)			SCD Endpoint (n = 14)		
	H.R. (95% C.I.)	p-Values	C-Index	H.R. (95% C.I.)	p-Values	C-Index
Age at CPET	–	NS	–	0.964 (0.934–0.996)	0.038	0.613
Male sex	–	NS	–	–	NS	–
Age at diagnosis	–	NS	–	0.944 (0.906–0.983)	0.006	0.729
FH-SCD	1.869 (1.010–3.460)	0.046	0.522	2.830 (0.892–8.979)	0.077	0.607
Unexplained Syncope	–	NS	–	–	NS	–
NSVT	1.917 (1.102–3.333)	0.021	0.548	–	NS	–
ABPRE	3.418 (1.769–6.605)	<0.001	0.641	–	NS	–
MWT > 30 mm	–	NS	–	3.956 (1.210–12.940)	0.023	0.569
MWT	–	NS	–	1.100 (1.012–1.195)	0.025	0.593
LVOTO	2.110 (1.215–3.664)	<0.01	0.641	–	NS	–
LAd	1.077 (1.039–1.116)	<0.001	0.704	1.054 (0.984–1.129)	0.112	0.660
LVOTG$_{max}$	1.016 (1.008–1.024)	<0.001	0.672	0.971 (0.937–1.007)	0.123	0.577
LVEF	0.929 (0.899–0.959)	<0.001	0.587	–	NS	–
pVO$_2$, mL/kg/min	0.851 (0.799–0.905)	<0.001	0.739	–	NS	–
pVO$_2$, % of predicted	0.851 (0.799–0.905)	<0.001	0.749	–	NS	–
VE/VCO$_2$ slope	1.017 (1.069–1.146)	<0.001	0.724	–	NS	–
CP%	0.998 (0.997–0.999)	<0.001	0.778	0.998 (0.997–1.000)	0.052	0.705
LP or P variants	2.395 (1.171–4.856)	0.013	0.609	–	NS	–

H.R.: hazard ratio; C.I.: confidence interval. See Table 1 for other abbreviations.

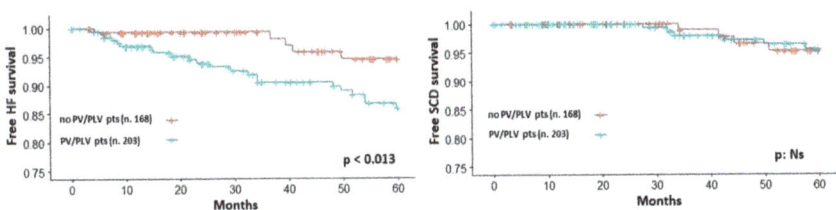

Figure 3. Kaplan–Meier estimator of survival free from heart failure (HF, **left panel**) and sudden cardiac death (SCD, **right panel**) related events according to the presence of likely pathogenic/pathogenic sarcomeric variants (PLV/PV).

Table 4. Significant multivariate Cox proportional survival analysis and test for proportional hazards assumption for the two study end-points.

	Multivariate Cox Proportional Survival Analysis					
	HF Endpoint			SCD Endpoint		
	H.R. (95% C.I.)	p-Values	C-Index	H.R. (95% C.I.)	p-Values	C-Index
LAd	1.083 (1.039–1.130)	<0.001	0.839	1.078 (1.005–1.163)	0.0485	0.738
CP%	0.998 (0.997–0.999)	<0.001		0.998 (0.9996–1.000)	0.0488	
VE/VCO$_2$ slope	1.044 (0.999–1.090)	0.05				

See Tables 1 and 2 for other abbreviations.

4. Discussion

The present multicenter retrospective study, conducted on a suitable cohort of consecutive HCM outpatients regularly followed at three Italian tertiary HCM centers, shows that HCM patients with LP/P sarcomeric variants tend to present a more aggressive form of disease with an earlier onset, a worse functional status and a greater risk of HF development and HF-related complications, compared to HCM patients with VUS or any variants. However, contextually, our data do not support a strict role of genetic testing over HCM patients' comprehensive clinical assessment. Indeed, the LP/P variants presence does not emerge at multivariate analysis as an independent risk factor, being other instrumental variables (i.e., LAd, CP% and VE/VCO$_2$ slope) much stronger outcome predictors.

Over the last decades a number of clinical features were investigated in order to identify those HCM patients at high risk of adverse events, both arrhythmic and HF-related. Indeed, albeit most of the cases show a benign course with a life expectancy equal to the general population [1], the SCD remains a rare but devastating event which is still the leading cause of death in the young population and athletes [2,3,6]. Furthermore, proper due to the improvement in the HCM management, both pharmacological and nonpharmacological (i.e., ICD, myectomy, LVAD/heart transplantation), there is a growing percentage of HCM patients who develop HF as well as HF-related complications [1,5,29]. The present study, as an ancillary result, confirms the abovementioned concern by showing a significant rate of HF-related events ($n = 114$ events) with a relatively low number of SCD and SCD-equivalent ($n = 14$ events) at a midterm follow-up.

Given the wide HCM clinical spectrum, its genetic nature and the need for targeted prevention strategies, previous studies sought to investigate and weigh the influence of sarcomere variants on the HCM clinical phenotype and outcome [7–13,16]. Indeed, HCM represents a sarcomeric disease with LP/P variants in *MYBPC3* and *MYH7* genes (thick filaments) together accounting for about 50% of the HCM families whereas LP/P variants in *TNNT2*, *TNNI3* (thin filaments) accounting for less than 10% [1,6]. In such a context, an old study by Olivotto and colleagues, conducted in the pre-NGS scenario on a cohort of 203 HCM patients with a median follow-up of 4.5 years, suggested that HCM patients with sarcomere variants had a greater probability of a worse outcome (i.e., cardiac death, nonfatal stroke, end-stage progression) compared to those with nonsarcomeric variants [8]. A more recent study by Li and colleagues, on a sample of 558 HCM patients with a median follow-up of 4.5 years, demonstrated that LP/P variants were associated to an early disease onset, to a high burden of established risk factors and, mainly, to a composite HF end-points (i.e., HF-related hospitalization, heart transplantation, HF-related death, progression to an end-stage phase) [10]. Further support to a possible role of genetic testing in the HCM risk stratification comes from Velzen and colleagues that, on a population of 626 HCM patients with a long-term follow-up (>10 years), confirmed that patients with LP/P variants had a more aggressive phenotype (i.e., young age, high prevalence of SCD risk factors) and found an independent association with all-cause mortality, HF-related and SCD mortality [12]. Eventually, the recent SHARE study, conducted on a large cohort of 2763 HCM patients followed-up for a median of 2.9 years, confirmed that patients carrying sarcomeric LP/P variants had an earlier disease onset and a greater risk of developing the overall composite outcome (SCD or SCD-equivalent, LVAD/cardiac transplantation, progression to an end-stage phase, all-cause mortality, atrial fibrillation and stroke) [13]. The present study confirms that HCM patients carrying LP/P variants have a worse clinical feature in terms of disease onset as well as of historical risk factors [29]. However, we proved just a univariate association between the HCM-mutated status and a composite HF end-point. Although a close comparison with the abovementioned studies remains difficult because of different methodological approaches (i.e., number of genes screened, variants classification, end-points' construction), the most likely reason underlying this negative datum could be the optimal clinical and functional characterization of our study cohort. Indeed, we specifically challenged the prognostic impact of LP/P variants not only with the historical variables but also, and specifically, with the CPET-derived parameters. Thus, we showed originally that patients with LP/P variants, although younger than the counterpart, exhibited also a more severe functional limitation both in terms of pVO$_2$ and ventilatory efficiency values. Furthermore, due to a concomitant blunted increase of SBP during exercise, HCM patients with LP/P variants showed significantly lower values of CP%. Each of the three abovementioned CPET-derived variables has a specific pathophysiological meaning in the HCM patients' context [30,31] and a possible capability as an outcome predictor. Particularly, the pVO$_2$ is a multidimensional parameter dependent on cardiac output (heart rate * stroke volume) and artero-venous O$_2$ extraction [24,32] and it has been extensively shown to be a strong predictor of poor outcome in HCM [14–18] as well as in HF patients [33,34]. The CP%, according to its formula [23,24], magnifies the prognostic power of the pVO$_2$ through the ABPRE [17,18] which, in turn, depends on the intrinsic myocardial function/geometry as well on abnormal peripheral autonomic reflexes [35,36]. Eventually, the ventilatory efficiency (i.e., VE/VCO$_2$ slope) has been shown to correlate with pulmonary capillary wedge pressure and left ventricular diastolic properties in HCM [37]. Although usually preserved in HCM patients, the VE/VCO$_2$ slope tends to worsen significantly only in the late systolic dysfunction phase but it is conceivable that it could mirror also an early exercise-induced left ventricular diastolic functional derangement [16,31,37–39].

5. Limitations

The relatively small number of patients enrolled, together with the low number of hard events, represents a certain limitation that does not allow us to define the true weight of the genetic analysis results in terms of HCM risk prediction when compared to a full clinical assessment. However, it should be noted that our data do not argue against the overall importance of genetic testing in HCM management. Indeed, the identification of unaffected mutated relatives can be possible only after the detection of P/LP variants in affected HCM probands by gene sequencing [40]. Furthermore, molecular analysis of HCM genes remains one of the pivotal approaches in distinguishing the so-called HCM phenocopies where early diagnosis is crucial to managing it optimally [2,3]. On the other hand, whenever a P/LP variant is not found in HCM patients, the HCM diagnosis should be carefully re-evaluated. Again, concerning risk stratification, a comprehensive clinical assessment might be essential.

Another limitation that needs to be acknowledged is that, apart from the main four genes (*MYBPC3*, *MYH7*, *TNNI3*, *TNNT2*) that were tested in all patients, other genes known to be HCM-related (i.e., *ACTC1*, *TPM1*, *TNNC1*, or *MYL2* and *MYL3*) were tested in most but not all patients. However, it should be remarked that these variants are rarely detected in HCM patients [6,7]. Moreover, given the few numbers of patients carrying variants in thin filaments genes (<15%) as well patients with multiple variants (6%) in our study sample, our survival analysis considered the overall impact of the LP/P sarcomeric variants without distinguishing the type of compromised filaments or a possible "gene dosage effect". Similarly, growing data report possible relationships between specific variants location in functional domains of sarcomeric proteins and prognostic implications. Particularly, pathogenic missense variants located in the converter domain of the *MYH7* gene were found associated with a worse outcome [41,42]. Furthermore, Garcia-Giustiniani and colleagues found a significant association between p.(Gly716Arg), p.(Arg719Trp) and p.(Arg719Gln) variants with a high risk of events (i.e., 50-year survival of only 20% of carriers) [43]. In the present study cohort, although six different pathogenic missense variants falling within the converter domain (p.(Gly716Arg), p.(Arg719Trp), p.(Arg719Gln), p.(Ile736Thr), p.(Gly741Arg) and p.(Arg723Cys)) were found, the small number of patients carrying these variants as well as their relatively young age unable us to support their specific prognostic power. For the same underlying reasons (i.e., small number of patients carrying VUS only), we cannot speculate about an intermediate prognosis in this subset of patients as hypothesized in the SHARE study [13]. Eventually, we found multiple variants in the same gene in 10 patients and in this specific setting, we cannot determinate whether the genetic alterations were on the same chromosome (heterozygous state) or not (compound heterozygous state).

Finally, besides the genetic profile per se, we examined the prognostic effect of several clinical and instrumental variables at a single time point. Accordingly, we cannot exclude that changes in some variables, as for instance an upgrading of treatment during follow-up or upcoming risk factors, altered our survival analysis. However, it is reasonable that seriate clinical and functional evaluations in HCM patients at the highest risk could further magnify our findings rather than rebut them.

6. Conclusions

Our data underline the importance of a multidimensional clinical assessment over the genetic testing analysis in the HCM risk stratification. This unexpected finding, different from other literature reports, might be likely explained by the limited size of the sample cohort. The LP/P variants were anyway associated with a more aggressive HCM phenotype in terms of early disease onset, high burden of historical risk factor and, for the first time, poor functional status. Of note, within a number of clinical and instrumental variables, the present study reaffirms the pivotal role of the variables derived from a CPET assessment.

Supplementary Materials: The following are available online at http://www.mdpi.com/2077-0383/9/6/1636/s1, Figure S1: Type of unique gene variants, Table S1: List of pathogenic (P) and likely pathogenic (LP) gene variants identified, Table S2: List of variants of uncertain significance (VUS) identified, Table S3: HCM patients with multiple sarcomeric genes variants (at least one LP/P variants).

Author Contributions: Conceptualization, D.M., M.P., S.R., C.A. and B.M.; methodology, M.P., A.M., M.R.T., C.S., S.P., A.G., M.F. and M.C.; formal analysis, D.M., V.M., G.G., M.P., S.R. and A.M.; investigation, D.M., V.M., G.G., D.G., E.Z., F.R., C.A., B.M., S.R., M.P., C.S., A.G. and S.P.; resources, D.M., S.R., C.A. and M.V.; data curation, D.M., V.M., G.G, M.P. and S.R.; writing—original draft preparation, D.M., V.M. and G.G; writing—review and editing, D.M., S.R., E.Z., F.R., C.A., M.V. and P.A.; visualization, D.M., V.M. and G.G.; supervision, C.A., S.R. and M.V.; project administration, D.M., C.A., B.M., S.R., E.Z. and F.R.; funding acquisition, D.M., S.R., C.A. and M.V. All authors have read and agreed to the published version of the manuscript.

Funding: This research received no external funding. The APC was funded by Sapienza, University of Rome.

Conflicts of Interest: The authors declare no conflicts of interest. The funders had no role in the design of the study; in the collection, analyses, or interpretation of data; in the writing of the manuscript, or in the decision to publish the results.

References

1. Maron, B.J.; Maron, M.S. Hypertrophic cardiomyopathy. *Lancet* **2013**, *381*, 242–255. [CrossRef]
2. Gersh, B.J.; Maron, B.J.; Bonow, R.O.; Dearani, J.A.; Fifer, M.A.; Link, M.S.; Naidu, S.S.; Nishimura, R.A.; Ommen, S.R.; Rakowski, H.; et al. 2011 ACCF/AHA Guideline for the Diagnosis and Treatment of Hypertrophic Cardiomyopathy: Executive Summary: A Report of the American College of Cardiology Foundation/American Heart Association Task Force on Practice Guidelines. *Circulation* **2011**, *124*, 2761–2796. [CrossRef]
3. Elliott, P.M.; Anastasakis, A.; Borger, M.A.; Borggrefe, M.; Cecchi, F.; Charron, P.; Hagege, A.A.; Lafont, A.; Limongelli, G.; Mahrholdt, H.; et al. 2014 ESC Guidelines on diagnosis and management of hypertrophic cardiomyopathy: The Task Force for the Diagnosis and Management of Hypertrophic Cardiomyopathy of the European Society of Cardiology (ESC). *Eur. Heart J.* **2014**, *35*, 2733–2779. [CrossRef]

4. Maron, B.J.; Ommen, S.R.; Semsarian, C.; Spirito, P.; Olivotto, I.; Maron, M.S. Hypertrophic cardiomyopathy: Present and future, with translation into contemporary cardiovascular medicine. *J. Am. Coll. Cardiol.* **2014**, *64*, 83–99. [CrossRef]
5. Musumeci, M.B.; Russo, D.; Limite, L.R.; Canepa, M.; Tini, G.; Casenghi, M.; Francia, P.; Adduci, C.; Pagannone, E.; Magrì, D.; et al. Long-Term Left Ventricular Remodeling of Patients with Hypertrophic Cardiomyopathy. *Am. J. Cardiol.* **2018**, *122*, 1924–1931. [CrossRef]
6. Marian, A.J.; Braunwald, E. Hypertrophic Cardiomyopathy: Genetics, Pathogenesis, Clinical Manifestations, Diagnosis, and Therapy. *Circ. Res.* **2017**, *121*, 749–770. [CrossRef]
7. Rubattu, S.; Bozzao, C.; Pennacchini, E.; Pagannone, E.; Musumeci, M.B.; Piane, M.; Germani, A.; Savio, C.; Francia, P.; Volpe, M.; et al. A Next-Generation Sequencing Approach to Identify Gene Mutations in Early- and Late-Onset Hypertrophic Cardiomyopathy Patients of an Italian Cohort. *Int. J. Mol. Sci.* **2016**, *17*, 1239. [CrossRef]
8. Olivotto, I.; Girolami, F.; Ackerman, M.J.; Nistri, S.; Bos, J.M.; Zachara, E.; Ommen, S.R.; Theis, J.L.; Vaubel, R.A.; Re, F.; et al. Myofilament protein gene mutation screening and outcome of patients with hypertrophic cardiomyopathy. *Mayo Clin. Proc.* **2008**, *83*, 630–638. [CrossRef]
9. Selvi Rani, D.; Nallari, P.; Dhandapany, P.S.; Rani, J.; Meraj, K.; Ganesan, M.; Narasimhan, C.; Thangaraj, K. Coexistence of Digenic Mutations in Both Thin (TPM1) and Thick (MYH7) Filaments of Sarcomeric Genes Leads to Severe Hypertrophic Cardiomyopathy in a South Indian FHCM. *DNA Cell Biol.* **2015**, *34*, 350–359. [CrossRef]
10. Li, Q.; Gruner, C.; Chan, R.H.; Care, M.; Siminovitch, K.; Williams, L.; Woo, A.; Rakowski, H. Genotype-positive status in patients with hypertrophic cardiomyopathy is associated with higher rates of heart failure events. *Circ. Cardiovasc. Genet.* **2014**, *7*, 416–422. [CrossRef]
11. Lopes, L.R.; Syrris, P.; Guttmann, O.P.; O'Mahony, C.; Tang, H.C.; Dalageorgou, C.; Jenkins, S.; Hubank, M.; Monserrat, L.; McKenna, W.J.; et al. Novel genotype-phenotype associations demonstrated by high-throughput sequencing in patients with hypertrophic cardiomyopathy. *Heart* **2015**, *101*, 294–301. [CrossRef]
12. Van Velzen, H.G.; Vriesendorp, P.A.; Oldenburg, R.A.; van Slegtenhorst, M.A.; van der Velden, J.; Schinkel, A.F.L.; Michels, M. Value of Genetic Testing for the Prediction of Long-Term Outcome in Patients with Hypertrophic Cardiomyopathy. *Am. J. Cardiol.* **2016**, *118*, 881–887. [CrossRef]
13. Ho, C.Y.; Day, S.M.; Ashley, E.A.; Michel, M.; Pereira, A.C.; Jacoby, D.; Cirino, A.L.; Fox, J.C.; Lakdawala, N.K.; Ware, J.S.; et al. Genotype and Lifetime Burden of Disease in Hypertrophic Cardiomyopathy: Insights from the Sarcomeric Human Cardiomyopathy Registry (SHaRe). *Circulation* **2018**, *138*, 1387–1398. [CrossRef]
14. Masri, A.; Pierson, L.M.; Smedira, N.G.; Agarwal, S.; Lytle, B.W.; Naji, P.; Thamilarasan, M.; Lever, H.M.; Cho, L.S.; Desai, M.Y. Predictors of longterm outcomes in patients with hypertrophic cardiomyopathy undergoing cardiopulmonary stress testing and echocardiography. *Am. Heart J.* **2015**, *169*, 684–692. [CrossRef]
15. Coats, C.J.; Rantell, K.; Bartnik, A.; Patel, A.; Mist, B.; McKenna, W.J.; Elliott, P.M. Cardiopulmonary exercise testing and prognosis in hypertrophic cardiomyopathy. *Circ. Heart Fail.* **2015**, *8*, 1022–1031. [CrossRef]
16. Finocchiaro, G.; Haddad, F.; Knowles, J.W.; Caleshu, C.; Pavlovic, A.; Homburger, J.; Shmargad, Y.; Sinagra, G.; Magavern, E.; Wong, M.; et al. Cardiopulmonary responses and prognosis in hypertrophic cardiomyopathy: A potential role for comprehensive noninvasive hemodynamic assessment. *JACC Heart Fail.* **2015**, *3*, 408–418. [CrossRef]
17. Magrì, D.; Re, F.; Limongelli, G.; Agostoni, P.; Zachara, E.; Correale, M.; Mastromarino, V.; Santolamazza, C.; Casenghi, M.; Pacileo, G.; et al. Heart Failure Progression in Hypertrophic Cardiomyopathy—Possible Insights From Cardiopulmonary Exercise Testing. *Circ. J.* **2016**, *80*, 2204–2211. [CrossRef]
18. Magrì, D.; Limongelli, G.; Re, F.; Agostoni, P.; Zachara, E.; Correale, M.; Mastromarino, V.; Santolamazza, C.; Casenghi, M.; Pacileo, G.; et al. Cardiopulmonary exercise test and sudden cardiac death risk in hypertrophic cardiomyopathy. *Heart* **2016**, *102*, 602–609. [CrossRef]
19. Lang, R.M.; Badano, L.P.; Mor-Avi, V.; Afilalo, J.; Armstrong, A.; Ernande, L.; Flachskampf, F.A.; Foster, E.; Goldstein, S.A.; Kuznetsova, T.; et al. Recommendations for cardiac chamber quantification by echocardiography in adults: An update from the American Society of Echocardiography and the European Association of Cardiovascular Imaging. *J. Am. Soc. Echocardiogr.* **2015**, *28*, 1–39. [CrossRef]

20. Autore, C.; Bernabò, P.; Barillà, C.S.; Bruzzi, P.; Spirito, P. The prognostic importance of left ventricular outflow obstruction in hypertrophic cardiomyopathy varies in relation to the severity of symptoms. *J. Am. Coll. Cardiol.* **2005**, *45*, 1076–1080. [CrossRef]
21. Agostoni, P.; Bianchi, M.; Moraschi, A.; Palermo, P.; Cattadori, G.; La Gioia, R.; Bussotti, M.; Wasserman, K. Work-rate affects cardiopulmonary exercise test results in heart failure. *Eur. J. Heart Fail.* **2005**, *7*, 498–504. [CrossRef]
22. Magrì, D.; Agostoni, P.; Sinagra, G.; Re, F.; Correale, M.; Limongelli, G.; Zachara, E.; Mastromarino, V.; Santolamazza, C.; Casenghi, M.; et al. Clinical and prognostic impact of chronotropic incompetence in patients with hypertrophic cardiomyopathy. *Int. J. Cardiol.* **2018**, *271*, 125–131. [CrossRef]
23. Corrà, U.; Mezzani, A.; Giordano, A.; Bosimini, E.; Giannuzzi, P. Exercise haemodynamic variables rather than ventilatory efficiency indexes contribute to risk assessment in chronic heart failure patients treated with carvedilol. *Eur. Heart J.* **2009**, *30*, 3000–3006. [CrossRef]
24. Wasserman, K.; Hansen, J.E.; Sue, D.Y.; Stringer, W.; Whipp, B.J. Normal Values. In *Principles of Exercise Testing and Interpretation*, 4th ed.; Weinberg, R., Ed.; Lippincott Williams and Wilkins: Philadelphia, PA, USA, 2005; pp. 160–182.
25. Richards, S.; Aziz, N.; Bale, S.; Bick, D.; Das, S.; Gastier-Foster, J.; Grody, W.W.; Hegde, M.; Lyon, E.; Spector, E.; et al. Standards and guidelines for the interpretation of sequence variants: A joint consensus recommendation of the American College of Medical Genetics and Genomics and the Association for Molecular Pathology. *Genet. Med.* **2015**, *17*, 405–424. [CrossRef]
26. Hershberger, R.E.; Givertz, M.M.; Ho, C.Y.; Judge, D.P.; Kantor, P.; McBride, K.L.; Morales, A.; Taylor, M.R.G.; Vatta, M.; Ware, S.M.; et al. Genetic evaluation of cardiomyopathy: A clinical practice resource of the American College of Medical Genetics and Genomics (ACMG). *Genet. Med.* **2018**, *20*, 899–909. [CrossRef]
27. O'Mahony, C.; Jichi, F.; Pavlou, M.; Monserrat, L.; Anastasakis, A.; Rapezzi, C.; Biagini, E.; Gimeno, J.R.; Limongelli, G.; McKenna, W.J.; et al. A novel clinical risk prediction model for sudden cardiac death in hypertrophic cardiomyopathy (HCM Risk-SCD). *Eur. Heart J.* **2014**, *35*, 2010–2020. [CrossRef]
28. O'Mahony, C.; Akhtar, M.M.; Anastasiou, Z.; Guttmann, O.P.; Vriesendorp, P.A.; Michels, M.; Magrì, D.; Autore, C.; Fernández, A.; Ochoa, J.P.; et al. Effectiveness of the 2014 European Society of Cardiology guideline on sudden cardiac death in hypertrophic cardiomyopathy: A systematic review and meta-analysis. *Heart* **2019**, *105*, 623–631. [CrossRef]
29. Biagini, E.; Olivotto, I.; Iascone, M.; Parodi, M.I.; Girolami, F.; Frisso, G.; Autore, C.; Limongelli, G.; Cecconi, M.; Maron, B.J.; et al. Significance of sarcomere gene mutations analysis in the end-stage phase of hypertrophic cardiomyopathy. *Am. J. Cardiol.* **2014**, *114*, 769–776. [CrossRef]
30. Magrì, D.; Santolamazza, C. Cardiopulmonary Exercise Test in Hypertrophic Cardiomyopathy. *Ann. Am. Thorac. Soc.* **2017**, *14* (Suppl. 1), 102–109. [CrossRef]
31. Magrì, D.; Agostoni, P.; Cauti, F.M.; Musumeci, B.; Egidy Assenza, G.; De Cecco, C.N.; Muscogiuri, G.; Maruotti, A.; Ricotta, A.; Pagannone, E.; et al. Determinants of peak oxygen uptake in patients with hypertrophic cardiomyopathy: A single-center study. *Intern. Emerg. Med.* **2014**, *9*, 293–302. [CrossRef]
32. Magrì, D. Peak oxygen uptake in heart failure: Look behind the number! *Eur. J. Prev. Cardiol.* **2018**, *25*, 1934–1936. [CrossRef]
33. Agostoni, P.; Corrà, U.; Cattadori, G.; Veglia, F.; La Gioia, R.; Scardovi, A.B.; Emdin, M.; Metra, M.; Sinagra, G.; Limongelli, G.; et al. Metabolic exercise test data combined with cardiac and kidney indexes, the MECKI score: A multiparametric approach to heart failure prognosis. *Int. J. Cardiol.* **2013**, *167*, 2710–2718. [CrossRef]
34. Paolillo, S.; Veglia, F.; Salvioni, E.; Corrà, U.; Piepoli, M.; Lagioia, R.; Limongelli, G.; Sinagra, G.; Cattadori, G.; Scardovi, A.B.; et al. Heart failure prognosis over time: How the prognostic role of oxygen consumption and ventilatory efficiency during exercise has changed in the last 20 years. *Eur. J. Heart Fail.* **2019**, *21*, 208–217. [CrossRef]
35. Ciampi, Q.; Betocchi, S.; Lombardi, R.; Manganelli, F.; Storto, G.; Losi, M.A.; Pezzella, E.; Finizio, F.; Cuocolo, A.; Chiariello, M. Hemodynamic determinants of exercise-induced abnormal blood pressure response in hypertrophic cardiomyopathy. *J. Am. Coll. Cardiol.* **2002**, *40*, 278–284. [CrossRef]
36. Kawasaki, T.; Azuma, A.; Kuribayashi, T.; Akakabe, Y.; Yamano, M.; Miki, S.; Sawada, T.; Kamitani, T.; Matsubara, H.; Sugihara, H. Vagal enhancement due to subendocardial ischemia as a cause of abnormal blood pressure response in hypertrophic cardiomyopathy. *Int. J. Cardiol.* **2008**, *129*, 59–64. [CrossRef]

37. Arena, R.; Owens, D.S.; Arevalo, J.; Smith, K.; Mohiddin, S.A.; McAreavey, D.; Ulisney, K.L.; Tripodi, D.; Fananapazir, L.; Plehn, J.F. Ventilatory efficiency and resting hemodynamics in hypertrophic cardiomyopathy. *Med. Sci. Sports Exerc.* **2008**, *40*, 799–805. [CrossRef]
38. Salvioni, E.; Corrà, U.; Piepoli, M.; Rovai, S.; Correale, M.; Paolillo, S.; Pasquali, M.; Magrì, D.; Vitale, G.; Fusini, L.; et al. Gender and age normalization and ventilation efficiency during exercise in heart failure with reduced ejection fraction. *ESC Heart Fail.* **2020**, *7*, 371–380. [CrossRef]
39. Musumeci, M.B.; Mastromarino, V.; Casenghi, M.; Tini, G.; Francia, P.; Maruotti, A.; Romaniello, A.; Magrì, D.; Lillo, R.; Adduci, C.; et al. Pulmonary hypertension and clinical correlates in hypertrophic cardiomyopathy. *Int. J. Cardiol.* **2017**, *248*, 326–332. [CrossRef]
40. Maron, B.J.; Maron, M.S.; Semsarian, C. Genetics of hypertrophic cardiomyopathy after 20 years: Clinical perspectives. *J. Am. Coll. Cardiol.* **2012**, *60*, 705–715. [CrossRef]
41. Homburger, J.R.; Green, E.M.; Caleshu, C.; Sunitha, M.S.; Taylor, R.E.; Ruppel, K.M.; Prasad Rao Metpally, R.; Colan, S.D.; Michels, M.; Day, S.M.; et al. Multidimensional Structure-Function Relationships in Human β-Cardiac Myosin from Population-Scale Genetic Variation. *Proc. Natl. Acad. Sci. USA* **2016**, *113*, 6701–6706. [CrossRef]
42. Alamo, L.; Ware, J.S.; Pinto, A.; Gillilan, R.E.; Seidman, J.G.; Seidman, C.E.; Padrón, R. Effects of Myosin Variants on Interacting-Heads Motif Explain Distinct Hypertrophic and Dilated Cardiomyopathy Phenotypes. *eLife* **2017**, *6*, e24634. [CrossRef]
43. García-Giustiniani, D.; Arad, M.; Ortíz-Genga, M.; Barriales-Villa, R.; Fernández, X.; Rodríguez-García, I.; Mazzanti, A.; Veira, E.; Maneiro, E.; Rebolo, P.; et al. Phenotype and Prognostic Correlations of the Converter Region Mutations Affecting the β Myosin Heavy Chain. *Heart* **2015**, *101*, 1047–1053. [CrossRef]

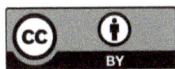

© 2020 by the authors. Licensee MDPI, Basel, Switzerland. This article is an open access article distributed under the terms and conditions of the Creative Commons Attribution (CC BY) license (http://creativecommons.org/licenses/by/4.0/).

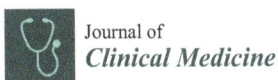

Review

Complexity of TNF-α Signaling in Heart Disease

Filip Rolski [1] and Przemysław Błyszczuk [1,2,*]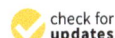

[1] Department of Clinical Immunology, Jagiellonian University Medical College, 30-663 Cracow, Poland; filip.rolski@uj.edu.pl
[2] Center of Experimental Rheumatology, Department of Rheumatology, University Hospital Zurich, 8952 Schlieren, Switzerland
* Correspondence: przemyslaw.blyszczuk@uj.edu.pl; Tel.: +48-12-658-24-86

Received: 13 August 2020; Accepted: 9 October 2020; Published: 12 October 2020

Abstract: Heart disease is a leading cause of death with unmet clinical needs for targeted treatment options. Tumor necrosis factor alpha (TNF-α) represents a master pro-inflammatory cytokine that plays an important role in many immunopathogenic processes. Anti-TNF-α therapy is widely used in treating autoimmune inflammatory disorders, but in case of patients with heart disease, this treatment was unsuccessful or even harmful. The underlying reasons remain elusive until today. This review summarizes the effects of anti-TNF-α treatment in patients with and without heart disease and describes the involvement of TNF-α signaling in a number of animal models of cardiovascular diseases. We specifically focused on the role of TNF-α in specific cardiovascular conditions and in defined cardiac cell types. Although some mechanisms, mainly in disease development, are quite well known, a comprehensive understanding of TNF-α signaling in the failing heart is still incomplete. Published data identify pathogenic and cardioprotective mechanisms of TNF-α in the affected heart and highlight the differential role of two TNF-α receptors pointing to the complexity of the TNF-α signaling. In the light of these findings, it seems that targeting the TNF-α pathway in heart disease may show therapeutic benefits, but this approach must be more specific and selectively block pathogenic mechanisms. To this aim, more research is needed to better understand the molecular mechanisms of TNF-α signaling in the failing heart.

Keywords: TNF-α; TNFR1; TNFR2; heart; cardiovascular disease; inflammation; cardiac fibrosis

---

1. Introduction

Heart disease refers to a group of diseases characterized by the affected function of the heart muscle. Epidemiologic data suggest that heart disease is a leading cause of death in the world. Heart failure affects 26 million people worldwide and causes 1 million annual hospitalizations in the United States and Europe [1]. Insufficient blood supply of the heart muscle by coronary arteries, which is termed coronary artery disease, represents the most common cause of heart disease. Extended ischemia in the myocardium is a life-threating condition that can lead to myocardial infarction or sudden cardiac death. Aberrant or impaired cardiac function (heart failure) can also develop in the absence of coronary artery disease. Such non-ischemic heart disease is a consequence of pathological changes in the structure of the cardiac muscle. In case of heart failure, the heart is unable to efficiently pump the blood due to ineffective muscle contraction (systolic heart failure) or relaxation (diastolic heart failure). From a clinical point of view, the type of heart failure depends on the left ventricular ejection fraction (LVEF) parameter. For LVEF < 40%, systolic heart function is impaired, and this condition is referred to as heart failure with reduced ejection fraction (HFrEF). Diastolic heart failure patients are often characterized by LVEF > 50% (or sometimes >40%); therefore, this type of heart failure is currently defined as heart failure with preserved ejection fraction (HFpEF). Both HFrEF and HFpEF patients show reduced life expectancy [2,3].

Inflammation plays an important role in the progression of many types of cardiovascular disease. On the one hand, the systemic inflammatory condition enhances atherogenesis, leading to coronary artery disease, but it also can promote the development of diastolic heart failure. On the other hand, cardiac inflammation occurs in post-ischemic myocardial events, and in more rare cases, it develops as a response to non-ischemic cardiac injury that often causes pathogenic changes in the cardiac tissue resulting in systolic dysfunction [4]. Thus, anti-inflammatory treatment has been suggested to protect the heart and cardiovascular system [5].

Tumor necrosis factor α (TNF-α) represents one of the most potent pro-inflammatory cytokines, and therefore, it was selected as the first target in the cytokine-targeted approach. Currently, TNF-α inhibitors are clinically used anti-inflammatory drugs to treat mainly patients with systemic inflammatory diseases. Roughly 1 million patients receive this type of treatment, and TNF-α antagonists are currently the most profitable class of drugs in the world, accounting for 25 billion US dollars in sales annually [6]. In case of heart failure, clinical data indicated that TNF-α inhibitors were not effective and even could worsen disease outcomes. However, the reasons of these disappointing results remain elusive.

2. TNF-α Biosynthesis

In humans, TNF-α is encoded by the *TNFA* gene located on chromosome 6 and shares locus with major histocompatibility complex (MHC) class II genes, which plays a central role in antigen presentation [7]. The *TNFA* gene consists of 200 nucleotide promoters with binding sites for several transcription factors, resulting in a high plasticity of transcription and responsiveness to various types of stimuli, which also vary between cell types [8].

At the post-transcript stage, the biosynthesis of TNF-α is controlled mainly through the competitive binding of the mRNA 3′ AU-rich untranslated region by RNA-binding proteins tristetraprolin (TTP) and stabilizing factor human antigen R (HuR). The dephosphorylated form of TTP effectively binds to mRNA and degrades it. The phosphorylation of TTP weakens its affinity to mRNA preventing its degradation. This allows the binding of HuR to mRNA and enables a more efficient translation of *TNFA* transcripts. Pro-inflammatory stimuli, such as lipopolysaccharide (LPS), regulate the activity of TTP and the translocation of HuR from the nucleus to cytoplasm, thereby enhancing TNF-α biosynthesis. TTP activity is regulated by p38 mitogen-activated protein kinases (MAPK), which controls TTP target genes at the post-transcriptional level and the binding of nuclear factor kappa B (NF-κB) to the promoter of TTP, which positively regulates its translation [9–11]. The deficiency of TTP in mice leads to increased TNF-α production that results in growth retardation, cachexia, arthritis, and autoimmune response [12]. The biosynthesis of TNF-α is regulated by a number of inflammatory mediators such as LPS, interleukin (IL)-1β, IL-6, interferon gamma (IFN-γ), tissue trauma, or hypoxia [13–15].

Upon translation, TNF-α is synthesized as a 17 kDa type II (i.e., possessing a single, uncleavable transmembrane segment, which anchors the protein in a cell membrane with the C-terminal end oriented toward cytoplasm) transmembrane protein. This membrane form of TNF-α (mTNF-α) can function as a ligand. The extracellular domain of mTNF-α can be cleaved by TNF-α cleaving enzyme (TACE; ADAM17) and released as soluble TNF-α (sTNF-α) [16]. mTNF-α and sTNF-α assemble as noncovalently bound homotrimers and in this form exert their biological functions [17].

3. TNF-α Receptors

TNF-α represents a ligand for two types of TNF-α receptors (TNFRs), namely TNFR1 (CD120a, p55) and TNFR2 (CD120b, p75). TNFRs represent single transmembrane glycoproteins with extracellular TNF-α binding domains characterized by four tandem-repeated cysteine-rich motifs [18]. TNFRs are typically located on the cell membrane, but they can be shed and released in soluble forms with the ability to bind and neutralize the activity of circulating sTNF-α. In the body, most cells constitutively express TNFR1. In contrast, the expression of TNFR2 is often induced by pro-inflammatory factors and is restricted mainly to immune cells, but it can be also upregulated by endothelial cells or cardiomyocytes [19,20]. The activation of TNFR1 or TNFR2 depends on the bioavailability of the soluble and membrane-bound forms of TNF-α. sTNF-α shows a far greater affinity to TNFR1, whereas TNFR2 is activated mainly by mTNF-α [21]. The stimulation of TNFR1 and TNFR2 activates a distinct molecular response resulting in different effector outputs in the affected cell. Furthermore, mTNF-α is capable of transmitting reverse signaling and therefore must be considered as a receptor, too [22]. In this case, TNFRs (membrane and soluble) serve as ligands for mTNF-α. The mTNF-α reverse signaling is mainly triggered by TNFR2 [22]. A schematic presentation of TNF-α signaling is shown in Figure 1.

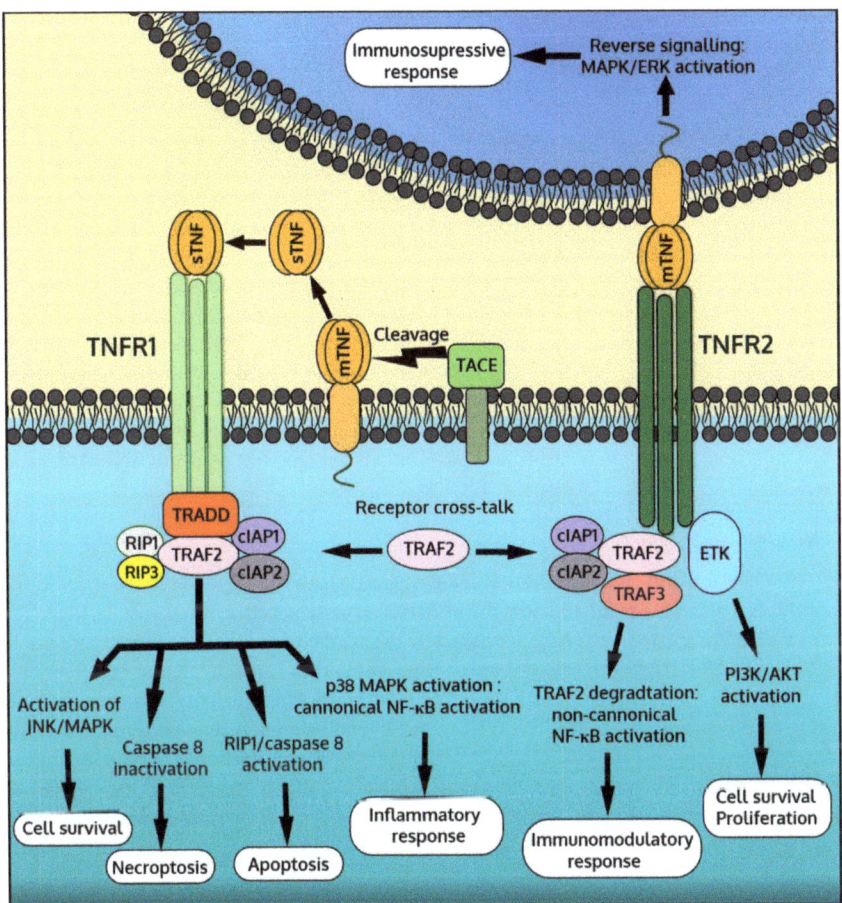

Figure 1. Overview of tumor necrosis factor-α (TNF-α) downstream signaling pathway mediated by two TNF-α receptors, TNFR1 and TNFR2, and by membrane form of TNF-α (mTNF-α) reverse signaling.

3.1. TNFR1 Signaling

In the presence of the ligand, TNFR1 recruits a number of adaptor proteins including TNFR-associated death domain (TRADD), TNF-α receptor associated factor 2 (TRAF2), receptor-interacting protein (RIP) kinase, inhibitors of apoptosis proteins (IAPs), Fas-associated death domain (FADD) and MAPK activating death domain (MADD) [19,21]. The newly formed TNFR1/TRADD/TRAF2/RIP/IAPs complex activates MAPKs, mainly c-Jun N-terminal kinase (JNK) and the p38 isoforms, and inhibitor of kappa B (IκB) kinases (IKKs). MAPKs transduce a signal into the nucleus through activation protein-1 (AP-1) and other transcription factors that bind to the specific DNA motifs of the target genes. IKKs activate the

NF-κB response by degrading the IκB complex and thus releasing the p50 subunit, which translocates to the nucleus and directly regulates gene expression. These MAPK- and IKK-dependent responses contribute mainly to pro-inflammatory cytokine production and cell survival, but they also mediate other processes [19,23]. Alternatively, TNFR1 can be internalized, and due to its intracellular death domain, it can form the TNFR1/TRADD/FADD complex with pro-caspase-8. Activated caspase-8 initiates a proteolytic cascade causing cell apoptosis. Of note, TNF-α-induced apoptosis is also mediated by MAPK/JNK [24]. Furthermore, TNFR1 can induce necroptosis through mitochondrial fission. Necroptosis is independent of other caspases, and the process occurs under conditions of caspase-8 inhibitor or depletion. TNF-α mediated necrosome formation critically depends on RIP1, RIP3, and mixed lineage kinase domain like (MLKL) pseudokinase [25,26].

3.2. TNFR2 Signaling

Unlike TNFR1, TNFR2 lacks the intracellular death domain and is unable to bind TRADD and initiate caspase-mediated apoptosis. Instead, activated TNFR2 recruits adaptor proteins TRAF2 and IAPs, activating the canonical NF-κB signaling through IKK. In addition, TNFR2, TRAF2, and IAPs form a complex with NF-κB-inducing kinase (NIK). As a result, NIK is released from the complex and activated. Active NIK induces the non-canonical NF-κB pathway through IKKα that ultimately produces a transcriptionally active p52 subunit [27]. TNFR2 can also activate phosphatidylinositol-3-kinase (PI3K)-dependent signaling. In this pathway, activated PI3K phosphorylates protein kinase B, also known as Akt, which in turn modulates several downstream effectors [28]. TNFR2-mediated activation of the canonical and non-canonical NF-κB and PI3K/Akt pathways typically promotes cell proliferation and survival. In cells expressing both TNFRs, the cross-talk between TNFR1 and TNFR2 may occur, which is mediated by TRAF2 [19,29]. As prolonged TNFR2 activation leads to TRAF2 degradation, this negatively regulates transcription factors and the immune response but enhances TNFR1-dependent caspase-mediated apoptosis and necroptosis [21,30].

3.3. mTNF-α Reverse Signaling

mTNF-α acts not only as a ligand for TNFRs triggering forward signaling in the target cells but also transduces a reverse signaling back to the mTNF-α expressing cell. Physiologically, the mTNF-α reverse signaling is triggered by TNFR2 expressed by the neighboring cells [31]. Furthermore, soluble TNFRs (mainly TNFR2) or even selected anti-TNF-α antibodies can activate the mTNF-α reverse signaling [32,33]. The intracellular domain of mTNF-α shows no kinase activity; however, the binding of TNFR to mTNF-α can activate MAPKs JNK and p38 signaling and the downstream transcriptional activities in the nucleus. mTNF-α reverse signaling regulates the production of certain inflammatory cytokines, but it is also involved in the modulation of other immune processes [34]. It should be noted that the role and mechanisms of mTNF-α reverse signal transduction are not well understood.

4. Anti-TNF-α Therapy and Cardiovascular Diseases in Humans

In the 20th century, TNF-α has been recognized as the key pro-inflammatory cytokine in humans. This led to the development of the first cytokine-targeted therapy with etanercept approved by the Food and Drug Administration (FDA) in 1998. Anti-TNF-α therapy has revolutionized the treatment of autoimmune inflammatory diseases by offering an alternative for non-specific immunosuppressive drugs, which cause multiple adverse effects for a long-term use [35]. To date, five FDA-approved TNF-α inhibitors are being used in routine clinical practice to treat patients with rheumatoid and psoriatic arthritis, psoriasis, ankylosing spondylitis, or Crohn's disease. TNF-α inhibitors represent the fusion protein of TNF-α receptors linked to the Fc region of human antibody (etanercept) or chimeric (infliximab), fully human (adalimumab and golimumab), or modified human (certolizumab–pegol) anti-TNF-α antibodies [36]. Although all these inhibitors neutralize TNF-α bioactivity, their therapeutic effect may vary [37,38].

The positive effects of anti-TNF-α therapy in autoimmune inflammatory diseases encouraged testing its therapeutic value in patients with systolic heart failure. These patients are characterized by elevated plasma levels of TNF-α and other pro-inflammatory cytokines [39–42], and improvement of their cardiac functions has been associated with decreasing TNF-α levels [43]. In fact, heart failure patients show also elevated cardiac TNF-α levels associated with dynamic changes in TNFR1 and TNFR2 expression [44]. Furthermore, genetic studies suggested that polymorphism in the *TNFA* gene was associated with increased risk of coronary heart disease development [45] and in case of coronary heart disease with increased risk of gastrointestinal complications [46]. Pilot studies suggested that a higher dose of etanercept increased the ejection fraction and quality-of-life scores [47,48], as well as improved systemic endothelial vasoreactivity in patients with advanced heart failure [49]. Nonetheless, randomized, double-blind, placebo-controlled studies failed to prove the therapeutic effect of etanercept in heart failure patients with reduced ejection fraction. In fact, the RECOVER (Research into Etanercept: Cytokine Antagonism in Ventricular Dysfunction) and RENAISSANCE (Randomized Etanercept North American Strategy to Study Antagonism of Cytokines) clinical trials were terminated early due to a general lack of improvement in composite clinical score and due to the dose-dependent toxicity observed in some patients [50]. Furthermore, the ATTACH (Anti-Tnf alpha Therapy Against Chronic Heart failure) study showed that high doses of infliximab in HFrEF patients increased the risk of death or heart failure-related hospitalization [51]. The injection of a single high dose of etanercept did not improve outcomes of patients following acute myocardial infarction [52]. In conclusion, continuous anti-TNF-α therapy in patients with systolic heart failure show no evident benefits and may even be harmful and exacerbate the disease. Consequently, the use of TNF-α inhibitors is not recommended for HFrEF patients.

Unlike for HFrEF patients, a long-term anti-TNF-α therapy in patients with autoimmune inflammatory diseases is generally not harmful, and it may even protect from enhanced cardiovascular complications and cardiovascular death [53,54]. Although heart failure cases have been reported in patients treated with TNF-α inhibitors [55], the risk of new onset of heart failure in patients under age 50 receiving etanercept or infliximab is low [56]. Anti-TNF-α treatment is most commonly used to treat rheumatoid arthritis. Importantly, these patients are characterized by a more rapid development of subclinical changes in diastolic function [57], and in case of incident heart failure, they are more likely to show the HFpEF phenotype [58]. In fact, rheumatoid arthritis patients with preserved left ventricular function treated with infliximab showed improvement in cardiac function [59] and decreased the left ventricular torsion [60]. A growing body of evidence suggests that anti-TNF-α therapy could effectively protect from the development of vascular diseases and atherosclerosis in particular. Standard anti-TNF-α treatment employed in treating rheumatoid arthritis has been demonstrated to decrease levels of soluble endothelial adhesions molecules [61] as well as improve arterial stiffness [62] and endothelial functions [63]. The use of TNF-α antagonists has been associated with a decreased risk of myocardial infarction [64] and development of acute coronary syndrome [65] pointing to anti-TNF-α treatment as an effective anti-atherosclerotic therapy in rheumatoid arthritis. In line with these data, large cohort clinical studies reported the unchanged or reduced overall cardiovascular-related death of rheumatoid arthritis patients receiving TNF-α inhibitors [66–69]. Importantly, in rheumatoid arthritis, anti-TNF-α therapy protects from the development of ischemic cardiac events, but it shows no cardioprotective effects in the post-ischemic heart [64]. Noteworthy, anti-TNF-α therapy in elderly rheumatoid arthritis patients might exacerbate heart failure and reduce survival [70].

Psoriasis represents another autoimmune inflammatory disease associated with increased serum levels of TNF-α [71]. Similarly to other systemic inflammatory diseases, psoriasis patients are at increased risk of developing cardiovascular diseases [72]. In psoriasis, patients treated with adalimumab showed improvement in vascular functions [73]. A large retrospective cohort study has demonstrated a significantly reduced incidence of myocardial infarction in psoriasis patients receiving TNF-α inhibitors [74]. In line with these findings, the use of TNF-α inhibitors in psoriasis lowered the occurrence of major cardiovascular events [75]. Reductions of cardiovascular events due to treatment with TNF-α inhibitors were also observed in ankylosing spondylitis and psoriatic arthritis [76,77].

Summarizing, in the light of published clinical data (summarized in the Table 1), anti-TNF-α treatment seems to reduce the risk of cardiovascular episodes mainly by inhibiting systemic inflammation and thereby suppressing the development of atherosclerosis and ischemic events. On the other hand, in the failing heart, TNF-α plays more of a cardioprotective role, but the mechanism remains unknown.

Table 1. Effects of anti-TNF-α treatments on cardiovascular outcomes in heart failure and in systemic inflammatory disease patients.

Type of Trial	Disease	Intervention	Outcomes	Ref.
Single-center clinical trial (18 patients)	Class III NYHA heart failure	Single infusion of etanercept (1, 4, or 10 mg/m^2) or placebo	Dose-dependent increased quality-of-life scores and ejection fraction measured at 14th day	[47]
Single-center clinical trial (47 patients)	Class III-IV NYHA heart failure	Biweekly injections of etanercept for 3 months (5 or 12 mg/m^2) or placebo	Dose-dependent increase in functional status, LV functions, and remodeling after 3 months	[48]
Single-center clinical trial (13 patients)	Class III NYHA heart failure	Single injection of etanercept (25 mg) in combination with standard treatment	Major improvement in systemic endothelial vasodilator capacity 7 days from intervention when compared to standard treatment group	[49]
Multi-center, double-blind clinical trial RECOVER (1123 patients)	Class II-IV NYHA heart failure	Weekly or biweekly injections of 25 mg etanercept for 6 months or placebo	Prematurely terminated due to lack of improvement in clinical outcome. No change in hospitalization or death occurrence	[50]
Multi-center, double-blind clinical trial RENAISSANCE (925 patients)	Class II-IV NYHA heart failure	Biweekly or 3 times a week injections of 25 mg etanercept for 6 months or placebo	Prematurely terminated due to lack of improvement in clinical outcome. Worsened clinical composite score in some patients	[50]
Multi-center, double-blind clinical trial ATTACH (150 patients)	Class III-IV NYHA heart failure	Injections of 5 or 10 mg/kg infliximab at 0, 2, and 6 weeks or placebo	After 14 weeks modest improvement in ejection fraction at 5 mg/kg dose. No improvement in composite clinical score at either dose, increased hospitalization and death occurrence at 10 mg/kg dose	[51]
Randomized controlled trial (26 patients)	Acute myocardial infarction	Single infusion of 10 mg etanercept in combination with standard treatment	Reduced systemic inflammation, increased platelet activation. No effect on peripheral vasomotor or fibrinolytic function when compared to standard treatment	[52]
Single-center clinical trial (23 patients)	Rheumatoid arthritis	3 mg/kg infliximab infusions every 2 months	Improvement in LV ejection fraction, reduction in IL-6, endothelin 1, and NT-proBNP serum levels	[59]
Single-center clinical trial (68 patients)	Rheumatoid arthritis	180 days of infliximab or prednisolone treatment	Improvement in LV longitudinal and radial systolic deformation and decreased LV torsion in comparison to prednisolone treatment	[60]
Multi-center comparative study (14258 patients)	Rheumatoid arthritis	90+ days of adalimumab, etanercept, or infliximab treatment with median of 5 years follow-up	Significantly decreased risk of myocardial infarction in comparison to patients receiving synthetic DMARD	[64]
Multi-center comparative study (7704 patients)	Rheumatoid arthritis	Long-term treatment (average of 2 years) with adalimumab, etanercept, and infliximab	Significantly decreased risk of acute coronary syndrome compared to biologic-naïve RA patients or DMARD treatment	[65]
Multi-center comparative study (10,156 patients)	Rheumatoid arthritis	Long-term treatment (median exposure period of 22,9 months) with adalimumab, etanercept, and infliximab	Reduced risk of cardiovascular-related death compared to patients receiving DMARD	[66]
Multi-center retrospective comparative study (20,811 patients)	Rheumatoid arthritis	Long-term treatment (median duration of 20 months) with TNF-α inhibitors	No change in cardiovascular-related death risk, improved cardiovascular outcomes in younger patients	[67]

Table 1. Cont.

Type of Trial	Disease	Intervention	Outcomes	Ref.
Multi-center retrospective comparative study (7077 patients)	Rheumatoid arthritis	Long term (up to 5 years) treatment with TNF-α inhibitors	Reduction in cardiovascular-related death in women	[68]
Multi-center retrospective comparative study (20,243 patients)	Rheumatoid arthritis	Switch from non-biological disease modifying antirheumatic drug to TNF antagonists	No change in risk of cardiovascular event (including in patients with heart failure history)	[69]
Multi-center retrospective comparative study (7077 patients)	Rheumatoid arthritis	Long-term treatment (1–2 years) with TNF-α inhibitors or methotrexate	Increased risk of heart failure onset and exacerbation of existent heart failure in elderly patients treated with TNF-α inhibitors	[70]
Multi-center comparative study (8845 patients)	Psoriasis	At least 2 months of adalimumab, etanercept, or infliximab treatment	Reduced risk of myocardial infarction in comparison to TNF-α inhibitor naïve patients	[74]
Multi-center comparative study (17,729)	Psoriasis	150 days of adalimumab, etanercept, infliximab, or methotrexate treatment	Treatment with TNF-α inhibitors was shown to reduce overall cardiovascular event risk in comparison to methotrexate	[75]
Multi-center retrospective comparative study (4140 patients)	Rheumatoid arthritis, psoriasis, ankylosing spondylitis	Long-term treatment (at least 1 year) with TNF-α inhibitors	Continuous use of TNF-α inhibitors reduced the incidence of major cardiovascular events in comparable manner in all studied diseases	[76]
Multi-center comparative study (319)	Psoriatic arthritis	Long-term treatment (2–3 years) with TNF-α inhibitors	Reduced atherosclerosis in men, but not women, receiving TNF-α inhibitors. Reduction of vascular inflammation in both sexes	[77]

LV: left ventricle, NT-proBNP: N-terminal prohormone of brain natriuretic peptide, DMARD-disease-modifying antirheumatic drugs.

5. TNF-α in Animal Models of Cardiovascular Diseases

Results of anti-TNF-α treatments in patients with heart failure or with autoimmune inflammatory diseases demonstrated the relevance and a dual role of TNF-α in cardiovascular diseases in humans. However, these clinical data are insufficient to elucidate the underlaying mechanisms. Animal models of cardiovascular diseases, on the other hand, can be used to specifically define the role of gene of interest and to study cellular and molecular mechanisms. In the case of TNF-α signaling, there is a number of available transgenic mouse models allowing for the systemic or cell type-specific overexpression or genetic knockdown of selected components of the TNF-α pathway. The results of these animal studies are summarized in the Table 2. A growing body of experimental data confirmed a dual role of TNF-α and pointed to the opposing effects of TNFR1 and TNFR2. Thus, experimental data from transgenic mouse models might explain the failure of clinical application of anti-TNF-α inhibitors in heart failure patients. Prospectively, these data suggest that targeting TNFRs, rather than TNF-α, with selective agonists or antagonists might represent a more promising cardioprotective strategy in the post-ischemic heart.

5.1. TNF-α in Gain-of-Function Approaches

A gain-of-function approach is based on the overexpression of the gene of interest in a cell or in an organism and represents one strategy to study its function. A popular knock-in mice model non-specifically overexpressing human TNF-α shows high TNF-α production mainly in synovial fibroblasts and in endothelial cells (without evident effects in other cell types) and develops severe erosive arthritis [78,79]. Therefore, these mice are used as a mouse model of rheumatoid arthritis. Instead, transgenic mice overexpressing TNF-α in cardiomyocytes are considered as a better model to address the role of TNF-α in the heart. An initial study showed that the cardiac-restricted overexpression of TNF-α caused lethal myocarditis with diffuse lymphohistiocytic infiltrates and interstitial edema that led to cardiac death at the age of 7–11 days [80]. In contrast, in other cardiac-restricted TNF-α overexpressing models (TNF1.6 and MHCsTNF strains), most of the transgenic mice survived and developed mild inflammation and dilated cardiomyopathy phenotype with cardiac tissue remodeling as well as systolic and diastolic dysfunction associated with atrial and ventricular arrhythmias [81–83]. Mathematical modeling suggested that the reentrant arrhythmias spontaneously occurring in these mice are caused by a reduced intercellular coupling [84]. Yet, it needs to be noted that cardiac tissue levels of TNF-α in these models were elevated up to 200-fold comparing native myocardium. The pathogenic effect caused by cardiac-restricted TNF-α overexpression depended mainly on the TNFR1 signaling. Accordingly, left ventricular dysfunction was preserved by the adenoviral-mediated expression of soluble TNFR1 [83], and the genetic deletion of *Tnfrsf1a* (gene encoding TNFR1) improved cardiac functions and completely protected from cardiac death [85]. On the contrary, *Tnfrsf1b* (gene encoding TNFR2) genetic deficiency exacerbated heart failure and increased the lethality of TNF-α overexpressing mice pointing to the cardioprotective role of TNFR2 [85]. Interestingly, the overexpression of non-cleavable mTNF-α in cardiomyocytes led to a concentric cardiac hypertrophy phenotype without evidence of myocarditis or systolic dysfunction [86]. This may suggest that in the TNF-α overexpressing heart, the mTNF-α reverse signaling regulates different processes than TNFR1 and TNFR2.

5.2. Atherosclerosis and Ischemic Heart Disease Models

Atherosclerosis is a pathogenic condition of arteries characterized by the development of atherosclerotic plaques. A rupture of atherosclerotic plaques and the subsequent blood clot formation can cause life-threatening ischemic events, such as myocardial infarction or sudden cardiac death. In a typical clinical scenario of myocardial infarction, atherosclerotic plaque rupture and the subsequent thrombosis blocks blood flow in larger coronary arteries, causing an ischemic condition in the myocardium and death of cardiomyocytes. Myocardial infarct size depends on the time and the extent of ischemia as well as the subsequent inflammatory response. In animal models, myocardial infarction is typically performed in non-atherosclerotic condition.

5.3. Atherosclerosis

Experimental atherosclerosis is typically induced by feeding animals an atherogenic high-fat, high-cholesterol diet over at least 3 months. The development of atherosclerotic plaques is significantly enhanced in mice with naturally elevated plasma cholesterol levels, such as $Apoe^{-/-}$ or $Ldlr^{-/-}$ mouse strains. In mice, TNF-α has been recognized as one of the most potent proatherogenic cytokines, and the formation of atherosclerotic lesions was preceded by an increased expression of TNF-α, TNFR1, and TNFR2, which were elevated even further during plaque growth [87]. Knockout of the *Tnfa* gene in $Apoe^{-/-}$ mice fed a high-fat diet retarded the progression of plaque growth and decreased levels of pro-atherosclerotic factors without affecting cholesterol levels [88,89]. Experiments with the APOE*3-Leiden $Tnfa^{-/-}$ strain fed a high-cholesterol diet also demonstrated that TNF-α promoted necrosis in plaque-infiltrating cells and enhanced advanced lesion formation [90]. Data obtained from bone marrow chimeric mice suggested that TNF-α expressed by the bone marrow cells played a key role in an $Apoe^{-/-}$ mouse model of atherosclerosis [91]. In line with this data, $Apoe^{-/-}$ mice on a high-fat, high-cholesterol diet receiving recombinant TNF-α developed an enhanced atherosclerotic phenotype, which could be reversed by NF-κB inhibitors [92].

In contrast to data from transgenic models, the results of the pharmacological inhibition of TNF-α in mouse models were less consistent. It has been demonstrated that recombinant soluble TNFR1 successfully attenuated the formation of aortic lesions in an $Apoe^{-/-}$ model [91]. Beneficial effects of infliximab on endothelial reactive oxygen species (ROS) production and plaque formation were further confirmed in $Apoe^{-/-}$ mice kept in hypoxia conditions and fed a high-fat diet [93]. However, in $Ldlr^{-/-}$ mice, monotherapy with etanercept failed to reduce the development of atherosclerotic plaques, and the atheroprotective effect of etanercept was observed only in combination with cholesterol-lowering drugs [94]. Instead, treatment with anti-TNF-α monoclonal antibody CNTO5048 (neutralizing specifically murine TNF-α) surprisingly increased plaque burden, the expression of vascular inflammatory genes, and the pro-atherogenic lipid profile in hypercholesterolemic $Ldlr^{-/-}$ mice [95]. These inconsistent findings could potentially be explained by the involvement of mTNF-α, because most of the anti-TNF-α antibodies neutralize exclusively sTNF-α. Indeed, the proatherogenic effect of mTNF-α has been associated with its presence on exosomes produced by dendritic cells and the activation of the pro-inflammatory NF-κB pathway in endothelial cells [96]. Although experiments with transgenic mice expressing an exclusively non-cleavable form of mTNF-α demonstrated the involvement of mTNF-α, these findings pointed primarily to the key role of sTNF-α in mouse atherogenesis [97–99]. On the other hand, mice with an increased expression of mTNF-α (due to a reduced expression of *Adam17*) showed enhanced macrophage adhesion and atherosclerosis in an $Ldlr^{-/-}$ mouse model [98]. It should be noticed that in this model, an increased expression of mTNF-α was associated with the constitutive activation of TNFR2 signaling. Mouse models have been also used to elucidate the role of TNFR1 in the pathogenesis of atherosclerosis. $Tnfrsf1a^{-/-}$ were initially reported to develop enhanced atherogenesis when fed an atherogenic diet [100]. However, $Tnfrsf1a^{-/-}$ mice on a proatherogenic $Apoe^{-/-}$ background showed reduced atherosclerosis, and the data pointed to the key role of TNFR1 expressed in arteries [101]. Summarizing, the proatherogenic role of TNF-α has been generally confirmed in animal studies, but there is a surprisingly high discrepancy in results obtained from different models. It seems that $Apoe^{-/-}$, rather than $Ldlr^{-/-}$ or non-transgenic mice, represents the most relevant animal model to study TNF-α signaling in atherosclerosis.

5.4. Myocardial Infarction

Experimental acute myocardial infarction is typically achieved by permanent or temporary mechanical ligation of the left anterior descending coronary artery. Animals surviving this procedure eventually develop fibrotic scars (that replaces necrotic myocardium), and their hearts show impaired function and hemodynamic abnormalities. Published data report elevated sTNF-α levels in the serum of post-infarcted mice and increased mTNF-α expression in the infarct and peri-infarct zones [102]. In a permanent occlusion model, $Tnfa^{-/-}$ mice showed a significantly smaller infarct area, decreased expression of intercellular adhesion molecule 1 (ICAM-1), and lower numbers of heart-infiltrating neutrophils and macrophages [103]. However, in the same model, a lack of both TNFRs led to a significant increase in the infarction size and to an increased apoptosis of cardiomyocytes [104]. A smaller infarct size, better cardiac function, and reduced inflammatory response were observed in $Tnfa^{-/-}$ mice also in a myocardial ischemia–reperfusion injury model [105]. Similarly, the blockade of TNF-α with etanercept 10 min prior to ischemia–reperfusion injury improved cardiac functions, reduced infarct size, and cardiomyocyte apoptosis [106]. Moreover, a single dose of etanercept injected at the time of myocardial infarction improved long-term cardiac function and reduced cardiac tissue remodeling in rats [107]. In another study, pharmacological inhibitor preventing TNF-α binding to its receptor (CAS1049741-03-8) reduced post-infarction inflammatory response but worsened cardiac function due to enhanced cardiomyocyte apoptosis [108]. The injection of anti-TNF-α antibody 3 h prior to ischemia–reperfusion was also shown to reduce endothelial dysfunction by reducing the production of endothelial ROS [109]. Pathogenic processes over a long term are primary mediated by TNFR1-dependent pathways, as $Tnfrsf1a^{-/-}$ mice were consistently reported to develop less impaired cardiac contractile functions and showed better survival rates up to several weeks after infarction [110–113]. This phenotype was associated with the reduced expression of inflammatory cytokines, matrix metalloproteinase activity, and diminished NF-κB and MAPK activation in the cardiac tissue. Data from mice lacking an NF-κB p50 subunit confirmed the involvement of this TNFR1-downstream pathway in the pathogenesis of myocardial infarction [114]. The pathogenic role of TNFR1 in myocardial infarction is not limited to its signaling in the heart. Cardiovascular homeostasis is regulated by the subfornical organ located in the forebrain, which controls cardiac sympathetic excitation. The targeted inactivation of TNFR1 in the subfornical organ reduced left ventricular dysfunction induced by coronary artery ligation in rats [115]. Unlike TNFR1 signaling, TNFR2-dependent pathways mainly activate cardioprotective processes in the post-infarction heart. Accordingly, $Tnfrsf1b^{-/-}$ mice showed exacerbated cardiomyocyte apoptosis and fibrosis as well as worsened cardiac function and long-term survival in a permanent occlusion model [110,111].

Of note, ischemia–reperfusion experiments on isolated hearts confirmed the deteriorating effect of TNF-α [116] and cardioprotective role of TNFR2 on myocardial function recovery [117]. Summarizing, mouse data underlined the activation of TNF-α signaling in the infarcted myocardium and highlighted the counteractive effects mediated by both TNFRs.

5.5. Non-Ischemic Heart Failure Models

Non-ischemic heart diseases refer to cardiac abnormalities occurring in the absence of coronary artery diseases. Cardiomyopathies represent the most common type of non-ischemic heart disease, in which ventricles become enlarged and stiff. Cardiomyopathies may be caused by an abnormally thick myocardium (hypertrophic cardiomyopathy) or by the dilatation of the ventricles (dilated cardiomyopathy) [118]. Hypertrophic cardiomyopathy may be genetic or can be caused by chronic hypertension or stress, and it is characterized by ineffective muscle relaxation. On the other hand, the phenotype of dilated cardiomyopathy, which is associated with left ventricular or biventricular dilatation and systolic and diastolic dysfunction, can be a consequence of the ongoing inflammatory processes in the heart. Cardiomyopathies are often progressive pathologies causing not only impaired blood pumping but also heart valve problems, blood clots, and arrhythmias, leading to heart and secondary organ failures. There is a number of established animal models that reproduce both hypertrophic and dilated cardiomyopathy conditions [119].

5.6. Hypertrophic Cardiomyopathy

Experimental hypertension in rodents is commonly achieved by the partial occlusion of the aorta (transverse aortic constriction model) or by continuous infusion of the vasoconstrictor angiotensin II using osmotic minipumps. In these models, increased blood pressure in the heart induces a compensatory mechanism, by which the left ventricle becomes over time thicker and thereby less effective in muscle relaxation. On the cellular level, cardiac tissue is characterized by cardiomyocyte hypertrophy and interstitial fibrosis. Data from a mouse model of pressure overload induced by aortic banding pointed to the active role of TNF-α–TNFR1 signaling in the development of hypertensive cardiomyopathy, as initially suggested by the correlation between progressive hypertrophy and increasing myocardial levels of TNF-α, TNFR1, and TACE [120,121]. In line with this suggestion, $Tnfa^{-/-}$ mice developed significantly lower inflammatory response, cardiac hypertrophy, and left ventricular remodeling, showing preserved cardiac functions in several studies [120–123]. This phenotype was attributed to the abrogated production of superoxide in a TNF-α/PI3K-dependent manner in cardiomyocytes and in cardiac fibroblasts [122], changes in the expression and activity of metalloproteinases [120], decreased cardiac inflammation, and abrogated cardiomyocyte apoptosis [121]. Interestingly, in this model of hypertension, cardiac TACE activity and TNF-α levels were controlled by tissue inhibitor of metalloproteinase (TIMP)-3 [120]. The pathogenic mechanism is mainly mediated by TNFR1. Accordingly, $Tnfrsf1a^{-/-}$ mice are partially protected from transverse aortic constriction-induced hypertrophy and are characterized by better survival rates [124]. In the same model, mice lacking the TNFR1 adaptor molecule TRADD also developed significantly attenuated fibrosis with better cardiac functions, suggesting a key role of the TNFR1–TRADD-dependent cell death in hypertrophic cardiomyopathy [125]. This pathogenic TNFR1 signaling seems to be counter-regulated by TNFR2. In response to the increased blood pressure induced by transverse aortic constriction, mice lacking $Tnfrsf1b$ showed worsened survival rates and increased cardiac hypertrophy, and the cardioprotective TNFR2 signaling has been linked to its effects in mitochondria [124]. Moreover, mice with cardiac-specific TRAF2 deletion developed exacerbated heart failure with pathological remodeling and cardiomyocyte necroptosis [30].

Similar data were obtained in another model of hypertrophic cardiomyopathy. In an angiotensin II osmotic minipump model, $Tnfa^{-/-}$ and $Tnfrsf1a^{-/-}$ mice showed significantly attenuated phenotype [126,127]. In-depth analysis demonstrated reduced immunofibrotic changes in the myocardium of $Tnfrsf1a^{-/-}$ mice, but there was no protective effect on diastolic dysfunction in this model [127]. In contrast, $Tnfrsf1b^{-/-}$ mice receiving angiotensin II infusion developed fibrosis and showed only slight changes in expression of pro-fibrotic genes [128]. Thus, it seems that also in this model of hypertrophy, TNF-α–TNFR1 signaling is involved in disease progression.

Cardiac hypertrophy associated with diastolic dysfunction can be alternatively induced by the continuous delivery of β-adrenergic agonist isoproterenol. In this model, mice lacking TNFR1 developed reduced inflammatory response, but this was insufficient to protect them from isoproterenol-induced hypertrophy, whereas mice deficient of TNFR2 showed an increased pro-inflammatory response and exacerbated cardiac hypertrophy [129]. Of note, in vitro experiments confirmed that TNF-α indeed could enhance isoproterenol-induced cardiomyocyte hypertrophy, but surprisingly, this effect was completely blocked by anti-TNFR2 antibody [130].

Mice consuming increasing doses of ethanol over longer periods of time develop a specific type of alcoholic cardiomyopathy with fibrotic and structural changes in the left ventricle. In this model, mice showed TNFR1-dependent elevated serum levels of TNF-α, left ventricle dysfunction, and increased cardiac ROS and pro-inflammatory cytokine production [131]. Increased TNF-α levels have been also observed in a rat model of adriamycin-induced cardiomyopathy. Animals with higher serum TNF-α levels showed worse heart function and increased mortality [132].

Summarizing, data from hypertrophic cardiomyopathy models suggest that targeting TNF-α indeed might successfully prevent from disease development. It should be noted that as in other cardiovascular diseases, pathogenic TNF-α signaling is mainly mediated by TNFR1.

5.7. Inflammatory Heart Diseases

In animal models, heart-specific inflammation is induced either by infection with cardiotropic virus (mainly coxsackievirus B3) or by the active induction of heart-specific autoimmunity [133]. In the infectious model, myocarditis is triggered by the immune response to the virus infecting and replicating in cardiomyocytes, whereas in the autoimmune model, myocarditis is mainly mediated by the activated heart-specific CD4$^+$ T lymphocytes. Published data suggest that the TNF-α–TNFR1 axis plays an active role in the development of myocarditis. In a coxsackievirus B3 model, $Tnfa^{-/-}$ and $Tnfrsf1a^{-/-}$ but not $Tnfrsf1b^{-/-}$ mice showed strikingly reduced cardiac inflammation [134]. Interestingly, defects in TNF-α signaling showed no effect on viral titers. In a mouse model of experimental autoimmune myocarditis induced by immunization with cardiac myosin, TNF-α/β neutralizing antibodies delivered prior to but not after immunization reduced the incidence of myocarditis [135]. Furthermore, $Tnfrsf1a^{-/-}$ mice were completely protected from the development of myocarditis induced by immunization with cardiac myosin or by an adoptive transfer of autoreactive T lymphocytes [136]. Although published data point to the pathogenic role of TNF-α signaling in the development of inflammatory heart disease, it should be noted that current knowledge is based on a few studies only and that the role of TNF-α signaling in the transition from myocarditis to dilated cardiomyopathy remains unknown.

Table 2. Summary of phenotypes observed in animal models of cardiovascular diseases in relation to modification of the TNF-α signaling pathway.

Model	Transgene/Intervention	Phenotype	Ref.
		Overexpression	
Cardiomyocyte-specific TNF-α overexpression	none	Lethal myocarditis with interstitial edema	[80]
	none	Progressive heart failure with severe LV remodeling	[81]
	none	Calcium-dependent atrial and ventricular arrhythmias	[82]
	sTNFR1 overexpression	Preservation of LV function	[83]
	$Tnfrsf1a^{-/-}$	Improved cardiac function, reduced mortality	[85]
	$Tnfrsf1b^{-/-}$	Exacerbated heart failure, increased mortality	
Cardiomyocyte-specific mTNF-α overexpression	none	Cardiac hypertrophy without inflammation and systolic dysfunction	[86]

Table 2. Cont.

Model	Transgene/Intervention	Phenotype	Ref.
Atherosclerosis			
Atherogenic diet	$Tnfa^{-/-}$	Protection from atherosclerotic lesion formation, lowered atherogenic lipid profile, decreased IL-6 levels	[99]
	Exclusive expression of mTNF-α	Partial protection from atherosclerosis. Lower lipid deposition and macrophage accumulation, no changes in atherogenic lipid profile and IL-6	
$Apoe^{-/-}$ on atherogenic diet	$Tnfa^{-/-}$	Slower plaque growth, decreased atherosclerotic markers, no changes in cholesterol levels	[88,89]
	$Tnfa^{-/-}$	Reduced plaque growth	[91]
	sTNFR1 treatment	Reduced plaque growth	
	Transplantation of $Tnfa^{-/-}$ bone marrow	Reduced plaque growth	
	$Tnfrsf1a^{-/-}$ grafted arteries	Reduced plaque growth and adhesion molecule expression	[101]
	Weekly infliximab injections	Improved endothelial functions, reduced atherosclerotic plaques, and decreased ROS	[93]
	Single injection of DC-derived mTNF-bearing exosomes	Increased levels of adhesion molecules in lesions, increased plaque formation	[96]
Apoe*3-Leiden on atherogenic diet	$Tnfa^{-/-}$	Higher number of early lesions and lower number of advanced lesions. Decreased necroptosis and increased apoptosis in lesion area. No changes in inflammatory parameters and lipid profiles	[90]
$Ldlr^{-/-}$ on atherogenic diet	ADAM17 deficiency (increased mTNF and permanent TNFR2 activation)	Faster plaque growth, enhanced macrophage adhesion, increased macrophage, and smooth muscle proliferation	[98]
	Etanercept in combination with pravastatin/saprogrelate therapy	Decrease in aortic lesion area, endothelial adhesion molecules, and improved lipid profile in comparison to pravastatin/saprogrelate	[94]
	Monoclonal anti-mouse TNF-α antibody administration	Reduced plaque stability, increased vascular pro-inflammatory gene expression, and larger plaque area	[95]
	Recombinant TNF-α administration	Increased plaque burden and endothelial LDL transcytosis. Prevented by pharmacological NF-κB inhibitors	[92]
Myocardial Infarction			
Permanent occlusion	$Tnfa^{-/-}$	Lower infarct area, less infiltrating mononuclear cells, reduced expression of endothelial adhesion molecules at day 1 and 7	[103]
		Improved cardiac functions up to 3 days, but not at day 7	[113]
		Improved contractile functions, diminished hypertrophy and remodeling, reduced NF-κB activation after 4 weeks	[110]
	$Tnfrsf1a^{-/-}$	Lower infarct area and fibrosis, preserved cardiac functions at day 7	[113]
		Improved contractile functions, increased survival rate after 4 weeks	[111]
		Protection for infarction-induced death, improved LV functions, and decreased hypertrophy after 6 weeks	[112]
		Reduced mortality 24 h post infarction, lower inflammation, and improved cardiac recovery after 28 days	[123]
	Pharmacological TNFR1 inactivation in subfornical organ	Reduced LV dysfunction after 4 weeks	[115]
	$Tnfrsf1b^{-/-}$	Worsened remodeling, hypertrophy and contractile functions, increased fibrosis and apoptosis at day 28	[110]
		Worsened cardiac functions, increased infarct size, exacerbated fibrosis at day 3 and 7	[113]
		Exacerbated hypertrophy, fibrosis, ventricular dilatation, and dysfunction after 4 weeks	[111]
		Increased mortality during the first 7 days, reduced number of functional blood vessels in infarct area after 28 days	[123]
	Daily monoclonal anti-TNF-α antibody administration during the first week after myocardial infarction	Reduced inflammation, worsened cardiac functions, inhibited autophagy and increased apoptosis in cardiomyocytes after 1, 2, 3, and 4 weeks	[108]
	Single etanercept injection directly after myocardial infarction	Reduced inflammation, improved remodeling, and preserved LV functions after 4 days	[107]

Table 2. Cont.

Model	Transgene/Intervention	Phenotype	Ref.
Myocardial Infarction			
Ischemia-reperfusion	$Tnfa^{-/-}$	Lower infarct area, improved cardiac functions, reduced cardiac NF-κB activation measured 120 min from reperfusion	[105]
	Etanercept administration 10 min prior to myocardial infarction	Lower infarct area, improved cardiac functions, 3 h, 24 h, or 14 days after reperfusion	[106]
	Anti-mouse TNF-α antibody injection 3 h prior myocardial infarction	Preserved endothelial functions, reduced endothelial production of ROS 90 min after reperfusion	[109]
Hypertrophic Cardiomyopathy			
Transverse aortic constriction	$Tnfa^{-/-}$	Reduced inflammatory response, decreased hypertrophy, improved cardiac functions	[121]
	$Tnfa^{-/-}Timp3^{-/-}$	Attenuated LV dilation, improved cardiac functions, increased survival after 7 weeks. Complete prevention of heart disease upon additional MMP inhibitors administration	[120]
	$Tnfa^{-/-}$	Improved cardiac functions, suppression of MMPs expression, reduction in superoxide production	[122]
	$Tnfrsf1b^{-/-}$	Increased survival rates, decreased hypertrophy, improved mitochondrial functions	[124]
	$Tradd^{-/-}$	Reduced hypertrophy with improved cardiac functions, attenuated TAK1/p38 MAPK phosphorylation	[125]
	$Tnfrsf1a^{-/-}Tnfrsf1b^{-/-}$	Increased mortality, hypertrophy, and mitochondrial DNA damage	[124]
	$Traf2^{-/-}$	TNFR1-dependent pathological remodeling and increased cardiomyocyte death	[30]
Angiotensin II-induced hypertrophy	$Tnfa^{-/-}$	Reduced hypertrophy and hypertension	[126]
	$Tnfrsf1a^{-/-}$	Slower progression of hypertrophy, reduced fibrosis and immune response	[127]
	$Tnfrsf1a^{-/-}$	No effect on early inflammatory phase, increased uptake of bone marrow-derived fibroblasts progenitors and exacerbated fibrosis	[128]
	$Tnfrsf1b^{-/-}$	No effects	[128]
Isoproterenol-induced hypertrophy	$Tnfrsf1a^{-/-}$	Reduced inflammatory response at day 1, unchanged hypertrophy at day 7	[129]
	$Tnfrsf1b^{-/-}$	Increased inflammatory response at day 1, exacerbated hypertrophy at day 7	
Alcoholic cardiomyopathy	$Tnfrsf1a^{-/-}$	Preserved LV functions, decreased ROS in LV, lower serum levels of TNF-α	[131]
Inflammatory Heart Diseases			
Coxsackievirus B3 induced myocarditis	$Tnfa^{-/-}$	Reduced myocarditis, no changes in virus titers	[134]
	$Tnfrsf1a^{-/-}$	Reduced myocarditis, no changes in virus titers	
	$Tnfrsf1b^{-/-}$	Unaffected myocarditis, no changes in virus titers	
Myocarditis induced by cardiac myosin immunization	Anti-TNF-α/β before immunization	Reduced myocarditis	[135]
	Anti-TNF-α/β after immunization	Unaffected myocarditis	
	$Tnfrsf1a^{-/-}$	Protection from myocarditis despite of T cell activation	
Myocarditis induced by autoreactive T cell transfer	$Tnfrsf1a^{-/-}$	Protection from myocarditis	[136]

LDL: low-density lipoprotein LV: left ventricular, MMP: matrix metalloproteinase, ROS: reactive oxygen species, $Timp3^{-/-}$: metalloproteinase inhibitor 3 knockout, $Tnfa^{-/-}$: tumor necrosis factor-α knockout, $Tnfrsf1a^{-/-}$: TNFR1 knockout, $Tnfrsf1b^{-/-}$: TNFR2 knockout, $TRADD^{-/-}$: tumor necrosis factor receptor type 1-associated death domain protein knockout.

6. Cellular and Molecular Mechanisms of TNF-α Signaling in Cardiovascular Diseases

The heart is made up of three main cell types: cardiomyocytes, cardiac microvascular endothelial cells, and cardiac stromal cells (mainly fibroblasts). In addition, heart-resident macrophages represent a small but important cell population in the healthy heart. Furthermore, in response to injury, cardiac tissue is infiltrated by immune cells, such as inflammatory monocytes and lymphocytes. It should be noted that TNF-α can be produced by many cardiac cell types, but immune cells seem to represent a particularly important source of this cytokine in cardiac pathology. TNF-α signaling controls many biological processes ranging from pro-inflammatory and proapoptotic to regenerative and cardioprotective (Figure 2). The actual effect of TNF-α depends not only on the cell type and activation of other molecular pathways, but also on expression of inducible TNFR2 (TNFR1 is generally stably expressed in nearly all cell types). As demonstrated in animal models, the deleterious effects of TNF-α are mainly mediated by the prolonged or excessive activation of TNFR1, while the activation of TNFR2 often exerts cardioprotective results.

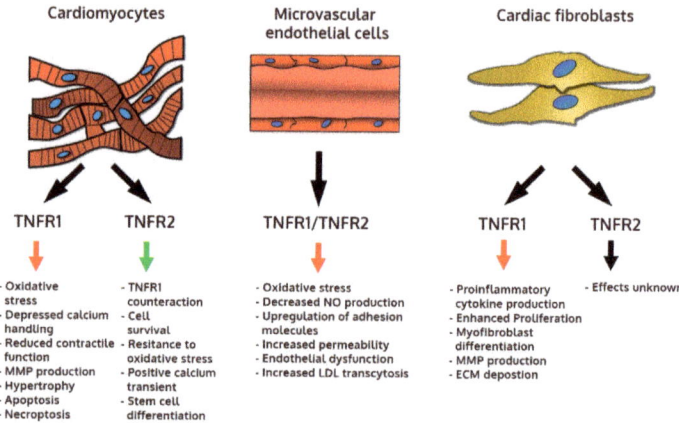

Figure 2. Biological effects mediated by TNFR1 and TNFR2 in main cellular components of the heart. ECM: extracellular matrix, LDL: low-density lipoprotein, MMP: matrix metalloproteinase, NO: nitric oxide.

6.1. Pathogenic Mechanisms

The activation of endothelial cells represents one of the best described pro-inflammatory mechanisms. Endothelial cells respond to TNF-α by an increased expression of adhesion molecules, which control the rolling and adhesion of inflammatory immune cells into the tissue. In this mechanism, both TNFRs are also critically engaged in the process of diapedesis [137]. TNF-α is also known to increase ROS levels and decrease nitric oxide production in blood vessels, which can lead to endothelial dysfunction: an initial step in atherogenesis [138]. In this process, TNF-α-induced ROS production depends on the activation of NADH oxidase [139,140]. TNF-α contributes also to the development of atherosclerotic plaques through an increase of LDL transcytosis in endothelial cells [91,92] and by regulating the activity of macrophage scavenger receptor and foam cell formation [141]. TNFR2 signaling contributes also to deleterious effects by increasing macrophage and smooth muscle proliferation [98].

In cardiomyocytes TNF-α triggers a hypertrophic response and induces apoptosis [131]. Endogenous TNF-α contributes to increased protein synthesis and hypertrophy [142] through the NF-κB-mediated production of ROS [143]. In cardiomyocytes, this process is dependent on TNFR1 activation, but it also negatively regulates calcium handling and cell contractility [144]. Moreover, TNF-α-induced superoxide production was shown to depend on NADPH oxidase activation by PI3K and to control the secretion of several matrix metalloproteinases (MMPs) [122]. Oxidative stress mediated by TNF-α is also responsible for mitochondrial DNA damage through the sphingomyelin–ceramide signaling pathway [145], which was also shown to induce apoptosis in cardiomyocytes [146]. TNFR1 promotes also cardiomyocyte apoptosis independently of NF-κB through RIP1–RIP3–MLKL axis activation by apoptosis signal-regulating kinase 1 (ASK1) [20,30].

Cardiac fibroblasts represent another heart-resident cell type that can be activated by TNF-α. In response to TNF-α, cardiac fibroblasts contribute to the inflammatory cascade by secreting monocyte chemoattractant proteins (MCP)-1 and MCP-3, which control monocyte recruitment but also positively regulate TNF-α production [147]. Furthermore, TNF-α mediates ROS production and MMP secretion in cardiac fibroblasts via the activation of PI3Kγ [122]. TNF-α contributes to hearts fibrosis also by stimulating cardiac fibroblasts proliferation and fibronectin deposition [148]. Moreover, TNF-α induces MMP9 production and promotes the transition of cardiac fibroblasts into pathogenic myofibroblasts [149]. Excessive collagen deposition and the expression of pro-fibrotic genes in these cells leading to pathological heart remodeling is controlled by TNFR1 [128,149]. TNFR1 is also important to induce fibroblast maturation from myeloid cells [150]. All these data demonstrate a wide spectrum of pathogenic effects of TNF-α in all cardiac cell types.

6.2. Cardioprotective Mechanisms

Most of the cardioprotective mechanisms are mediated by TNFR2. It seems that one of the most important effects of TNFR2-dependent signaling is to suppress activation of the pathogenic TNFR1 downstream pathways. It has been observed that in the absence of TNFR2, there is an increased activity of TNFR1 downstream effector molecules NF-κB [110] and MAPK p38 [129] as well as an increased production of pro-inflammatory cytokines IL-1β and IL-6 [111]. The TNFR2 cardioprotective mechanism has been described to counter-regulate the deleterious effects of TNFR1-mediated signaling in cardiomyocytes. Accordingly, the activation of TNFR2 protected cardiomyocytes from apoptosis and promoted cell cycle entry by activating endothelial/epithelial tyrosine kinase (ETK) [20], enhanced resistance to oxidative stress [130,144], and mediated positive calcium transient [144]. Of interest, TNFR2 was also shown to be critically involved in the differentiation of cardiomyocytes from stem cells in vitro [151] and in promoting cell cycle entry in resident cardiac stem cells [152]. Furthermore, TNFR2 signaling plays an important role in immunosuppression. In particular, the activation of TNFR2 on regulatory T cells stimulated their expansion [153] and suppressed effector T cell differentiation [31]. TNFR2 signaling plays also a crucial role in the recruitment of myeloid suppressor cells [154], which exert cardioprotective functions in heart failure [155]. It should be noted that the immunomodulatory effect of TNF-α in heart failure is not well understood, mostly because of its involvement in the activation of endothelial cells and pro-inflammatory role during the early inflammatory phase.

7. Clinical Perspectives

TNF-α is undoubtedly an important pro-inflammatory cytokine playing a key role during the early inflammatory phase. Clinical studies and data from animal models confirmed that TNF-α enhanced the development of a number of cardiovascular pathologies. However, preventive anti-TNF-α therapy would not be recommended due to side effects and economic reasons. Instead, such targeted immunomodulatory therapeutic intervention was considered in heart failure patients, but the failure of anti-TNF-α therapy could be explained by the cardioprotective properties of TNF-α in the failing heart. Currently, our knowledge on the beneficial activity of TNF-α is limited; therefore, more experimental research is needed to uncover these processes and the underlying mechanisms. Available data suggest that most of the cardioprotective activity is mediated by TNFR2, whereas the activation of TNFR1 initiates pathogenic processes. So far, most of these findings have been obtained in mouse models using transgenic mice lacking one or the other TNFR. In the next step, targeting these receptors, either by blocking TNFR1 or activating TNFR2, should be performed pharmacologically. The development of drugs selectively targeting TNFRs, rather than blocking TNF-α activity, might represent a novel and more effective therapeutic concept in the treatment of heart disease.

Funding: Funding Information National Science Centre (Poland): 2016/21/B/NZ5/01397.

Conflicts of Interest: The authors declare no conflict of interest.

References

1. Savarese, G.; Lund, L.H. Global Public Health Burden of Heart Failure. *Card. Fail. Rev.* **2017**, *3*, 7–11. [CrossRef]
2. Bloom, M.W.; Greenberg, B.; Jaarsma, T.; Januzzi, J.L.; Lam, C.S.P.; Maggioni, A.P.; Trochu, J.N.; Butler, J. Heart failure with reduced ejection fraction. *Nat. Rev. Dis. Prim.* **2017**, *3*, 1–19. [CrossRef]
3. Dunlay, S.M.; Roger, V.L.; Redfield, M.M. Epidemiology of heart failure with preserved ejection fraction. *Nat. Rev. Cardiol.* **2017**, *14*, 591–602. [CrossRef] [PubMed]
4. Van Linthout, S.; Tschöpe, C. Inflammation – Cause or Consequence of Heart Failure or Both? *Curr. Heart Fail. Rep.* **2017**, *14*, 251–265. [CrossRef] [PubMed]
5. Dick, S.A.; Epelman, S. Chronic heart failure and inflammation. *Circ. Res.* **2016**, *119*, 159–176. [CrossRef] [PubMed]
6. Monaco, C.; Nanchahal, J.; Taylor, P.; Feldmann, M. Anti-TNF therapy: Past, present and future. *Int. Immunol.* **2015**, *27*, 55–62. [CrossRef] [PubMed]
7. Shiina, T.; Blancher, A.; Inoko, H.; Kulski, J.K. Comparative genomics of the human, macaque and mouse major histocompatibility complex. *Immunology* **2017**, *150*, 127–138. [CrossRef]
8. Falvo, J.V.; Tsytsykova, A.V.; Goldfeld, A.E. Transcriptional control of the TNF Gene. *Curr. Dir. Autoimmun.* **2010**, *11*, 27–60. [CrossRef]
9. Tiedje, C.; Ronkina, N.; Tehrani, M.; Dhamija, S.; Laass, K.; Holtmann, H.; Kotlyarov, A.; Gaestel, M. The p38/MK2-Driven Exchange between Tristetraprolin and HuR Regulates AU-Rich Element-Dependent Translation. *PLoS Genet.* **2012**, *8*. [CrossRef]
10. Clark, A.R.; Dean, J.L.E. The control of inflammation via the phosphorylation and dephosphorylation of tristetraprolin: A tale of two phosphatases. *Biochem. Soc. Trans.* **2016**, *44*, 1321–1337. [CrossRef]
11. Chen, Y.L.; Jiang, Y.W.; Su, Y.L.; Lee, S.C.; Chang, M.S.; Chang, C.J. Transcriptional regulation of tristetraprolin by NF-κB signaling in LPS-stimulated macrophages. *Mol. Biol. Rep.* **2013**, *40*, 2867–2877. [CrossRef] [PubMed]
12. Taylor, G.A.; Carballo, E.; Lee, D.M.; Lai, W.S.; Thompson, M.J.; Patel, D.D.; Schenkman, D.I.; Gilkeson, G.S.; Broxmeyer, H.E.; Haynes, B.F.; et al. A pathogenetic role for TNF-α in the syndrome of cachexia, arthritis, and autoimmunity resulting from tristetraprolin (TTP) deficiency. *Immunity* **1996**, *4*, 445–454. [CrossRef]
13. Yimin; Kohanawa, M. A regulatory effect of the balance between TNF-alpha and IL-6 in the granulomatous and inflammatory response to Rhodococcus aurantiacus infection in mice. *J. Immunol.* **2006**, *177*, 642–650. [CrossRef] [PubMed]
14. Chung, I.Y.; Benveniste, E.N. Tumor necrosis factor-alpha production by astrocytes. Induction by lipopolysaccharide, IFN-gamma, and IL-1 beta. *J. Immunol.* **1990**, *144*, 2999–3007.
15. Li, D.L.; Liu, J.J.; Liu, B.H.; Hu, H.; Sun, L.; Miao, Y.; Xu, H.F.; Yu, X.J.; Ma, X.; Ren, J.; et al. Acetylcholine inhibits hypoxia-induced tumor necrosis factor-α production via regulation of MAPKs phosphorylation in cardiomyocytes. *J. Cell. Physiol.* **2011**, *226*, 1052–1059. [CrossRef]
16. Moss, M.L.; Jin, S.-L.C.; Milla, M.E.; Bickett, D.M.; Burkhart, W.; Carter, H.L.; Chen, W.-J.; William, C.; Didsbury, J.R.; Hassler, D.; et al. Erratum: Cloning of a disintegrin metalloproteinase that processes precursor tumour-necrosis factor-α. *Nature* **2003**, *386*, 738. [CrossRef]
17. Grell, M.; Douni, E.; Wajant, H.; Löhden, M.; Clauss, M.; Maxeiner, B.; Georgopoulos, S.; Lesslauer, W.; Kollias, G.; Pfizenmaier, K.; et al. The transmembrane form of tumor necrosis factor is the prime activating ligand of the 80 kDa tumor necrosis factor receptor. *Cell* **1995**, *83*, 793–802. [CrossRef]
18. MacEwan, D.J. TNF ligands and receptors—A matter of life and death. *Br. J. Pharmacol.* **2002**, *135*, 855–875. [CrossRef]
19. Cabal-Hierro, L.; Lazo, P.S. Signal transduction by tumor necrosis factor receptors. *Cell. Signal.* **2012**, *24*, 1297–1305. [CrossRef]
20. Al-Lamki, R.S.; Brookes, A.P.; Wang, J.; Reid, M.J.; Parameshwar, J.; Goddard, M.J.; Tellides, G.; Wan, T.; Min, W.; Pober, J.S.; et al. TNF receptors differentially signal and are differentially expressed and regulated in the human heart. *Am. J. Transplant.* **2009**, *9*, 2679–2696. [CrossRef]
21. Wajant, H.; Pfizenmaier, K.; Scheurich, P. Tumor necrosis factor signaling. *Cell Death Differ.* **2003**, *10*, 45–65. [CrossRef] [PubMed]
22. Ardestani, S.; Deskins, D.L.; Young, P.P. Membrane TNF-alpha-activated programmed necrosis is mediated by Ceramide-induced reactive oxygen species. *J. Mol. Signal.* **2013**, *8*, 1–10. [CrossRef] [PubMed]

23. Liu, T.; Zhang, L.; Joo, D.; Sun, S.-C. NF-κB signaling in inflammation. *Signal Transduct. Target. Ther.* **2017**, *2*, 17023. [CrossRef] [PubMed]
24. Schneider-Brachert, W.; Heigl, U.; Ehrenschwender, M. Membrane trafficking of death receptors: Implications on signalling. *Int. J. Mol. Sci.* **2013**, *14*, 14475–14503. [CrossRef] [PubMed]
25. Remijsen, Q.; Goossens, V.; Grootjans, S.; Van den Haute, C.; Vanlangenakker, N.; Dondelinger, Y.; Roelandt, R.; Bruggeman, I.; Goncalves, A.; Bertrand, M.J.; et al. Depletion of RIPK3 or MLKL blocks TNF-driven necroptosis and switches towards a delayed RIPK1 kinase-dependent apoptosis. *Cell Death Dis.* **2014**, *5*, e1004. [CrossRef] [PubMed]
26. Vanlangenakker, N.; Bertrand, M.J.M.; Bogaert, P.; Vandenabeele, P.; Vanden Berghe, T. TNF-induced necroptosis in L929 cells is tightly regulated by multiple TNFR1 complex i and II members. *Cell Death Dis.* **2011**, *2*, e230. [CrossRef] [PubMed]
27. Wajant, H.; Siegmund, D. TNFR1 and TNFR2 in the control of the life and death balance of macrophages. *Front. Cell Dev. Biol.* **2019**, *7*, 91. [CrossRef] [PubMed]
28. Yang, S.; Wang, J.; Brand, D.D.; Zheng, S.G. Role of TNF-TNF Receptor 2 Signal in Regulatory T Cells and Its Therapeutic Implications. *Front. Immunol.* **2018**, *9*, 784. [CrossRef]
29. Borghi, A.; Verstrepen, L.; Beyaert, R. TRAF2 multitasking in TNF receptor-induced signaling to NF-κB, MAP kinases and cell death. *Biochem. Pharmacol.* **2016**. [CrossRef]
30. Guo, X.; Yin, H.; Li, L.; Chen, Y.; Li, J.; Doan, J.; Steinmetz, R.; Liu, Q. Cardioprotective Role of Tumor Necrosis Factor Receptor-Associated Factor 2 by Suppressing Apoptosis and Necroptosis. *Circulation* **2017**, *136*, 729–742. [CrossRef]
31. Miller, P.G.; Bonn, M.B.; McKarns, S.C. Transmembrane TNF-TNFR2 Impairs Th17 Differentiation by Promoting Il2 Expression. *J. Immunol.* **2015**, *195*, 2633–2647. [CrossRef] [PubMed]
32. Van den Brande, J.M.H.; Braat, H.; Van den Brink, G.R.; Versteeg, H.H.; Bauer, C.A.; Hoedemaeker, I.; Van Montfrans, C.; Hommes, D.W.; Peppelenbosch, M.P.; Van Deventer, S.J.H. Infliximab but not etanercept induces apoptosis in lamina propria T-lymphocytes from patients with Crohn's disease. *Gastroenterology* **2003**, *124*, 1774–1785. [CrossRef]
33. Zhang, M.; Wang, J.; Jia, L.; Huang, J.; He, C.; Hu, F.; Yuan, L.; Wang, G.; Yu, M.; Li, Z. Transmembrane TNF-α promotes activation-induced cell death by forward and reverse signaling. *Oncotarget* **2017**, *8*, 63799–63812. [CrossRef] [PubMed]
34. Rossol, M.; Meusch, U.; Pierer, M.; Kaltenhäuser, S.; Häntzschel, H.; Hauschildt, S.; Wagner, U. Interaction between Transmembrane TNF and TNFR1/2 Mediates the Activation of Monocytes by Contact with T Cells. *J. Immunol.* **2007**, *179*, 4239–4248. [CrossRef] [PubMed]
35. Elliott, M.J.; Maini, R.N.; Feldmann, M.; Kalden, J.R.; Antoni, C.; Smolen, J.S.; Leeb, B.; Breedveld, F.C.; Macfarlane, J.D.; Bijl, J.A.; et al. Randomised double-blind comparison of chimeric monoclonal antibody to tumour necrosis factor α (cA2) versus placebo in rheumatoid arthritis. *Lancet* **1994**, *344*, 1105–1110. [CrossRef]
36. Willrich, M.A.V.; Murray, D.L.; Snyder, M.R. Tumor necrosis factor inhibitors: Clinical utility in autoimmune diseases. *Transl. Res.* **2015**, *165*, 270–282. [CrossRef]
37. Meroni, P.L.; Valentini, G.; Ayala, F.; Cattaneo, A.; Valesini, G. New strategies to address the pharmacodynamics and pharmacokinetics of tumor necrosis factor (TNF) inhibitors: A systematic analysis. *Autoimmun. Rev.* **2015**, *14*, 812–829. [CrossRef]
38. Singh, J.A.; Saag, K.G.; Bridges, S.L.; Akl, E.A.; Bannuru, R.R.; Sullivan, M.C.; Vaysbrot, E.; McNaughton, C.; Osani, M.; Shmerling, R.H.; et al. 2015 American College of Rheumatology Guideline for the Treatment of Rheumatoid Arthritis. *Arthritis Care Res.* **2016**, *68*, 1–25. [CrossRef]
39. Ghigo, A.; Franco, I.; Morello, F.; Hirsch, E. Myocyte signalling in leucocyte recruitment to the heart. *Cardiovasc. Res.* **2014**, *102*, 270–280. [CrossRef]
40. Javed, Q.; Murtaza, I. Therapeutic Potential of Tumour Necrosis Factor-alpha Antagonists in Patients with Chronic Heart Failure. *Heart Lung Circ.* **2013**, *22*, 323–327. [CrossRef]
41. Xing, J.; Liu, Y.; Chen, T. Correlations of chemokine CXCL16 and TNF-α with coronary atherosclerotic heart disease. *Exp. Ther. Med.* **2018**, *15*, 773–776. [CrossRef] [PubMed]
42. Li, X.; Zhang, F.; Zhou, H.; Hu, Y.; Guo, D.; Fang, X.; Chen, Y. Interplay of TNF-α, soluble TNF receptors and oxidative stress in coronary chronic total occlusion of the oldest patients with coronary heart disease. *Cytokine* **2020**, *125*. [CrossRef] [PubMed]

43. Shao, T.; Zhang, Y.; Tang, R.; Zhang, H.; Wang, Q.; Yang, Y.; Liu, T. Effects of milrinone on serum IL-6, TNF-α, Cys-C and cardiac functions of patients with chronic heart failure. *Exp. Ther. Med.* **2018**, *16*, 4162–4166. [CrossRef] [PubMed]
44. Torre-Amione, G.; Kapadia, S.; Lee, J.; Durand, J.B.; Bies, R.D.; Young, J.B.; Mann, D.L. Tumor necrosis factor-α and tumor necrosis factor receptors in the failing human heart. *Circulation* **1996**, *93*, 704–711. [CrossRef]
45. Pulido-Gómez, K.; Hernández-Díaz, Y.; Tovilla-Zárate, C.A.; Juárez-Rojop, I.E.; González-Castro, T.B.; López-Narváez, M.L.; Alpuin-Reyes, M. Association of G308A and G238A Polymorphisms of the TNF-α Gene with Risk of Coronary Heart Disease: Systematic Review and Meta-analysis. *Arch. Med. Res.* **2016**, *47*, 557–572. [CrossRef]
46. Wang, T. ping Association between TNF-α polymorphisms and the risk of upper gastrointestinal bleeding induced by aspirin in patients with coronary heart disease. *Ann. Hum. Genet.* **2019**, *83*, 124–133. [CrossRef]
47. Deswal, A.; Bozkurt, B.; Seta, Y.; Parilti-Eiswirth, S.; Hayes, F.A.; Blosch, C.; Mann, D.L. Safety and efficacy of a soluble P75 tumor necrosis factor receptor (Enbrel, etanercept) in patients with advanced heart failure. *Circulation* **1999**, *99*, 3224–3226. [CrossRef]
48. Bozkurt, B.; Torre-Amione, G.; Warren, M.S.; Whitmore, J.; Soran, O.Z.; Feldman, A.M.; Mann, D.L. Results of targeted anti-tumor necrosis factor therapy with etanercept (ENBREL) in patients with advanced heart failure. *Circulation* **2001**, *103*, 1044–1047. [CrossRef]
49. Fichtlscherer, S.; Rössig, L.; Breuer, S.; Vasa, M.; Dimmeler, S.; Zeiher, A.M. Tumor necrosis factor antagonism with etanercept improves systemic endothelial vasoreactivity in patients with advanced heart failure. *Circulation* **2001**, *104*, 3023–3025. [CrossRef]
50. Mann, D.L.; McMurray, J.J.V.; Packer, M.; Swedberg, K.; Borer, J.S.; Colucci, W.S.; Djian, J.; Drexler, H.; Feldman, A.; Kober, L.; et al. Targeted Anticytokine Therapy in Patients with Chronic Heart Failure: Results of the Randomized Etanercept Worldwide Evaluation (RENEWAL). *Circulation* **2004**, *109*, 1594–1602. [CrossRef]
51. Chung, E.S.; Packer, M.; Lo, K.H.; Fasanmade, A.A.; Willerson, J.T. Randomized, double-blind, placebo-controlled, pilot trial of infliximab, a chimeric monoclonal antibody to tumor necrosis factor-α, in patients with moderate-to-severe heart failure: Results of the anti-TNF therapy against congestive heart failure (ATTACH). *Circulation* **2003**, *107*, 3133–3140. [CrossRef] [PubMed]
52. Padfield, G.J.; Din, J.N.; Koushiappi, E.; Mills, N.L.; Robinson, S.D.; Le May Cruden, N.; Lucking, A.J.; Chia, S.; Harding, S.A.; Newby, D.E. Cardiovascular effects of tumour necrosis factor α antagonism in patients with acute myocardial infarction: A first in human study. *Heart* **2013**, *99*, 1330–1335. [CrossRef] [PubMed]
53. Roubille, C.; Richer, V.; Starnino, T.; McCourt, C.; McFarlane, A.; Fleming, P.; Siu, S.; Kraft, J.; Lynde, C.; Pope, J.; et al. The effects of tumour necrosis factor inhibitors, methotrexate, non-steroidal anti-inflammatory drugs and corticosteroids on cardiovascular events in rheumatoid arthritis, psoriasis and psoriatic arthritis: A systematic review and meta-analysis. *Ann. Rheum. Dis.* **2015**, *74*, 480–489. [CrossRef] [PubMed]
54. Błyszczuk, P.; Szekanecz, Z. Pathogenesis of ischaemic and non-ischaemic heart diseases in rheumatoid arthritis. *RMD Open* **2020**, *6*, 1–7. [CrossRef] [PubMed]
55. Keating, E.; Kelleher, T.B.; Lahiff, C. De novo Anti-TNF-α-induced Congestive Heart Failure in a Patient with Turner Syndrome and Crohn's Disease. *Inflamm. Bowel Dis.* **2020**. [CrossRef]
56. Curtis, J.R.; Kramer, J.M.; Martin, C.; Saag, K.G.; Patkar, N.; Shatin, D.; Burgess, M.; Xie, A.; Braun, M.M. Heart failure among younger rheumatoid arthritis and Crohn's patients exposed to TNF-α antagonists. *Rheumatology* **2007**, *46*, 1688–1693. [CrossRef]
57. Davis, J.M.; Lin, G.; Oh, J.K.; Crowson, C.S.; Achenbach, S.J.; Therneau, T.M.; Matteson, E.L.; Rodeheffer, R.J.; Gabriel, S.E. Five-year changes in cardiac structure and function in patients with rheumatoid arthritis compared with the general population. *Int. J. Cardiol.* **2017**, *240*, 379–385. [CrossRef]
58. Davis, J.M.; Roger, V.L.; Crowson, C.S.; Kremers, H.M.; Therneau, T.M.; Gabriel, S.E. The presentation and outcome of heart failure in patients with rheumatoid arthritis differs from that in the general population. *Arthritis Rheum.* **2008**, *58*, 2603–2611. [CrossRef]
59. Kotyla, P.J.; Owczarek, A.; Rakoczy, J.; Lewicki, M.; Kucharz, E.J.; Emery, P. Infliximab treatment increases left ventricular ejection fraction in patients with rheumatoid arthritis: Assessment of heart function by echocardiography, endothelin 1, interleukin 6, and NT-pro brain natriuretic peptide. *J. Rheumatol.* **2012**, *39*, 701–706. [CrossRef]

60. Ayyildiz, Y.O.; Vural, M.G.; Efe, T.H.; Ertem, A.G.; Koseoglu, C.; Ayturk, M.; Yeter, E.; Keskin, G.; Akdemir, R. Effect of Long-Term TNF-α Inhibition with Infliximab on Left Ventricular Torsion in Patients with Rheumatoid Arthritis. *Hellenic J. Cardiol.* **2015**, *56*, 406–413.
61. Hürlimann, D.; Forster, A.; Noll, G.; Enseleit, F.; Chenevard, R.; Distler, O.; Béchir, M.; Spieker, L.E.; Neidhart, M.; Michel, B.A.; et al. Anti-tumor necrosis factor-α treatment improves endothelial function in patients with rheumatoid arthritis. *Circulation* **2002**, *106*, 2184–2187. [CrossRef] [PubMed]
62. Wong, M.; Oakley, S.P.; Young, L.; Jiang, B.Y.; Wierzbicki, A.; Panayi, G.; Chowienczyk, P.; Kirkham, B. Infliximab improves vascular stiffness in patients with rheumatoid arthritis. *Ann. Rheum. Dis.* **2009**, *68*, 1277–1284. [CrossRef] [PubMed]
63. Ursini, F.; Leporini, C.; Bene, F.; D'Angelo, S.; Mauro, D.; Russo, E.; De Sarro, G.; Olivieri, I.; Pitzalis, C.; Lewis, M.; et al. Anti-TNF-alpha agents and endothelial function in rheumatoid arthritis: A systematic review and meta-analysis. *Sci. Rep.* **2017**, *7*. [CrossRef] [PubMed]
64. Low, A.S.L.; Symmons, D.P.M.; Lunt, M.; Mercer, L.K.; Gale, C.P.; Watson, K.D.; Dixon, W.G.; Hyrich, K.L. Relationship between exposure to tumour necrosis factor inhibitor therapy and incidence and severity of myocardial infarction in patients with rheumatoid arthritis. *Ann. Rheum. Dis.* **2017**, *76*, 654–660. [CrossRef]
65. Ljung, L.; Askling, J.; Rantapää-Dahlqvist, S.; Jacobsson, L.; Klareskog, L.; Lindblad, S.; von Vollenhoven, R.; Baecklund, E.; Cöster, L.; Forsblad, H.; et al. The risk of acute coronary syndrome in rheumatoid arthritis in relation to tumour necrosis factor inhibitors and the risk in the general population: A national cohort study. *Arthritis Res. Ther.* **2014**, *16*. [CrossRef]
66. Greenberg, J.D.; Kremer, J.M.; Curtis, J.R.; Hochberg, M.C.; Reed, G.; Tsao, P.; Farkouh, M.E.; Nasir, A.; Setoguchi, S.; Solomon, D.H. Tumour necrosis factor antagonist use and associated risk reduction of cardiovascular events among patients with rheumatoid arthritis. *Ann. Rheum. Dis.* **2011**, *70*, 576–582. [CrossRef]
67. Al-Aly, Z.; Pan, H.; Zeringue, A.; Xian, H.; McDonald, J.R.; El-Achkar, T.M.; Eisen, S. Tumor necrosis factor-α blockade, cardiovascular outcomes, and survival in rheumatoid arthritis. *Transl. Res.* **2011**, *157*, 10–18. [CrossRef]
68. Jacobsson, L.T.H.; Turesson, C.; Nilsson, J.Å.; Petersson, I.F.; Lindqvist, E.; Saxne, T.; Geborek, P. Treatment with TNF blockers and mortality risk in patients with rheumatoid arthritis. *Ann. Rheum. Dis.* **2007**, *66*, 670–675. [CrossRef]
69. Solomon, D.H.; Rassen, J.A.; Kuriya, B.; Chen, L.; Harrold, L.R.; Graham, D.J.; Lewis, J.D.; Lii, J.; Liu, L.; Griffin, M.R.; et al. Heart failure risk among patients with rheumatoid arthritis starting a TNF antagonist. *Ann. Rheum. Dis.* **2013**, *72*, 1813–1818. [CrossRef]
70. Setoguchi, S.; Schneeweiss, S.; Avorn, J.; Katz, J.N.; Weinblatt, M.E.; Levin, R.; Solomon, D.H. Tumor necrosis factor-α antagonist use and heart failure in elderly patients with rheumatoid arthritis. *Am. Heart J.* **2008**, *156*, 336–341. [CrossRef]
71. Arican, O.; Aral, M.; Sasmaz, S.; Ciragil, P. Serum levels of TNF-α, IFN-γ, IL-6, IL-8, IL-12, IL-17, and IL-18 in patients with active psoriasis and correlation with disease severity. *Mediators Inflamm.* **2005**, *2005*, 273–279. [CrossRef]
72. Wakkee, M.; Thio, H.B.; Prens, E.P.; Sijbrands, E.J.G.; Neumann, H.A.M. Unfavorable cardiovascular risk profiles in untreated and treated psoriasis patients. *Atherosclerosis* **2007**, *190*, 1–9. [CrossRef] [PubMed]
73. Bissonnette, R.; Tardif, J.-C.; Harel, F.; Pressacco, J.; Bolduc, C.; Guertin, M.-C. Effects of the tumor necrosis factor-α antagonist adalimumab on arterial inflammation assessed by positron emission tomography in patients with psoriasis: Results of a randomized controlled trial. *Circ. Cardiovasc. Imaging* **2013**, *6*, 83–90. [CrossRef] [PubMed]
74. Wu, J.J.; Poon, K.Y.T.; Channual, J.C.; Shen, A.Y.J. Association between tumor necrosis factor inhibitor therapy and myocardial infarction risk in patients with psoriasis. *Arch. Dermatol.* **2012**, *148*, 1244–1250. [CrossRef] [PubMed]
75. Wu, J.J.; Guérin, A.; Sundaram, M.; Dea, K.; Cloutier, M.; Mulani, P. Cardiovascular event risk assessment in psoriasis patients treated with tumor necrosis factor-α inhibitors versus methotrexate. *J. Am. Acad. Dermatol.* **2017**, *76*, 81–90. [CrossRef] [PubMed]
76. Lee, J.L.; Sinnathurai, P.; Buchbinder, R.; Hill, C.; Lassere, M.; March, L. Biologics and cardiovascular events in inflammatory arthritis: A prospective national cohort study. *Arthritis Res. Ther.* **2018**, *20*, 171. [CrossRef]

77. Eder, L.; Joshi, A.A.; Dey, A.K.; Cook, R.; Siegel, E.L.; Gladman, D.D.; Mehta, N.N. Association of Tumor Necrosis Factor Inhibitor Treatment with Reduced Indices of Subclinical Atherosclerosis in Patients with Psoriatic Disease. *Arthritis Rheumatol.* **2018**, *70*, 408–416. [CrossRef]
78. Butler, D.M.; Malfait, A.M.; Mason, L.J.; Warden, P.J.; Kollias, G.; Maini, R.N.; Feldmann, M.; Brennan, F.M. DBA/1 mice expressing the human TNF-alpha transgene develop a severe, erosive arthritis: Characterization of the cytokine cascade and cellular composition. *J. Immunol.* **1997**, *159*, 2867–2876.
79. Li, G.; Wu, Y.; Jia, H.; Tang, L.; Huang, R.; Peng, Y.; Zhang, Y. Establishment and evaluation of a transgenic mouse model of arthritis induced by overexpressing human tumor necrosis factor alpha. *Biol. Open* **2016**, *5*, 418–423. [CrossRef]
80. Kubota, T.; McTiernan, C.F.; Frye, C.S.; Demetris, A.J.; Feldman, A.M. Cardiac-specific overexpression of tumor necrosis factor-alpha causes lethal myocarditis in transgenic mice. *J. Card. Fail.* **1997**, *3*, 117–124. [CrossRef]
81. Sivasubramanian, N.; Coker, M.L.; Kurrelmeyer, K.M.; MacLellan, W.R.; DeMayo, F.J.; Spinale, F.G.; Mann, D.L. Left ventricular remodeling in transgenic mice with cardiac restricted overexpression of tumor necrosis factor. *Circulation* **2001**, *104*, 826–831. [CrossRef] [PubMed]
82. London, B.; Baker, L.C.; Lee, J.S.; Shusterman, V.; Choi, B.R.; Kubota, T.; McTiernan, C.F.; Feldman, A.M.; Salama, G. Calcium-dependent arrhythmias in transgenic mice with heart failure. *Am. J. Physiol. Heart Circ. Physiol.* **2003**, *284*. [CrossRef]
83. Li, Y.Y.; Feng, Y.Q.; Kadokami, T.; McTiernan, C.F.; Draviam, R.; Watkins, S.C.; Feldman, A.M. Myocardial extracellular matrix remodeling in transgenic mice overexpressing tumor necrosis factor α can be modulated by anti-tumor necrosis factor α therapy. *Proc. Natl. Acad. Sci. USA* **2000**, *97*, 12746–12751. [CrossRef]
84. Petkova-Kirova, P.S.; London, B.; Salama, G.; Rasmusson, R.L.; Bondarenko, V.E. Mathematical modeling mechanisms of arrhythmias in transgenic mouse heart overexpressing TNF-α. *Am. J. Physiol. Heart Circ. Physiol.* **2012**, *302*, H934. [CrossRef] [PubMed]
85. Higuchi, Y.; McTiernan, C.F.; Frye, C.B.; McGowan, B.S.; Chan, T.O.; Feldman, A.M. Tumor Necrosis Factor Receptors 1 and 2 Differentially Regulate Survival, Cardiac Dysfunction, and Remodeling in Transgenic Mice with Tumor Necrosis Factor-α-Induced Cardiomyopathy. *Circulation* **2004**, *109*, 1892–1897. [CrossRef] [PubMed]
86. Dibbs, Z.I.; Diwan, A.; Nemoto, S.; DeFreitas, G.; Abdellatif, M.; Carabello, B.A.; Spinale, F.G.; Feuerstein, G.; Sivasubramanian, N.; Mann, D.L.; et al. Targeted overexpression of transmembrane tumor necrosis factor provokes a concentric cardiac hypertrophic phenotype. *Circulation* **2003**, *108*, 1002–1008. [CrossRef] [PubMed]
87. Niemann-Jönsson, A.; Söderberg, I.; Lindholm, M.W.; Jovinge, S.; Nilsson, J.; Fredrikson, G.N. Medial Expression of TNF-α and TNF Receptors Precedes the Development of Atherosclerotic Lesions in Apolipoprotein E/LDL Receptor Double Knockout Mice. *Int. J. Biomed. Sci.* **2007**, *3*, 116–122. [PubMed]
88. Xiao, N.; Yin, M.; Zhang, L.; Qu, X.; Du, H.; Sun, X.; Mao, L.; Ren, G.; Zhang, C.; Geng, Y.; et al. Tumor necrosis factor-alpha deficiency retards early fatty-streak lesion by influencing the expression of inflammatory factors in apoE-null mice. *Mol. Genet. Metab.* **2009**, *96*, 239–244. [CrossRef] [PubMed]
89. Ohta, H.; Wada, H.; Niwa, T.; Kirii, H.; Iwamoto, N.; Fujii, H.; Saito, K.; Sekikawa, K.; Seishima, M. Disruption of tumor necrosis factor-α gene diminishes the development of atherosclerosis in ApoE-deficient mice. *Atherosclerosis* **2005**, *180*, 11–17. [CrossRef] [PubMed]
90. Boesten, L.S.M.; Zadelaar, A.S.M.; Van Nieuwkoop, A.; Gijbels, M.J.J.; De Winther, M.P.J.; Havekes, L.M.; Van Vlijmen, B.J.M. Tumor necrosis factor-α promotes atherosclerotic lesion progression in APOE*3-leiden transgenic mice. *Cardiovasc. Res.* **2005**, *66*, 179–185. [CrossRef]
91. Brånén, L.; Hovgaard, L.; Nitulescu, M.; Bengtsson, E.; Nilsson, J.; Jovinge, S. Inhibition of tumor necrosis factor-α reduces atherosclerosis in apolipoprotein E knockout mice. *Arterioscler. Thromb. Vasc. Biol.* **2004**, *24*, 2137–2142. [CrossRef] [PubMed]
92. Zhang, Y.; Yang, X.; Bian, F.; Wu, P.; Xing, S.; Xu, G.; Li, W.; Chi, J.; Ouyang, C.; Zheng, T.; et al. TNF-α promotes early atherosclerosis by increasing transcytosis of LDL across endothelial cells: Crosstalk between NF-κB and PPAR-γ. *J. Mol. Cell. Cardiol.* **2014**, *72*, 85–94. [CrossRef] [PubMed]
93. Tuleta, I.; Fran a, C.N.; Wenzel, D.; Fleischmann, B.; Nickenig, G.; Werner, N.; Skowasch, D. Hypoxia-induced endothelial dysfunction in apolipoprotein E-deficient mice; effects of infliximab and L-glutathione. *Atherosclerosis* **2014**, *236*, 400–410. [CrossRef] [PubMed]

94. Park, K.-Y.; Heo, T.-H. Critical role of TNF inhibition in combination therapy for elderly mice with atherosclerosis. *Cardiovasc. Ther.* **2017**, *35*, e12280. [CrossRef]
95. Oberoi, R.; Vlacil, A.K.; Schuett, J.; Schösser, F.; Schuett, H.; Tietge, U.J.F.; Schieffer, B.; Grote, K. Anti-tumor necrosis factor-α therapy increases plaque burden in a mouse model of experimental atherosclerosis. *Atherosclerosis* **2018**, *277*, 80–89. [CrossRef]
96. Gao, W.; Liu, H.; Yuan, J.; Wu, C.; Huang, D.; Ma, Y.; Zhu, J.; Ma, L.; Guo, J.; Shi, H.; et al. Exosomes derived from mature dendritic cells increase endothelial inflammation and atherosclerosis via membrane TNF-α mediated NF-κB pathway. *J. Cell. Mol. Med.* **2016**, *20*, 2318–2327. [CrossRef]
97. Canault, M.; Peiretti, F.; Poggi, M.; Mueller, C.; Kopp, F.; Bonardo, B.; Bastelica, D.; Nicolay, A.; Alessi, M.C.; Nalbone, G. Progression of atherosclerosis in ApoE-deficient mice that express distinct molecular forms of TNF-alpha. *J. Pathol.* **2008**, *214*, 574–583. [CrossRef]
98. Nicolaou, A.; Zhao, Z.; Northoff, B.H.; Sass, K.; Herbst, A.; Kohlmaier, A.; Chalaris, A.; Wolfrum, C.; Weber, C.; Steffens, S.; et al. Adam17 Deficiency promotes atherosclerosis by enhanced TNFR2 signaling in Mice. *Arterioscler. Thromb. Vasc. Biol.* **2017**, *37*, 247–257. [CrossRef]
99. Canault, M.; Peiretti, F.; Mueller, C.; Kopp, F.; Morange, P.; Rihs, S.; Portugal, H.; Juhan-Vague, I.; Nalbone, G. Exclusive expression of transmembrane TNF-α in mice reduces the inflammatory response in early lipid lesions of aortic sinus. *Atherosclerosis* **2004**, *172*, 211–218. [CrossRef]
100. Schreyer, S.A.; Peschon, J.J.; LeBoeuf, R.C. Accelerated atherosclerosis in mice lacking tumor necrosis factor receptor p55. *J. Biol. Chem.* **1996**, *271*, 26174–26178. [CrossRef]
101. Zhang, L.; Peppel, K.; Sivashanmugam, P.; Orman, E.S.; Brian, L.; Exum, S.T.; Freedman, N.J. Expression of tumor necrosis factor receptor-1 in arterial wall cells promotes atherosclerosis. *Arterioscler. Thromb. Vasc. Biol.* **2007**, *27*, 1087–1094. [CrossRef] [PubMed]
102. Irwin, M.W.; Mak, S.; Mann, D.L.; Qu, R.; Penninger, J.M.; Yan, A.; Dawood, F.; Wen, W.-H.; Shou, Z.; Liu, P. Tissue Expression and Immunolocalization of Tumor Necrosis Factor-α in Postinfarction Dysfunctional Myocardium. *Circulation* **1999**, *99*, 1492–1498. [CrossRef] [PubMed]
103. Sato, T.; Suzuki, H.; Shibata, M.; Kusuyama, T.; Omori, Y.; Soda, T.; Shoji, M.; Iso, Y.; Koba, S.; Geshi, E.; et al. Tumor-necrosis-factor-alpha-gene-deficient mice have improved cardiac function through reduction of intercellular adhesion molecule-1 in myocardial infarction. *Circ. J.* **2006**, *70*, 1635–1642. [CrossRef] [PubMed]
104. Kurrelmeyer, K.M.; Michael, L.H.; Baumgarten, G.; Taffet, G.E.; Peschon, J.J.; Sivasubramanian, N.; Entman, M.L.; Mann, D.L. Endogenous tumor necrosis factor protects the adult cardiac myocyte against ischemic-induced apoptosis in a murine model of acute myocardial infarction. *Proc. Natl. Acad. Sci. USA* **2000**, *97*, 5456–5461. [CrossRef]
105. Maekawa, N.; Wada, H.; Kanda, T.; Niwa, T.; Yamada, Y.; Saito, K.; Fujiwara, H.; Sekikawa, K.; Seishima, M. Improved myocardial ischemia/reperfusion injury in mice lacking tumor necrosis factor-α. *J. Am. Coll. Cardiol.* **2002**, *39*, 1229–1235. [CrossRef]
106. Gao, C.; Liu, Y.; Yu, Q.; Yang, Q.; Li, B.; Sun, L.; Yan, W.; Cai, X.; Gao, E.; Xiong, L.; et al. TNF-α antagonism ameliorates myocardial ischemia-reperfusion injury in mice by upregulating adiponectin. *Am. J. Physiol. Heart Circ. Physiol.* **2015**, *308*, H1583–H1591. [CrossRef] [PubMed]
107. Berry, M.F.; Woo, Y.J.; Pirolli, T.J.; Bish, L.T.; Moise, M.A.; Burdick, J.W.; Morine, K.J.; Jayasankar, V.; Gardner, T.J.; Sweeney, H.L. Administration of a tumor necrosis factor inhibitor at the time of myocardial infarction attenuates subsequent ventricular remodeling. *J. Heart Lung Transplant.* **2004**, *23*, 1061–1068. [CrossRef]
108. Wang, X.; Guo, Z.; Ding, Z.; Mehta, J.L. Inflammation, autophagy, and apoptosis after myocardial infarction. *J. Am. Heart Assoc.* **2018**, *7*. [CrossRef]
109. Zhang, C.; Xu, X.; Potter, B.J.; Wang, W.; Kuo, L.; Michael, L.; Bagby, G.J.; Chilian, W.M. TNF-α contributes to endothelial dysfunction in ischemia/reperfusion injury. *Arterioscler. Thromb. Vasc. Biol.* **2006**, *26*, 475–480. [CrossRef]
110. Hamid, T.; Gu, Y.; Ortines, R.V.; Bhattacharya, C.; Wang, G.; Xuan, Y.T.; Prabhu, S.D. Divergent TNF Receptor-Related Remodeling Responses in Heart Failure: Role of NF-κB and Inflammatory Activation. *Circulation* **2009**, *119*, 1386–1397. [CrossRef]
111. Monden, Y.; Kubota, T.; Inoue, T.; Tsutsumi, T.; Kawano, S.; Ide, T.; Tsutsui, H.; Sunagawa, K. Tumor necrosis factor-α is toxic via receptor 1 and protective via receptor 2 in a murine model of myocardial infarction. *Am. J. Physiol. Heart Circ. Physiol.* **2007**, *293*, 743–753. [CrossRef] [PubMed]

112. Ramani, R.; Mathier, M.; Wang, P.; Gibson, G.; Tögel, S.; Dawson, J.; Bauer, A.; Alber, S.; Watkins, S.C.; McTiernan, C.F.; et al. Inhibition of tumor necrosis factor receptor-1-mediated pathways has beneficial effects in a murine model of postischemic remodeling. *Am. J. Physiol. Heart Circ. Physiol.* **2004**, *287*, 1369–1377. [CrossRef] [PubMed]
113. Zhang, Y.; Zhao, J.; Lau, W.B.; Jiao, L.Y.; Liu, B.; Yuan, Y.; Wang, X.; Gao, E.; Koch, W.J.; Ma, X.L.; et al. Tumor Necrosis Factor-α and Lymphotoxin-α Mediate Myocardial Ischemic Injury via TNF Receptor 1, but Are Cardioprotective When Activating TNF Receptor 2. *PLoS ONE* **2013**, *8*. [CrossRef] [PubMed]
114. Frantz, S.; Hu, K.; Bayer, B.; Gerondakis, S.; Strotmann, J.; Adamek, A.; Ertl, G.; Bauersachs, J. Absence of NF-κB subunit p50 improves heart failure after myocardial infarction. *FASEB J.* **2006**, *20*, 1918–1920. [CrossRef]
115. Yu, Y.; Wei, S.G.; Weiss, R.M.; Felder, R.B. TNF-α receptor 1 knockdown in the subfornical organ ameliorates sympathetic excitation and cardiac hemodynamics in heart failure rats. *Am. J. Physiol. Heart Circ. Physiol.* **2017**, *313*, 744–756. [CrossRef]
116. Jude, B.; Vetel, S.; Giroux-Metges, M.A.; Pennec, J.P. Rapid negative inotropic effect induced by TNF-α in rat heart perfused related to PKC activation. *Cytokine* **2018**, *107*, 65–69. [CrossRef]
117. Wang, M.; Crisostomo, P.R.; Markel, T.A.; Wang, Y.; Meldrum, D.R. Mechanisms of sex differences in TNFR2-mediated cardioprotection. *Circulation* **2008**, *118*, 38–45. [CrossRef]
118. Braunwald, E. Cardiomyopathies: An overview. *Circ. Res.* **2017**, *121*, 711–721. [CrossRef]
119. Carlson, W.D. Animal models of heart failure. In *Heart Failure*, 2nd ed.; CRC Press: Boca Raton, FL, USA, 2012; Volume 111, pp. 78–94, ISBN 9781420077018.
120. Kassiri, Z.; Oudit, G.Y.; Sanchez, O.; Dawood, F.; Mohammed, F.F.; Nuttall, R.K.; Edwards, D.R.; Liu, P.P.; Backx, P.H.; Khokha, R. Combination of tumor necrosis factor-α ablation and matrix metalloproteinase inhibition prevents heart failure after pressure overload in tissue inhibitor of metalloproteinase-3 knock-out mice. *Circ. Res.* **2005**, *97*, 380–390. [CrossRef]
121. Sun, M.; Chen, M.; Dawood, F.; Zurawska, U.; Li, J.Y.; Parker, T.; Kassiri, Z.; Kirshenbaum, L.A.; Arnold, M.; Khokha, R.; et al. Tumor necrosis factor-α mediates cardiac remodeling and ventricular dysfunction after pressure overload state. *Circulation* **2007**, *115*, 1398–1407. [CrossRef]
122. Awad, A.E.; Kandalam, V.; Chakrabarti, S.; Wang, X.; Penninger, J.M.; Davidge, S.T.; Oudit, G.Y.; Kassiri, Z. Tumor necrosis factor induces matrix metalloproteinases in cardiomyocytes and cardiofibroblasts differentially via superoxide production in a PI3Kγ-dependent manner. *Am. J. Physiol.-Cell Physiol.* **2010**, *298*, 679–692. [CrossRef] [PubMed]
123. Kishore, R.; Tkebuchava, T.; Sasi, S.P.; Silver, M.; Gilbert, H.Y.; Yoon, Y.S.; Park, H.Y.; Thorne, T.; Losordo, D.W.; Goukassian, D.A. Tumor necrosis factor-α Signaling via TNFR1/p55 is deleterious whereas TNFR2/p75 signaling is protective in adult infarct myocardium. In *Proceedings of the Advances in Experimental Medicine and Biology*; Springer Nature Switzerland AG: Cham, Switzerland, 2011; Volume 691, pp. 433–448.
124. Nan, J.; Hu, H.; Sun, Y.; Zhu, L.; Wang, Y.; Zhong, Z.; Zhao, J.; Zhang, N.; Wang, Y.; Wang, Y.; et al. TNFR2 Stimulation Promotes Mitochondrial Fusion via Stat3- and NF-kB-Dependent Activation of OPA1 Expression. *Circ. Res.* **2017**, *121*, 392–410. [CrossRef] [PubMed]
125. Wu, L.; Cao, Z.; Ji, L.; Mei, L.; Jin, Q.; Zeng, J.; Lin, J.; Chu, M.; Li, L.; Yang, X. Loss of TRADD attenuates pressure overload-induced cardiac hypertrophy through regulating TAK1/P38 MAPK signalling in mice. *Biochem. Biophys. Res. Commun.* **2017**, *483*, 810–815. [CrossRef] [PubMed]
126. Sriramula, S.; Haque, M.; Majid, D.S.; Francis, J. Involvement of tumor necrosis factor-α in angiotensin II-mediated effects on salt appetite, hypertension, and cardiac hypertrophy. *Hypertension* **2008**, *51*, 1345–1351. [CrossRef]
127. Mayr, M.; Duerrschmid, C.; Medrano, G.; Taffet, G.E.; Wang, Y.; Entman, M.L.; Haudek, S.B. TNF/Ang-II synergy is obligate for fibroinflammatory pathology, but not for changes in cardiorenal function. *Physiol. Rep.* **2016**, *4*, 1–15. [CrossRef]
128. Duerrschmid, C.; Crawford, J.R.; Reineke, E.; Taffet, G.E.; Trial, J.A.; Entman, M.L.; Haudek, S.B. TNF receptor 1 signaling is critically involved in mediating angiotensin-II-induced cardiac fibrosis. *J. Mol. Cell. Cardiol.* **2013**, *57*, 59–67. [CrossRef]
129. Garlie, J.B.; Hamid, T.; Gu, Y.; Ismahil, M.A.; Chandrasekar, B.; Prabhu, S.D. Tumor necrosis factor receptor 2 signaling limits β-adrenergic receptor-mediated cardiac hypertrophy in vivo. *Basic Res. Cardiol.* **2011**, *106*, 1193–1205. [CrossRef]

130. Keck, M.; Flamant, M.; Mougenot, N.; Favier, S.; Atassi, F.; Barbier, C.; Nadaud, S.; Lompré, A.M.; Hulot, J.S.; Pavoine, C. Cardiac inflammatory CD11b/c cells exert a protective role in hypertrophied cardiomyocyte by promoting TNFR 2- and Orai3- dependent signaling. *Sci. Rep.* **2019**, *9*, 1–19. [CrossRef]
131. Nakashima, M.A.; Silva, C.B.P.; Gonzaga, N.A.; Simplicio, J.A.; Omoto, A.C.M.; Tirapelli, L.F.; Tanus-Santos, J.E.; Tirapelli, C.R. Chronic ethanol consumption increases reactive oxygen species generation and the synthesis of pro-inflammatory proteins in the heart through TNFR1-dependent mechanisms. *Cytokine* **2019**, *121*, 154734. [CrossRef]
132. Tang, J.; Xie, Q.; Ma, D.; Wang, W. Effects of ET-1 and TNF-α levels on the cardiac function and prognosis in rats with chronic heart failure. *Eur. Rev. Med. Pharmacol. Sci.* **2019**, *23*, 11004–11010. [CrossRef]
133. Błyszczuk, P. Myocarditis in Humans and in Experimental Animal Models. *Front. Cardiovasc. Med.* **2019**, *6*, 64. [CrossRef]
134. Huber, S.A.; Sartini, D. Roles of Tumor Necrosis Factor Alpha (TNF-α) and the p55 TNF Receptor in CD1d Induction and Coxsackievirus B3-Induced Myocarditis. *J. Virol.* **2005**, *79*, 2659–2665. [CrossRef]
135. Smith, S.C.; Allen, P.M. Neutralization of endogenous tumor necrosis factor ameliorates the severity of myosin-induced myocarditis. *Circ. Res.* **1992**, *70*, 856–863. [CrossRef]
136. Bachmaier, K.; Pummerer, C.; Kozieradzki, I.; Pfeffer, K.; Mak, T.W.; Neu, N.; Penninger, J.M. Low-molecular-weight tumor necrosis factor receptor p55 controls induction of autoimmune heart disease. *Circulation* **1997**, *95*, 655–661. [CrossRef]
137. Chandrasekharan, U.M.; Siemionow, M.; Unsal, M.; Yang, L.; Poptic, E.; Bohn, J.; Ozer, K.; Zhou, Z.; Howe, P.H.; Penn, M.; et al. Tumor necrosis factor α (TNF-α) receptor-II is required for TNF-α-induced leukocyte-endothelial interaction in vivo. *Blood* **2007**, *109*, 1938–1944. [CrossRef] [PubMed]
138. Lee, J.; Lee, S.; Zhang, H.; Hill, M.A.; Zhang, C.; Park, Y. Interaction of IL-6 and TNF-α contributes to endothelial dysfunction in type 2 diabetic mouse hearts. *PLoS ONE* **2017**, *12*, 1–17. [CrossRef]
139. Gao, X.; Belmadani, S.; Picchi, A.; Xu, X.; Potter, B.J.; Tewari-Singh, N.; Capobianco, S.; Chilian, W.M.; Zhang, C. Tumor necrosis factor-α induces endothelial dysfunction in Lepr db mice. *Circulation* **2007**, *115*, 245–254. [CrossRef]
140. De Keulenaer, G.W.; Alexander, R.W.; Ushio-Fukai, M.; Ishizaka, N.; Griendling, K.K. Tumour necrosis factor α activates a p22phox-based NADH oxidase in vascular smooth muscle. *Biochem. J.* **1998**, *329*, 653–657. [CrossRef] [PubMed]
141. Hsu, H.Y.; Twu, Y.C. Tumor necrosis factor-α-mediated protein kinases in regulation of scavenger receptor and foam cell formation on macrophage. *J. Biol. Chem.* **2000**, *275*, 41035–41048. [CrossRef] [PubMed]
142. Yokoyama, T.; Nakano, M.; Bednarczyk, J.L.; McIntyre, B.W.; Entman, M.; Mann, D.L. Tumor necrosis factor-α provokes a hypertrophic growth response in adult cardiac myocytes. *Circulation* **1997**, *95*, 1247–1252. [CrossRef] [PubMed]
143. Higuchi, Y.; Otsu, K.; Nishida, K.; Hirotani, S.; Nakayama, H.; Yamaguchi, O.; Matsumura, Y.; Ueno, H.; Tada, M.; Hori, M. Involvement of reactive oxygen species-mediated NF-κB activation in TNF-α-induced cardiomyocyte hypertrophy. *J. Mol. Cell. Cardiol.* **2002**, *34*, 233–240. [CrossRef] [PubMed]
144. Defer, N.; Azroyan, A.; Pecker, F.; Pavoine, C. TNFR1 and TNFR2 signaling interplay in cardiac myocytes. *J. Biol. Chem.* **2007**, *282*, 35564–35573. [CrossRef] [PubMed]
145. Suematsu, N.; Tsutsui, H.; Wen, J.; Kang, D.; Ikeuchi, M.; Ide, T.; Hayashidani, S.; Shiomi, T.; Kubota, T.; Hamasaki, N.; et al. Oxidative stress mediates tumor necrosis factor-α-induced mitochondrial DNA damage and dysfunction in cardiac myocytes. *Circulation* **2003**, *107*, 1418–1423. [CrossRef] [PubMed]
146. Krown, K.A.; Page, M.T.; Nguyen, C.; Zechner, D.; Gutierrez, V.; Comstock, K.L.; Glembotski, C.C.; Quintana, P.J.E.; Sabbadini, R.A. Tumor necrosis factor alpha-induced apoptosis in cardiac myocytes: Involvement of the sphingolipid signaling cascade in cardiac cell death. *J. Clin. Investig.* **1996**, *98*, 2854–2865. [CrossRef]
147. Lindner, D.; Zietsch, C.; Tank, J.; Sossalla, S.; Fluschnik, N.; Hinrichs, S.; Maier, L.; Poller, W.; Blankenberg, S.; Schultheiss, H.P.; et al. Cardiac fibroblasts support cardiac inflammation in heart failure. *Basic Res. Cardiol.* **2014**, *109*, 1–16. [CrossRef]
148. Jacobs, M.; Staufenberger, S.; Gergs, U.; Meuter, K.; Brandstätter, K.; Hafner, M.; Ertl, G.; Schorb, W. Tumor necrosis factor-α at acute myocardial infarction in rats and effects on cardiac fibroblasts. *J. Mol. Cell. Cardiol.* **1999**, *31*, 1949–1959. [CrossRef]

149. Porter, K.E.; Turner, N.A.; O'Regan, D.J.; Ball, S.G. Tumor necrosis factor α induces human atrial myofibroblast proliferation, invasion and MMP-9 secretion: Inhibition by simvastatin. *Cardiovasc. Res.* **2004**, *64*, 507–515. [CrossRef]
150. Bunney, P.E.; Zink, A.N.; Holm, A.A.; Billington, C.J.; Kotz, C.M. Tumor Necrosis Factor: A Mechanistic Link between Angiotensin-II-Induced Cardiac Inflammation and Fibrosis. *Physiol. Behav.* **2017**, *176*, 139–148. [CrossRef]
151. Aker, S.; Belosjorow, S.; Konietzka, I.; Duschin, A.; Martin, C.; Heusch, G.; Schulz, R. Serum but not myocardial TNF-α concentration is increased in pacing-induced heart failure in rabbits. *Am. J. Physiol.-Regul. Integr. Comp. Physiol.* **2003**, *285*, R463–R469. [CrossRef]
152. Al-Lamki, R.S.; Lu, W.; Wang, J.; Yang, J.; Sargeant, T.J.; Wells, R.; Suo, C.; Wright, P.; Goddard, M.; Huang, Q.; et al. TNF, acting through inducibly expressed TNFR2, drives activation and cell cycle entry of c-Kit+ cardiac stem cells in ischemic heart disease. *Stem Cells* **2013**, *31*, 1881–1892. [CrossRef]
153. Wang, J.; Ferreira, R.; Lu, W.; Farrow, S.; Downes, K.; Jermutus, L.; Minter, R.; Al-Lamki, R.S.; Pober, J.S.; Bradley, J.R. TNFR2 ligation in human T regulatory cells enhances IL2-induced cell proliferation through the non-canonical NF-κB pathway. *Sci. Rep.* **2018**, *8*, 1–11. [CrossRef] [PubMed]
154. Ba, H.; Li, B.; Li, X.; Li, C.; Feng, A.; Zhu, Y.; Wang, J.; Li, Z.; Yin, B. Transmembrane tumor necrosis factor-α promotes the recruitment of MDSCs to tumor tissue by upregulating CXCR4 expression via TNFR2. *Int. Immunopharmacol.* **2017**, *44*, 143–152. [CrossRef] [PubMed]
155. Zhou, L.; Miao, K.; Yin, B.; Li, H.; Fan, J.; Zhu, Y.; Ba, H.; Zhang, Z.; Chen, F.; Wang, J.; et al. Cardioprotective Role of Myeloid-Derived Suppressor Cells in Heart Failure. *Circulation* **2018**, *138*, 181–197. [CrossRef] [PubMed]

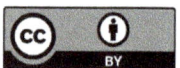

© 2020 by the authors. Licensee MDPI, Basel, Switzerland. This article is an open access article distributed under the terms and conditions of the Creative Commons Attribution (CC BY) license (http://creativecommons.org/licenses/by/4.0/).

Article
Levosimendan Improves Oxidative Balance in Cardiogenic Shock/Low Cardiac Output Patients

Elena Grossini [1,*], Serena Farruggio [1], Daniele Pierelli [2], Virginia Bolzani [3], Lidia Rossi [3], Piero Pollesello [4] and Carolina Monaco [2]

1. Laboratory of Physiology, Department of Translational Medicine, UPO, 28100 Novara, Italy; serefar@live.it
2. Cardiothoracic Intensive Care Unit, AOU, 28100 Novara, Italy; daniele.pierelli@gmail.com (D.P.); carolina.monaco@maggioreosp.novara.it (C.M.)
3. Cardiology Division, AOU, 28100 Novara, Italy; virgi.bolzani@gmail.com (V.B.); rossilidia7@gmail.com (L.R.)
4. Critical Care, OrionPharma, 02101 Espoo, Finland; piero.pollesello@orionpharma.com
* Correspondence: elena.grossini@med.uniupo.it; Tel.: +390321660526; Fax: +3903213733537

Received: 18 December 2019; Accepted: 25 January 2020; Published: 30 January 2020

Abstract: The beneficial effects exerted by levosimendan against cardiac failure could be related to the modulation of oxidative balance. We aimed to examine the effects of levosimendan in patients with cardiogenic shock or low cardiac output on cardiac systo-diastolic function and plasma oxidants/antioxidants (glutathione, GSH; thiobarbituric acid reactive substances, TBARS). In four patients undergoing coronary artery bypass grafting or angioplasty, cardiovascular parameters and plasma GSH and TBARS were measured at T0 (before levosimendan infusion), T1 (1 h after the achievement of the therapeutic dosage of levosimendan), T2 (end of levosimendan infusion), T3 (72 h after the end of levosimendan infusion), and T4 (end of cardiogenic shock). We found an improvement in the indices of systolic (ejection fraction, cardiac output, cardiac index) and diastolic (E to early diastolic mitral annular tissue velocity, E/′; early to late diastolic transmitral flow velocity, EA) cardiac function at early T2. A reduction of central venous pressure and pulmonary wedge pressure was also observed. Plasma levels of GSH and TBARS were restored by levosimendan at T1, as well. The results obtained indicate that levosimendan administration can regulate oxidant/antioxidant balance as an early effect in cardiogenic shock/low cardiac output patients. Modulation of oxidative status on a mitochondrial level could thus play a role in exerting the cardio-protection exerted by levosimendan in these patients.

Keywords: antioxidants; calcium sensitizer; heart failure; mitochondria function; peroxidation

1. Introduction

Levosimendan is an inotrope used for the treatment of acutely decompensated heart failure patients with low cardiac output or cardiogenic shock [1–4].

Among its mechanisms of action, the sensitization of cardiac troponin C to calcium in cardiac muscle [5–7] and the opening adenosine triphosphate-sensitive potassium (K_{ATP}) channels in vascular smooth muscle cells [8,9] have been described. Due to these pharmacological actions, levosimendan improves atrio-ventricular coupling and cardiac mechanical efficiency without increasing myocardial oxygen consumption [10–13]. Moreover, levosimendan has been shown to have a direct effect on mitochondria [14–19].

Preliminary data obtained in vitro, ex vivo, and in vivo in animal models have shown that levosimendan could improve endothelial and mitochondrial function, and protect against peroxidation, as well. In anesthetized pigs subjected to renal ischemia/reperfusion, the intrarenal levosimendan administration was able to increase renal function and keep the oxidant balance, as shown by the increased plasma levels of glutathione (GSH) and the reduced release of peroxidation markers, like thiobarbituric acid reactive substances (TBARS) [20]. Similar nominally beneficial effects against peroxidation were observed in anesthetized rats subjected to hepatic ischemia/reperfusion and treated with levosimendan [21].

TBARS, which reflect the release of malon(MDA) generated through the peroxidation of polyunsaturated fatty acids, have been widely adopted as indicators of oxidative stress in various cardiovascular diseases [22]. GSH plays an important role in the maintenance of the thiol-redox status of the cell, and for this reason could act as antioxidant. GSH deficiency might manifest itself through an increased susceptibility to oxidative stress and to the augmented onset and progression of many diseases, including the cardiovascular diseases [23].)

Similar beneficial effects against peroxidation, as were observed in the renal model of ischemia/reperfusion, have been observed in anesthetized rats subjected to hepatic ischemia/reperfusion and treated with levosimendan [21]. Finally, in rat hepatocytes, the administration of levosimendan dose-dependently counteracted the injuries caused by oxidative stress, as evidenced by the keeping GSH content and the reduction of TBARS release [24]. In all the above conditions, endothelial and mitochondrial function were found to be ameliorated by levosimendan, which prevented the fall of mitochondrial membrane potential and restored nitric oxide (NO) release.

The beneficial effects elicited by levosimendan against oxidative stress could represent a further mechanism of protection in heart failure (HF) patients. The implication of oxidative stress in the pathophysiology of HF is well established. Oxidative stress may impair cardiac functions through damage to the cellular proteins and membranes by initiation of lipid peroxidation, thereby inducing cellular death and apoptosis. Moreover, it could exert direct negative inotropic effects through the reduction of cytosolic intracellular free calcium [25]. Thus, there is strong circumstantial evidence that oxidative stress is a prognostic factor in HF patients. Keith et al. showed that circulating MDA, a marker of lipid peroxidation, was significantly different between control subjects and patients with HF [26]. In addition, MDA plasma levels have been positively correlated not only with the presence of HF, but also with New York Heart Association (NYHA) functional class [27].

It is worth noting that levosimendan administration to decompensated HF subjects was able to improve oxidative damage, as shown by the TBARS measurement, by five days [28]. To date, however, the information available about the effects of levosimendan on oxidative stress and cardiac systo-diastolic function in cardiogenic shock/low cardiac output patients for ischemic disease, is scarce.

For this reason, in the present study, we aimed to examine, at the same time, the effects of intravenous levosimendan treatment on (1) systolic and diastolic functions, (2) hemodynamic variables, and (3) oxidant/antioxidant systems, in patients admitted to the cardiothoracic intensive care unit (ICU) for cardiogenic shock or decompensated heart failure after coronary artery bypass grafting (CABG) or percutaneous transluminal coronary angioplasty (PTCA). To our knowledge, this is the first time these parallel assessments have been performed in a clinical setting.

2. Materials and Methods

This was a prospective, longitudinal study approved by the Ethical Committee of Azienda Ospedaliero Universitaria (AOU) Maggiore della Carità of Novara (655/CE; Studio n. CE 107/17; approval date 16/06/2017). All procedures were compliant with the ethical standards of the Helsinki Declaration and conformed to standards currently applied in Italy. Patients' informed written consent was collected before starting the study.

In this pilot study, 4 adult patients admitted to the cardiothoracic ICU of AOU Maggiore della Carità of Novara were enrolled.

Inclusion criteria were: Aged over 18 years, reduced systolic function (ejection fraction, EF, < 30%) due to cardiogenic shock post-CABG or decompensated heart failure after PTCA.

Exclusion criteria: Acute renal or liver failure, septic condition.

Two male patients underwent CABG for three vessel-diseases. In PTCA patients (one male and one female), three arterial grafts were positioned on the left anterior descending coronary artery, and intra-aortic balloon pumps (IABP) were used. Demographic data are reported in Table 1.

Table 1. Demographic data of patients.

Males/Females	3/1
Age (years)	63 ± 13.5
BMI (body mass index)	26.63 ± 1.2
Diabetes	1/4
Hypertension	0
Smoker (>1 cigarette)	0
Dyslipidemia	0

Hemodynamic variables were monitored by means of a Swan–Ganz pulmonary artery catheter in all patients [29,30].

The central venous pressure (CVP), mean pulmonary arterial pressure (PAP), cardiac output (CO), cardiac index (CI), systemic vascular resistance index (SVRI), pulmonary vascular resistance index (PVRI), and the pulmonary capillary wedge pressure (PCWP) were continuously measured. Heart rate (HR), and systolic (SAP) and diastolic (DAP) arterial blood pressure were also recorded. Arterial and venous oxygen partial pressure (pO_2), and arterial and venous oxygen saturation (SO_2) were examined by hemogasanalyis (Radiometer ABL 90 Flex).

In all patients, systo-diastolic cardiac function was examined by an expert cardiologist through echocardiography (GE Vivid-i), following the time-course reported below, and as recommended by international guidelines [31–33].

After baseline data evaluation, levosimendan was administered intravenously at the dose of 0.1 µg/kg/min without a loading dose, which is adopted in the ICU for the treatment of cardiogenic shock or low cardiac output patients [34,35]. In all patients, vasopressor support was implemented by epinephrine (0.01–0.1 µg/kg/min) and in one patient with dopamine (2 µg/kg/min), as well. Mechanically assisted ventilation was provided to CABG patients.

Venous samples were taken for GSH and TBARS measurements, following the time-course reported below.

2.1. Collection of Samples

For the determination of GSH and TBARS, 10 mL of blood samples were taken from each donor using BD Vacutainer tubes (sodium heparin as anticoagulant). Each sample was immediately centrifuged by a refrigerated centrifuge (Eppendorf, mod. 5702 with rotor A-4-38) for 10 min, at a speed of 3100 g at 4 °C. The plasma obtained was divided into 5 tubes that were stored at −20 °C at the Physiology laboratory of the University of Eastern Piedmont of Novara.

2.2. GSH Quantification

GSH measurement was performed by using the Glutathione Assay Kit (Cayman Chemical, Ann Arbor, MI, USA), as previously described [36,37]. Each plasma sample was deproteinated by adding an equal volume of MPA solution to the sample which was then centrifuged at 2000 g for 2 min. The supernatant was collected, and 50 µL/mL of TEAM reagent was added to each sample in order to increase the pH. Fifty microliters of the samples were transferred to a 96-well plate where GSH was detected following the manufacturer's instructions through a spectrophotometer (VICTOR™ X Multilabel Plate Reader), at excitation/emission wavelengths of 405–414 nm. Glutathione was expressed as µM. The measurements were performed in triplicate.

2.3. TBARS Quantification

TBARS were determined as MDA release. The MDA measurement was performed by using the TBARS assay Kit (Cayman Chemical), as previously [36,38]. For the assays, 100 µL of each plasma sample was added to 100 µL of sodium dodecyl sulfate (SDS) solution and 2 mL of the Color Reagent, following the manufacturer's instructions. Each sample was boiled for 1 h and then transferred to ice for 10 min in order to stop the reaction. Each sample was centrifuged for 10 min at 1600 g at 4 °C and 150 µL was transferred to a 96-well plate where MDA was detected following the manufacturer's instructions through a spectrophotometer (VICTOR™ X Multilabel Plate Reader), at excitation/emission wavelengths of 530–540 nm. MDA production was expressed in µM. The measurements were performed in triplicate.

2.4. Time-Course of Measurements

T0, before the beginning of levosimendan administration: Hemodynamic variable measurements and cardiac systo-diastolic evaluation, GSH and TBARS sampling.

T1, at the end of 0.1 µg/kg/min levosimendan infusion (duration 24 h): Hemodynamic variable measurements and cardiac systo-diastolic evaluation, GSH and TBARS sampling.

T2, 24 h after the end of levosimendan infusion: Hemodynamic variable measurements and cardiac systo-diastolic evaluation, GSH and TBARS sampling.

T3, at 72 h after the end of levosimendan administration: Hemodynamic variable measurements and cardiac systo-diastolic evaluation, GSH and TBARS sampling.

T4, at the end of inotropic support: Hemodynamic variable measurements and cardiac systo-diastolic evaluation, GSH and TBARS sampling.

2.5. Statistical Analysis

All data were recorded using the Institution's database. Statistical analysis was performed by using GraphPad Prism 6.0. Non-nominal variables were checked for normality before statistical analysis. ANOVA for repeated measurements was used to compare results obtained in each patient at various timings. All non-nominal data were expressed as means ± standard deviation (SD). A p value lower than 0.05 was taken for statistical significance.

3. Results

The patients were overweight, and one patient was diabetic, but major cardiovascular risk factors like hypertension, smoking, or dyslipidemia were not identified (Table 1). At T0, mean EF amounted to 25%. In the two patients who underwent cardiothoracic surgery, extracorporeal circulation lasted 145 ± 21 min.

Improvements were recorded in CO, CI, and SAP, as shown in Figures 1 and 2A,B.

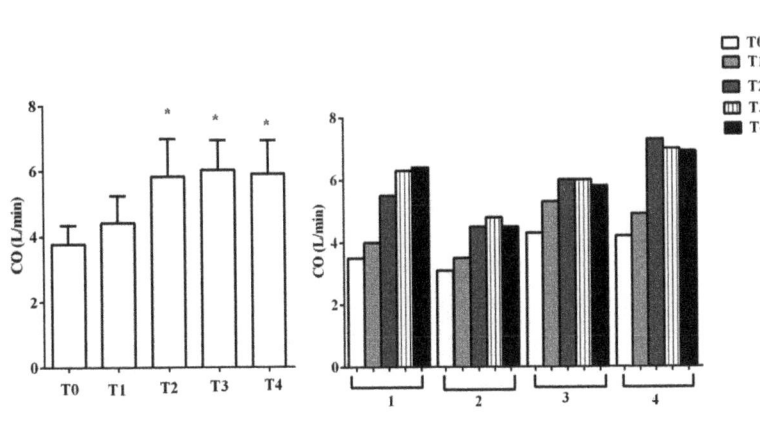
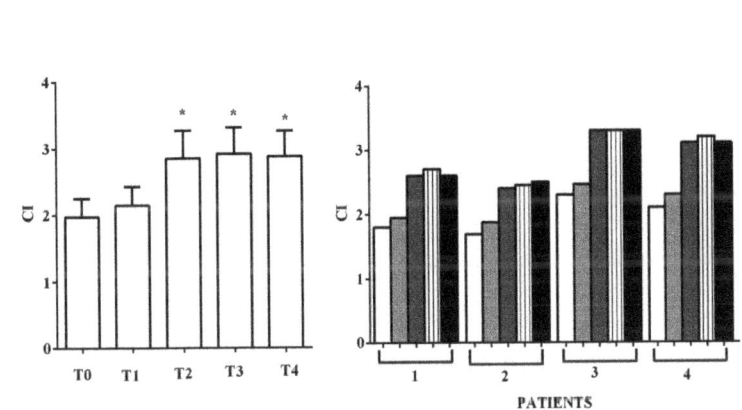

Figure 1. In (**A**,**B**), effects of levosimendan on cardiac output (CO) and in (**C**,**D**), on cardiac index (CI). In A and C, values are means ± SD. In B and D, columns represent single patients. * $p < 0.05$ vs. T0.

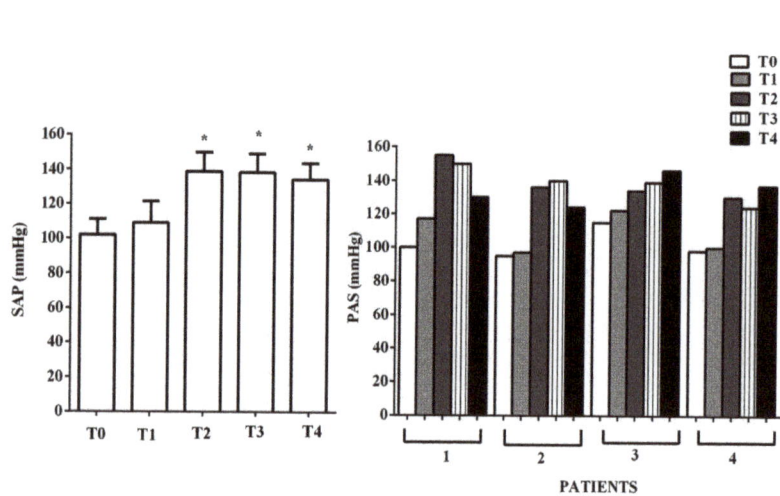

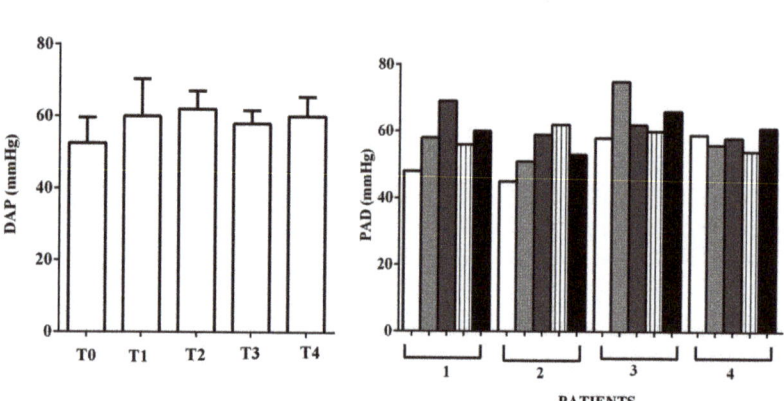

Figure 2. In (**A**,**B**), effects of levosimendan on systolic (SAP) and in (**C**,**D**), diastolic (DAP) arterial blood pressure. In A and C, values are means ± SD. In B and D, columns represent single patients. * $p < 0.05$ vs. T0.

EF increased from mean 26.25% ± 2.2 to 43.7% ± 2.9 at early T2, and to 48% ± 1.4 at T4 ($p < 0.05$). A reduction of CVP, pulmonary capillary wedge pressure (wedge), and PVRI was also observed (Figure 3A,B and Figure 4B,D). PAP at T4 was lower than PAP at T0 (Figure 3C,D).

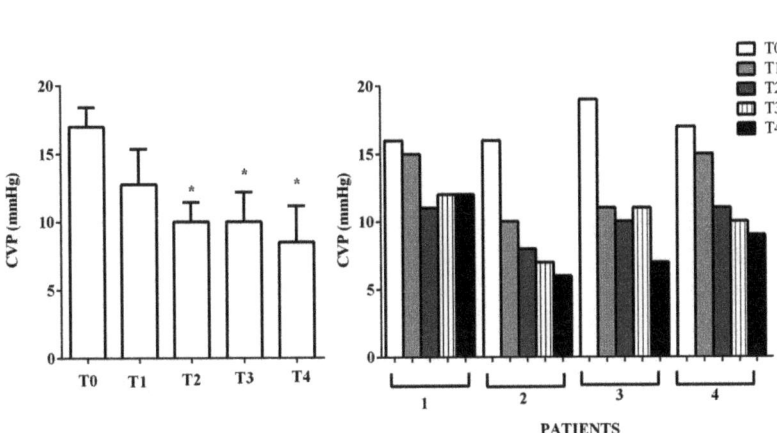

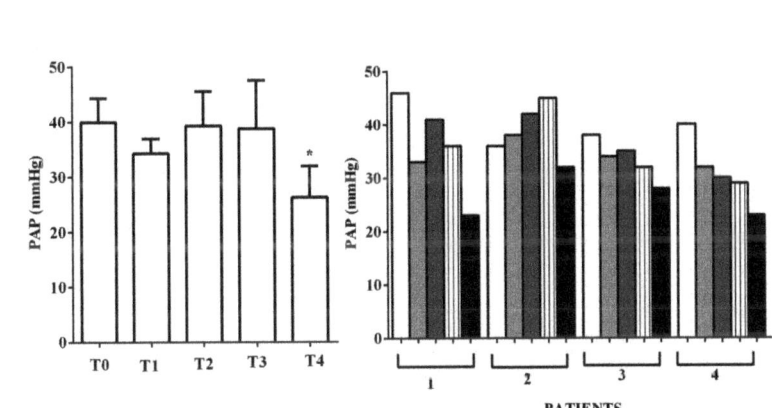

Figure 3. In (**A**,**B**), effects of levosimendan on central venous pressure (CVP) and in (**C**,**D**) on mean pulmonary arterial pressure (PAP). In A and C, values are means ± SD. In B and D, columns represent single patients. * $p < 0.05$ vs. T0.

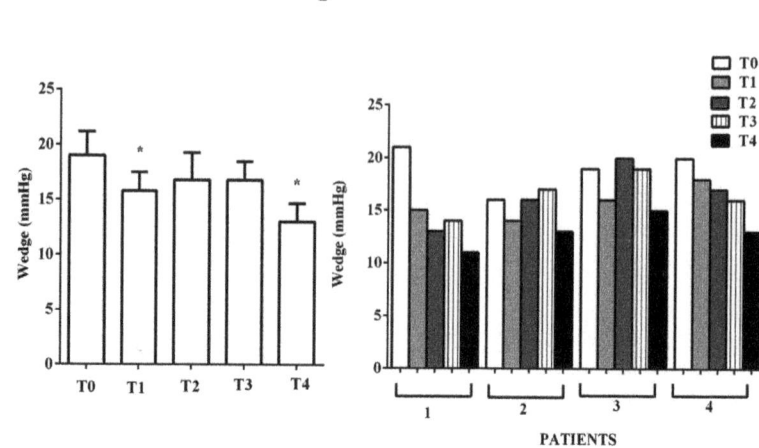

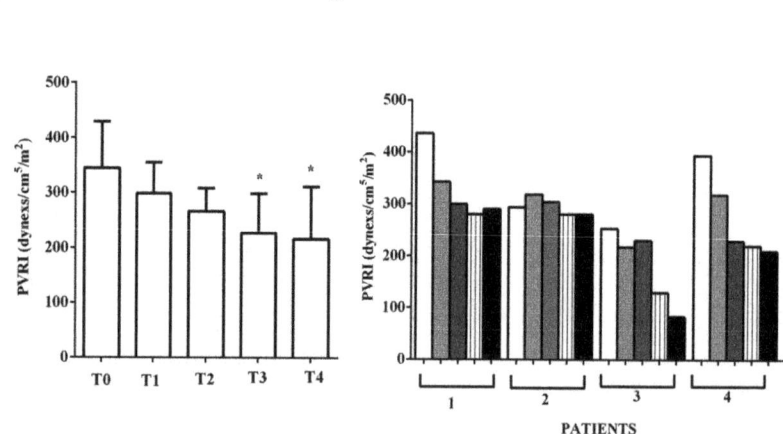

Figure 4. In (**A,B**), effects of levosimendan on pulmonary capillary wedge pressure (wedge) and in (**C,D**), on pulmonary vascular resistance index (PVRI). In A and C, values are means ± SD. In B and D, columns represent single patients. * $p < 0.05$ vs. T0.

Indices of diastolic function (E/E′, E/A) were improved by levosimendan administration (E to early diastolic mitral annular tissue velocity, E/, from mean 14.5 ± 1.3 at T0, to mean 11 ± 1.4 at T2, to mean 6.7 ± 1.7 at T4; early to late diastolic transmitral flow velocity, E/A, from >1 at T0 to <1 at T4; $p < 0.05$). No significant changes of HR were observed (mean values at T0 to T4, respectively: 96.75, 90.75, 95.75, 88, 91 beats/min), nor in DAP (Figure 2C,D). In the two PTCA patients, IABP was removed at T2 and mechanical ventilation was suspended after 1 and 3 days, respectively. In all patients, epinephrine was reduced from mean 0.06 ± 0.04 µg/kg/min at T0, to 0.04 ± 0.02 µg/kg/min at T2, to 0.001 ± 0.009 µg/kg/min at T3; at T4 it was suspended. Dopamine was reduced from 2 µg/kg/min at T0, to 1 µg/kg/min at T2; at T4 it was suspended.

Arterial oxygen saturation and oxygen partial pressure amounted to about 98% and 96 mmHg at T0 and did not vary significantly throughout the time-course (Figure 5).

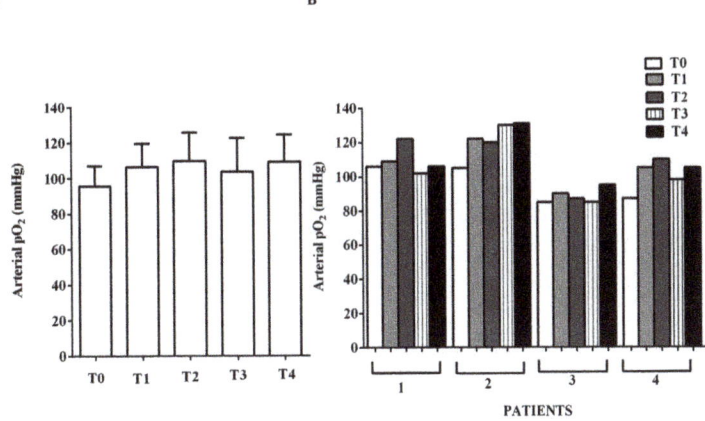

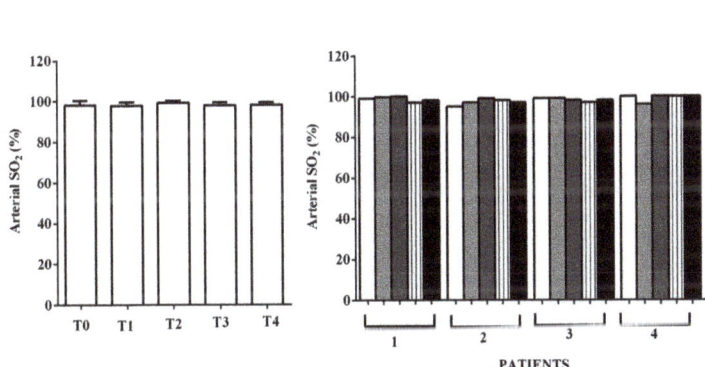

Figure 5. In (**A**,**B**), effects of levosimendan on arterial partial pressure (pO$_2$) and in (**C**,**D**), on arterial oxygen saturation (SO$_2$). In A and C, values are means ± SD. In B and D, columns represent single patients.

ygen venous partial pressure and venous oxygen saturation amounted to about 37 mmHg and 63% at T0 and did not show any changes (Figure 6).

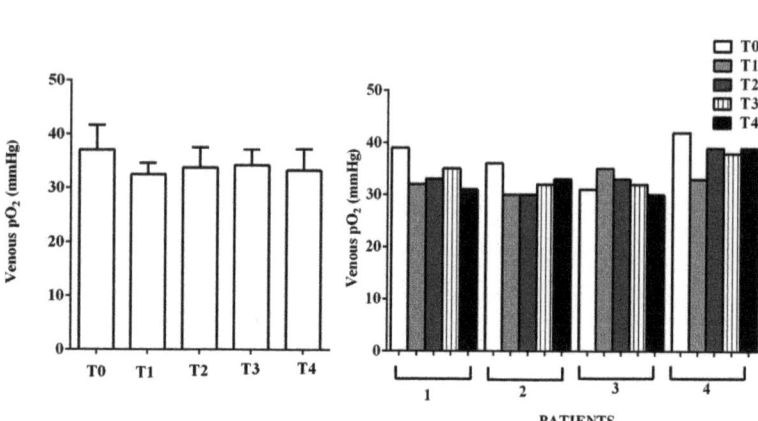
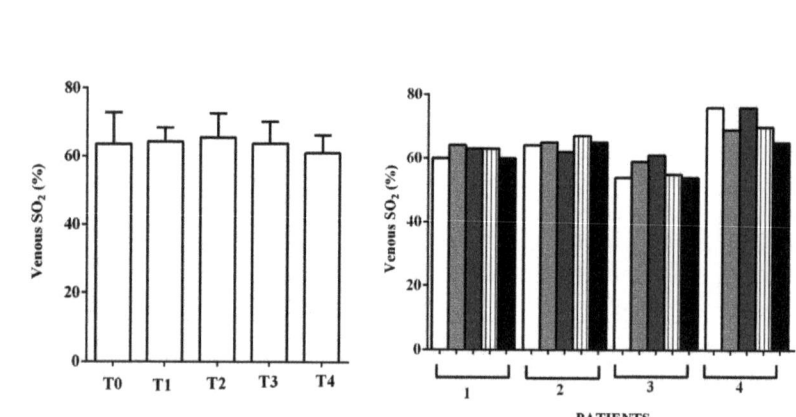

Figure 6. In (**A**,**B**), effects of levosimendan on venous oxygen partial pressure (pO$_2$) and in (**C**,**D**), on venous oxygen saturation (SO$_2$). In A and C, values are means ± SD. In B and D, columns represent single patients.

As depicted in Figure 7, at T0, the levels of GSH and MDA were 0.21 ± 0.16 µM and 7.1 ± 1.9 µM, respectively. Immediately after levosimendan administration, an improvement of the above parameters was observed. GSH at T1 rose to 1.16 ± 0.5 µM, whereas MDA declined to 4.3 ± 1.1 µM (both $p < 0.05$ vs. T0). At T2, T3, and T4, the levels of GSH increased (3.1 ± 1.3; 3.8 ± 1.2; 2.8 ± 1.2 µM, respectively; all $p < 0.05$ vs. T0) and those of MDA decreased progressively (2.5 ± 0.9; 2.4 ± 0.9; 2.1 ± 0.8 µM; all $p < 0.05$ vs. T0).

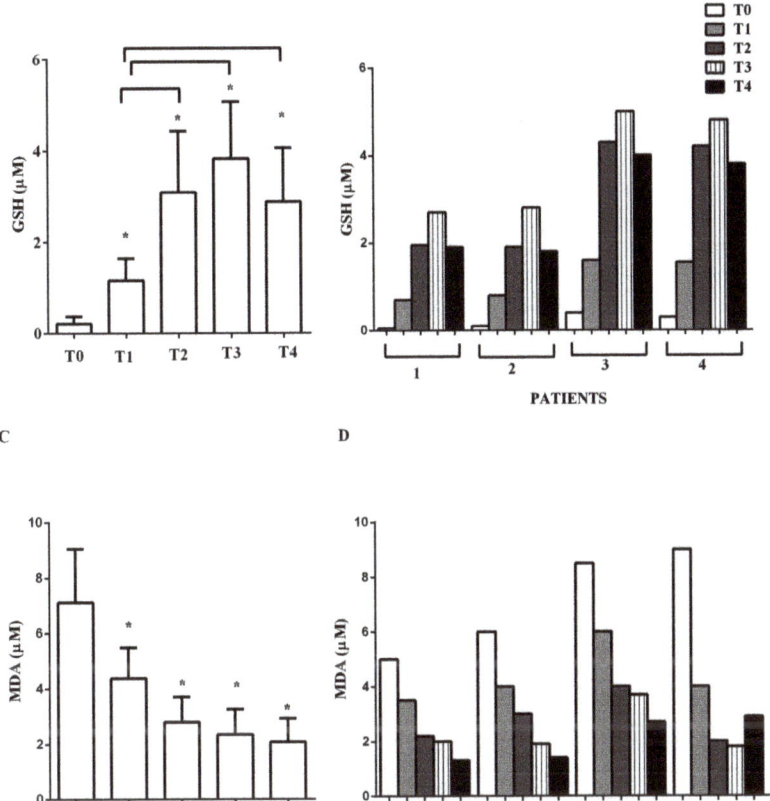

Figure 7. In (**A,B**), effects of levosimendan on plasma glutathione (GSH) and in (**C,D**), on plasma malonyldialdeide (MDA) concentration. In A and C, values are means ± SD. In B and D, columns represent single patients. * $p < 0.05$ vs. T0.

4. Discussion

The results obtained in the present study show protective effects elicited by levosimendan administration in cardiogenic shock or low cardiac output patients post-CABG or PTCA, through the modulation of oxidant/antioxidant balance.

The balance between ROS production and their removal by antioxidant systems is described as the "redox state". Oxidative stress arises any time the production of ROS exceeds the levels of antioxidants. In HF, an increased production of ROS, originating mainly by mitochondria from failing hearts, has been widely evidenced [39]. Chronic increases in ROS production may lead to a cycle of mitochondrial DNA damage, leading to a functional decline, further ROS generation, and cellular injury. ROS can directly impair contractile function by modifying proteins central to excitation–contraction coupling, ion transporters, and Ca^{2+} cycling, as well [40].

It is noteworthy that cardiac oxidative stress has been associated with diastolic dysfunction, as well [41], via changes in Ca^{2+} handling. Hence, increased ROS production can impair the activity of Ca^{2+}/calmodulin kinase (CaMK) II or SERCA2, or affect Ca^{2+} sensitivity of myofilaments. As a result, a diastolic SR Ca^{2+} leak and a reduction of relaxation stiffness of cardiomyocytes would happen [42].

In addition, changes of mitochondrial function could lead to increased intracellular Ca^{2+}, resulting in cardiomyocyte super-contracture, disruption of plasmalemma and therefore necrotic cell death. Although it was not clearly shown, at the basis of the above effects there could be the increased mitochondrial ROS generation [43].

Furthermore, K_{ATP} channels could represent a target for ROS in HF [44]. It has been shown that ROS-dependent modification of mitochondrial K_{ATP} channels, in particular, could represent a feedback mechanism for the regulation of mitochondrial K_{ATP} channel activity itself. Moreover, K_{ATP} channels have been widely shown to play important roles in protection of the heart from ischemic injury [45]. The opening of K_{ATP} channels could contribute to the regulation of cardiac mitochondrial function [46] and cardioprotection induced by ischemic preconditioning, as well.

For this reason, any factor able to affect K_{ATP} channel activity could represent a rescue method against cardiac damage.

The mechanisms of action of levosimendan are mainly related to the increase of Ca^{2+} sensitivity of troponin C and the opening of K_{ATP} channels in myocardium and vessels. Being a calcium sensitizer and not a calcium mobilizer, levosimendan does not increase myocardial oxygen consumption nor prevent myocardial apoptosis and remodeling [1].

For those reasons, levosimendan is widely used for the treatment of low cardiac output conditions for its effects on systemic and pulmonary hemodynamics and for the relief of symptoms of HF [47].

Recent evidence indicates that levosimendan could reduce oxidative markers and increase the antioxidant system. In decompensated HF patients, a reduction of TBARS levels was observed after 5 days from the start of levosimendan administration [28], while, in the animal model of renal and liver ischemia/reperfusion plasma, TBARS and GSH concentration was restored by levosimendan infusion [20,21]. A role for the modulation of the "redox state", as a possible mechanism of action of levosimendan in the protection against HF, might therefore be hypothesized.

In our study, the infusion of levosimendan in cardiogenic shock or low cardiac output patients post-CABG or PTCA improved GSH and reduced TBARS early at the achievement of the therapeutic levosimendan dosage. Those effects preceded those on hemodynamics and cardiac systo-diastolic function, which were evidenced by the improvement of EF, CO, CI, E/E', and E/A.

Our data confirm previous data about the protective effects exerted by levosimendan against peroxidation, and highlight their potential as further mechanisms through which levosimendan could exert its action on cardiac function. Although it was not examined, the maintenance of mitochondria function by levosimendan could be presumed to play a role in its antioxidant effects.

Hence, mitochondria have emerged as a central factor in the pathogenesis and progression of HF. It is widely accepted that mitochondrial dysfunction can contribute to impaired myocardial energetics and increased oxidative stress in cardiomyopathies, cardiac ischemic damage, and HF. Mitochondrial permeability transition pore opening has been shown to act as a critical trigger of myocyte death and myocardial remodeling. Increased mitochondrial permeabilization is a mechanistic pathway at the basis of myocardial apoptosis [48].

Previous findings have evidenced that levosimendan is able to prevent the fall of mitochondrial membrane potential and transition pore opening in cardiomyocytes [49]. In this way, it could modulate ROS release and apoptotic signaling. Thus, it could be hypothesized that the keeping mitochondrial function by levosimendan could represent the starting mechanism for the reduction of ROS release and the restoration of myocardial energetics and cell viability. These events would be followed by the improvement of cardiac systole and diastole and hemodynamics.

In conclusion, the results obtained have shown that levosimendan improved GSH and reduced TBARS early before the onset of the cardiovascular effects.

The main limitation of this study is the low number of patients and the different etiologies. However, the aim of this pilot study was to evaluate if levosimendan could exert its protective effects in patients with cardiac low output syndrome or cardiogenic shock on cardiovascular function and hemodynamics as a result of its ability to prevent the GSH reduction and TBARS increase, regardless of the etiology. Moreover, no comparison was performed with a "control" group. However, in this study, all patients were in control of themselves and we analyzed, at different time points, the concomitant changes of hemodynamic variables and cardiac systo-diastolic function, as well as the changes in the levels of oxidants and antioxidants. The results obtained have shown that levosimendan improved GSH and reduced TBARS early before the onset of the cardiovascular effects. Thus, in spite of the low number of cases, levosimendan infusion was able to significantly exert beneficial effects on both the oxidant and antioxidant system, hemodynamics, and cardiac function in cardiogenic shock/low cardiac output patients. A larger number of cases will be necessary to perform a more detailed analysis of the protective effects of levosimendan and evaluation of any differences among various patients.

Overall, the results obtained in this pilot study set the rationale for a clinical trial in a larger population, whose number will be established through a power calculation, and stratified for age, sex, BMI, comorbidities, and etiologies. In this regard, the role of IABP as a modulator of oxidative stress could be further analyzed. In addition, it would be interesting to collect more data about the "redox state" and inflammation and compare the effects of levosimendan with those of other inotropes.

Finally, it seems important to follow the putative anti-inflammatory effects of this drug, not only in cardiac patients, but also in patients with conditions such as pulmonary hypertension or amyotrophic lateral sclerosis, in which levosimendan is currently being clinically evaluated [50,51].

Author Contributions: Author Contributions: Conception and design: E.G., C.M. and P.P.; patient data and samples: D.P., L.R. and V.B.; experiments, collection and assembly of data: S.F., C.M., D.P., L.R. and V.B.; data analysis and interpretation: E.G. and P.P.; manuscript writing and editing: e.g., S.F., C.M., D.P., L.R., V.B. and P.P. All authors have read and agreed to the published version of the manuscript.

Funding: This research received no external funding.

Acknowledgments: We thank Azienda Ospedaliera Universitaria AOU Maggiore della Carità for its help. We thank Hughes Associated, Oxford, for the language check of the document

Conflicts of Interest: P.P. is full time employee of Orion Pharma, where levosimendan has been discovered and developed; the other authors declare no conflict of interest.

References

1. Farmakis, D.; Alvarez, J.; Gal, T.B.; Brito, D.; Fedele, F.; Fonseca, C.; Gordon, A.C.; Gotsman, I.; Grossini, E.; Guarracino, F.; et al. Levosimendan beyond inotropy and acute heart failure: Evidence of pleiotropic effects on the heart and other organs: An expert panel position paper. *Int. J. Cardiol.* **2016**, *222*, 303–312. [CrossRef] [PubMed]
2. Follath, F.; Cleland, J.G.; Just, H.; Papp, J.G.; Scholz, H.; Peuhkurinen, K.; Harjola, V.P.; Mitrovic, V.; Abdalla, M.; Sandell, E.P.; et al. Steering Committee and Investigators of the Levosimendan Infusion versus Dobutamine (LIDO) Study. Efficacy and safety of intravenous levosimendan compared with dobutamine in severe low-output heart failure (the LIDO study): A randomised double-blind trial. *Lancet* **2002**, *360*, 196–202. [CrossRef]
3. Moiseyev, V.S.; Põder, P.; Andrejevs, N.; Ruda, M.Y.; Golikov, A.P.; Lazebnik, L.B.; Kobalava, Z.D.; Lehtonen, L.A.; Laine, T.; et al. Nieminen MSRUSSLAN Study Investigators. Safety and efficacy of a novel calcium sensitizer, levosimendan, in patients with left ventricular failure due to an acute myocardial infarction. A randomized, placebo-controlled, double-blind study (RUSSLAN). *Eur. Heart J.* **2002**, *23*, 1422–1432. [CrossRef] [PubMed]
4. Herpain, A.; Bouchez, S.; Girardis, M.; Guarracino, F.; Knotzer, J.; Levy, B.; Liebregts, T.; Pollesello, P.; Ricksten, S.E.; Riha, H.; et al. Use of Levosimendan in Intensive Care Unit Settings: An Opinion Paper. *J. Cardiovasc. Pharmacol.* **2019**, *73*, 3–14. [CrossRef]

5. Pollesello, P.; Ovaska, M.; Kaivola, J.; Tilgmann, C.; Lundström, K.; Kalkkinen, N.; Ulmanen, I.; Nissinen, E.; Taskinen, J. Binding of a new Ca^{2+} sensitizer, levosimendan, to recombinant human cardiac troponin C. A molecular modelling, fluorescence probe, and proton nuclear magnetic resonance study. *J. Biol. Chem.* **1994**, *269*, 28584–28590.
6. Pääkkönen, K.; Annila, A.; Sorsa, T.; Pollesello, P.; Tilgmann, C.; Kilpeläinen, I.; Karisola, P.; Ulmanen, I.; Drakenberg, T. Solution structure and main chain dynamics of the regulatory domain (Residues 1-91) of human cardiac troponin C. *J. Biol. Chem.* **1998**, *273*, 15633–15638. [CrossRef]
7. Sorsa, T.; Heikkinen, S.; Abbott, M.B.; Abusamhadneh, E.; Laakso, T.; Tilgmann, C.; Serimaa, R.; Annila, A.; Rosevear, P.R.; Drakenberg, T. Binding of levosimendan, a calcium sensitizer, to cardiac troponin C. *J. Biol. Chem.* **2001**, *276*, 9337–9343. [CrossRef]
8. Yokoshiki, H.; Katsube, Y.; Sunagawa, M.; Sperelakis, N. The novel calcium sensitizer levosimendan activates the ATP-sensitive K+ channel in rat ventricular cells. *J. Pharmacol. Exp. Ther.* **1997**, *283*, 375–383.
9. Paturicza, J.; Krassói, I.; Höhn, J.; Kun, A.; Papp, J.G. Functional role of potassium channels in the vasodilating mechanism of levosimendan in porcine isolated coronary artery. *Cardiovasc. Drugs Ther.* **2003**, *17*, 115–121. [CrossRef]
10. Kaheinen, P.; Pollesello, P.; Levijoki, J.; Haikala, H. Effects of levosimendan and milrinone on oxygen consumption in isolated guinea-pig heart. *J. Cardiovasc. Pharmacol.* **2004**, *43*, 555–561. [CrossRef]
11. Eriksson, O.; Pollesello, P.; Haikala, H. Effect of levosimendan on balance between ATP production and consumption in isolated perfused guinea-pig heart before ischemia or after reperfusion. *J. Cardiovasc. Pharmacol.* **2004**, *44*, 316–321. [CrossRef] [PubMed]
12. Ukkonen, H.; Saraste, M.; Akkila, J.; Knuuti, M.J.; Lehikoinen, P.; Någren, K.; Lehtonen, L.; Voipio-Pulkki, L.M. Myocardial efficiency during calcium sensitization with levosimendan: A noninvasive study with positron emission tomography and echocardiography in healthy volunteers. *Clin. Pharmacol. Ther.* **1997**, *61*, 596–607. [CrossRef]
13. Ukkonen, H.; Saraste, M.; Akkila, J.; Knuuti, J.; Karanko, M.; Iida, H.; Lehikoinen, P.; Någren, K.; Lehtonen, L.; Voipio-Pulkki, L.M. Myocardial efficiency during levosimendan infusion in congestive heart failure. *Clin. Pharmacol. Ther.* **2000**, *68*, 522–531. [CrossRef] [PubMed]
14. Kopustinskiene, D.M.; Pollesello, P.; Saris, N.E. Levosimendan is a mitochondrial K(ATP) channel opener. *Eur. J. Pharmacol.* **2001**, *428*, 311–314. [CrossRef]
15. Kopustinskiene, D.M.; Pollesello, P.; Saris, N.E. Potassium-specific effects of levosimendan on heart mitochondria. *Biochem. Pharmacol.* **2004**, *68*, 807–812. [CrossRef]
16. Soeding, P.F.; Crack, P.J.; Wright, C.E.; Angus, J.A.; Royse, C.F. Levosimendan preserves the contractile responsiveness of hypoxic human myocardium via mitochondrial K(ATP) channel and potential pERK 1/2 activation. *Eur. J. Pharmacol.* **2011**, *655*, 59–66. [CrossRef]
17. Torraco, A.; Carrozzo, R.; Piemonte, F.; Pastore, A.; Tozzi, G.; Verrigni, D.; Assenza, M.; Orecchioni, A.; D'Egidio, A.; Marraffa, E.; et al. Effects of levosimendan on mitochondrial function in patients with septic shock: A randomized trial. *Biochimie* **2014**, *102*, 166–173. [CrossRef]
18. Sommer, S.; Leistner, M.; Aleksic, I.; Schimmer, C.; Alhussini, K.; Kanofsky, P.; Leyh, R.G.; Sommer, S.P. Impact of levosimendan and ischaemia-reperfusion injury on myocardial subsarcolemmal mitochondrial respiratory chain, mitochondrial membrane potential, Ca^{2+} cycling and ATP synthesis. *Eur. J. Cardiothorac. Surg.* **2016**, *49*, 54–62. [CrossRef]
19. Bunte, S.; Behmenburg, F.; Bongartz, A.; Stroethoff, M.; Raupach, A.; Heinen, A.; Minol, J.P.; Hollmann, M.W.; Huhn, R.; Sixt, S.U. Preconditioning by Levosimendan is Mediated by Activation of Mitochondrial Ca^{2+}-Sensitive Potassium (mBKCa) Channels. *Cardiovasc. Drugs Ther.* **2018**, *32*, 427–434. [CrossRef]
20. Grossini, E.; Molinari, C.; Pollesello, P.; Bellomo, G.; Valente, G.; Mary, D.; Vacca, G.; Caimmi, P. Levosimendan protection against kidney ischemia/reperfusion injuries in anesthetized pigs. *J. Pharmacol. Exp. Ther.* **2012**, *342*, 376–388. [CrossRef]
21. Grossini, E.; Pollesello, P.; Bellofatto, K.; Sigaudo, L.; Farruggio, S.; Origlia, V.; Mombello, C.; Mary, D.A.; Valente, G.; Vacca, G. Protective effects elicited by levosimendan against liver ischemia/reperfusion injury in anesthetized rats. *Liver Transpl.* **2014**, *20*, 361–375. [CrossRef]
22. Ho, E.; Karimi Galougahi, K.; Liu, C.C.; Bhindi, R.; Figtree, G.A. Biological markers of oxidative stress: Applications to cardiovascular research and practice. *Redox Biol.* **2013**, *1*, 483–491. [CrossRef]

23. Ballatori, N.; Krance, S.M.; Notenboom, S.; Shi, S.; Tieu, K.; Hammond, C.L. Glutathione dysregulation and the etiology and progression of human diseases. *Biol. Chem.* **2009**, *390*, 191–214. [CrossRef] [PubMed]
24. Grossini, E.; Bellofatto, K.; Farruggio, S.; Sigaudo, L.; Marotta, P.; Raina, G.; De Giuli, V.; Mary, D.; Pollesello, P.; Minisini, R.; et al. Levosimendan inhibits peroxidation in hepatocytes by modulating apoptosis/autophagy interplay. *PLoS ONE* **2015**, *10*, e0124742. [CrossRef] [PubMed]
25. López Farré, A.; Casado, S. Heart failure, redox alterations, and endothelial dysfunction. *Hypertension* **2001**, *38*, 1400–1405. [CrossRef] [PubMed]
26. Keith, M.; Geranmayegan, A.; Sole, M.J.; Kurian, R.; Robinson, A.; Omran, A.S.; Jeejeebhoy, K.N. Increased oxidative stress in patients with congestive heart failure. *J. Am. Coll. Cardiol.* **1998**, *31*, 1352–1356. [CrossRef]
27. Polidori, M.C.; Savino, K.; Alunni, G.; Freddio, M.; Senin, U.; Sies, H.; Stahl, W.; Mecocci, P. Plasma lipophilic antioxidants and malondialdehyde in congestive heart failure patients: Relationship to disease severity. *Free Radic. Biol. Med.* **2002**, *32*, 148–152. [CrossRef]
28. Avgeropoulou, C.; Andreadou, I.; Markantonis-Kyroudis, S.; Demopoulou, M.; Missovoulos, P.; Androulakis, A.; Kallikazaros, I. The Ca^{2+}-sensitizer levosimendan improves oxidative damage, BNP and pro-inflammatory cytokine levels in patients with advanced decompensated heart failure in comparison to dobutamine. *Eur. J. Heart Fail.* **2005**, *7*, 882–887. [CrossRef]
29. Delle Karth, G.; Buberl, A.; Geppert, A.; Neunteufl, T.; Huelsmann, M.; Kopp, C.; Nikfardjam, M.; Berger, R.; Heinz, G. Hemodynamic effects of a continuous infusion of levosimendan in critically ill patients with cardiogenic shock requiring catecholamines. *Acta Anaesthesiol. Scand.* **2003**, *47*, 1251–1256. [CrossRef]
30. Wilkman, E.; Kaukonen, K.M.; Pettilä, V.; Kuitunen, A.; Varpula, M. Association between inotrope treatment and 90-day mortality in patients with septic shock. *Acta Anaesthesiol. Scand.* **2013**, *57*, 431–442. [CrossRef]
31. Lang, R.M.; Badano, L.P.; Mor-Avi, V.; Afilalo, J.; Armstrong, A.; Ernande, L.; Flachskampf, F.A.; Foster, E.; Goldstein, S.A.; Kuznetsova, T. Guidelines and standrards. Recommendations for Cardiac Chamber Quantification by Echocardiography in Adults: An Update from the American Society of Echocardiography and the European Association of Cardiovascular Imaging. *J. Am. Soc. Echocardiogr.* **2015**, *28*, 1–39. [CrossRef] [PubMed]
32. Rudski, L.G.; Lai, W.W.; Afilalo, J.; Hua, L.; Handschumacher, M.D.; Chandrasekaran, K.; Solomon, S.D.; Louie, E.K.; Schiller, N.B. Guidelines and standards. Guidelines for the Echocardiographic Assessment of the Right Heart in Adults: A Report from the American Society of Echocardiography Endorsed by the European Association of Echocardiography, a registered branch of the European Society of Cardiology, and the Canadian Society of Echocardiography. *J. Am. Soc. Echocardiogr.* **2010**, *23*, 685–713.
33. Nagueh, S.F.; Smiseth, O.A.; Appleton, C.P.; Byrd, B.F.; Dokainish, H.; Edvardsen, T.; Flachskampf, F.A.; Gillebert, T.C.; Klein, A.L.; Lancellotti, P.; et al. Lancellotti PASE/EACVI Guidelines and standards. Recommendations for the Evaluation of Left Ventricular Diastolic Function by Echocardiography: An Update from the American Society of Echocardiography and the European Association of Cardiovascular Imaging. *J. Am. Soc. Echocardiogr.* **2016**, *29*, 277–314. [CrossRef]
34. Cholley, B.; Caruba, T.; Grosjean, S.; Amour, J.; Ouattara, A.; Villacorta, J.; Miguel, B.; Guinet, P.; Lévy, F.; Squara, P.; et al. Effect of Levosimendan on Low Cardiac Output Syndrome in Patients with Low Ejection Fraction Undergoing Coronary Artery Bypass Grafting with Cardiopulmonary Bypass: The LICORN Randomized Clinical Trial. *JAMA* **2017**, *318*, 548–556. [CrossRef] [PubMed]
35. Sangalli, F.; Avalli, L.; Laratta, M.; Formica, F.; Maggioni, E.; Caruso, R.; Cristina Costa, M.; Guazzi, M.; Fumagalli, R. Effects of Levosimendan on Endothelial Function and Hemodynamics During Weaning from Veno-Arterial Extracorporeal Life Support. *J. Cardiothorac. Vasc. Anesth.* **2016**, *30*, 1449–1453. [CrossRef] [PubMed]
36. De Cillà, S.; Vezzola, D.; Farruggio, S.; Vujosevic, S.; Clemente, N.; Raina, G.; Mary, D.; Casini, G.; Rossetti, L.; Avagliano, L.; et al. The subthreshold micropulse laser treatment of the retina restores the oxidant/antioxidant balance and counteracts programmed forms of cell death in the mice eyes. *Acta Ophthalmol.* **2017**, *42*, 1725–1738. [CrossRef]
37. Farruggio, S.; Raina, G.; Cocomazzi, G.; Librasi, C.; Mary, D.; Gentilli, S.; Grossini, E. Genistein improves viability, proliferation and mitochondrial function of cardiomyoblasts cultured in physiologic and peroxidative conditions. *Int. J. Mol. Med.* **2019**, *44*, 2298–2310. [CrossRef]

38. Surico, D.; Bordino, V.; Cantaluppi, V.; Mary, D.; Gentilli, S.; Oldani, A.; Farruggio, S.; Melluzza, C.; Raina, G.; Grossini, E. Preeclampsia and intrauterine growth restriction: Role of human umbilical cord mesenchymal stem cells-trophoblast cross-talk. *PLoS ONE* **2019**, *14*, e0218437. [CrossRef]
39. Leong, L.N. Targeting oxidative stress in HF. *Heart Metab.* **2009**, *42*, 21–24.
40. Mochizuki, M.; Yano, M.; Oda, T.; Tateishi, H.; Kobayashi, S.; Yamamoto, T.; Ikeda, Y.; Ohkusa, T.; Ikemoto, N.; Matsuzaki, M. Scavenging free radicals by low-dose carvedilol prevents redox-dependent Ca^{2+} leak via stabilization of ryanodine receptor in heart failure. *J. Am. Coll Cardiol.* **2007**, *49*, 1722–1732. [CrossRef]
41. Oe, H.; Nakamura, K.; Kihara, H.; Shimada, K.; Fukuda, S.; Takagi, T.; Miyoshi, T.; Hirata, K.; Yoshikawa, J.; Ito, H. FESC, for Effect of a DPP-4 inhibitor on left ventricular diastolic dysfunction in patients with type 2 diabetes and diabetic cardiomyopathy (3D) study investigators. Comparison of effects of sitagliptin and voglibose on left ventricular diastolic dysfunction in patients with type 2 diabetes: Results of the 3D trial. *Cardiovasc Diabetol.* **2015**, *14*, 83. [CrossRef] [PubMed]
42. Jeong, E.M.; Dudley, S.C. Diastolic dysfunction. *Circ. J.* **2015**, *79*, 470–477. [CrossRef] [PubMed]
43. Kuznetsov, A.V.; Javadov, S.; Margreiter, R.; Grimm, M.; Hagenbuchner, J.; Ausserlechner, M.J. The Role of Mitochondria in the Mechanisms of Cardiac Ischemia-Reperfusion Injury. *Antioxidants* **2019**, *8*, 454. [CrossRef] [PubMed]
44. Liang, W.; Chen, J.; Mo, L.; Ke, X.; Zhang, W.; Zheng, D.; Pan, W.; Wu, S.; Feng, J.; Song, M.; et al. ATP-sensitive K^+ channels contribute to the protective effects of exogenous hydrogen sulfide against high glucose-induced injury in H9c2 cardiac cells. *Int. J. Mol. Med.* **2016**, *37*, 763–772. [CrossRef]
45. Zhang, D.M.; Chai, Y.; Erickson, J.R.; Brown, J.H.; Bers, D.M.; Lin, Y.F. Intracellular signalling mechanism responsible for modulation of sarcolemmal ATP-sensitive potassium channels by nitric oxide in ventricular cardiomyocytes. *J. Physiol.* **2014**, *592*, 971–990. [CrossRef]
46. Holmuhamedov, E.L.; Jovanović, S.; Dzeja, P.P.; Jovanović, A.; Terzic, A. Mitochondrial ATP-sensitive K+ channels modulate cardiac mitochondrial function. *Am. J. Physiol.* **1998**, *275*, 1567–1576. [CrossRef]
47. Bouchez, S.; Fedele, F.; Giannakoulas, G.; Gustafsson, F.; Harjola, V.P.; Karason, K.; Kivikko, M.; Von Lewinski, D.; Oliva, F.; Papp, Z.; et al. Levosimendan in Acute and Advanced Heart Failure: An Expert Perspective on Posology and Therapeutic Application. *Cardiovasc. Drugs Ther.* **2018**, *32*, 617–624. [CrossRef]
48. Goldenthal, M.J. Mitochondrial involvement in myocyte death and heart failure. *Heart Fail. Rev.* **2016**, *21*, 137–155. [CrossRef]
49. Uberti, F.; Caimmi, P.P.; Molinari, C.; Mary, D.; Vacca, G.; Grossini, E. Levosimendan modulates programmed forms of cell death through K(ATP) channels and nitric oxide. *J. Cardiovasc. Pharmacol.* **2011**, *57*, 246–258. [CrossRef]
50. Hemodynamic Evaluation of Levosimendan in Patients with PH-HFpEF (HELP). Available online: https://clinicaltrials.gov/ct2/show/NCT03541603 (accessed on 4 December 2019).
51. Al-Chalabi, A.; Heunks, L.M.A.; Papp, Z.; Pollesello, P. Potential of the Cardiovascular Drug Levosimendan in the Management of Amyotrophic Lateral Sclerosis: An Overview of a Working Hypothesis. *J. Cardiovasc. Pharmacol.* **2019**, *74*, 389–399. [CrossRef]

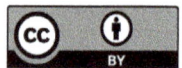

© 2020 by the authors. Licensee MDPI, Basel, Switzerland. This article is an open access article distributed under the terms and conditions of the Creative Commons Attribution (CC BY) license (http://creativecommons.org/licenses/by/4.0/).

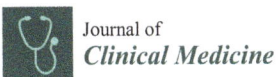

Article

Increased Lymphangiogenesis and Lymphangiogenic Growth Factor Expression in Perivascular Adipose Tissue of Patients with Coronary Artery Disease

Ioannis Drosos [1], Maria Pavlaki [2], Maria Del Pilar Ortega Carrillo [1], Adriani Kourkouli [2], Katja Buschmann [3], Fotios Konstantinou [4], Rajinikanth Gogiraju [1], Magdalena L. Bochenek [1,5], Georgios Chalikias [2], Christos Tortopidis [2], Christian F. Vahl [3], Dimitrios Mikroulis [4], Dimitrios Tziakas [2], Thomas Münzel [1], Stavros Konstantinides [2,5] and Katrin Schäfer [1,*]

1. Center for Cardiology, Cardiology 1, University Medical Center of the Johannes Gutenberg University Mainz, 55130 Mainz, Germany
2. Department of Cardiology, Democritus University of Thrace, 68100 Alexandroupolis, Greece
3. Department of Cardiothoracic and Vascular Surgery, University Medical Center of the Johannes Gutenberg University Mainz, 55130 Mainz, Germany
4. Department of Cardiothoracic Surgery, Democritus University of Thrace, 68100 Alexandroupolis, Greece
5. Center for Thrombosis and Hemostasis, University Medical Center of the Johannes Gutenberg University Mainz, 55130 Mainz, Germany
* Correspondence: katrin.schaefer@unimedizin-mainz.de; Tel.: +49-6131-17-4221

Received: 5 June 2019; Accepted: 4 July 2019; Published: 9 July 2019

Abstract: Experimental and human autopsy studies have associated adventitial lymphangiogenesis with atherosclerosis. An analysis of perivascular lymphangiogenesis in patients with coronary artery disease is lacking. Here, we examined lymphangiogenesis and its potential regulators in perivascular adipose tissue (PVAT) surrounding the heart (C-PVAT) and compared it with PVAT of the internal mammary artery (IMA-PVAT). Forty-six patients undergoing coronary artery bypass graft surgery were included. Perioperatively collected C-PVAT and IMA-PVAT were analyzed using histology, immunohistochemistry, real time PCR, and PVAT-conditioned medium using cytokine arrays. C-PVAT exhibited increased PECAM-1 (platelet endothelial cell adhesion molecule 1)-positive vessel density. The number of lymphatic vessels expressing lymphatic vessel endothelial hyaluronan receptor-1 or podoplanin was also elevated in C-PVAT and associated with higher inflammatory cell numbers, increased intercellular adhesion molecule 1 (ICAM1) expression, and fibrosis. Significantly higher expression of regulators of lymphangiogenesis such as vascular endothelial growth factor (VEGF)-C, VEGF-D, and VEGF receptor-3 was observed in C-PVAT compared to IMA-PVAT. 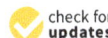 Cytokine arrays identified angiopoietin-2 as more highly expressed in C-PVAT vs. IMA-PVAT. Findings were confirmed histologically and at the mRNA level. Stimulation of human lymphatic endothelial cells with recombinant angiopoietin-2 in combination with VEGF-C enhanced sprout formation. Our study shows that PVAT surrounding atherosclerotic arteries exhibits more extensive lymphangiogenesis, inflammation, and fibrosis compared to PVAT surrounding a non-diseased vessel, possibly due to local angiopoietin-2, VEGF-C, and VEGF-D overexpression.

Keywords: coronary artery disease; human; inflammation; lymphangiogenesis; perivascular adipose tissue

1. Introduction

Accumulating clinical and experimental data suggest an active contribution of the adventitia to remodeling processes in the vascular wall, including neointima formation and atherosclerosis.

For example, preclinical studies in hypercholesterolemic animal models have shown that adventitial angiogenesis promotes atherosclerotic plaque progression, whereas inhibition of plaque neovascularization reduced lesion growth [1–3]. The expansion of thin-walled, leaky vasa vasorum and microvessels within atherosclerotic lesions has been pathophysiologically linked to plaque instability by increasing inflammatory cell infiltration and intraplaque hemorrhage [4–6], among others.

In addition to arteries and veins, lymphatic vessels exist and develop in parallel with blood vessels in most organs. Although the extent and complexity of the lymphatic vasculature has been known for more than a century [7], its role in the pathogenesis of cardiovascular disease processes has received little attention. Lymph vessels control the drainage of interstitial fluids and macromolecules (proteins, lipids) leaking from capillaries back to the venous circulation and are thus critical for the maintenance of tissue homeostasis [8]. In addition, they have an important function in immune surveillance and may accelerate the resolution of inflammation by removing inflammatory mediators or trafficking immune cells to draining lymph nodes. Lymph vessel dysfunction results in lymphedema, but also may play a role during inflammation, cancer, obesity, or hypertension (reviewed in [9]).

Regarding atherosclerosis, which is characterized by chronic inflammation and cholesterol accumulation in the arterial wall, the possibility of a direct contribution of adventitial lymphangiogenesis has only been recently addressed. Studies in animal models after experimentally induced lymphostasis or genetic modulation of lymphatic vessel formation suggested a protective role of the lymphatic vasculature during atherosclerosis [10,11]. Moreover, cardiac lymphangiogenesis has been shown to take part in the clearance of immune cells and resolution of inflammation after myocardial infarction [12,13]. A causal role of lymph vessel dysfunction in the pathophysiology of atherosclerosis is further supported by findings in mice that excessive cholesterol accumulation is associated with structural and functional alterations of lymphatic vessels [14], and that lymphatic dysfunction develops before atherosclerotic lesion formation [15]. As far as human atherosclerosis is concerned, the available knowledge is limited to autopsy studies of large arteries from organ donors and the clinical observation that (adventitial) lymphangiogenesis correlates with atherosclerosis severity [11,16–18]. Similar findings were obtained in 21 endarterectomy samples from patients with internal carotid artery stenosis showing a more developed lymphatic network in the adventitia of atherosclerotic lesions compared to healthy arteries [19]. Whether these observations reflect lymphatic dysfunction or the reactive enlargement of perivascular lymphatic networks to local cues or systemic differences between patients at risk and control individuals remains unknown.

Given the anatomical proximity of perivascular adipose tissue (PVAT) with the adventitia and its known paracrine activities on the underlying vessel, studied by our group [20] and others (reviewed in [21]), we hypothesized that differences may exist in the extent of the lymphatic vasculature and the expression of lymphangiogenic growth factors between PVAT surrounding the aortic root and coronaries of patients with coronary artery disease (CAD) and PVAT of the internal mammary artery (IMA), an artery protected from the development of atherosclerosis [22].

2. Materials and Methods

2.1. Study Patients

Forty-six patients (76% male; mean age, 68.6 ± 9.8 years; mean body mass index, 29.1 ± 5.4 kg/m^2) undergoing elective coronary artery bypass graft surgery in two university medical centers were included in the study. All patients had been diagnosed with multivessel CAD via coronary angiography. The left (and in some cases also the right) IMA was used as an aortocoronary bypass in all patients. The study complied with the declaration of Helsinki and was approved by the Ethics Committee of the University General Hospital of Alexandroupolis, Greece, and the University Medical Center of the Johannes Gutenberg University Mainz, Germany, respectively. All patients signed a written informed consent prior to inclusion in the study. Due to the limited amount of tissue from each patient, not all analyses could be performed in all patients, and samples had to be split into groups.

2.2. Tissue Specimen Collection

'Cardiac' perivascular adipose tissue (C-PVAT), located adjacent to the aortic root and around the coronary arteries, and PVAT surrounding the IMA (IMA-PVAT) was collected perioperatively and immediately transferred to the laboratory in ice-cold sterile saline solution (Braun). IMA-PVAT was collected immediately after preparation of the arterial bypass graft and before establishing the extracorporeal circulation. C-PVAT was collected during extracorporeal circulation, immediately after removing the aortic cross-clamp, from the same position in all patients, regardless of the localization of atherosclerotic lesions within the coronary tree. PVAT specimens were briefly rinsed with sterile saline and visible connective tissue or blood vessels removed. PVAT samples were then either directly processed under sterile conditions for the preparation of conditioned medium (CM) or stored at −80 °C pending protein or RNA isolation. Specimens intended for RNA isolation were transferred to TRI Reagent®Solution (ThermoFisher Scientific; Dreieich, Germany) before storage at −80 °C. PVAT samples intended for histology/immunohistochemistry were fixed in 10% zinc formalin (Sigma-Aldrich; Darmstadt, Germany), embedded in paraffin wax (Leica; Wetzlar, Germany) and cut into 5-µm-thick sections.

2.3. Generation of Perivascular Adipose Tissue Conditioned Medium

For the generation of PVAT-derived CM, C-PVAT and IMA-PVAT specimens were cut into pieces under sterile conditions and then transferred into Dulbecco's Modified Eagle's medium (ThermoFisher Scientific) supplemented with 1% penicillin/streptomycin and 0.5% fetal bovine serum (both Biosera). A standard culture medium volume/tissue mass proportion of 2 µL per mg of tissue was employed. Culture medium and PVAT were then incubated in a cell culture incubator (New Brunswick, Eppendorf; Wesseling-Berzdorf, Germany; 37 °C, 5% CO_2) for 24 h. Control medium was prepared in parallel by incubating medium without PVAT tissue. After removal of PVAT pieces, CM was centrifuged at 20,000 g for 10 min and the supernatant kept at −80°C pending analysis.

2.4. Membrane-Based Protein Array

C-PVAT- and IMA-PVAT-derived CM (1 mL) from five patients with CAD was examined for secreted proteins using a customized RayBio®membrane-based antibody array against 29 target proteins (RayBiotech, Hölzel Diagnostika Handels GmbH; Köln, Germany), following the instructions of the manual. Chemiluminescence detection was performed using a ChemiDoc™ MP imaging system (Bio-Rad; Rüdigheim, Germany). Semi-quantitative analysis was performed by densitometry using ImageJ software (version 1.52, NIH) and Gilles Carpentier's Protein Array Analyser for ImageJ macro (rsb.info.nih.gov/ij/macros/toolsets/ProteinArrayAnalyzer.txt). Negative control dots were used for background subtraction and positive control dots to normalize values and to allow comparison among array membranes. Quantitative data were expressed as fold change vs. IMA-PVAT.

2.5. Reverse Transcription Quantitative Real-time PCR

PVAT was homogenized in TRI Reagent®solution using a rotating homogenizer (ART Prozess and Labortechnik GmbH; Müllheim, Germany). For RNA isolation from human dermal lymphatic endothelial cells (HDLECs), cells were directly harvested from the culture plate using TRI Reagent®solution and a cell scraper. RNA isolation was performed using a standard protocol. For PVAT samples, an additional purification step was performed using NucleoSpin®RNA columns (Macherey-Nagel; Düren, Germany). The amount of RNA was quantified on a NanoDrop™ 2000 spectrophotometer (ThermoFisher Scientific). Reverse transcription was performed using M-MLV reverse transcriptase (Promega; Mannheim, Germany) or iScript™ cDNA Synthesis Kit (Bio-Rad). For quantitative real-time PCR (qPCR), SsoAdvanced™ Universal SYBR®Green Supermix (Bio-Rad) and a CFX Connect™ Real-Time PCR Detection System (Bio-Rad) were used. Two technical replicates were prepared for each sample. For PVAT gene expression analysis, LRP10 was used as endogenous reference gene [20]. For HDLECs, preliminary analysis of common reference genes indicated 18S as the most stably expressed gene. The sequences of all primers that were used are shown in Table S1. Data were normalized to the respective reference gene and are expressed as $2^{(-DCq)}$ values for C-PVAT and IMA-PVAT or as $2^{(-DDCq)}$ (fold change vs. control-treated samples) for HDLECs.

2.6. Spheroid Lymphangiogenesis Assay

HDLECs were cultured in Endothelial Cell Growth Medium MV2 (PromoCell; Heidelberg, Germany) and analyzed up to passage 5. Spheroids of HDLECs were prepared on day one following a standard protocol. In short, cultured HDLECs were detached using 0.05% trypsin-EDTA (ThermoFisher Scientific) and resuspended at a density of 400 cells per 100 µL Endothelial Cell Growth Medium MV2 containing 20% methylcellulose in Medium 199 (both Sigma-Aldrich). Subsequently, 100 µL of the cell suspension were transferred to the wells of a round-bottom 96-well suspension culture plate and incubated for 24 h at 5% CO_2, 37 °C in order for HDLEC spheroids to form. On day two, spheroids were collected from the 96-well plate. After centrifugation at 390 g for three minutes, the supernatant was discarded and spheroids resuspended at a 1:1 mixture of 50% rat tail collagen I (Corning; Wiesbaden, Germany), 0.05% acetic acid (in Medium 199) and 5% fetal bovine serum in methylcellulose/Medium 199 solution. The suspension was transferred to the wells of a 24-well plate and incubated for 30 min before adding Endothelial Cell Growth Medium MV2. Spheroids were stimulated with recombinant human angiopoietin-2 (ANGPT2; 100 ng/mL) and/or recombinant human vascular endothelial growth factor (VEGF)-C (100 ng/mL; both from R&D Systems) for 24 h. Images of five randomly selected spheroids per well were captured using an inverted microscope (Motic AE31; Wetzlar, Germany). The number of sprouts was manually counted and the cumulative sprout length measured using ImageJ software.

2.7. Histology and Immunohistochemistry

Masson's trichrome stain was used for the histological examination of PVAT specimens. For the immunohistochemical staining of the paraffin-embedded tissue sections, a standardized protocol was used. Briefly, paraffin sections were deparaffinized and epitopes were retrieved by heating in 10 mM Tris buffer containing 1 mM EDTA or in 0.1 M citrate buffer (pH 6.0), depending on the target epitope. Unspecific binding sites were blocked using 10% normal goat serum (Abcam; Cambridge, UK). Vessel endothelium was stained using an anti-PECAM-1 antibody (mouse monoclonal; Dako; Santa Clara, CA, USA). Anti-podoplanin (PDPN; rabbit polyclonal; Novus Biologicals) and anti-lymphatic vessel endothelial hyaluronan receptor 1 (LYVE-1; rabbit polyclonal; Novus Biologicals) antibodies were used to selectively stain lymphatic endothelium. Tissue macrophages were visualized using anti-CD68 antibodies (mouse monoclonal; Dako), ANGPT2-expressing cells using anti-ANGPT2 antibody (rabbit polyclonal; Novus Biologicals; Wiesbaden, Germany). After incubating with biotinylated secondary goat anti-mouse or anti-rabbit antibodies (ThermoFisher Scientific), sections were incubated with avidin–biotin complex (Vector Laboratories; Burlingame, CA, USA). Diaminobenzidine or aminoethylcarbazole (Vector Laboratories) substrate was used for visualization, followed by brief counterstaining using Gill's hematoxyline (Sigma-Aldrich). Negative controls were prepared for all immunohistochemical stainings by omitting the primary antibody (representative images shown in Figure S1).

2.8. Image Acquisition and Analysis

Histology and immunohistochemistry sections were examined and representative images were captured using an Olympus BX51 microscope (Hamburg, Germany). The number of total vessels and lymphatic collector vessels was quantified by manually counting PECAM-1- and PDPN-immunopositive vessel-like structures per 200× microscope field, respectively. The number of lymphatic capillaries was quantified by manually counting LYVE-1-immunopositive structures per 200× microscope field. The number of tissue macrophages was determined by manually counting

CD68-immunopositive cells per 400× microscope field. Results were expressed as number of immunopositive vessel-like structures or cells per mm². Sections stained with Masson's trichrome stain were used for the assessment of fibrosis, which was performed by quantifying the blue-stained collagen area relative to total tissue area at 100× magnification. For all quantitative image analyses, three optical fields were randomly selected and measurements averaged.

2.9. Statistical Analysis

Data are presented as mean ± standard deviation (SD), if normally distributed, or as median (25% and 75% interquartile range (IQR)), if not. Normal distribution was examined with the D'Agostino–Pearson omnibus normality test. Paired comparison analyses between PVAT samples from one patient were performed using Student's paired t-test if values were normally distributed, or the Wilcoxon matched-pairs signed rank test if not. Multiple comparisons were performed using one-way ANOVA with Turkey's multiple comparisons test. Differences were considered statistically significant if $p < 0.05$. All statistical analyses were performed using GraphPad PRISM version 8.0.

3. Results

3.1. C-PVAT Contains More Lymphatic Vessels than IMA-PVAT

We had previously shown that C-PVAT from patients with CAD is characterized by more pronounced angiogenesis and higher numbers of blood vessels compared to IMA-PVAT [20]. Immunohistochemical detection of PECAM-1 in paired PVAT tissue specimens from 10 patients with CAD confirmed those previous findings by showing a significantly higher density of PECAM-1-immunopositive vessels in C-PVAT compared to IMA-PVAT (25.4 ± 2.75 vs. 12.9 ± 1.79 per mm², $p = 0.004$; Figure 1A,D; for findings in negative controls please see Figure S1A). To distinguish lymphatic vessels, we used markers expressed on lymphatic endothelium, namely LYVE-1 and PDPN. LYVE-1 has been shown to be mainly expressed in lymphatic capillaries, PDPN in lymphatic collector vessels [23]. These analyses revealed that both the number of LYVE-1 (24.7 (0.61–32.3) vs. 2.97 (0–6.58) per mm², $p = 0.027$; Figure 1B,E; Figure S1B) and PDPN (5.45 ± 1.54 vs. 0.74 ± 0.34 per mm², $p = 0.023$; Figure 1C,F; Figure S1C) -immunopositive vessels was significantly increased in C-PVAT compared to IMA-PVAT. Of note, neither the anti-LYVE-1 nor the anti-PDPN antibody showed any immunoreactivity for endothelium lining blood vessels. Interestingly, the mean diameter of PDPN-positive vessels was significantly increased in C-PVAT compared to IMA-PVAT ($p = 0.008$), in line with lymphatic dysfunction [14,15].

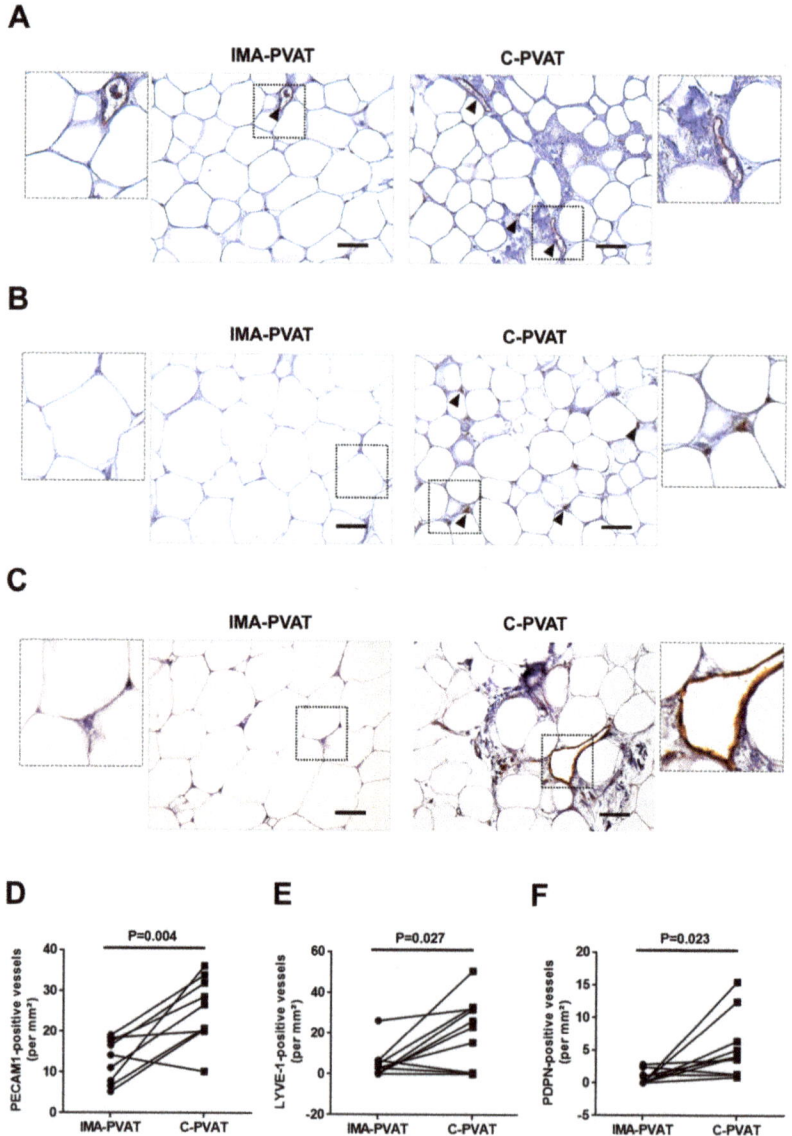

Figure 1. Angiogenesis and lymphangiogenesis in perivascular adipose tissue (PVAT). (**A–C**) Immunohistochemical detection of platelet endothelial cell adhesion molecule 1 (PECAM-1) (**A**), anti-lymphatic vessel endothelial hyaluronan receptor 1 (LYVE-1) (**B**), and anti-podoplanin (PDPN) (**C**) in internal mammary artery (IMA)-PVAT and cardiac (C)-PVAT. Inserts show higher magnification. Size bars represent 100 μm. (**D–F**) Quantification of the number of PECAM-1 (**D**), LYVE-1 (**E**), and PDPN (**F**) immunopositive vessels per mm^2 in $n = 10$ patients with coronary artery disease (CAD). Paired IMA-PVAT (●) and C-PVAT (■) values in individual patients are connected with a line. Statistical analysis was performed using Student's paired t-test (**D**,**F**) or Wilcoxon matched-pairs signed rank test (**E**).

3.2. Lymphangiogenic Growth Factors and Their Receptors Are Expressed at Higher Levels in C-PVAT Compared to IMA-PVAT

To examine whether the more extensive lymphatic network in C-PVAT is accompanied by a higher expression of growth factors known to mediate (lymph-) angiogenesis, qPCR analysis was employed to determine gene expression levels of vascular endothelial growth factor (VEGF)-A, VEGF-B, VEGF-C, and VEGF-D in C-PVAT and IMA-PVAT (paired tissue samples from 16–18 patients). These analyses revealed no significant differences in the mRNA levels of *VEGF-A* (0.85 (0.68–1.21) vs. 0.72 (0.41–1.02), $p = 0.421$; Figure 2A), whereas the expression of *VEGF-C* (0.83 (0.55–1.25) vs. 0.36 (0.22–0.72), $p = 0.022$; Figure 2C) and *VEGF-D* (0.58 (0.42–0.87) vs. 0.25 (0.21–0.31), $p = 0.007$; Figure 2D) was significantly increased in C-PVAT compared to IMA-PVAT. On the other hand, *VEGF-B* mRNA levels were significantly reduced in C-PVAT compared to IMA-PVAT (5.38 (3.92–7.53) vs. 2.99 (2.72–4.13), $p = 0.002$; Figure 2B).

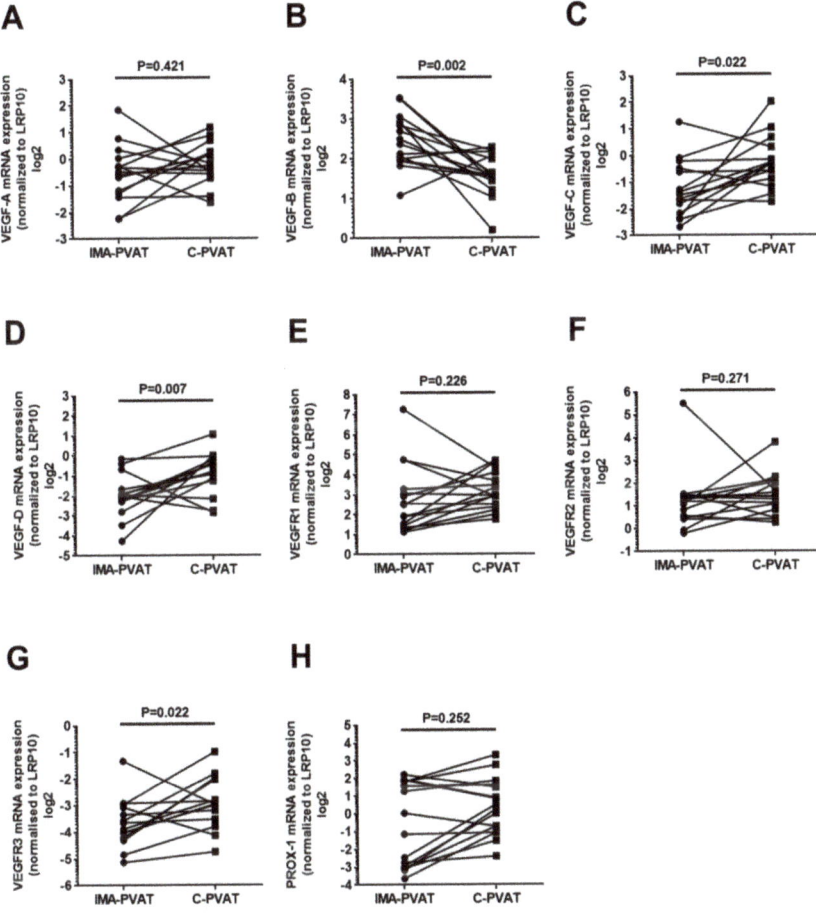

Figure 2. Analysis of growth factors involved in angiogenesis and lymphangiogenesis. Quantification of mRNA expression of vascular endothelial growth factor (*VEGF*)-*A* (**A**), *VEGF-B* (**B**), *VEGF-C* (**C**), *VEGF-D* (**D**), VEGF receptor (*VEGFR*)-*1* (**E**), *VEGFR2* (**F**), *VEGFR3* (**G**), and prospero homeobox-1 (*PROX-1*) (**H**) in IMA-PVAT and C-PVAT of $n = 15$–16 patients with CAD. Paired IMA-PVAT (●) and C-PVAT (■) values in individual patients are connected with a line. Statistical analysis was performed using Wilcoxon matched-pairs signed rank test.

We then also examined the mRNA expression of the receptors for VEGF, namely VEGF receptor (VEGFR)-1, VEGFR2, and VEGFR3. In agreement with our findings of a significantly higher VEGF-C and VEGF-D expression in C-PVAT, mRNA levels of *VEGFR3* were significantly increased in C-PVAT compared to IMA-PVAT (0.13 (0.09–0.25) vs. 0.07 (0.05–0.12), $p = 0.022$; Figure 2G), whereas no differences in the mRNA expression of *VEGFR1* (7.78 (5.29–16.2) vs. 4.70 (2.59–9.37), $p = 0.226$; Figure 2E) and *VEGFR2* (2.68 (1.85–4.15) vs. 2.38 (1.41–2.79), $p = 0.271$; Figure 2F) were observed between both PVAT depots. These results suggested a higher state of VEGF-C/VEGF-D-mediated VEGFR3 signaling which may be responsible for the observed differences in the lymphatic endothelial cell density between C-PVAT and IMA-PVAT.

Analysis of the transcription factor prospero-related homeobox (PROX)-1, a master regulator of embryonic lymphatic development [24,25], revealed similar *PROX-1* mRNA levels in C-PVAT and IMA-PVAT (1.31 (0.51–3.01) vs. 0.74 (0.12–3.50), $p = 0.252$; Figure 2H) suggesting that the observed differences in the number of lymphatic vessels was not the result of a different embryonically defined lymphangiogenic potential in both adipose tissue depots.

3.3. Increased Inflammation and Fibrosis in PVAT Surrounding Atherosclerotic Arteries

Previous studies have shown that inflammation triggers lymphangiogenesis and identified macrophages as main cellular source of VEGF-C and VEGF-D [26,27]. Higher numbers of CD68-immunopositive macrophages were observed in human C-PVAT compared to IMA-PVAT of patients with CAD (207 ± 35.8 vs. 52.9 ± 7.32 per mm^2, $p = 0.001$; Figure 3A,C; Figure S1D). Because of the complex interplay between lymphangiogenesis, inflammation and fibrosis, we next examined both PVAT depots after staining with Masson's trichrome stain. These analyses revealed a significantly higher degree of fibrosis in C-PVAT compared to IMA-PVAT (0.83 (0.02–4.63) vs. 0.02 (0.01–0.11) % per microscope field, $p = 0.027$; Figure 3B,D). Of note, real time PCR analysis did not reveal differences of transforming growth factor-beta (*TGFβ*) mRNA levels between both adipose tissue depots ($p = 0.151$).

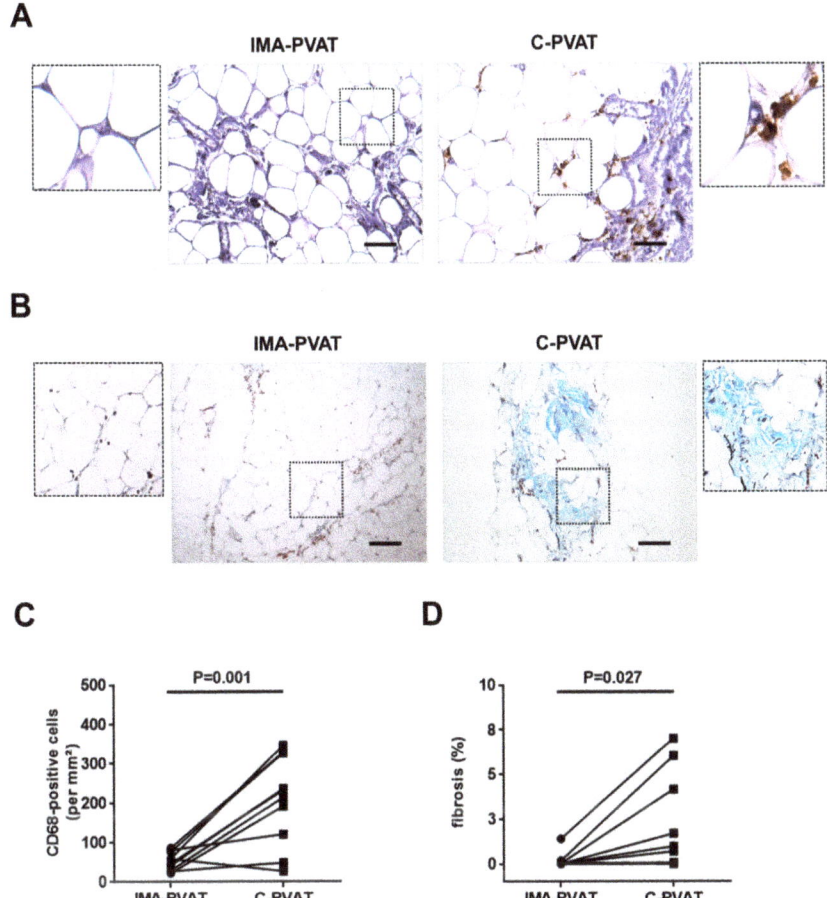

Figure 3. Fibrosis and inflammation in PVAT. (**A**) Immunohistochemical detection of CD68 in IMA-PVAT and C-PVAT. Size bars represent 50 µm. (**B**) Masson trichrome stain in IMA-PVAT and C-PVAT. Size bars represent 200 µm. (**C**) Quantification of the number of CD68-immunopositive cells per mm^2. (**D**) Quantification of the percentage of fibrotic area in $n = 10$ patients with coronary artery disease (CAD). Paired IMA-PVAT (●) and C-PVAT (■) values in individual patients are connected with a line. Statistical analysis was performed using Student's paired t-test (**C**) or Wilcoxon matched-pairs signed rank test (**D**).

3.4. Protein Array Analysis Reveals Significantly Higher Angiopoietin-2 and Intercellular Adhesion Molecule-1 Levels in C-PVAT Compared to IMA-PVAT

PVAT has been shown to express and secrete a number of cytokines and other factors, which may act locally or in a paracrine manner on the neighboring vessel wall (reviewed in [28]). For this reason and given our findings, we next aimed at investigating a broader spectrum of PVAT-secreted factors, with particular focus on potential candidates involved in (lymph)angiogenesis, inflammation and fibrosis. A semiquantitative paired expression analysis of 29 target proteins was performed in conditioned medium (CM) derived from C-PVAT and IMA-PVAT of five patients with CAD using a membrane-based antibody array (representative results are shown in Figure 4A, the position of all target proteins on the membranes is given in Figure S2). Among those, inflammatory factors (interleukin-6, interleukin-8, monocyte chemoattractant protein-1), matrix metalloproteinases (MMP1, MMP9) and their inhibitors (tissue inhibitor of metalloproteinases TIMP1, TIMP2), adipokines (adiponectin, leptin) and growth factors (angiopoietin-1 and -2, basic fibroblast growth factor) were detected in CM from both adipose tissue depots (heat map in Figure 4B, quantitative analyses for all 29 target proteins in Figure S3A–D).

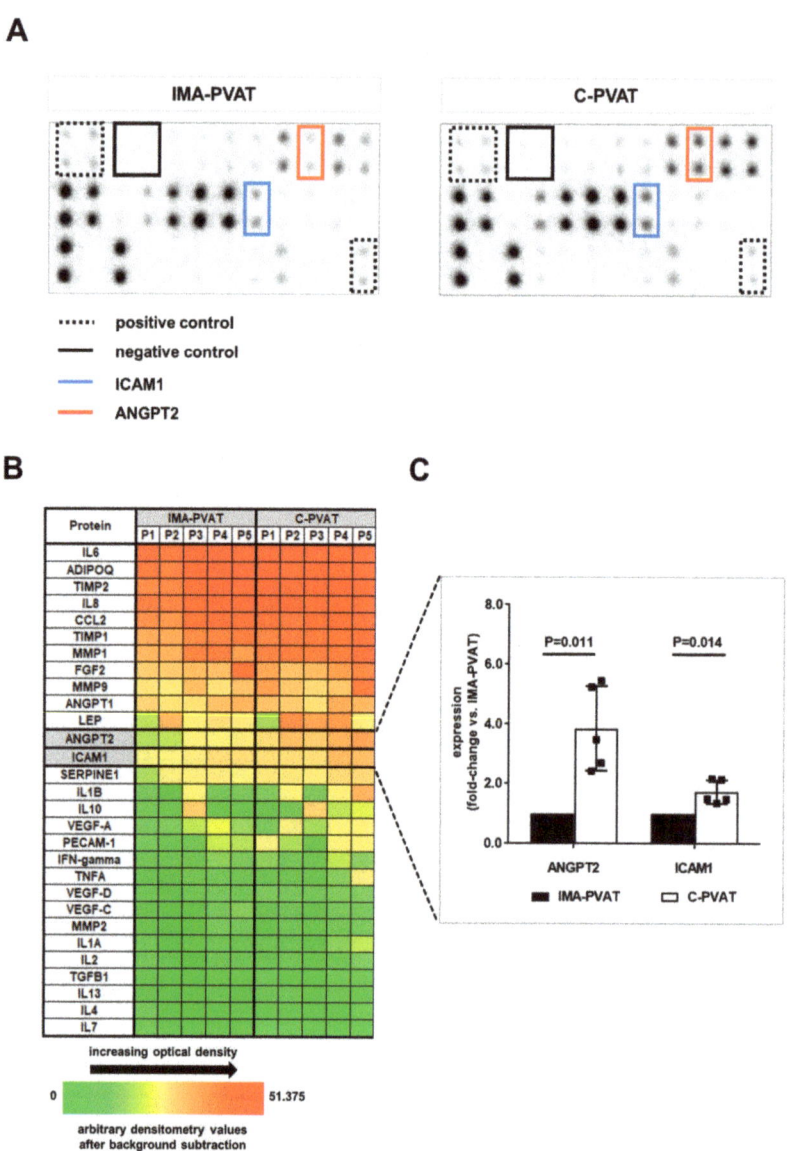

Figure 4. Protein array analysis of factors potentially involved in perivascular lymphangiogenesis. (**A**) Representative chemiluminescence detection images of a protein membrane array in IMA-PVAT- and C-PVAT-derived conditioned medium from one patient with CAD. A commercially available membrane-based antibody protein array was used. Each vertical pair of dots represents one protein.

Boxes of the same color on both membranes mark the respective dot pairs for each protein. Positive and negative control dots are also marked. (**B**) Heat map representation of the expression of 29 proteins quantified using membrane-based protein array analysis in IMA-PVAT- and C-PVAT-derived conditioned medium of $n = 5$ patients with CAD. Each column represents one patient (P1, P2, etc.). (**C**) Quantitative analysis shown for proteins exhibiting a statistically significant difference in expression between IMA-PVAT and C-PVAT. Bars represent fold change of mean protein expression compared to IMA-PVAT. Error bars represent standard deviation. Statistical analysis was performed using Student's paired t-test.

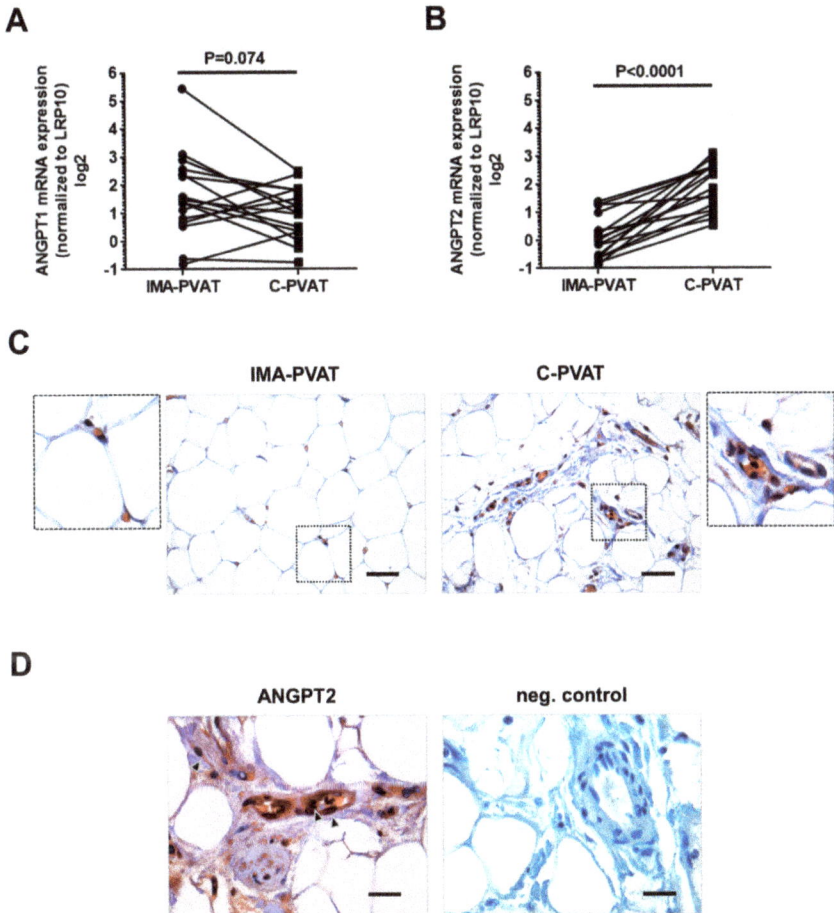

Figure 5. Expression of angiopoietin-1 and -2 in PVAT. (**A**) Quantification of mRNA expression of angiopoietin-1 (ANGPT1) (**A**) and angiopoietin-2, ANGPT2 (**B**) in IMA-PVAT and C-PVAT of $n = 16$ patients with CAD. Paired IMA-PVAT (●) and C-PVAT (■) values of individual patient are connected with a line. (**C**) Representative image after immunohistochemical detection of ANGPT2 in IMA-PVAT and C-PVAT. Size bars represent 50 µm. (**D**) Higher magnification showing ANGPT2-positive cells (arrows). Negative control after omitting the primary antibody is also shown. Size bars represent 20 µm. Statistical analysis was performed using Wilcoxon matched-pairs signed rank test.

Among the most abundant factors, ANGPT2 ($p = 0.011$) and ICAM1 ($p = 0.014$) protein levels were found to significantly differ, with higher levels in C-PVAT compared to IMA-PVAT (Figure 4B). ANGPT2 overexpression in C-PVAT could be confirmed on the transcriptional level by qPCR analysis in 16 patients with CAD, showing significantly higher *ANGPT2* mRNA levels in C-PVAT compared to IMA-PVAT (1.31 (0.51–3.01) vs. 0.74 (0.12–3.50), $p < 0.0001$; Figure 5B). On the other hand, *ANGPT1* mRNA levels did not significantly differ between C-PVAT and IMA-PVAT (2.18 (1.28–5.73) vs. 2.70 (1.63–5.73), $p = 0.074$; Figure 5A). Immunohistochemical staining of ANGPT2 identified endothelium, but also infiltrating immune cells and fibroblasts as possible cellular source of ANGPT2 in PVAT specimens (Figure 5D), both of which were more abundant in C-PVAT (Figure 5C). These findings suggested that the increased expression of ANGPT2 in C-PVAT compared to IMA-PVAT represents the composite result of increased vascularization, inflammation, and fibrosis. Protein levels of ICAM1 were significantly elevated in C-PVAT compared to IMA-PVAT (Figure 4B), in line with the presence of inflamed lymphatic endothelium [29]. Moreover, VEGF-D levels were also significantly increased in C-PVAT compared to IMA-PVAT, in accordance with the difference at mRNA level, whereas no statistically significant increase was detected for VEGF-C (Figure S3A). The expression of MMP9 was also found to be increased in C-PVAT compared to IMA-PVAT, the difference approaching but not reaching statistical significance ($p = 0.057$).

3.5. Recombinant ANGPT2 Stimulates Sprouting Angiogenesis of Human Lymphatic Endothelial Cells

To further study the importance of the above observations for perivascular adipose tissue lymphangiogenesis, the effect of recombinant human ANGPT2 was examined employing the three-dimensional spheroid angiogenesis assay in human lymphatic endothelial cells (HDLECs). Of note, total CM from C-PVAT and IMA-PVAT did not differ in its ability to promote HDLECs angiogenesis in the matrigel™ (Figure S4A–C) or the spheroid assay (Figure S4D–F); however, due to the fact that PVAT-derived conditioned medium contains a mixture of numerous factors, the effects of one specific factor on cultivated cells in vitro may have been obscured.

Flow cytometry analysis confirmed that HDLECs express (lymphatic) endothelial cell markers, including VEGFR3, the receptor for VEGF-C, and TIE2 (TEK receptor tyrosine kinase), the receptor for ANGPT2 (Figure S5). Stimulation of HDLEC spheroids with ANGPT2 (100 ng/mL) for 24 h did not alter the number of sprouts (Figure 6A,B) or the cumulative sprout length (Figure 6A,C) compared to control-treated spheroids. Stimulation of HDLECs spheroids with ANGPT2 together with VEGF-C (100 ng/mL each), both overexpressed (ANGPT2 on the mRNA and the protein level, VEGF-C on the mRNA level) in C-PVAT, significantly increased both the number of sprouts ($p = 0.005$ vs. control, $p = 0.021$ vs. VEGF-C; Figure 6B) and the cumulative sprout length ($p = 0.004$ vs. control and ANGPT2, $p = 0.006$ vs. VEGF-C; Figure 6C). These findings are in agreement with the more extended lymphatic network in C-PVAT compared to IMA-PVAT observed in this study and previous findings on the role of ANGPT2 and VEGF-C as important regulators of functional lymphatic vessel formation [30–32].

Previous studies have shown that inflammatory cytokines, in particular TNFα, is capable of inducing ANPGT2, but also ICAM1 expression suggesting a role of ANGPT2 in inflammatory lymphangiogenesis [33]. Because TNFα levels did not differ in CM from either of the PVAT depots (Figure S3C), we examined the possible role of perivascular hypoxia in the observed overexpression of ANGPT2 and ICAM1. Chemical hypoxia was induced on cultured HDLECs by stimulation with 1 mM cobalt chloride ($CoCl_2$) for 4 h (eight independent experiments). The mRNA expression of ICAM1 was found to be significantly increased in $CoCl_2$-treated compared to control-treated HDLECs (5.4 fold increase vs. control; $p < 0.0001$; Figure 6D). VEGF-D mRNA levels were also significantly increased (8.7 fold increase vs. control; $p = 0.001$; Figure 6E), whereas no significant differences were found in the mRNA expression of ANGPT2, VEGF-C, TIE2 and VEGFR3.

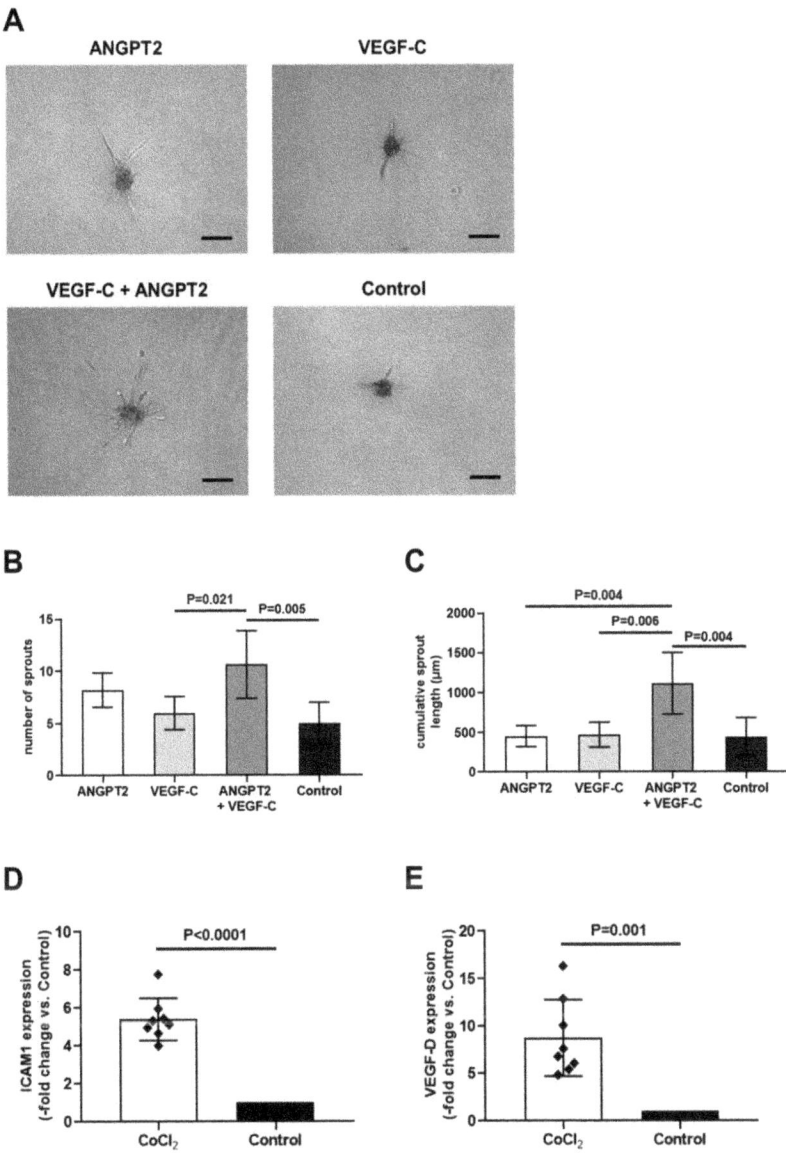

Figure 6. Effects of ANGPT2 and VEGF-C on human sprouting lymphangiogenesis. Representative images of human dermal lymphatic endothelial cell (HDLEC) spheroids (**A**) as well as the results after quantitative analysis of the number of sprouts (per spheroid) (**B**) and the cumulative sprout length (μm) in $n = 5$ spheroids (**C**) after stimulation with recombinant human ANGPT2; (100 ng/mL) and/or VEGF-C (100 ng/mL) or control (CTL). Size bars represent 200 μm. (**D**–**E**) Quantification of mRNA expression of ICAM1 (**D**) and VEGF-D (**E**) in HDLECs, after induction of chemical hypoxia using 1 mM of $CoCl_2$ for 4 h in $n = 8$ independent experiments. Bars represent fold change of mean mRNA expression compared to Control. Error bars represent standard deviation. Statistical analysis was performed using one-way ANOVA with Turkey's multiple comparisons test (**B**,**C**) and Student's paired *t*-test (**D**,**E**).

4. Discussion

The main findings of our study are that (1) PVAT surrounding the aortic root and the coronary arteries of patients with CAD exhibits a denser lymphatic vessel network compared to PVAT surrounding the IMA, an 'atherosclerosis-resistant' artery; (2) The expression of lymphangiogenic growth factors (VEGF-C and VEGF-D) and their primary receptor (VEGFR3) is significantly increased in C-PVAT compared to IMA-PVAT, both at the mRNA (VEGF-C and VEGF-D) and the protein level (VEGF-D); (3) Increased lymphangiogenesis was accompanied with increased expression of ICAM1, infiltration with macrophages and more extensive fibrosis; and (4) Elevated levels of ANGPT2 in C-PVAT could be identified as one potential factor contributing to the observed increase in perivascular lymphangiogenesis. To the best of our knowledge, the present study is the first to compare lymphangiogenesis and its regulators in the perivascular fat surrounding an atherosclerotic and a non-diseased vessel in patients with coronary artery disease. Regarding the use of the IMA as 'control' artery it should be noted that, although the reason for the observed resistance of this artery to atherosclerosis is unclear [34], PVAT surrounding the IMA has been reported to exert vasodilatatory effects on the underlying vessel [35], which supports the hypothesis that IMA-PVAT may in part be responsible for the protection of this artery against atherosclerosis. Previous findings of marked gene expression heterogeneity between PVAT surrounding the coronary artery and the IMA in patients with CAD also support the contribution of differences in perivascular fat composition to the susceptibility to atherosclerosis [36,37]. On the other hand, C-PVAT from healthy individuals cannot be surgically obtained and is therefore not available as 'control' PVAT depot in patients with CAD undergoing bypass surgery.

The possible role of the adventitia and perivascular adipose tissue in the pathophysiology of atherosclerosis has only recently received attention. Several studies, including from our own group, identified factors expressed and released in the perivascular fat as important local mediators of vascular repair processes and atherosclerotic lesion formation (reviewed in [28]). Some of the factors overexpressed in PVAT possess angiogenic activities, such as leptin [38] or CCL2 [39], and adventitial neoangiogenesis may contribute to atherosclerotic plaque progression and instability [1–6]. In contrast to perivascular networks created by blood endothelial cells, studies on the possible role of adventitial lymphangiogenesis in atherosclerosis are limited. For example, dissection of the plaque draining lymph node in apolipoprotein E-knockout mice aggravated atherosclerotic burden [11], whereas restoration of lymphatic drainage in hypercholesterolemic mice improved reverse cholesterol transport. On the other hand, and to the best of our knowledge, animal studies have so far not addressed the importance of coronary perivascular lymphangiogenesis during atherosclerosis. On the other hand, post-mortem analyses in humans and a clinical study found a more extended lymphatic vasculature in the adventitia of atherosclerotic vessels [11,16–19]. Although contradictory at first, both observations may reflect different stages of a chronic disease process in which perivascular lymph vessels reactively develop to accelerate the removal of lipids and the exit of inflammatory cells, but become exhausted and dysfunctional at later stages due to chronic overactivation [8,15]. Although our study cannot provide a definite answer to the important question of whether the observed increased lymphangiogenesis in C-PVAT is the consequence of the existing atherosclerosis in human coronary arteries or one of its causes, the increased expression of ICAM1, infiltration with macrophages, and fibrosis observed in C-PVAT appear to be in accordance with the concept of reactive, i.e. inflammation- or fibrosis-induced, adventitial lymphangiogenesis.

Overall, the findings of this and previous studies emphasize that the connections among (peri)vascular inflammation, fibrosis and (lymph)angiogenesis are rather complex and that the pathophysiological pathways underlying our observations are probably not unidirectional. Available data rather propose a circular mechanism with multiple shortcuts among various biological processes (schematically depicted in Figure 7), in which advanced atherosclerosis with arterial wall inflammation and fibrosis promote perivascular angiogenesis and lymphangiogenesis.

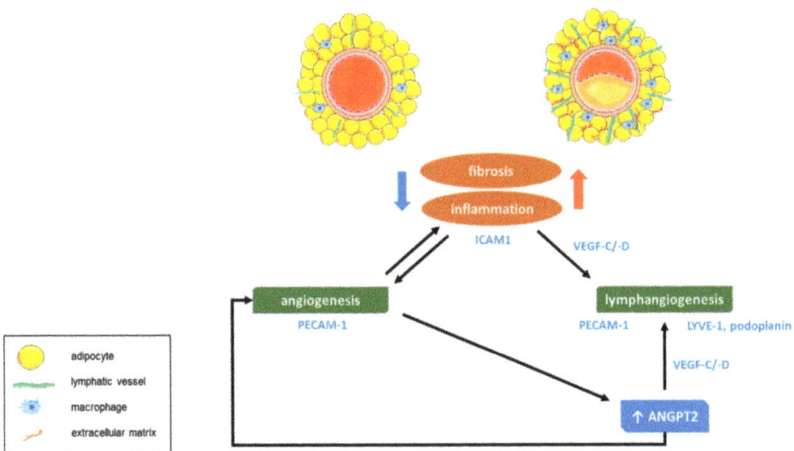

Figure 7. Schematic drawing depicting the main findings of this study.

Regarding the signals mediating perivascular lymphangiogenesis, the increase in lymphatic vessels in C-PVAT compared to IMA-PVAT was accompanied with elevated mRNA levels of two major regulators of lymphangiogenesis, namely VEGF-C and VEGF-D, as well as their receptor VEGFR3. Increased numbers of intimal cells expressing VEGF-C were also reported in patients with atherosclerosis of the iliac arteries and found to correlate with atherosclerotic lesion severity and the number of LYVE1-positive lymphatic vessels, whereas similar associations were not observed for VEGF-D [18]. Macrophages are an important source of VEGF-C and VEGF-D, as shown in tumors [26,27,40], and both growth factors may also act as chemoattractant by upregulating the expression of VEGFR3 on M1 polarized macrophages, as shown in visceral adipose tissue of mice [41]. TGFβ [42,43] and proinflammatory cytokines, such as interleukin (IL) 1β and TNFα [44], have been shown to further enhance the expression of VEGF-C and to promote lymphangiogenesis, although we did not detect differences in their expression levels between both adipose tissue depots.

The importance of VEGF-C–VEGFR3 in the regulation of lymphangiogenesis is well established [31,45,46]. However, under some circumstances VEGF-C may also bind to VEGFR2, expressed on lymphatic and blood endothelial cells [47,48]. VEGF-C was shown to promote angiogenesis in the developing embryo [49] or following ischemia [50]. Others found that VEGF-C overexpression selectively induced lymphangiogenesis without altering accompanying angiogenesis [45,51]. The net result of VEGF-C signaling in terms of (lymph)angiogenesis may depend on the local abundance of VEGFR2 and VEGFR3 receptors, as findings in mice expressing a VEGFR3-specific mutant of VEGF-C exhibited growth of lymphatic, but not of blood vessels [52]. VEGF-D also binds both VEGFR2 and VEGFR3 with high affinity [53] and has angiogenic as well as lymphangiogenic activities [54,55]. On the other hand, the expression of VEGF-A, an essential hemangiogenic factor, did not significantly differ between C-PVAT and IMA-PVAT, whereas VEGF-B, a specific ligand for VEGFR1 with limited angiogenic potential, was markedly reduced in our study. Although VEGF-B is dispensable for blood vessel growth, it was found to have pro-survival effects on endothelial cells, vascular smooth muscle cells and pericytes [56]. Interestingly, VEGF-B is highly expressed in brown adipose tissue [57] and was shown to control endothelial fatty acid uptake [58]. The significantly reduced expression observed in C-PVAT may reflect the loss of protective (brown) adipose tissue properties compared to IMA-PVAT, as suggested by findings in rodents [59].

ANGPT2 holds a significant role in postnatal angiogenic remodeling, but also the proper development of lymphatic vessels [30,60]. Here, we show that the expression of ANGPT2 is increased in C-PVAT compared to IMA-PVAT in patients with CAD, and findings could be confirmed at the protein level in the secretome of C-PVAT and IMA-PVAT. Others have shown that ANGPT2 overexpression leads to lymphatic hyperplasia [30], suggesting that increased ANGPT2 levels may have contributed to the enhanced lymphangiogenic vessel density observed in this PVAT depot. In agreement with the described synergistic effect of VEGF and ANGPT2 in promoting lymphangiogenesis [60,61], we could show that stimulation of HDLEC spheroids using a combination of ANGPT2 and VEGF-C results in lymphangiogenic sprouting, whereas stimulation with ANPGT2 or VEGF-C alone had weak or no effects at all. Although ANGPT2 is mainly expressed in endothelial cells [62], immunohistochemical analysis revealed ANGPT2 protein expression also in infiltrating immune cells and myofibroblasts, in line with their role as important source of lymphangiogenic growth factors. Binding of ANGPT2 to TIE2 receptors may activate NFκB (nuclear factor 'kappa-light-chain-enhancer' of activated B-cells) signaling and the expression of adhesion receptors on endothelial cells, including ICAM1 [63]. NFkB may also upregulate the expression of VEGFR3 on lymphatic endothelial cells and increase their sensitivity to VEGF-C and -D [64], and analyses in mice or human endothelial cells lacking ANGPT2 showed that it may increase the responsiveness of vascular endothelial cells to inflammatory stimuli [65].

In addition to inflammatory signals, hypoxia may be a relevant factor underlying the observed elevated lymphangiogenic growth factor levels in C-PVAT. Hypoxic cells, such as those present in tumors or atherosclerotic plaques, may release angiogenic growth factors, and we have previously shown that hypoxia levels are higher in C-PVAT compared to IMA-PVAT and that this difference may underlie the increased expression of leptin, an adipokine with proangiogenic properties, in the C-PVAT of CAD patients [20]. Hypoxia is also a major stimulus inducing the expression of VEGF. In the present study, inhibition of hypoxia-inducible factor 1-alpha (HIF1α) degradation by $CoCl_2$ did not alter the expression of ANGPT2 and VEGF-C or their receptors, but significantly increased the expression of VEGF-D and ICAM-1. A previous study showed that the VEGF-C promotor does not contain hypoxia-responsive elements, and that hypoxia may induces VEGF-C via HIF1α-independent mechanisms [66]. Interestingly, lymphatic vessels respond to the same angiogenic cues as endothelial cells lining blood vessels, although they exhibit unidirectional flow and do not transport erythrocytes and thus will not improve oxygen supply to hypoxic tissues. The parallel increase of blood and lymph vessel formation could represent a mechanism to remove excess interstitial fluid and cells extravasated from immature and leaky angiogenic blood vessels during hypoxia.

Our study has some limitations. Due to the small amount of tissue available from each patient, the total study collective had to be split into groups for different types of assays, which may have influenced our observations. It should also be noted that 'only' PVAT but not specimens from the underlying vascular wall were available for analysis, and that we could not directly associate our findings in PVAT with the severity of the atherosclerotic lesion in the underlying artery. Also, perioperative C-PVAT sampling was performed in a standardized manner (near the aortic root), regardless of the localization of atherosclerotic lesions within the coronary tree. All individuals included in the present study were diagnosed with advanced coronary atherosclerosis with indication for a bypass graft surgery, and our study could therefore not examine earlier stages of this chronic vascular wall disease evolving over many years. Also, C-PVAT from healthy individuals is not available for analysis and thus the distribution of lymphatic vessels in C-PVAT under 'normal' conditions is unknown. On the other hand, using the IMA as an internal 'healthy' control artery may have helped to provide additional insights into the pathophysiological role of local processes, in particular perivascular lymphangiogenesis during atherosclerosis, whereas the possible impact of systemic effects on the composition and expression patterns should have been minimized by the direct comparison of these two PVAT depots from the same patient. However, it cannot be excluded that differences in the local microenvironment between the two PVAT depots may have contributed to the observed differences.

In conclusion, our findings show an increased lymphangiogenic activity in PVAT surrounding atherosclerotic coronary arteries compared to PVAT surrounding the IMA, an artery free of atherosclerosis, in patients with CAD. Increased ANGPT2 expression and activated VEGF-C/VEGF-D-mediated VEGFR3 signaling, in combination with a local proinflammatory and hypoxic environment, may pathophysiologically underlie these observations.

Supplementary Materials: The following are available online at http://www.mdpi.com/2077-0383/8/7/1000/s1; Figure S1: Immunohistochemical analysis of PVAT: negative controls; Figure S2: Cytokine antibody array map; Figure S3: Quantitative analysis of protein expression in PVAT using cytokine antibody arrays; Figure S4: Analysis of paracrine effects of PVAT-derived conditioned medium on human dermal lymphatic endothelial cells; Figure S5: Flow cytometry analysis of (lymphatic) endothelial cell markers in HDLECs; Table S1: Primer sequences used for gene expression analysis of human PVAT.

Author Contributions: Conceptualization of the study, I.D., S.K., and K.S.; validation, I.D., M.P., and K.S.; formal analysis, I.D., G.C., and K.S.; investigation, I.D., M.P., M.O.C., A.K., R.G., M.L.B., G.C., and C.T.; resources, K.B., F.K., C.F.V., D.M., D.T., and T.M.; data curation, I.D., M.P., M.O.C., and A.K.; writing—original draft preparation, I.D. and K.S.; writing—review and editing, I.D., M.P., K.B., S.K., and K.S.; visualization, I.D.; supervision, S.K. and K.S.; project administration, K.S.; funding acquisition, I.D., S.K., and K.S.

Funding: This work was supported by grants from the German Research Foundation (Deutsche Forschungsgemeinschaft; Scha 808/7-1) to K.S., by the National and European Union funds from the 'Operational Programme Education and Lifelong Learning (NSRF 2007-2013) MIS 379527' to S.K. and K.S., and by a fellowship from the Margarethe Waitz Foundation to I.D. Data shown are part of the medical thesis of M.O.C.

Acknowledgments: The authors acknowledge the expert technical assistance of Marina Janocha, Anna Kern, and Michaela Moisch.

Conflicts of Interest: The authors declare no conflict of interest.

References

1. Moulton, K.S.; Vakili, K.; Zurakowski, D.; Soliman, M.; Butterfield, C.; Sylvin, E.; Lo, K.M.; Gillies, S.; Javaherian, K.; Folkman, J. Inhibition of plaque neovascularization reduces macrophage accumulation and progression of advanced atherosclerosis. *Proc. Natl. Acad. Sci. USA* **2003**, *100*, 4736–4741. [CrossRef] [PubMed]
2. Tanaka, K.; Nagata, D.; Hirata, Y.; Tabata, Y.; Nagai, R.; Sata, M. Augmented angiogenesis in adventitia promotes growth of atherosclerotic plaque in apolipoprotein E-deficient mice. *Atherosclerosis* **2011**, *215*, 366–373. [CrossRef] [PubMed]
3. Xu, X.; Mao, W.; Chai, Y.; Dai, J.; Chen, Q.; Wang, L.; Zhuang, Q.; Pan, Y.; Chen, M.; Ni, G.; et al. Angiogenesis Inhibitor, Endostar, Prevents Vasa Vasorum Neovascularization in a Swine Atherosclerosis Model. *J. Atheroscler. Thromb.* **2015**, *22*, 1100–1112. [CrossRef] [PubMed]
4. Dunmore, B.J.; McCarthy, M.J.; Naylor, A.R.; Brindle, N.P. Carotid plaque instability and ischemic symptoms are linked to immaturity of microvessels within plaques. *J. Vasc. Surg.* **2007**, *45*, 155–159. [CrossRef] [PubMed]
5. Sluimer, J.C.; Kolodgie, F.D.; Bijnens, A.P.; Maxfield, K.; Pacheco, E.; Kutys, B.; Duimel, H.; Frederik, P.M.; van Hinsbergh, V.W.; Virmani, R.; et al. Thin-walled microvessels in human coronary atherosclerotic plaques show incomplete endothelial junctions relevance of compromised structural integrity for intraplaque microvascular leakage. *J. Am. Coll. Cardiol.* **2009**, *53*, 1517–1527. [CrossRef] [PubMed]
6. Michel, J.B.; Virmani, R.; Arbustini, E.; Pasterkamp, G. Intraplaque haemorrhages as the trigger of plaque vulnerability. *Eur. Heart J.* **2011**, *32*, 1977–1985. [CrossRef]
7. Hoggan, G.; Hoggan, F.E. The Lymphatics of the Walls of the Larger Blood-Vessels and Lymphatics. *J. Anat. Physiol.* **1882**, *17*, 1–23. [PubMed]
8. Lim, H.Y.; Thiam, C.H.; Yeo, K.P.; Bisoendial, R.; Hii, C.S.; McGrath, K.C.; Tan, K.W.; Heather, A.; Alexander, J.S.; Angeli, V. Lymphatic vessels are essential for the removal of cholesterol from peripheral tissues by SR-BI-mediated transport of HDL. *Cell Metab.* **2013**, *17*, 671–684. [CrossRef]
9. Coso, S.; Bovay, E.; Petrova, T.V. Pressing the right buttons: Signaling in lymphangiogenesis. *Blood* **2014**, *123*, 2614–2624. [CrossRef]
10. Martel, C.; Li, W.; Fulp, B.; Platt, A.M.; Gautier, E.L.; Westerterp, M.; Bittman, R.; Tall, A.R.; Chen, S.H.; Thomas, M.J.; et al. Lymphatic vasculature mediates macrophage reverse cholesterol transport in mice. *J. Clin. Invest.* **2013**, *123*, 1571–1579. [CrossRef]
11. Rademakers, T.; van der Vorst, E.P.; Daissormont, I.T.; Otten, J.J.; Theodorou, K.; Theelen, T.L.; Gijbels, M.; Anisimov, A.; Nurmi, H.; Lindeman, J.H.; et al. Adventitial lymphatic capillary expansion impacts on plaque T cell accumulation in atherosclerosis. *Sci. Rep.* **2017**, *7*. [CrossRef] [PubMed]

12. Santulli, G. The lymphatic border patrol outwits inflammatory cells in myocardial infarction. *Sci. Transl. Med.* **2018**, *10*. [CrossRef] [PubMed]
13. Vieira, J.M.; Norman, S.; Villa Del Campo, C.; Cahill, T.J.; Barnette, D.N.; Gunadasa-Rohling, M.; Johnson, L.A.; Greaves, D.R.; Carr, C.A.; Jackson, D.G.; et al. The cardiac lymphatic system stimulates resolution of inflammation following myocardial infarction. *J. Clin. Invest.* **2018**, *128*, 3402–3412. [CrossRef] [PubMed]
14. Lim, H.Y.; Rutkowski, J.M.; Helft, J.; Reddy, S.T.; Swartz, M.A.; Randolph, G.J.; Angeli, V. Hypercholesterolemic mice exhibit lymphatic vessel dysfunction and degeneration. *Am. J. Pathol.* **2009**, *175*, 1328–1337. [CrossRef] [PubMed]
15. Milasan, A.; Dallaire, F.; Mayer, G.; Martel, C. Effects of LDL Receptor Modulation on Lymphatic Function. *Sci. Rep.* **2016**, *6*. [CrossRef] [PubMed]
16. Kholova, I.; Dragneva, G.; Cermakova, P.; Laidinen, S.; Kaskenpaa, N.; Hazes, T.; Cermakova, E.; Steiner, I.; Yla-Herttuala, S. Lymphatic vasculature is increased in heart valves, ischaemic and inflamed hearts and in cholesterol-rich and calcified atherosclerotic lesions. *Eur. J. Clin. Invest.* **2011**, *41*, 487–497. [CrossRef] [PubMed]
17. Drozdz, K.; Janczak, D.; Dziegiel, P.; Podhorska, M.; Piotrowska, A.; Patrzalek, D.; Andrzejak, R.; Szuba, A. Adventitial lymphatics and atherosclerosis. *Lymphology* **2012**, *45*, 26–33.
18. Grzegorek, I.; Drozdz, K.; Chmielewska, M.; Gomulkiewicz, A.; Jablonska, K.; Piotrowska, A.; Karczewski, M.; Janczak, D.; Podhorska-Okolow, M.; Dziegiel, P.; et al. Arterial wall lymphangiogenesis is increased in the human iliac atherosclerotic arteries: Involvement of CCR7 receptor. *Lymphat. Res. Biol.* **2014**, *12*, 222–231. [CrossRef]
19. Drozdz, K.; Janczak, D.; Dziegiel, P.; Podhorska, M.; Patrzalek, D.; Ziolkowski, P.; Andrzejak, R.; Szuba, A. Adventitial lymphatics of internal carotid artery in healthy and atherosclerotic vessels. *Folia. Histochem. Cytobiol.* **2008**, *46*, 433–436. [CrossRef]
20. Drosos, I.; Chalikias, G.; Pavlaki, M.; Kareli, D.; Epitropou, G.; Bougioukas, G.; Mikroulis, D.; Konstantinou, F.; Giatromanolaki, A.; Ritis, K.; et al. Differences between perivascular adipose tissue surrounding the heart and the internal mammary artery: Possible role for the leptin-inflammation-fibrosis-hypoxia axis. *Clin. Res. Cardiol.* **2016**, *105*, 887–900. [CrossRef]
21. Tanaka, K.; Sata, M. Roles of Perivascular Adipose Tissue in the Pathogenesis of Atherosclerosis. *Front. Physiol.* **2018**, *9*. [CrossRef] [PubMed]
22. Sims, F.H. A comparison of coronary and internal mammary arteries and implications of the results in the etiology of arteriosclerosis. *Am. Heart J.* **1983**, *105*, 560–566. [CrossRef]
23. Kilarski, W.W. Physiological Perspective on Therapies of Lymphatic Vessels. *Adv. Wound Care* **2018**, *7*, 189–208. [CrossRef] [PubMed]
24. Hong, Y.K.; Harvey, N.; Noh, Y.H.; Schacht, V.; Hirakawa, S.; Detmar, M.; Oliver, G. Prox1 is a master control gene in the program specifying lymphatic endothelial cell fate. *Dev. Dyn.* **2002**, *225*, 351–357. [CrossRef] [PubMed]
25. Wigle, J.T.; Harvey, N.; Detmar, M.; Lagutina, I.; Grosveld, G.; Gunn, M.D.; Jackson, D.G.; Oliver, G. An essential role for Prox1 in the induction of the lymphatic endothelial cell phenotype. *EMBO J.* **2002**, *21*, 1505–1513. [CrossRef] [PubMed]
26. Schoppmann, S.F.; Birner, P.; Stockl, J.; Kalt, R.; Ullrich, R.; Caucig, C.; Kriehuber, E.; Nagy, K.; Alitalo, K.; Kerjaschki, D. Tumor-associated macrophages express lymphatic endothelial growth factors and are related to peritumoral lymphangiogenesis. *Am. J. Pathol.* **2002**, *161*, 947–956. [CrossRef]
27. Gousopoulos, E.; Proulx, S.T.; Bachmann, S.B.; Dieterich, L.C.; Scholl, J.; Karaman, S.; Bianchi, R.; Detmar, M. An Important Role of VEGF-C in Promoting Lymphedema Development. *J. Invest. Dermatol.* **2017**, *137*, 1995–2004. [CrossRef]
28. Schäfer, K.; Drosos, I.; Konstantinides, S. Perivascular adipose tissue: Epiphenomenon or local risk factor? *Int. J. Obes. (Lond.)* **2017**, *41*, 1311–1323. [CrossRef]
29. Podgrabinska, S.; Kamalu, O.; Mayer, L.; Shimaoka, M.; Snoeck, H.; Randolph, G.J.; Skobe, M. Inflamed lymphatic endothelium suppresses dendritic cell maturation and function via Mac-1/ICAM-1-dependent mechanism. *J. Immunol.* **2009**, *183*, 1767–1779. [CrossRef]

30. Zheng, W.; Nurmi, H.; Appak, S.; Sabine, A.; Bovay, E.; Korhonen, E.A.; Orsenigo, F.; Lohela, M.; D'Amico, G.; Holopainen, T.; et al. Angiopoietin 2 regulates the transformation and integrity of lymphatic endothelial cell junctions. *Genes Dev.* **2014**, *28*, 1592–1603. [CrossRef]
31. Kuchler, A.M.; Gjini, E.; Peterson-Maduro, J.; Cancilla, B.; Wolburg, H.; Schulte-Merker, S. Development of the zebrafish lymphatic system requires VEGFC signaling. *Curr. Biol.* **2006**, *16*, 1244–1248. [CrossRef] [PubMed]
32. Sweat, R.S.; Sloas, D.C.; Murfee, W.L. VEGF-C induces lymphangiogenesis and angiogenesis in the rat mesentery culture model. *Microcirculation* **2014**, *21*, 532–540. [CrossRef] [PubMed]
33. Yan, Z.X.; Jiang, Z.H.; Liu, N.F. Angiopoietin-2 promotes inflammatory lymphangiogenesis and its effect can be blocked by the specific inhibitor L1-10. *Am. J. Physiol. Heart Circ. Physiol.* **2012**, *302*, H215–H223. [CrossRef] [PubMed]
34. Otsuka, F.; Yahagi, K.; Sakakura, K.; Virmani, R. Why is the mammary artery so special and what protects it from atherosclerosis? *Ann. Cardiothorac. Surg.* **2013**, *2*, 519–526. [CrossRef]
35. Malinowski, M.; Deja, M.A.; Janusiewicz, P.; Golba, K.S.; Roleder, T.; Wos, S. Mechanisms of vasodilatatory effect of perivascular tissue of human internal thoracic artery. *J. Physiol. Pharmacol.* **2013**, *64*, 309–316. [PubMed]
36. Lu, D.; Wang, W.; Xia, L.; Xia, P.; Yan, Y. Gene expression profiling reveals heterogeneity of perivascular adipose tissues surrounding coronary and internal thoracic arteries. *Acta. Biochim. Biophys. Sin. (Shanghai)* **2017**, *49*, 1075–1082. [CrossRef]
37. Numaguchi, R.; Furuhashi, M.; Matsumoto, M.; Sato, H.; Yanase, Y.; Kuroda, Y.; Harada, R.; Ito, T.; Higashiura, Y.; Koyama, M.; et al. Differential Phenotypes in Perivascular Adipose Tissue Surrounding the Internal Thoracic Artery and Diseased Coronary Artery. *J. Am. Heart Assoc.* **2019**, *8*. [CrossRef]
38. Schroeter, M.R.; Stein, S.; Heida, N.M.; Leifheit-Nestler, M.; Cheng, I.F.; Gogiraju, R.; Christiansen, H.; Maier, L.S.; Shah, A.M.; Hasenfuss, G.; et al. Leptin promotes the mobilization of vascular progenitor cells and neovascularization by NOX2-mediated activation of MMP9. *Cardiovasc. Res.* **2012**, *93*, 170–180. [CrossRef]
39. Salcedo, R.; Ponce, M.L.; Young, H.A.; Wasserman, K.; Ward, J.M.; Kleinman, H.K.; Oppenheim, J.J.; Murphy, W.J. Human endothelial cells express CCR2 and respond to MCP-1: Direct role of MCP-1 in angiogenesis and tumor progression. *Blood* **2000**, *96*, 34–40.
40. Nakano, T.; Nakashima, Y.; Yonemitsu, Y.; Sumiyoshi, S.; Chen, Y.X.; Akishima, Y.; Ishii, T.; Iida, M.; Sueishi, K. Angiogenesis and lymphangiogenesis and expression of lymphangiogenic factors in the atherosclerotic intima of human coronary arteries. *Hum. Pathol.* **2005**, *36*, 330–340. [CrossRef]
41. Karaman, S.; Hollmen, M.; Robciuc, M.R.; Alitalo, A.; Nurmi, H.; Morf, B.; Buschle, D.; Alkan, H.F.; Ochsenbein, A.M.; Alitalo, K.; et al. Blockade of VEGF-C and VEGF-D modulates adipose tissue inflammation and improves metabolic parameters under high-fat diet. *Mol. Metab.* **2015**, *4*, 93–105. [CrossRef] [PubMed]
42. Kinashi, H.; Falke, L.L.; Nguyen, T.Q.; Bovenschen, N.; Aten, J.; Leask, A.; Ito, Y.; Goldschmeding, R. Connective tissue growth factor regulates fibrosis-associated renal lymphangiogenesis. *Kidney Int.* **2017**, *92*, 850–863. [CrossRef] [PubMed]
43. Kinashi, H.; Ito, Y.; Sun, T.; Katsuno, T.; Takei, Y. Roles of the TGF-beta(-)VEGF-C Pathway in Fibrosis-Related Lymphangiogenesis. *Int. J. Mol. Sci.* **2018**, *19*, 2487. [CrossRef]
44. Ristimaki, A.; Narko, K.; Enholm, B.; Joukov, V.; Alitalo, K. Proinflammatory cytokines regulate expression of the lymphatic endothelial mitogen vascular endothelial growth factor-C. *J. Biol. Chem.* **1998**, *273*, 8413–8418. [CrossRef] [PubMed]
45. Jeltsch, M.; Kaipainen, A.; Joukov, V.; Meng, X.; Lakso, M.; Rauvala, H.; Swartz, M.; Fukumura, D.; Jain, R.K.; Alitalo, K. Hyperplasia of lymphatic vessels in VEGF-C transgenic mice. *Science* **1997**, *276*, 1423–1425. [CrossRef] [PubMed]
46. Karkkainen, M.J.; Haiko, P.; Sainio, K.; Partanen, J.; Taipale, J.; Petrova, T.V.; Jeltsch, M.; Jackson, D.G.; Talikka, M.; Rauvala, H.; et al. Vascular endothelial growth factor C is required for sprouting of the first lymphatic vessels from embryonic veins. *Nat. Immunol.* **2004**, *5*, 74–80. [CrossRef]
47. Joukov, V.; Pajusola, K.; Kaipainen, A.; Chilov, D.; Lahtinen, I.; Kukk, E.; Saksela, O.; Kalkkinen, N.; Alitalo, K. A novel vascular endothelial growth factor, VEGF-C, is a ligand for the Flt4 (VEGFR-3) and KDR (VEGFR-2) receptor tyrosine kinases. *EMBO J.* **1996**, *15*, 1751. [CrossRef]

48. Kriehuber, E.; Breiteneder-Geleff, S.; Groeger, M.; Soleiman, A.; Schoppmann, S.F.; Stingl, G.; Kerjaschki, D.; Maurer, D. Isolation and characterization of dermal lymphatic and blood endothelial cells reveal stable and functionally specialized cell lineages. *J. Exp. Med.* **2001**, *194*, 797–808. [CrossRef]
49. Cao, Y.; Linden, P.; Farnebo, J.; Cao, R.; Eriksson, A.; Kumar, V.; Qi, J.H.; Claesson-Welsh, L.; Alitalo, K. Vascular endothelial growth factor C induces angiogenesis in vivo. *Proc. Natl. Acad. Sci. USA* **1998**, *95*, 14389–14394. [CrossRef]
50. Witzenbichler, B.; Asahara, T.; Murohara, T.; Silver, M.; Spyridopoulos, I.; Magner, M.; Principe, N.; Kearney, M.; Hu, J.S.; Isner, J.M. Vascular endothelial growth factor-C (VEGF-C/VEGF-2) promotes angiogenesis in the setting of tissue ischemia. *Am. J. Pathol.* **1998**, *153*, 381–394. [CrossRef]
51. Enholm, B.; Karpanen, T.; Jeltsch, M.; Kubo, H.; Stenback, F.; Prevo, R.; Jackson, D.G.; Yla-Herttuala, S.; Alitalo, K. Adenoviral expression of vascular endothelial growth factor-C induces lymphangiogenesis in the skin. *Circ. Res.* **2001**, *88*, 623–629. [CrossRef] [PubMed]
52. Veikkola, T.; Jussila, L.; Makinen, T.; Karpanen, T.; Jeltsch, M.; Petrova, T.V.; Kubo, H.; Thurston, G.; McDonald, D.M.; Achen, M.G.; et al. Signalling via vascular endothelial growth factor receptor-3 is sufficient for lymphangiogenesis in transgenic mice. *EMBO J.* **2001**, *20*, 1223–1231. [CrossRef] [PubMed]
53. Achen, M.G.; Jeltsch, M.; Kukk, E.; Makinen, T.; Vitali, A.; Wilks, A.F.; Alitalo, K.; Stacker, S.A. Vascular endothelial growth factor D (VEGF-D) is a ligand for the tyrosine kinases VEGF receptor 2 (Flk1) and VEGF receptor 3 (Flt4). *Proc. Natl. Acad. Sci. USA* **1998**, *95*, 548–553. [CrossRef] [PubMed]
54. Marconcini, L.; Marchio, S.; Morbidelli, L.; Cartocci, E.; Albini, A.; Ziche, M.; Bussolino, F.; Oliviero, S. c-fos-induced growth factor/vascular endothelial growth factor D induces angiogenesis in vivo and in vitro. *Proc. Natl. Acad. Sci. USA* **1999**, *96*, 9671–9676. [CrossRef] [PubMed]
55. Byzova, T.V.; Goldman, C.K.; Jankau, J.; Chen, J.; Cabrera, G.; Achen, M.G.; Stacker, S.A.; Carnevale, K.A.; Siemionow, M.; Deitcher, S.R.; et al. Adenovirus encoding vascular endothelial growth factor-D induces tissue-specific vascular patterns in vivo. *Blood* **2002**, *99*, 4434–4442. [CrossRef] [PubMed]
56. Zhang, F.; Tang, Z.; Hou, X.; Lennartsson, J.; Li, Y.; Koch, A.W.; Scotney, P.; Lee, C.; Arjunan, P.; Dong, L.; et al. VEGF-B is dispensable for blood vessel growth but critical for their survival, and VEGF-B targeting inhibits pathological angiogenesis. *Proc. Natl. Acad. Sci. USA* **2009**, *106*, 6152–6157. [CrossRef] [PubMed]
57. Asano, A.; Irie, Y.; Saito, M. Isoform-specific regulation of vascular endothelial growth factor (VEGF) family mRNA expression in cultured mouse brown adipocytes. *Mol. Cell Endocrinol.* **2001**, *174*, 71–76. [CrossRef]
58. Hagberg, C.E.; Falkevall, A.; Wang, X.; Larsson, E.; Huusko, J.; Nilsson, I.; van Meeteren, L.A.; Samen, E.; Lu, L.; Vanwildemeersch, M.; et al. Vascular endothelial growth factor B controls endothelial fatty acid uptake. *Nature* **2010**, *464*, 917–921. [CrossRef]
59. Berbee, J.F.; Boon, M.R.; Khedoe, P.P.; Bartelt, A.; Schlein, C.; Worthmann, A.; Kooijman, S.; Hoeke, G.; Mol, I.M.; John, C.; et al. Brown fat activation reduces hypercholesterolaemia and protects from atherosclerosis development. *Nat. Commun.* **2015**, *6*. [CrossRef]
60. Gale, N.W.; Thurston, G.; Hackett, S.F.; Renard, R.; Wang, Q.; McClain, J.; Martin, C.; Witte, C.; Witte, M.H.; Jackson, D.; et al. Angiopoietin-2 is required for postnatal angiogenesis and lymphatic patterning, and only the latter role is rescued by Angiopoietin-1. *Dev. Cell* **2002**, *3*, 411–423. [CrossRef]
61. Holash, J.; Maisonpierre, P.C.; Compton, D.; Boland, P.; Alexander, C.R.; Zagzag, D.; Yancopoulos, G.D.; Wiegand, S.J. Vessel cooption, regression, and growth in tumors mediated by angiopoietins and VEGF. *Science* **1999**, *284*, 1994–1998. [CrossRef] [PubMed]
62. Scholz, A.; Plate, K.H.; Reiss, Y. Angiopoietin-2: A multifaceted cytokine that functions in both angiogenesis and inflammation. *Ann. N. Y. Acad. Sci.* **2015**, *1347*, 45–51. [CrossRef] [PubMed]
63. Rathnakumar, K.; Savant, S.; Giri, H.; Ghosh, A.; Fisslthaler, B.; Fleming, I.; Ram, U.; Bera, A.K.; Augustin, H.G.; Dixit, M. Angiopoietin-2 mediates thrombin-induced monocyte adhesion and endothelial permeability. *J. Thromb. Haemost.* **2016**, *14*, 1655–1667. [CrossRef] [PubMed]
64. Flister, M.J.; Wilber, A.; Hall, K.L.; Iwata, C.; Miyazono, K.; Nisato, R.E.; Pepper, M.S.; Zawieja, D.C.; Ran, S. Inflammation induces lymphangiogenesis through up-regulation of VEGFR-3 mediated by NF-kappaB and Prox1. *Blood* **2010**, *115*, 418–429. [CrossRef] [PubMed]

65. Fiedler, U.; Reiss, Y.; Scharpfenecker, M.; Grunow, V.; Koidl, S.; Thurston, G.; Gale, N.W.; Witzenrath, M.; Rosseau, S.; Suttorp, N.; et al. Angiopoietin-2 sensitizes endothelial cells to TNF-alpha and has a crucial role in the induction of inflammation. *Nat. Med.* **2006**, *12*, 235–239. [CrossRef] [PubMed]
66. Morfoisse, F.; Kuchnio, A.; Frainay, C.; Gomez-Brouchet, A.; Delisle, M.B.; Marzi, S.; Helfer, A.C.; Hantelys, F.; Pujol, F.; Guillermet-Guibert, J.; et al. Hypoxia induces VEGF-C expression in metastatic tumor cells via a HIF-1alpha-independent translation-mediated mechanism. *Cell Rep.* **2014**, *6*, 155–167. [CrossRef] [PubMed]

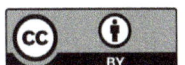 © 2019 by the authors. Licensee MDPI, Basel, Switzerland. This article is an open access article distributed under the terms and conditions of the Creative Commons Attribution (CC BY) license (http://creativecommons.org/licenses/by/4.0/).

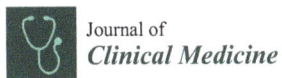

Article

The Impact of the Circadian Genes *CLOCK* and *ARNTL* on Myocardial Infarction

Ivana Škrlec [1,*], Jakov Milić [2] and Robert Steiner [2,3]

1. Histology, Genetics, Cellular, and Molecular Biology Laboratory, Department of Biology and Chemistry, Faculty of Dental Medicine and Health, Josip Juraj Strossmayer University of Osijek, Crkvena 21, HR-31000 Osijek, Croatia
2. Faculty of Medicine, Josip Juraj Strossmayer University of Osijek, Josipa Huttlera 4, HR-31000 Osijek, Croatia; milic.jakov@gmail.com (J.M.); steiner_robert5@hotmail.com (R.S.)
3. Clinical Department of Cardiovascular Diseases and Intensive Care, Clinic for Internal Medicine, University Hospital Osijek, Josipa Huttlera 4, HR-31000 Osijek, Croatia
* Correspondence: iskrlec@fdmz.hr

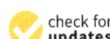

Received: 6 January 2020; Accepted: 5 February 2020; Published: 10 February 2020

Abstract: The circadian rhythm regulates various physiological mechanisms, and its disruption can promote many disorders. Disturbance of endogenous circadian rhythms enhances the chance of myocardial infarction (MI), showing that circadian clock genes could have a crucial function in the onset of the disease. This case-control study was performed on 1057 participants. It was hypothesized that the polymorphisms of one nucleotide (SNP) in three circadian clock genes (*CLOCK*, *ARNTL*, and *PER2*) could be associated with MI. Statistically significant differences, estimated by the Chi-square test, were found in the distribution of alleles and genotypes between MI and no-MI groups of the *CLOCK* (rs6811520 and rs13124436) and *ARNTL* (rs3789327 and rs12363415) genes. According to the results of the present study, the polymorphisms in the *CLOCK* and *ARNTL* genes could be related to MI.

Keywords: cardiovascular diseases; circadian rhythm; clock genes; myocardial infarction; polymorphisms

---

1. Introduction

Today, there is a global epidemic of cardiovascular diseases (CVDs). The World Health Organization (WHO) data for 2017 shows that CVDs caused 19.9 million deaths globally, and around 80% of CVDs deaths were because of stroke and myocardial infarction (MI) [1]. In recent decades, mortality from CVDs has decreased in developed countries, but CVDs remains one of the principal causes of death worldwide [2]. However, CVDs continue to be the third major cause of death in Croatia, with 45% of total mortality in 2016 [3,4]. Various pathophysiological processes stimulate and lead to the onset of MI. MI is an inflammatory disease. Thrombotic obstruction of the coronary arteries occurs at the position of initiated atherosclerotic plaque. It promotes total coronary circulation arrest, which leads to the death of cardiomyocytes and MI [5]. The etiology of MI is mainly unknown, in spite of the many studies conducted.

The circadian rhythm regulates many physiological mechanisms, and its disruption can result in many physiopathological disorders [6]. The circadian clock is integrated within approximately 24 h [7]. It regulates physiological processes at several levels, from gene transcription to sophisticated performance [8]. Cardiovascular incidents happen in a circadian fashion, with a significant incidence in the morning after rising [9]. Many cardiovascular events show morning circadian preferences, such as myocardial infarction [10], dissection of aortic aneurysms [11], and stroke [12]. Additionally, the incidence of MI is higher during the winter months, especially in the elderly [13]. The circadian rhythm adjusts the feedback of endothelial cells to damage the circulatory system [14]. Some physiological factors that oscillate with the circadian rhythms might trigger the onset of MI [15]. Those physiological factors are glucose homeostasis, blood pressure [16], myocardial contractions, vascular endothelial function, fibrinolytic activity, and metabolism [17,18].

In the peripheral clocks of cardiovascular cells or tissue, the central clock synchronizes and controls the everyday transcription of clock-controlled genes (CCGs) [19]. The primary circadian clock is placed in the SCN (suprachiasmatic nucleus) in the hypothalamus and is controlled by many circadian rhythm genes. Light drives the central clock. Decreased daylight exposure and overexposure to light at night impairs the circadian organization of sleep. Sleep disorders can lead to increased energy input, decreased energy expenditure, and insulin resistance [20]. Short sleep is associated with hypertension, diabetes mellitus, obesity, and mortality. Daylight saving time also causes a modest increase in MI occurrence [21]. Peripheral clocks are found in the cardiomyocyte, blood vessels, and vascular endothelial cells [22]. The circadian clock within cardiomyocytes regulates cardiac metabolic gene expression. It has the function of synchronizing cardiomyocyte metabolic activity with the availability of nutrients [22,23]. Polymorphisms in clock genes are associated with obesity, sleep disturbances, psychological and metabolic complications, plus cardiovascular disorders, such as stroke, vascular death, and myocardial infarction [6]. Desynchronization of the circadian rhythm can cause metabolic disorders and various other issues. Some of those are dyslipidemia, glucose intolerance, hypertension, type 2 diabetes mellitus (T2DM), and CVDs [24,25]. Whole-genome studies have detected numerous genes variants related to the elevated risk of myocardial infarction [26]. Genes included in the metabolic processes of lipid metabolism and the progress of T2DM have been the most investigated genes so far in relation to an enhanced risk of myocardial infarction [7].

Through the transcription and translation feedback loops, circadian rhythm genes control the cyclic transcription of mRNA and protein synthesis. There are some essential proteins in the SCN. The activators are CLOCK (Circadian Locomotor Output Cycles Kaput) and ARNTL (Aryl Hydrocarbon Receptor Nuclear Translocator-Like), while the inhibitors of transcription are PER (Period) and CRY (Cryptochrome) proteins. The day-to-night shift is generated by circadian oscillations that are maintained at the transcriptional and posttranscriptional levels in a single cell by the feedback loop of the circadian clock genes. ARNTL/CLOCK protein heterodimers trigger the expression of PER, CRY, and other clock-controlled genes. CRY/PER protein heterodimers serve as a negative feedback loop and repress the action of ARNTL and CLOCK [8,27]. The entire procedure of activating and suppressing gene transcription in a loop persists for approximately 24 h. Transcription factors stimulate the transcription of clock genes and other clock-controlled genes, initiating numerous physiological processes [7,28].

This research is a continuation of the preliminary study from 2018 [29]. The present study was aimed at searching for a potential correlation between the SNPs of the *CLOCK*, *ARNTL*, and *PER2* genes in patients with myocardial infarction. It was carried out as a case-referent study, comparing participants with myocardial infarction versus the participants without myocardial infarction.

2. Experimental Section

2.1. Participants

The data presented here were collected as part of previously reported studies on circadian rhythm variations in patients with myocardial infarction [25,29,30]. The sample included 431 patients (243 males, 188 females) of Croatian origin with non-fatal acute myocardial infarction at the Clinical Department of Cardiovascular Diseases and Intensive Care at the University Hospital Osijek, from August 2012 to December 2018. Inclusion criteria for type 1 and 2 MI patients, according to Thygesen et al., were elevated cardiac troponin T above the 99th percentile and one of the following factors: symptoms of myocardial ischemia, electrocardiogram (ECG) changes, pathological Q waves, evidence of loss of viable myocardium, and coronary thrombus [31,32]. Patients were eliminated from the analysis if they did not satisfy these requirements. Patients were excluded if they had undergone percutaneous coronary intervention or a coronary artery bypass, because those are not clinical characteristics of acute MI. Patients with type 4 and 5 MI were excluded, and also patients with type 1 and 2 MI who underwent PCI (percutaneous coronary intervention). A total of 125 patients were eliminated from the study: 35 due to percutaneous coronary intervention, 42 due to coronary artery bypass, 37 refused to participate, and 11 withdrew from the study (Figure 1).

Participants (total of 626) whose medical records did not present a history of cardiovascular disease were included in the control no-MI group. Their general physician selected them in the outpatient clinic after a checkup. Patients with cardiovascular disease or MI were eliminated. Due to the complex inheritance of cardiovascular risk factors identified in monozygotic twins, the relatives of the patient were eliminated from the no-MI group [33].

Systematic data on their medical history were obtained from all participants. Data on age, smoking, hypertension, and diabetes mellitus were included in the questionnaire. The patient's medical record confirms all of the above information.

This study was authorized by the Ethics Committees of the University Hospital Osijek (No. 25-1:3160-3/2012) and the Faculty of Medicine Osijek (No. 2158-61-07-12-2). It was performed following the Declaration of Helsinki and its amendments. All participants signed informed consent.

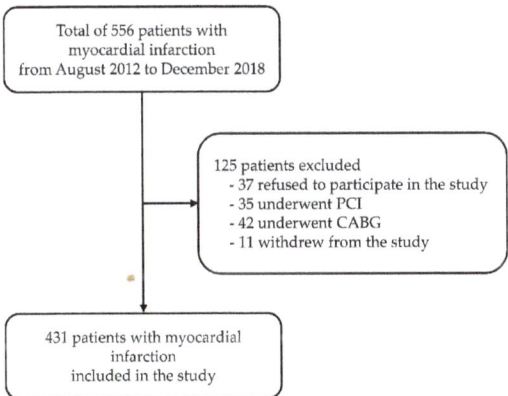

Figure 1. Patient selection flow chart. CABG—coronary artery bypass grafting, PCI—percutaneous coronary intervention.

2.2. SNP Selection and Genotyping

SNPs in three circadian rhythm genes, CLOCK, ARNTL, and PER2, were genotyped in this study. SNPs were selected on the basis of the familiar genetic linkage, consistent with HapMap Phase 3 (http://www.hapmap.org). The collection of the most specific polymorphisms for *CLOCK* (rs11932595, rs6811520, and rs13124436), *ARNTL* (rs3789327, rs4757144, and rs12363415), and *PER2* (rs35333999 and rs934945) genes were acquired using the Tagger algorithm accessible within the Haploview software (Haploview, version 4.2) [34]. Additionally, selected circadian rhythm gene SNPs had been associated with cardiovascular risk factors in previous studies [14,16,18].

The extraction of genomic DNA was made from lymphocytes using conventional methods (QIAamp DNA Blood Mini Kit, Qiagen, Hilden, Germany). Genotyping was performed using TaqMan SNP genotyping assays by the real-time PCR method, performed using a 7500 Real-Time PCR System (Applied Biosystems, Foster City, CA, USA). Details of the selected TaqMan probes are shown in Table 1. Allele discrimination analyses were carried out using SDS 7500 Software Version 2.3 (Applied Biosystems, Foster City, CA, USA).

Table 1. Selected TaqMan probe details.

Gene	SNP	SNP ID	Location	SNP Type
ARNTL	rs3789327	C_2160503_20	Chromosome 11	intronic region
ARNTL	rs4757144	C_1870683_20	Chromosome 11	intronic region
ARNTL	rs12363415	C_31248677_10	Chromosome 11	intronic region
CLOCK	rs11932595	C_296556_10	Chromosome 4	intronic region
CLOCK	rs6811520	C_31137409_30	Chromosome 4	intronic region
CLOCK	rs13124436	C_11821304_10	Chromosome 4	intronic region
PER2	rs35333999	C_25992030_10	Chromosome 2	Coding (Iso/Val)
PER2	rs934945	C_8740718_20	Chromosome 2	Coding (Glu/Gly)

2.3. Statistical Analysis

All analyses were performed using SPSS software (version 22.0, SPSS Inc., Chicago, IL, USA) for Windows). Quantitative demographic and clinical variables are presented as mean and standard deviation, while categorical variables are presented as frequency and percentages. Chi-square tests (χ^2) on contingency tables were applied to analyze allele and genotype frequencies in both groups. By comparing the distribution of genotypes with those expected by the Hardy–Weinberg equilibrium, a further level of quality control of genotyping was accomplished applying the Chi-square goodness-of-fit test. Analyses were performed using SNPStats [35] and the SHEsis web tools [36]. The relationship between genotypes and cardiovascular risk factors were studied applying the Mann–Whitney U test. Logistic regression, for the likelihood of a patient having a manifestation of myocardial infarction, was applied to evaluate the outcome of CLOCK (rs11932595, rs6811520, rs13124436), ARNTL (rs3789327, rs4757144, rs12363415), and PER2 (rs35333999 and rs934945) genotypes. Age, hypertension history, diastolic and systolic blood pressure, and BMI were applied as covariates. The Kruskal–Wallis test was applied to establish the association within genotypes and risk factors. When the p-value was equal to or less than 0.05, the associations were marked significant. Appling the Benjamini–Hochberg (false detection rate—FDR value) correction method, significant value corrections were made due to the many SNPs studied. Q-values less than 0.05 were deemed significant. Pairwise linkage disequilibrium (LD) and haplotypes were calculated applying the SHEsis web tool [37] and Haploview (version 4.2) because the participants in the present study were not related.

3. Results

Table 2 shows the prevalence of cardiovascular risk factors in the 1057 study participants. In the present study, the mean age of all participants was 64 ± 10 years, and 53.4% were males. Table 3 presents allele frequencies, while Table 4 shows the genotype distribution of the CLOCK, ARNTL, and PER2 SNPs. In the patients' group, the ARNTL gene SNPs rs3789327 and rs12363415, and rs6811520 and rs13124436 of the CLOCK gene deviated from the Hardy–Weinberg equilibrium.

Table 2. Prevalence of cardiovascular risk factors of myocardial infarction (MI) and no-MI participants.

	MI	no-MI	p-Value *
Number	431	626	
Male sex (%)	243 (56.4%)	321 (51.3%)	0.102
Age (years)	66 ±11	62 ± 10	<0.001
History of hypertension (%)	351 (73.1%)	408 (65.2%)	0.007
Smokers (%)	119 (27.6%)	193 (30.8%)	<0.001
History of type 2 diabetes mellitus (%)	275 (63.8%)	426 (68.1%)	0.151
Diastolic blood pressure (mm Hg)	79.12 ± 11.39	83.46 ± 11.13	<0.001
Systolic blood pressure (mm Hg)	140.04 ± 22.20	142.3 ± 21.42	0.085
BMI (kg/m^2)	29.78 ± 4.46	29.37 ± 4.59	0.198

BMI, body mass index. *Mann–Whitney U test p-value.

Table 3. Allele frequencies of the ARNTL, CLOCK, and PER2 polymorphisms (N = 1057).

Gene	SNP	Minor Allele	MAF MI	MAF no-MI	p-Value	q-Value
ARNTL	rs3789327 *	G	0.425	0.518	2.27×10^{-5}	6.05×10^{-5}
	rs4757144	G	0.420	0.442	0.324	0.432
	rs12363415 *	A	0.413	0.338	4.37×10^{-4}	8.74×10^{-4}
	rs11932595	G	0.428	0.437	0.685	0.782
CLOCK	rs6811520 *	C	0.444	0.620	7.11×10^{-15}	5.68×10^{-14}
	rs13124436 *	A	0.200	0.301	1.72×10^{-7}	6.88×10^{-7}
PER2	rs35333999	T	0.038	0.055	0.077	0.123
	rs934945	T	0.172	0.174	0.885	0.885

MAF, minor allele frequency; q-value, corrected significant p-value by the Benjamini–Hochberg method. * Deviation from the Hardy–Weinberg equilibrium in the MI group.

Table 4. Genotype distribution and frequencies of the ARNTL, CLOCK, and PER2 polymorphisms.

Gene	SNP	Genotype	Genotype Frequency, N (%)				
			MI	no-MI	p-value	χ^2	q-Value
ARNTL	rs3789327 *	AA	161 (37.4%)	164 (26.3%)	2.7×10^{-4}	16.46	7.2×10^{-4}
		AG	174 (40.4%)	237 (43.8%)			
		GG	96 (22.3%)	187 (30%)			
	rs4757144	AA	153 (35.5%)	199 (31.8%)	0.456	1.57	0.608
		AG	194 (45%)	300 (48%)			
		GG	84 (19.5%)	126 (20.2%)			
	rs12363415 *	AA	142 (32.9%)	151 (24.1%)	0.007	9.95	0.014
		AG	72 (16.7%)	121 (19.3%)			
		GG	217 (50.3%)	354 (56.5%)			
	rs11932595	AA	142 (33%)	191 (30.6%)	0.589	1.06	0.673
		AG	208 (48.4%)	322 (51.5%)			
		GG	80 (18.6%)	112 (17.9%)			
CLOCK	rs6811520 *	CC	123 (28.5%)	255 (40.8%)	3.44×10^{-15}	69.33	2.75×10^{-14}
		CT	137 (31.8%)	265 (42.4%)			
		TT	171 (39.7%)	105 (16.8%)			
	rs13124436 *	AA	39 (9%)	123 (19.6%)	1.26×10^{-5}	22.61	5.04×10^{-5}
		AG	94 (21.8%)	131 (20.9%)			
		GG	298 (69.1%)	372 (59.4%)			
PER2	rs35333999	CC	399 (92.8%)	560 (89.6%)	0.208	3.14	0.333
		CT	29 (6.7%)	61 (9.8%)			
		TT	2 (0.5%)	4 (0.6%)			
	rs934945	CC	296 (68.7%)	427 (68.2%)	0.986	0.03	0.986
		CT	122 (28.3%)	180 (28.8%)			
		TT	13 (3%)	19 (3%)			

χ^2, Chi-square; q-value, corrected significant p value by the Benjamini–Hochberg method. * Deviation from the Hardy–Weinberg equilibrium in the MI group.

Logistic regression was adjusted to evaluate the independent impact of the chosen polymorphism after modification for cardiovascular risk factors. All tested SNPs showed a significant interaction between age, diastolic blood pressure, and the risk of myocardial infarction ($p < 0.001$) (Table 5). Under the dominant genotype model, a considerable difference was for the rs3789327 and rs12363415 SNPs in the ARNTL gene (AA + AG versus GG, $p = 0.003$, OR = 1.52 with 95% CI = 1.12–1.95, and AA + AG versus GG, $p < 0.001$, OR = 3.14 with 95% CI = 2.13–4.62, respectively). Under the recessive genotype model notable difference was for the rs6811520 and rs13124436 SNPs in the CLOCK gene (CC versus CT + TT, $p < 0.001$, OR = 0.35 with 95% CI = 0.26–0.47, and GG versus AG + AA, $p = 0.006$, OR = 1.76 with 95% CI = 1.17–2.65, respectively). The significant difference was detected under the dominant genotype model for the *PER2* gene polymorphism rs35333999 (TT + CT versus CC, $p = 0.005$, OR = 1.93 with 95% CI = 1.19-3.11).

Table 5. Odds ratios for myocardial infarction adjusted for cardiovascular risk factors included in the logistic regression model.

Risk Factor	OR (95% CI)	*p*-Value
Age	0.96 (0.95–0.97)	**<0.001**
History of hypertension	1.23 (0.91–1.68)	0.182
Diastolic blood pressure	1.36 (1.02–1.05)	**<0.001**
Systolic blood pressure	1.01 (0.99–1.01)	0.217
BMI	0.98 (0.95–1.07)	0.114

OR, odds ratio; CI, confidence interval.

The association between circadian rhythm gene polymorphisms and cardiovascular risk factors in patients with MI is shown in Table 6.

Table 6. The association between cardiovascular risk factors and circadian rhythm gene polymorphisms in patients with MI.

Gene	Sex	Age	History of Hypertension	Smoking	History of T2DM	Diastolic Blood Pressure	Systolic Blood Pressure	BMI
ARNTL								
rs3789327	**0.045**	0.953	0.247	0.133	**0.006**	0.309	0.113	0.561
rs4757144	0.844	0.818	0.319	0.273	0.537	0.129	0.121	0.777
rs12363415	0.071	0.872	**<0.001**	0.168	**<0.001**	**0.005**	**<0.001**	**<0.001**
CLOCK								
rs11932595	0.177	0.487	0.263	0.319	0.118	0.266	**0.029**	0.229
rs6811520	**<0.001**	0.641	**<0.001**	0.950	**<0.001**	0.820	**<0.001**	0.200
rs13124436	**0.003**	0.665	**<0.001**	0.309	**<0.001**	0.402	**<0.001**	**0.028**
PER2								
rs35333999	0.956	**0.002**	0.720	0.422	0.102	0.521	0.934	0.772
rs934945	0.156	0.104	0.085	**0.048**	0.518	0.734	0.589	0.302

Kruskal–Wallis test *p*-values. T2DM, type 2 diabetes mellitus; BMI, body mass index.

The completed haplotypes were analyzed in the three circadian rhythm genes. The frequencies of the predicted haplotypes of the tested circadian rhythm gene genetic variants in MI and no-MI participants are presented in Table S1.

There was no linkage disequilibrium (LD) between SNPs in the *ARNTL* gene. The LD between rs3789327 and rs4757144 was D′ = 0.039, R^2 = 0.001, between rs3789327 and rs12363415 D′ = 0.216, R^2 = 0.025, and between rs4757144 and rs12363415 D′ = 0.109, R^2 = 0.005. The LD for the *CLOCK* gene polymorphisms was as follows: the LD between rs1192595 and rs6811520 was D′ = 0.414, R^2 = 0.108, between rs1192595 and rs13124436 D′ = 0.062, R^2 = 0.001, and between rs6811520 and rs13124436 D′ = 0.596, R^2 = 0.103. The LD calculated for polymorphisms in the *PER2* gene (rs35333999 and rs934945) was D′ = 0.986, R^2 = 0.010 (Figure S1).

4. Discussion

In the present study, given the findings of the investigated SNPs of the *CLOCK*, *ARNTL*, and *PER2* genes, it was noted that polymorphisms in those clock genes might be an extra risk factor for myocardial infarction. An association between MI and polymorphisms of the *CLOCK* (rs6811520 and rs13124436) and *ARNTL* (rs37389327 and rs12363415) genes were found in a sample of 1057 participants in this case-referent study. *ARNTL*, rs3789327, was connected with T2DM in MI patients, while rs13124436 and rs6811520 of the *CLOCK* gene were connected with hypertension, T2DM, and systolic blood pressure in MI patients. In the present study, patients with MI had substantially reduced diastolic blood pressure as opposed to the no-MI group.

The circadian rhythm is a network that enables a person to manage environmental variations and adjust to them. Accordingly, the circadian rhythm controls a range of physiological and metabolic activities, and any obstruction of that rhythm may impact a person's health. The role of circadian rhythm in MI has been investigated in several studies. Cardiomyocyte circadian gene expression regulates the myocardial contractile purpose, metabolism, and gene expression [38]. The fundamental idea is that acute cardiovascular events do not happen randomly throughout the day but are accelerated partially by circadian controlled factors [39]. An increasing amount of experimental and clinical evidence shows an essential connection between cardiac dysfunction and intrinsic circadian biology. Virtually all tissues of the body have a circadian clock that regulates the timing of many critical biological reactions in response to a diversity of environmental signals. The molecular machinery for the regulation of circadian rhythms is very conserved and found in virtually every cell type [40].

Human research has recognized polymorphisms and transcription motifs of circadian rhythm genes, such as CRY2, CLOCK, ARNTL, PER2, or NPAS2, which are linked with hypertension, metabolic syndrome, or T2DM [30,41]. Circadian rhythm genes play a significant part in homeostatic equilibrium. They adjust the fibrinolytic system, and the CRY and CLOCK genes are precisely engaged in this action and, accordingly, raise the CVD risk. The purpose of the circadian clock in cardiovascular activity has been strongly emphasized in many studies. However, this research showed an association of MI with some circadian clock polymorphisms. This is relevant because approximately 43% of all protein-coding genes have circadian transcription in an organ-specific way [40].

Circadian rhythm genes play a crucial role in many physiological activities. The ARNTL gene is an integral part of lipid metabolism due to its influences on the transcription of genes included in lipogenesis in adipocytes in a circadian fashion, as shown in animal models [24]. In humans, CLOCK gene SNPs are connected to body weight, metabolic syndrome risk, and insomnia [24,42], while PER2 and PER3 gene SNPs are linked to sleep disturbances [43]. Different polymorphisms of circadian clock genes are connected with various cardiovascular disease risk factors [44]. Thus, metabolic syndrome, T2DM, and stroke are associated with CLOCK gene variants [29,45,46], while myocardial infarction is associated with CRY2 and PER2 gene variations [29]. Metabolic syndrome in humans is associated with the transcription of CRY1 and PER2 in adipose tissue [41,47]. Patients with diabetes have more severe atherosclerotic changes in their blood vessels [48] and have a two to three times higher risk of developing cardiovascular disease than healthy subjects [46]. Lifestyle and metabolic disorders are directly related, as indicated by biological and epidemiological studies [49], although the biochemical and genetic connection of the circadian clock with metabolic disorders has not been investigated in detail. Therefore, the significance of the circadian rhythm in the preservation of "energetic" equilibrium and metabolism is obvious.

Tsai et al. showed the significance of the circadian clock in cardiomyocytes in mice with mutated clock genes. They pointed out that the circadian rhythm is a primary controller of cardiac triglyceride metabolism [50], whereas ARNTL gene deletion in adipocyte causes obesity [51]. Polymorphisms of the BMAL1 gene, which is the mouse equivalent of the human ARNTL gene, are connected with hypertension and T2DM [52,53], just as in this study where we found an association of rs3789327 and rs12363415 with T2DM in MI patients. All these data confirm the responsibility of ARNTL polymorphisms in the metabolic disorders in humans. The ARNTL gene SNPs are associated with hypertension, diabetes mellitus, and metabolic syndrome. All these conditions increase the risk of MI [54]. BMAL1 was shown to be responsible for the daily variations in blood pressure [40], and here, we found an association of rs12363415 with diastolic and systolic blood pressure. Physiological rhythms of heart rate and blood pressure are lost in Bmal1 knockout mice [55], and such mice developed dilated cardiomyopathy [56]. BMAL1 knockout mice had depressed cardiovascular circadian rhythms and developed age-dependent dilated cardiomyopathy. The knockout of BMAL1 or deletion of all three isoforms of Cry in mice contributed to arterial stiffness and the impairment of extracellular matrix composition [40].

Genetic variations in the CLOCK gene are connected with T2DM and cardiovascular disorders in humans [29,30,41,53,57]. Here, an association of rs6811520 and rs13124436 with T2DM was found in MI patients. Studies using CLOCK mutant mice show the crucial function of the CLOCK in myocardial contractility, basal metabolism, and daily pulse rate control [41]. Mutation of the *Clock* gene in mouse cardiomyocytes only disrupts circadian rhythm in cardiomyocytes. This *Clock* mutation leads to physiological changes in cardiomyocytes. Some of these are heart rate, cardiac metabolism, response to external signals, contractility, and cardiac growth and regeneration [38]. CLOCK is a transcription factor and one of the primary regulators of the transcription of the circadian clock gene. It is also the regulator of expression of the various transcription factors required for control of the diverse physiological and behavioral processes that occur in a circadian fashion [58]. In this study, rs11932595 SNP of the *CLOCK* gene was connected with systolic blood pressure in MI patients. CLOCK, thrombomodulin, and plasminogen activator-1 inhibitor are required for the endothelial homeostasis. The circadian rhythm regulates genes in vascular endothelial cells [41], and disorder of clock could cause atherosclerosis and MI. Specific *CLOCK* gene polymorphisms are linked to excess weight [59,60], metabolic syndrome, and CVD [61]. A mutation in *CLOCK* leads to the development of age-dependent cardiomyopathy in male mice [40].

PER2 polymorphisms could be connected with myocardial infarction [29]. In this study, the *PER2* genetic variant rs35333999 is connected with age in MI patients. PER2 in the heart plays a crucial part in myocardial ischemia and fatty acid metabolism [62]. In contrast, mutations in the *PER2* gene are connected with a shortened circadian period during constant darkness [63]. In the mouse heart, PER2 has a protective function during myocardial ischemia [62,64]. It is included in the control of fatty acid metabolism with raised utilization of oxygen. In the hearts of mice with clock gene mutations, lipolysis is considerably reduced, which can accelerate the development of metabolic disorders, such as atherosclerosis, which could result in MI [50]. *PER2* knockout mice had more extensive infarct sizes, and the *PER2* in the heart exhibits an essential function during inflammation in myocardial ischemia and reperfusion [64]. The reduction of glycogen storage leads to enlarged infarct areas in mice with *PER2* mutation as a result of lowered glycolysis during myocardial ischemia. Suarez-Barrientos et al. observed that the infarct area was more extensive early in the morning [61], which is similar to the conclusion of Eckle et al. that PER2 stabilization dependent on light had a cardioprotective function in ischemia [65]. The deletion of the *Per2* gene in mice reduces the severity of MI because it limits inflammatory processes, reduces apoptosis, and promotes cardiomyocyte hypertrophy. Therefore, *Per2* gene disruption has a protective function in MI [66]. Activation of PER2 at the time of ischemia controls the beta-oxidation of fatty acids and inflammatory processes. Inflammation and metabolism are related, and inflammation might be an outcome of a disturbed metabolism [61]. Patients with raised inflammatory markers and metabolic syndrome have a higher chance of developing CVD. Disturbance of the circadian rhythm is involved in the development of a CVD, and hypertension is an essential element [30,53]. Furthermore, a mutation in the *PER2* gene was connected with aortic endothelial dysfunction, it reduces the production of nitric oxide, and other vasodilatory prostaglandins [40]. Per1 was also found to control the expression of many genes linked to sodium transport in the kidneys [40].

Genetic factors may explain, at least in part, some susceptibility to MI in individuals exposed to chronic or even short-term disorders. Thus, shift work is associated with a small but significant increase in the risk of developing CVD, which means that sleep disorders make an essential contribution to the risk of developing CVD [67]. Shift work and physical inactivity are associated with CVD risk factors such as increased triglyceride levels, which can lead to increased risk for MI [68]. A family history of CVD is another risk factor for developing CVD, especially premature CVD, and sudden cardiac death. In addition to genetic factors, a lifestyle passed on from generation to generation has a significant impact on the development of CVD. The increased genetic predisposition for MI, along with inherited life patterns of physical inactivity, may explain to some extent the increase in the incidence of MI [69]. Studies have shown an association between daylight saving time and the incidence of myocardial infarction. A particularly significant increase in the incidence of MI was observed in the first week after the spring shift [21]. The shift to daylight saving time causes circadian rhythm disturbance and sleep disruption, thereby increasing the risk of MI. Therefore, the abolition of daylight saving time is considered to be good for human health and might reduce the risk of CVD [70].

Cardiovascular disease and metabolic disorders are associated with circadian rhythm disturbances in humans [71]. It is crucial to know the ethnic structure of the investigated population since the frequency of circadian rhythm gene polymorphisms differs significantly between different populations [72]. This study investigated the relationship between myocardial infarction patients and various circadian clock genes polymorphisms. The present study examined the prevalence of genetic variants and several genotype models within two groups, patients with myocardial infarction and no-MI participants. Specific genetic variants of circadian rhythm genes might affect the ability of individuals to adapt their circadian rhythm to changing environmental conditions. The results of the present study are compatible with new presumptions, where circadian rhythm aberrations play an essential part in the onset of MI.

A possible explanation for the lack of correlation of all the studied polymorphisms of the circadian rhythm genes with MI is that individual SNPs have a minor input in the onset of MI. Only when certain combinations of specific SNPs are considered together, a significant association might be obtained. It is significant because the circadian rhythm genes are closely connected in a complex clock mechanism. As MI is a complex trait, the humble contributions of numerous genes affect the phenotypic presentation.

Limitations of the Study

The sample size is a limitation of this research. A more significant association between phenotype and genotype might be obtained with more patients involved. The number of participants was limited and might produce a false-positive result. The inadequate statistical capability to distinguish positive relationships is a result of the small frequency of some genotypes, as well as the excessive ORs and an extensive range of 95% CI. There is a chance of developing some of the CVDs in the no-MI group. A limitation of the study might be the age discrepancy between the MI patients and the no-MI group. However, a significant association only exists for age and one SNP in the *PER2* gene, rs35333999, in MI patients. Moreover, it is plausible that the *CLOCK*, *ARNTL*, and *PER2* gene SNPs studied are not usefully associated with MI. In the present case, useful polymorphisms or a collection of usefully relevant SNPs that could be better related to MI should be identified. This strategy of approaching the MI problem produces the chance to proceed with the investigation in multicenter studies with more participants. An advantage of the sample in this research is that it was nearly homogeneous in demographic variables such as sex, ethnicity, and cultural background.

5. Conclusions

The physiological activities of the individual are coordinated daily by the circadian rhythm. The circadian rhythm plays a significant part in numerous features of normal cardiovascular homeostasis and disease pathogenesis and pathophysiology. Circadian clock gene SNPs might be valuable in assessing the risk, prediction, or evaluating the feedback to therapy of CVD patients. Data are presented here indicating that the *ARNTL* and *CLOCK* gene polymorphisms could be associated with MI and therefore suggest the involvement of the circadian clock in the development of MI. These findings might increase knowledge of the physiopathological processes implicated in MI, and need replication in different individuals with MI. Additional confirmation and systematic study of the circadian rhythm in MI are achievable. In this age of personalized medicine, understanding of the genetic background of the circadian rhythm of a person could be essential for therapy and should be incorporated into diagnostic procedures.

Supplementary Materials: The following are available online at http://www.mdpi.com/2077-0383/9/2/484/s1, Figure S1: Linkage disequilibrium (LD) analysis among single nucleotide polymorphisms (SNPs) within the same chromosome and gene, Table S1: Frequencies and distribution of probable haplotypes in the MI and no-MI groups.

Author Contributions: I.Š. and J.M. performed experiments, analyzed data, and managed the specimens. I.Š. and R.S. were responsible for the design, collection, and quality control of the human specimen. R.S. supervised the study. I.Š. wrote the manuscript. All authors have read and agreed to the published version of the manuscript.

Funding: This research was partially supported by grant from the Faculty of Dental Medicine and Health, Osijek, Croatia dedicated to institutional funding of scientific activity – grant number FDMZ-2019-IP8.

Acknowledgments: The authors acknowledge the contribution of the medical staff who helped with this study.

Conflicts of Interest: The authors declare no conflicts of interest. The funders had no role in the design of the study; in the collection, analyses, or interpretation of data; in the writing of the manuscript, or in the decision to publish the results.

References

1. World Health Organization. *Noncommunicable Diseases Progress Monitor, 2017*; WHO: Geneva, Switzerland, 2017.
2. Kralj, V.; Brkić Biloš, I. Cardiovascular diseases – mortality and morbidity trends in Croatia, Europe and worldwide. *Cardiol. Croat.* **2016**, *11*, 504. [CrossRef]
3. World Health Organization. *Noncommunicable Diseases Country Profiles 2018*; WHO: Geneva, Switzerland, 2018.
4. Stevanovic, R.; Capak, K.; Brkic, K. *Croatian Health Statistics Yearbook 2016*; Croatian Institute of Public Health: Zagreb, Croatia, 2017.
5. Thygesen, K.; Alpert, J.S.; White, H.D. Universal definition of myocardial infarction. *Eur. Heart J.* **2007**, *28*, 2525–2538. [CrossRef]
6. Škrlec, I. Circadian rhythm and myocardial infarction. *Med. Flum.* **2019**, *55*, 32–42. [CrossRef]
7. Škrlec, I.; Marić, S.; Včev, A. Myocardial infarction and circadian rhythm. In *Visions Cardiomyocyte-Fundamental Concepts of Heart and Life Disease*; Tsipis, A., Ed.; IntechOpen: London, UK, 2019; pp. 60–75. [CrossRef]
8. Partch, C.L.; Green, C.B.; Takahashi, J.S. Molecular architecture of the mammalian circadian clock. *Trends Cell Biol.* **2014**, *24*, 90–99. [CrossRef]
9. Touitou, Y.; Bogdan, A. Circadian and seasonal variations of physiological and biochemical determinants of acute myocardial infarction. *Biol. Rhythm Res.* **2007**, *38*, 169–179. [CrossRef]
10. Muller, J.E.; Stone, P.H.; Turi, Z.G.; Rutherford, J.D.; Czeisler, C.A.; Parker, C.; Poole, W.K.; Passamani, E.; Roberts, R.; Robertson, T.; et al. Circadian variation in the frequency of onset of acute myocardial infarction. *N. Engl. J. Med.* **1985**, *313*, 1315–1322. [CrossRef]
11. Mehta, R.H.; Manfredini, R.; Hassan, F.; Sechtem, U.; Bossone, E.; Oh, J.K.; Cooper, J.V.; Smith, D.E.; Portaluppi, F.; Penn, M.; et al. Chronobiological patterns of acute aortic dissection. *Circulation* **2002**, *106*, 1110–1115. [CrossRef]
12. Elliott, W.J. Circadian variation in the timing of stroke onset: A meta-analysis. *Stroke* **1998**, *29*, 992–996. [CrossRef]
13. Manfredini, R.; Boari, B.; Smolensky, M.H.; Salmi, R.; Gallerani, M.; Guerzoni, F.; Guerra, V.; Malagoni, A.M.; Manfredini, F. Seasonal variation in onset of myocardial infarction—A 7-year single-center study in Italy. *Chronobiol. Int.* **2005**, *22*, 1121–1135. [CrossRef]
14. Garaulet, M.; Madrid, J.A. Chronobiology, genetics and metabolic syndrome. *Curr. Opin. Lipidol.* **2009**, *20*, 127–134. [CrossRef]
15. Virag, J.A.I.; Lust, R.M. Circadian influences on myocardial infarction. *Front. Physiol.* **2014**, *5*, 422. [CrossRef]
16. Leu, H.B.; Chung, C.M.; Lin, S.J.; Chiang, K.M.; Yang, H.C.; Ho, H.Y.; Ting, C.T.; Lin, T.H.; Sheu, S.H.; Tsai, W.C.; et al. Association of circadian genes with diurnal blood pressure changes and non-dipper essential hypertension: A genetic association with young-onset hypertension. *Hypertens. Res.* **2015**, *38*, 155–162. [CrossRef]
17. Kelly, M.A.; Rees, S.D.; Hydrie, M.Z.I.; Shera, A.S.; Bellary, S.; O'Hare, J.P.; Kumar, S.; Taheri, S.; Basit, A.; Barnett, A.H.; et al. Circadian gene variants and susceptibility to type 2 diabetes: A pilot study. *PLoS ONE* **2012**, *7*, e32670. [CrossRef]
18. Englund, A.; Kovanen, L.; Saarikoski, S.T.; Haukka, J.; Reunanen, A.; Aromaa, A.; Lönnqvist, J.; Partonen, T. NPAS2 and PER2 are linked to risk factors of the metabolic syndrome. *J. Circadian Rhythm.* **2009**, *7*, 5. [CrossRef]
19. Suzuki, S.; Ishii, H.; Ichimiya, S.; Kanashiro, M.; Watanabe, J.; Uchida, Y.; Yoshikawa, D.; Maeda, K.; Matsubara, T.; Murohara, T. Impact of the circadian rhythm on microvascular function in patients with ST-elevation myocardial infarction. *Int. J. Cardiol.* **2013**, *168*, 4948–4949. [CrossRef]

20. Poggiogalle, E.; Jamshed, H.; Peterson, C.M. Circadian regulation of glucose, lipid, and energy metabolism in humans. *Metabolism* **2018**, *84*, 11–27. [CrossRef]
21. Manfredini, R.; Fabbian, F.; Cappadona, R.; Modesti, P.A. Daylight saving time, circadian rhythms, and cardiovascular health. *Intern. Emerg. Med.* **2018**, *13*, 641–646. [CrossRef]
22. Martino, T.A.; Young, M.E. Influence of the cardiomyocyte circadian clock on cardiac physiology and pathophysiology. *J. Biol. Rhythm.* **2015**, *30*, 183–205. [CrossRef]
23. Durgan, D.J.; Young, M.E. The cardiomyocyte circadian clock: Emerging roles in health and disease. *Circ. Res.* **2010**, *106*, 647–658. [CrossRef]
24. Gómez-Abellán, P.; Madrid, J.A.; Ordovás, J.M.; Garaulet, M. Chronobiological aspects of obesity and metabolic syndrome. *Endocrinol. Nutr.* **2012**, *59*, 50–61. [CrossRef]
25. Škrlec, I.; Milić, J.; Heffer, M.; Steiner, R.; Peterlin, B.; Wagner, J. Association of Circadian Rhythm with Myocardial Infarction. *Acta Clin. Croat.* **2018**, *57*, 480–485. [CrossRef] [PubMed]
26. Erdmann, J.; Linsel-Nitschke, P.; Schunkert, H. Genetic causes of myocardial infarction: New insights from genome-wide association studies. *Dtsch. Arztebl. Int.* **2010**, *107*, 694–699. [CrossRef] [PubMed]
27. Takeda, N.; Maemura, K. Circadian clock and the onset of cardiovascular events. *Hypertens. Res.* **2016**, *39*, 383–390. [CrossRef] [PubMed]
28. Kelleher, F.C.; Rao, A.; Maguire, A. Circadian molecular clocks and cancer. *Cancer Lett.* **2014**, *342*, 9–18. [CrossRef] [PubMed]
29. Škrlec, I.; Milić, J.; Heffer, M.; Peterlin, B.; Wagner, J. Genetic variations in circadian rhythm genes and susceptibility for myocardial infarction. *Genet. Mol. Biol.* **2018**, *41*, 403–409. [CrossRef]
30. Škrlec, I.; Milić, J.; Heffer, M.; Wagner, J.; Peterlin, B. Circadian clock genes and circadian phenotypes in patients with myocardial infarction. *Adv. Med. Sci.* **2019**, *64*, 224–229. [CrossRef]
31. Thygesen, K.; Alpert, J.S.; Jaffe, A.S.; Simoons, M.L.; Chaitman, B.R.; White, H.D. Third universal definition of myocardial infarction. *Nat. Rev. Cardiol.* **2012**, *9*, 620–633. [CrossRef]
32. Thygesen, K.; Alpert, J.S.; Jaffe, A.S.; Chaitman, B.R.; Bax, J.J.; Morrow, D.A.; White, H.D.; Mickley, H.; Crea, F.; Van de Werf, F.; et al. Fourth universal definition of myocardial infarction (2018). *Eur. Heart J.* **2019**, *40*, 237–269. [CrossRef]
33. Elder, S.J.; Lichtenstein, A.H.; Pittas, A.G.; Roberts, S.B.; Fuss, P.J.; Greenberg, A.S.; McCrory, M.A.; Bouchard, T.J., Jr.; Saltzman, E.; Neale, M.C. Genetic and environmental influences on factors associated with cardiovascular disease and the metabolic syndrome. *J. Lipid Res.* **2009**, *50*, 1917–1926. [CrossRef]
34. de Bakker, P.I.W.; Yelensky, R.; Pe'er, I.; Gabriel, S.B.; Daly, M.J.; Altshuler, D. Efficiency and power in genetic association studies. *Nat. Genet.* **2005**, *37*, 1217–1223. [CrossRef]
35. Solé, X.; Guinó, E.; Valls, J.; Iniesta, R.; Moreno, V. SNPStats: A web tool for the analysis of association studies. *Bioinformatics* **2006**, *22*, 1928–1929. [CrossRef] [PubMed]
36. Shi, Y.Y.; He, L. SHEsis, a powerful software platform for analyses of linkage disequilibrium, haplotype construction, and genetic association at polymorphism loci. *Cell Res.* **2005**, *15*, 97–98. [CrossRef]
37. Li, Z.; Zhang, Z.; He, Z.; Tang, W.; Li, T.; Zeng, Z.; He, L.; Shi, Y.Y. A partition-ligation-combination-subdivision EM algorithm for haplotype inference with multiallelic markers: Update of the SHEsis (http://analysis.bio-x.cn). *Cell Res.* **2009**, *19*, 519–523. [CrossRef] [PubMed]
38. Bray, M.S.; Shaw, C.A.; Moore, M.W.S.; Garcia, R.A.P.; Zanquetta, M.M.; Durgan, D.J.; Jeong, W.J.; Tsai, Ju.; Bugger, H.; Zhang, D.; et al. Disruption of the circadian clock within the cardiomyocyte influences myocardial contractile function, metabolism, and gene expression. *Am. J. Physiol. Heart Circ. Physiol.* **2008**, *294*, H1036–H1047. [CrossRef] [PubMed]
39. Khaper, N.; Bailey, C.D.C.; Ghugre, N.R.; Reitz, C.; Awosanmi, Z.; Waines, R.; Martino, T.A. Implications of disturbances in circadian rhythms for cardiovascular health: A new frontier in free radical biology. *Free Radic. Biol. Med.* **2017**, *119*, 85–92. [CrossRef] [PubMed]
40. Rabinovich-Nikitin, I.; Lieberman, B.; Martino, T.A.; Kirshenbaum, L.A. Circadian-Regulated Cell Death in Cardiovascular Diseases. *Circulation* **2019**, *139*, 965–980. [CrossRef] [PubMed]
41. Scott, E.M. Circadian clocks, obesity and cardiometabolic function. *Diabetes Obes. Metab.* **2015**, *17*, 84–89. [CrossRef]
42. Huang, W.; Ramsey, K.M.; Marcheva, B.; Bass, J. Circadian rhythms, sleep, and metabolism. *J. Clin. Investig.* **2011**, *121*, 2133–2141. [CrossRef]

43. Pedrazzoli, M.; Secolin, R.; Esteves, L.O.B.; Pereira, D.S.; Koike, B.D.V.; Louzada, F.M.; Lopes-Cendes, I.; Tufik, S. Interactions of polymorphisms in different clock genes associated with circadian phenotypes in humans. *Genet. Mol. Biol.* **2010**, *33*, 627–632. [CrossRef]
44. Dashti, H.S.; Smith, C.E.; Lee, Y.C.; Parnell, L.D.; Lai, C.Q.; Arnett, D.K.; Ordovás, JM.; Garaulet, M. CRY1 circadian gene variant interacts with carbohydrate intake for insulin resistance in two independent populations: Mediterranean and North American. *Chronobiol. Int.* **2014**, *31*, 660–667. [CrossRef]
45. Prasai, M.J.; George, J.T.; Scott, E.M. Molecular clocks, type 2 diabetes and cardiovascular disease. *Diabetes Vasc. Dis. Res.* **2008**, *5*, 89–95. [CrossRef]
46. Martín-Timón, I.; Sevillano-Collantes, C.; Segura-Galindo, A.; Del Cañizo-Gómez, F.J. Type 2 diabetes and cardiovascular disease: Have all risk factors the same strength? *World J. Diabetes* **2014**, *5*, 444–470. [CrossRef]
47. Gómez-Abellán, P.; Hernández-Morante, J.J.; Luján, J.A.; Madrid, J.A.; Garaulet, M. Clock genes are implicated in the human metabolic syndrome. *Int. J. Obes.* **2008**, *32*, 121–128. [CrossRef]
48. Paneni, F.; Beckman, J.A.; Creager, M.A.; Cosentino, F. Diabetes and vascular disease: Pathophysiology, clinical consequences, and medical therapy: Part I. *Eur. Heart J.* **2013**, *34*, 2436–2443. [CrossRef]
49. Dibner, C.; Schibler, U. Circadian timing of metabolism in animal models and humans. *J. Intern. Med.* **2015**, *277*, 513–527. [CrossRef]
50. Tsai, J.Y.; Kienesberger, P.C.; Pulinilkunnil, T.; Sailors, M.H.; Durgan, D.J.; Villegas-Montoya, C.; Jahoor, A.; Gonzalez, R.; Garvey, M.E.; Boland, B.; et al. Direct Regulation of Myocardial Triglyceride Metabolism by the Cardiomyocyte Circadian Clock. *J. Biol. Chem.* **2010**, *285*, 2918–2929. [CrossRef]
51. Paschos, G.K.; Ibrahim, S.; Song, W.L.; Kunieda, T.; Grant, G.; Reyes, T.M.; Bradfield, C.A.; Vaughan, C.H.; Eiden, M.; Masoodi, M.; et al. Obesity in mice with adipocyte-specific deletion of clock component Arntl. *Nat. Med.* **2012**, *18*, 1768–1777. [CrossRef]
52. Woon, P.Y.; Kaisaki, P.J.; Bragança, J.; Bihoreau, M.; Levy, J.C.; Farrall, M.; Gauguier, D. Aryl hydrocarbon receptor nuclear translocator-like (BMAL1) is associated with susceptibility to hypertension and type 2 diabetes. *Proc. Natl. Acad. Sci. USA* **2007**, *104*, 14412–14417. [CrossRef]
53. Škrlec, I.; Milić, J.; Cilenšek, I.; Petrovič, D.; Wagner, J.; Peterlin, B. Circadian clock genes and myocardial infarction in patients with type 2 diabetes mellitus. *Gene* **2019**, *701*, 98–103. [CrossRef]
54. Crnko, S.; Du Pré, B.C.; Sluijter, J.P.G.; Van Laake, L.W. Circadian rhythms and the molecular clock in cardiovascular biology and disease. *Nat. Rev. Cardiol.* **2019**, *16*, 437–447. [CrossRef]
55. Curtis, A.M.; Cheng, Y.; Kapoor, S.; Reilly, D.; Price, T.S.; Fitzgerald, G.A. Circadian variation of blood pressure and the vascular response to asynchronous stress. *Proc. Natl. Acad. Sci. USA* **2007**, *104*, 3450–3455. [CrossRef]
56. Lefta, M.; Campbell, K.S.; Feng, H.Z.; Jin, J.P.; Esser, K.A. Development of dilated cardiomyopathy in Bmal1-deficient mice. *Am. J. Physiol.-Heart Circ. Physiol.* **2012**, *303*, H475–H485. [CrossRef]
57. Corella, D.; Asensio, E.M.; Coltell, O.; Sorlí, J.V.; Estruch, R.; Martínez-González, M.Á.; Salas-Salvadó, J.; Castañer, O.; Arós, F.; Lapetra, J.; et al. CLOCK gene variation is associated with incidence of type-2 diabetes and cardiovascular diseases in type-2 diabetic subjects: Dietary modulation in the PREDIMED randomized trial. *Cardiovasc. Diabetol.* **2016**, *15*, 4. [CrossRef]
58. Riestra, P.; Gebreab, S.Y.; Xu, R.; Khan, R.J.; Gaye, A.; Correa, A.; Min, N.; Sims, M.; Davis, S.K. Circadian CLOCK gene polymorphisms in relation to sleep patterns and obesity in African Americans: Findings from the Jackson heart study. *BMC Genet.* **2017**, *18*, 58. [CrossRef]
59. Bandín, C.; Martinez-Nicolas, A.; Ordovás, J.M.; Ros Lucas, J.A.; Castell, P.; Silvente, T.; Madrid, J.A.; Garaulet, M. Differences in circadian rhythmicity in CLOCK 3111T/C genetic variants in moderate obese women as assessed by thermometry, actimetry and body position. *Int. J. Obes.* **2013**, *37*, 1044–1050. [CrossRef]
60. Garcia-Rios, A.; Gomez-Delgado, F.J.; Garaulet, M.; Alcala-Diaz, J.F.; Delgado-Lista, F.J.; Marin, C.; Rangel-Zuniga, O.A.; Rodriguez-Cantalejo, F.; Gomez-Luna, P.; Ordovas, J.M.; et al. Beneficial effect of CLOCK gene polymorphism rs1801260 in combination with low-fat diet on insulin metabolism in the patients with metabolic syndrome. *Chronobiol. Int.* **2014**, *31*, 401–408. [CrossRef]
61. Suarez-Barrientos, A.; Lopez-Romero, P.; Vivas, D.; Castro-Ferreira, F.; Nunez-Gil, I.; Franco, E.; Ruiz-Mateos, B.; Garcia-Rubira, J.C.; Fernandez-Ortiz, A.; Macaya, C.; et al. Circadian variations of infarct size in acute myocardial infarction. *Heart* **2011**, *97*, 970–976. [CrossRef]

62. Bonney, S.; Kominsky, D.; Brodsky, K.; Eltzschig, H.; Walker, L.; Eckle, T. Cardiac Per2 functions as novel link between fatty acid metabolism and myocardial inflammation during ischemia and reperfusion injury of the heart. *PLoS ONE* **2013**, *8*, e71493. [CrossRef]
63. Vukolic, A.; Antic, V.; Van Vliet, B.N.; Yang, Z.; Albrecht, U.; Montani, J. Role of mutation of the circadian clock gene Per2 in cardiovascular circadian rhythms. *Am. J. Physiol.-Regul. Integr. Comp. Physiol.* **2010**, *298*, 627–634. [CrossRef]
64. Bonney, S.; Hughes, K.; Harter, P.N.; Mittelbronn, M.; Walker, L.; Eckle, T. Cardiac period 2 in myocardial ischemia: Clinical implications of a light dependent protein. *Int. J. Biochem. Cell Biol.* **2013**, *45*, 667–671. [CrossRef]
65. Eckle, T.; Hartmann, K.; Bonney, S.; Reithel, S.; Mittelbronn, M.; Walker, L.A.; Lowes, B.D.; Han, J.; Borchers, C.H.; Buttrick, P.M.; et al. Adora2b-elicited Per2 stabilization promotes a HIF-dependent metabolic switch crucial for myocardial adaptation to ischemia. *Nat. Med.* **2012**, *18*, 774–782. [CrossRef]
66. Virag, J.A.I.; Dries, J.L.; Easton, P.R.; Friesland, A.M.; Deantonio, J.H.; Chintalgattu, V.; DeAntonio, J.H.; Chintalgattu, V.; Cozzi, E.; Lehmann, B.D.; et al. Attenuation of myocardial injury in mice with functional deletion of the circadian rhythm gene mPer2. *Am. J. Physiol. Heart Cric. Physiol.* **2010**, *198*, H1088–H1095. [CrossRef]
67. Vetter, C.; Devore, E.E.; Wegrzyn, L.R.; Massa, J.; Speizer, F.E.; Kawachi, I.; Rosner, B.; Stampfer, M.J.; Schernhammer, E.S. Association between rotating night shiftwork and risk of coronary heart disease among women. *JAMA* **2016**, *315*, 1726–1734. [CrossRef]
68. Hermansson, J.; Bøggild, H.; Hallqvist, J.; Karlsson, B.; Knutsson, A.; Nilsson, T.; Reuterwall, C.; Gillander Gådin, K. Interaction between shift work and established coronary risk factors. *Int. J. Occup. Environ. Med.* **2019**, *10*, 57–65. [CrossRef]
69. Hermansson, J.; Hallqvist, J.; Karlsson, B.; Knutsson, A.; Gillander Gådin, K. Shift work, parental cardiovascular disease and myocardial infarction in males. *Occup. Med.* **2018**, *68*, 120–125. [CrossRef]
70. Manfredini, R.; Fabbian, F.; Cappadona, R.; De Giorgi, A.; Bravi, F.; Carradori, T.; Flacco, M.E.; Manzoli, L. Daylight Saving Time and Acute Myocardial Infarction: A Meta-Analysis. *J. Clin. Med.* **2019**, *8*, 404. [CrossRef]
71. Kurose, T.; Yabe, D.; Inagaki, N. Circadian rhythms and diabetes. *J. Diabetes Investig.* **2011**, *2*, 176–177. [CrossRef]
72. Allebrandt, K.V.; Roenneberg, T. The search for circadian clock components in humans: New perspectives for association studies. *Braz. J. Med. Biol. Res.* **2008**, *41*, 716–721. [CrossRef]

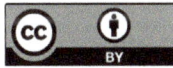

© 2020 by the authors. Licensee MDPI, Basel, Switzerland. This article is an open access article distributed under the terms and conditions of the Creative Commons Attribution (CC BY) license (http://creativecommons.org/licenses/by/4.0/).

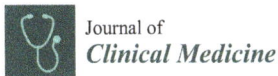

Review

Hypertension, Thrombosis, Kidney Failure, and Diabetes: Is COVID-19 an Endothelial Disease? A Comprehensive Evaluation of Clinical and Basic Evidence

Celestino Sardu [1,2,†], Jessica Gambardella [3,4,†], Marco Bruno Morelli [4,5,†], Xujun Wang [4], Raffaele Marfella [1] and Gaetano Santulli [3,4,5,*]

1. Department of Advanced Medical and Surgical Sciences, University of Campania "Luigi Vanvitelli", 80100 Naples, Italy; drsarducele@gmail.com (C.S.); raffaele.marfella@unicampania.it (R.M.)
2. Department of Medical Sciences, International University of Health and Medical Sciences "Saint Camillus", 00131 Rome, Italy
3. Department of Advanced Biomedical Sciences, International Translational Research and Medical Education Academic Research Unit (ITME), "Federico II" University, 80131 Naples, Italy; jessica.gambardella@einsteinmed.org
4. Department of Medicine, Division of Cardiology, Albert Einstein College of Medicine, Wilf Family Cardiovascular Research Institute, New York, NY 10461, USA; marco.morelli@einstein.yu.edu (M.B.M.); xujun.wang@einsteinmed.org (X.W.)
5. Department of Molecular Pharmacology, Fleischer Institute for Diabetes and Metabolism (FIDAM), Montefiore University Hospital, New York, NY 10461, USA
* Correspondence: gaetano.santulli@einsteinmed.org
† These authors equally contributed to this work.

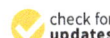

Received: 12 April 2020; Accepted: 4 May 2020; Published: 11 May 2020

Abstract: The symptoms most commonly reported by patients affected by coronavirus disease (COVID-19) include cough, fever, and shortness of breath. However, other major events usually observed in COVID-19 patients (e.g., high blood pressure, arterial and venous thromboembolism, kidney disease, neurologic disorders, and diabetes mellitus) indicate that the virus is targeting the endothelium, one of the largest organs in the human body. Herein, we report a systematic and comprehensive evaluation of both clinical and preclinical evidence supporting the hypothesis that the endothelium is a key target organ in COVID-19, providing a mechanistic rationale behind its systemic manifestations.

Keywords: ACE2, acute kidney injury; blood pressure; catepsin; coronavirus; COVID; cytokine storm; endothelium; heparin; Kawasaki disease

1. Introduction

Coronavirus disease (COVID-19) represents a public health crisis of global proportions [1]. Caused by the *severe acute respiratory syndrome corona virus 2* (SARS-CoV-2), COVID-19 was first announced in December 2019 in Wuhan, the capital of China's Hubei province [2,3].

The symptoms most commonly reported include cough, fever, and shortness of breath. The pathophysiology of the disease explains why respiratory symptoms are so common: indeed, the virus accesses host cells via the protein angiotensin-converting enzyme 2 (ACE2) [4,5], which is very abundant in the lungs [6].

Nevertheless, ACE2 is also expressed by endothelial cells [7,8], and other major clinical events usually observed in COVID-19 patients (e.g., high blood pressure [9–13], thrombosis [14–16] kidney disease [17,18], pulmonary embolism [19,20], cerebrovascular and neurologic disorders [21,22]) indicate that the virus is targeting the endothelium [23], one of the largest organs in the human body [24–26]. The cases of Kawasaki disease reported in young COVID-19 patients [27] support our view of a systemic vasculitis caused by SARS-CoV-2.

2. Pathogenesis of COVID-19

To access host cells, SARS-CoV-2 uses a surface glycoprotein (peplomer) known as spike; ACE2 has been shown to be a co-receptor for coronavirus entry [28–30]. Therefore, the density of ACE2 in each tissue may correlate with the severity of the disease in that tissue [31–36]. Other receptors on the surface of human cells have been suggested to mediate the entry of SARS-CoV-2 [5], including transmembrane serine protease 2 (TMPRSS2) [37,38], sialic acid receptors [39,40], and extracellular matrix metalloproteinase inducer (CD147, also known as basigin) [41]. Additionally, catepsin B and L have been shown to be critical entry factors in the pathogenesis of COVID-19 [38,42].

Intriguingly, all of these factors involved in the entry of SARS-CoV-2 in the host cell are known to be expressed by endothelial cells [43–49] (Figure 1).

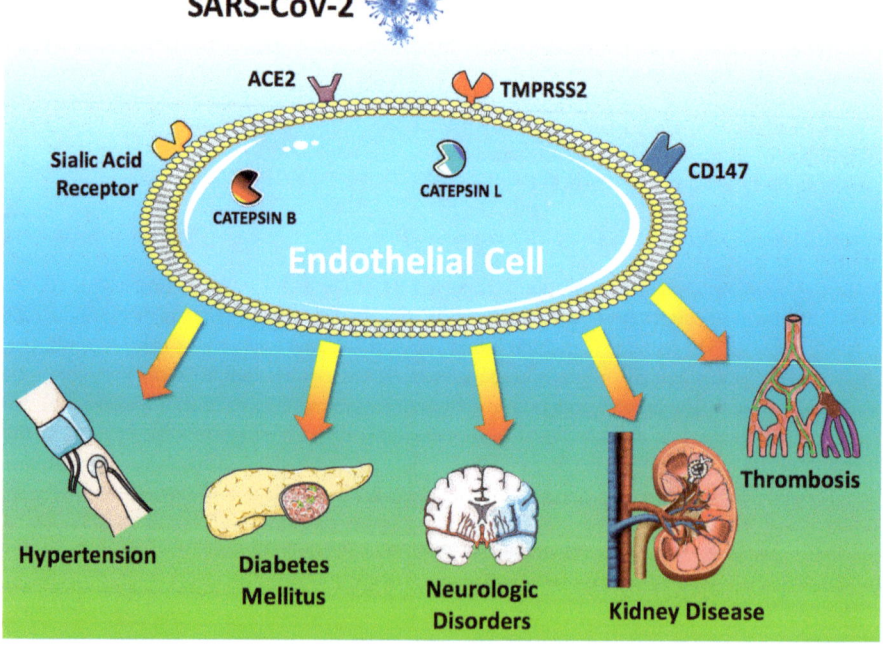

Figure 1. Endothelial dysfunction is a major determinant of COVID-19. The SARS-CoV-2 coronavirus accesses host cells via the binding of its spike glycoprotein to angiotensin-converting enzyme 2 (ACE2), sialic acid receptor, transmembrane serine protease 2 (TMPRSS2), and extracellular matrix metalloproteinase inducer (CD147); catepsin B and L also participate in virus entry. All of these factors are expressed in endothelial cells. Endothelial dysfunction is a common feature of the clinical manifestations observed in COVID-19 patients. All of the drugs proposed as a potential therapeutic strategy to treat COVID-19 patients have been shown to improve endothelial function, including tocilizumab, colchicine, chloroquine/hydroxychloroquine, azithromycin, and famotidine (see text for details and references).

ACE2 remains the most studied of these receptors [34,50–54]: for instance, its genetic inactivation has been shown to cause severe lung injury in H5N1-challenged mice [55], whereas administration of recombinant human ACE2 ameliorates H5N1 virus-induced lung injury in mice [55].

ACE2 is currently at the center of a heated debate among physicians [56–59], and there are concerns that medical management of hypertension, including the use of inhibitors of the renin-angiotensin-aldosterone system (RAAS), may contribute to the adverse health outcomes observed [34,60,61]; TMPRSS2 binds the viral spike glycoprotein [37]; recent structural assays have suggested that coronaviruses can bind sialic acid receptors [39]; CD147 has been shown to be essential for the entry of cytomegalovirus into endothelial cells [46]; both catepsin B [47] and L [49] are present in endothelial cells (Figure 1).

The endothelium prevents blood clotting by providing an antithrombotic surface, maintained by heparan sulphate present in the matrix surrounding the cells [62,63], by the expression of tissue factor inhibitor [64], thrombomodulin [65], and by the production of tissue-type plasminogen activator that promotes fibrinolysis [66,67].

Endothelial dysfunction refers to a systemic condition in which the endothelium loses its physiological properties, including the tendency to promote vasodilation, fibrinolysis, and anti-aggregation [68–72]; moreover, endothelial dysfunction appears to be a consistent finding in patients with diabetes [69,73–78]. Here we will discuss clinical and preclinical findings supporting our hypothesis [79] that COVID-19 impairs endothelial function (Figure 1).

3. Hypertension and COVID-19

Several investigators have called attention to the potential over-representation of hypertension among patients with COVID-19 [13,80–82]. Moreover, hypertension appears to track closely with advancing age, which is emerging as one of the strongest predictors of COVID-19–related death [14,83]. Specifically, observational trials and retrospectives studies conducted near Wuhan area have actually shown that hypertension is the most common co-morbidity observed in patients affected by COVID-19, ranging from 15% to over 30% [14,84–87].

One of the largest studies has been conducted by Guan et al. between December 11, 2019, and January 29, 2020, providing data on 1099 hospitalized patients and outpatients with laboratory-confirmed COVID-19 infection [84]; in this cohort, 165 (~15%) had high blood pressure [84]. The authors also evaluated the severity of disease, and the composite outcome of intensive care unit (ICU) admission, mechanical ventilation and death, concluding that 23.7% of hypertensive patients had disease severity (vs. 13.4% of normotensive subjects), and that 35.8% (vs. 13.7%) reached the composite endpoint of ICU admission, mechanical ventilation and death [84].

The high rate of hypertensive patients with COVID-19 was later confirmed in a prospective analysis on 41 patients admitted to hospital in Wuhan [85] as well as in a large study conducted on 138 hospitalized patients with confirmed COVID-19 infection [86]. In the latter report, the rate of hypertension was 31.2%, and 58.3% of hypertensive patients with COVID-19 infection were admitted to ICU compared to 21.6% of individuals with normal blood pressure [86], evidencing the hypertensive state as a common co-morbidity and cause of ICU admission in COVID-19 patients [86].

Similarly, among 191 COVID-19 patients from Jinyintan Hospital and Wuhan Pulmonary Hospital, 58 (30%) had hypertension, and 26 (48%) did not survive COVID-19, whereas 32 (23%) were survivors [14]. The 30% rate of hypertensive patients was further confirmed in an analysis based on the severity of COVID-19 conducted on 140 patients in Wuhan: 58 patients were classified as severe vs. 82 patients classified as not severe: hypertensive patients represented 37.9% of severe vs. 24.4% of not severe COVID-19 patients [87]. In a cohort of 1590 patients from 575 hospitals, underlying hypertension was independently associated with severe COVID-19 (hazard ratio 1.58, 95% CI: 1.07–2.32) [13]. Overall, these findings confirm a dual aspect of hypertension during COVID-19 pandemic: first, hypertension is the most common co-morbidity observed in COVID-19 patients; second, hypertension is evidenced in patients with worse prognosis and higher rate of death.

These studies also raise numerous questions regarding the association between hypertension and COVID-19. Indeed, hypertension is known to be one of most common diseases and co-morbidities worldwide, considered a silent killer for the worldwide population [88]. We speculate that the higher rate of hypertension and the worse prognosis in patients with COVID-19 infection could be seen as the spy of a cause-effect mechanism, more than as a casual pre-existing association between these two different diseases.

4. ACE2 and Anti-Hypertensive Drugs: What Do We Know?

ACE inhibitors (ACEi) and angiotensin II receptor blockers (ARB) represent very effective strategies for the treatment of hypertension [88]. These drugs reduce the effects of renin-angiotensin axis by inhibiting ACE (ACEi) or by blocking the angiotensin receptors (ARB), as shown in Figure 2. A growing question for the scientific community and physicians is to understand whether ACEi/ARB could affect the prognosis of hypertensive COVID-19 patients [34,89–91].

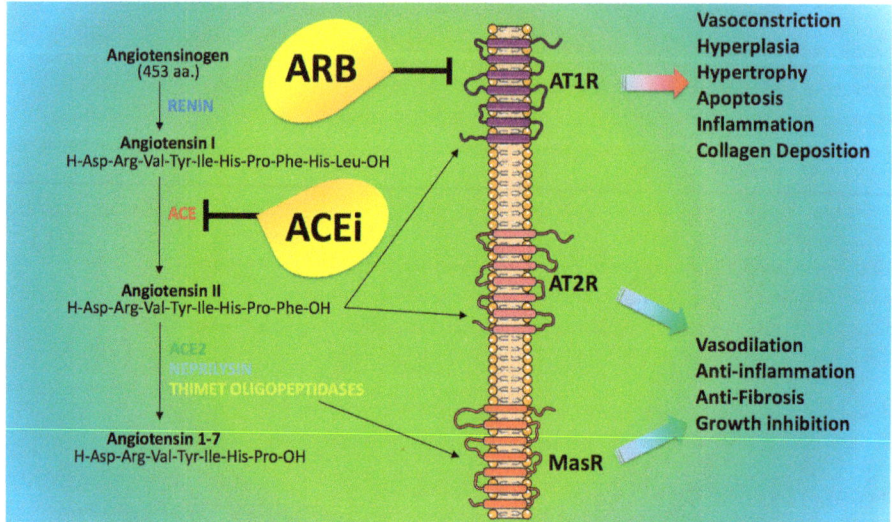

Figure 2. Angiotensin-converting enzyme inhibitors (ACEi) and blockers of the angiotensin receptor 1 (ARB). Angiotensin II and Angiotensin 1–7 binds heptahelical receptors; namely, angiotensin II can activate AT1R (type 1 angiotensin II receptor) and AT2R (type 2 angiotensin II receptor), whereas angiotensin 1–7 binds the Mas Receptor (MasR). The actions mediated by these receptors are depicted in the figure.

The exact role of ACEi/ARB in the control of ACE2 molecular pathways is controversial: indeed, preclinical studies evidenced that the selective blockade of either angiotensin II synthesis or activity in rats induces increases in ACE2 gene expression and activity [92–96]; similarly, treating infarcted rats with ARB increased plasma concentration of angiotensin 1–7 and ACE2 [97]. In mice, ARB treatment augmented ACE2 mRNA and protein levels [98,99] and prevented the decrease in ACE2 protein levels induced by Angiotensin II [100]. Equally important, mineralocorticoid receptor blockers prevented aldosterone-induced reduction in cardiac ACE2 mRNA expression in rat cardiomyocytes [101] and increased ACE2 expression and activity in murine hearts and in monocyte-derived macrophages obtained from ten patients with heart failure [102].

Nevertheless, there is no clinical evidence that ACEi could directly affect molecular pathways linked to ACE2 activity. For instance, urinary ACE2 levels were reported to be higher in patients treated with olmesartan vs. untreated controls, but this finding was not observed in patients treated with other ARB or enalapril [103]; instead, another study reported no difference in ACE2 activity in patients who were taking ACEi or ARB vs. untreated patients [89]. Of note, ACE2, which functions as a carboxypeptidase [104] is not inhibited by clinically prescribed ACEi.

In particular, ACE2 acts to counterbalance the effect of ACE [105]; indeed, whereas ACE generates angiotensin II from angiotensin I, ACE2 converts angiotensin II into an active heptapeptide (angiotensin 1-7), which binds the Mas receptor (MasR), triggering vasodilative, anti-oxidant, and anti-inflammatory properties [106–109] (Figure 2).

Some media sources have recently called for the discontinuation of ACEi and ARB, both prophylactically and in the context of suspected COVID-19 [110]. However, several associations have recommended not to suspend these therapies [61,111–114], and these recommendations have been confirmed by three recent studies: the first one performed on 362 hypertensive patients showed that ACEIs/ARBs are not associated with the severity or mortality of COVID-19 [91]; the second one verified the effects of ACEI/ARB on 1128 hypertensive COVID-19 patients, showing that the use of ACEI/ARB was associated with lower risk of all-cause mortality compared with ACEI/ARB non-users [115]; the third one demonstrated that without increasing the risk for SARS-CoV-2 infection, ACEI/ARB outcompeted other antihypertensive drugs in reducing inflammatory markers like C-reactive protein and procalcitonin levels in COVID-19 patients with preexisting hypertension [116]. Consistent with these findings, three observational studies performed in different populations and with different designs [117–119] (published in the same issue of the *New England Journal of Medicine*), arrived at the consistent message that the continued use of ACEI/ARB is unlikely to be harmful in COVID-19 patients. Notably, in one of these studies [117], the use of either ACEI or statins—two classes of drugs that are known to ameliorate endothelial function [120–123]—was found to be associated with a lower risk of in-hospital death than non-use.

The binding of the SARS-CoV-2 spike protein to ACE2 has been suggested to cause the down-regulation of ACE2 from the cell membrane [124]. Consequently, ACE2 down-regulation could lead to a loss of protective effects exerted by ACEi/ARB in humans [125]. Such down-regulation of ACE2 is an attractive research field [95,126–128]. Indeed, it could be a valid therapeutic target to ameliorate response and clinical prognosis in hypertensive patients affected by COVID-19. Moreover, some investigators proposed the restoration of ACE2 by administration of recombinant ACE2 to reverse the lung-injury process during viral infections [4]. Actually, these effects are being investigated in ongoing clinical trials (ClinicalTrials.gov NCT04287686), alongside the use of losartan as first therapy for COVID-19 in hospitalized (NCT04312009) or not hospitalized patients (NCT04311177). A major role in the pathogenesis of (as well as in the clinical response to) COVID-19 could also be played by ACE2 polymorphisms, which are relatively under-investigated if compared to ACE [129,130].

Finally, we have to consider the higher rate of cardiac injury and adverse outcomes in hypertensive patients during the COVID-19 pandemic [131–133]. Therefore, ACEi/ARB chronic therapy should not be discontinued in hypertensive patients with COVID-19. Indeed, the loss of their pneumo- and cardio-protective effects could be detrimental [88]. In addition, in the absence of adequate follow-up visits, switching from ACEi/ARB to another anti-hypertensive therapy could cause a suboptimal control of blood pressure.

Thus, as suggested by several medical associations [110], in the absence of definitive clinical studies and without clear evidence, hypertensive patients should avoid discontinuation and/or therapeutic switching during COVID-19 infection.

Another noteworthy feature of COVID-19 for cardiologists is the significant decrease in the rates of hospital admissions for acute coronary syndromes which has been reported both in Italy [134] and US [135] during the COVID-19 outbreak, and despite being initially attributed to reduced air pollution, better adherence to treatment, or absence of occupational stress during lockdown, this phenomenon seems to be most likely due to the fear of going to the hospital and/or seeking medical attention during a pandemic. Unfortunately, the current decline in hospitalization for acute coronary syndromes will trigger an increase in cases of heart failure in the near future.

5. Kidney Disease in COVID-19

Acute kidney injury (AKI) has been reported in > 20% of critically ill or deceased COVID-19 patients, a percentage that is consistent in studies from China [136], Italy [137] and United States [10]. It is important to note that AKI, proteinuria, and hematuria have been independently associated with a higher risk of death in COVID-19 patients [138]. Furthermore, in a meta-analysis including 1389 COVID-19 patients [139], the prevalence of underlying chronic kidney disease was significantly more frequent among those with a severe COVID-19 disease (3.3% vs. 0.4%; odds ratio 3.03, 95% CI: 1.09–8.47).

According to immunohistochemistry assays [140], ACE2 seems not to be expressed in renal endothelial cells; however, a study based on single-cell analysis has confirmed the expression of ACE2 and TMPRSS2 in human renal endothelial cells [141], and most recently the presence of viral particles was confirmed by electron microscopy in endothelial cells of the glomerular capillary loops of a COVID-19 patient [142]. Besides, endothelial damage was a common finding in renal histopathological analyses of 26 COVID-19 patients, in the absence of interstitial inflammatory infiltrates [143].

6. Diabetes and COVID-19

Diabetes mellitus is a frequent co-morbidity and a cause of worse prognosis in COVID-19 patients [12,144–148]. Indeed, evaluating pneumonia cases of unknown causes reported in Wuhan and in patients with history of exposure to Huanan seafood market before Jan 1, 2020, 20% had diabetes [85]. Similarly, among 1099 COVID-19 patients analyzed by Guan and colleagues, 7.4% had diabetes: this percentage goes up to 16.2% among patients with severe disease (vs. 5.7% in patients with non-severe disease) [84]; furthermore, 35.8% of patients experiencing the composite endpoint of ICU admission, mechanical ventilation and death, had diabetes (vs. 13.7% of patients that did not experience such endpoint) [84]. Data from Italy show that more than two-thirds of COVID-19 patients that did not survive had diabetes [149]. In summary, diabetes is a frequent co-morbidity, a risk factor, and an independent prognostic factor in COVID-19 patients. A strong evidence of the negative effects of diabetes in COVID-19 patients is also corroborated by two meta-analyses [150,151].

The worse prognosis in patients with diabetes and COVID-19 could be attributed to the fact that the pneumonia evolves towards clinical stages more refractory to medical therapies, oxygen administration and mechanical ventilation, with necessity of ICU care. These data have been investigated in a previous study conducted in patients with SARS [152], in which the relationship between a known history of diabetes and fasting plasma glucose (FPG) levels with death and morbidity rate was assessed, showing that the percentage of patients with diabetes was significantly higher in deceased vs. survivors (21.5% vs. 3.9%, $p < 0.01$) [152]. Moreover, diabetic subjects with hypoxemia ($SaO_2 < 93\%$) had higher FPG levels and FPG was independently associated with an increased hazard ratio of mortality (1.1, 95% CI: 1.0–1.1) and hypoxia (1.1, 95% CI: 1.0–1.1) after controlling for age and gender [152]; the authors concluded that both diabetes (3.0, 95% CI: 1.4–6.3) and FPG > or = 7.0 mmol/l (3.3, 95% CI: 1.4–7.7) were independent predictors of death [152].

In COVID-19 patients, the incidence of diabetes is two times higher in ICU/severe vs. non-ICU/severe cases [151]. Indeed, the diagnosis of diabetes in a cohort of patients with COVID-19 infection evidenced a sub-group of patients with a 2.26-fold higher risk of experiencing adverse disease outcome analyses [150]. Additionally, patients with obesity and/or glucose intolerance seem to be particularly vulnerable to COVID-19 [10,148,153,154]. Unfortunately, no data are hitherto available on anti-diabetic medications and glucose homeostasis in COVID-19 patients. This aspect is really limiting, because diabetes and altered glucose homeostasis during a condition of severe pneumonia with SARS are reported as main factors of worse prognosis and death [152]. COVID-19 could also induce new onset diabetes, by augmenting insulin resistance and/or by a direct action [155] on the islets of Langerhans; supporting this view, previous studies have shown that ACE2 can be a therapeutic target to ameliorate microcirculation in the islets [156], and ACE2 is known to be expressed by pancreatic beta cells [157–162].

Moreover, frequent cases of ketoacidosis in COVID-19 patients have been reported [163]. Therefore, the investigation of anti-diabetic medications and glucose homeostasis could be harnessed to evaluate patients with higher risk of experiencing worse prognosis and death by COVID-19. We speculate that the amelioration of glucose homeostasis in diabetic COVID-19 patients by specific hypoglycemic drugs could result in the amelioration of clinical outcomes with death reduction. However, these data are not reported in trials on COVID-19, and they need to be investigated in further studies [164].

7. Thromboembolism and COVID-19

Patients with COVID19 often show clotting disorders, with organ dysfunction and coagulopathy, resulting in higher mortality [15,165,166]. Critical data came from the analysis of coagulation tests including prothrombin time (PT), activated partial thromboplastin time (APTT), antithrombin activity (AT), fibrinogen, fibrin degradation product (FDP), and D-dimer, in samples collected on admission and during the hospital stay of COVID-19 patients [167]. Non-survivors had significantly higher D-dimer and FDP levels, and longer PT vs. survivors on admission [167]. Moreover, significant reduction and lowering of fibrinogen and AT levels were observed in non-survivors during late stages of hospitalization, which is compatible with a clinical diagnosis of disseminated intravascular coagulation (DIC) [167,168]. Specifically, among 191 COVID-19 patients seen at two hospitals in Wuhan, D-dimer levels over 1 µg/L at admission predicted an 18-fold increase in odds of dying before discharge [14]. Of note, when DIC is caused by a systemic infection, it features an acute systemic over-inflammatory response, strictly linked to endothelial dysfunction [169].

Most recently a case of a COVID-19 patient with an increase of Factor VIII clotting activity and a massive elevation of von Willebrand Factor (vWF) has been reported [170], further supporting our theory: indeed, vWF can be seen as a marker of endothelial damage, since it is normally stored in Weibel-Palade bodies within endothelial cells [171]. Equally important, angiotensin II level in the plasma of COVID-19 patients was markedly elevated and linearly associated to viral load and lung injury [172]; notably, angiotensin II is known to increase microvascular permeability [173,174], to induce the transcription of tissue factor in endothelial cells [175–177], and to activate platelets [178–180]. Additionally, angiotensin II can trigger the release of several components of the complement system from endothelial cells [181–187], further corroborating the key role of endothelium in the pathogenesis of venous and arterial thrombosis in COVID-19 patients [188,189].

A dysregulated immune response, as observed in COVID-19, especially in the late stages of the disease, plays a decisive role in endothelial dysfunction and thrombosis [190,191], and microvascular permeability is crucial in viral infections [192]. Indeed, pulmonary endothelium represent a fundamental barrier between the blood and interstitium and have vital regulatory functions; specifically, endothelial cells represent one-third of the cell population of the lung [193], and pulmonary endothelial damage is considered the hallmark of acute respiratory distress syndrome (ARDS) [194]. Animal models of coronavirus-induced severe ARDS have shown that reduced ACE2 activity and loss of ACE2 in the lungs is mirrored by enhanced vascular permeability, and exacerbated pulmonary edema [108]. The functional role of endothelium in pulmonary disease is also suggested by previous reports [195,196]; for instance, the H3N2 influenza virus has been shown to infect endothelial cells in vitro and to trigger endothelial cell apoptosis, which is known to enhance platelet adhesion [197]: endothelial cell death would cause exposure of the extracellular matrix to circulating blood, favoring platelet binding; similarly, the endothelium has been shown to contribute to the development of severe disease during H5N1 influenza infection [198].

Deep vein thrombosis and/or pulmonary embolism have been previously described in patients with SARS [199–202] and cases of thrombosis complicating influenza-associated pneumonia have also been reported [203–205]. Excessive activation of the immune system in response to pathogens can lead to pathological inflammatory consequences. In the case of highly virulent 1918 and avian H5N1 influenza virus infections, the recruitment of inflammatory leukocytes followed by excessive cytokine responses is considered to be the key contributor to morbidity and mortality of the infection [206,207].

Cytokine storm syndromes (CSS) are a group of disorders representing a variety of inflammatory etiologies with the final result of overwhelming systemic inflammation, hemodynamic instability, multiple organ dysfunction, and potentially death [208,209]. Specifically, macrophage activation syndrome [210] and hemophagocytic lymphohistiocytosis (HLH) [211] represent two clinically similar CSS with an unknown degree of etiopathogenic overlap [208]. The interaction between endothelial and immune cells could play a crucial role in COVID-19, especially in severe cases and in the late stages of the disease [212]. For instance, the cytokine storm might lead to an abrupt deterioration of the inflammatory response and hyper-coagulation; the increased vulnerability of patients with cardiovascular diseases and/or diabetes might therefore simply reflect the impact of the underlying chronic inflammation and its response during SARS-CoV-2 infection. If this is the case, endothelial alterations could just be seen as an epiphenomenon.

However, according to numerous investigators, the inflammatory response observed in COVID-19 patients can be considered mild if compared to the one observed in typical ARDS and in cytokine-release syndrome [212–215]: indeed, in ARDS patients, levels of interleukin-1β and interleukin-6 have been shown to be 10 to 60 fold higher than in COVID-19 [216,217]. Therefore, other mechanisms have to be involved in order to explain the systemic manifestations reported in COVID-19 patients, and endothelial cells, known orchestrators of cytokine amplification during viral infections [218], seem to be one of the best candidates in this sense. Further supporting our view, catecholamines are considered an essential component of the cytokine release syndrome [215] and we have demonstrated that endothelial cells are able to synthetize and release catecholamines [219].

Acute pulmonary embolism, reported in COVID-19 patients [20,220–222], has been shown to be a cause of clinical deterioration in viral pneumonias [205,223]. Endothelial dysfunction is known to be a key determinant in hypertension, thrombosis, and DIC [72,224–227]. Henceforth, it is important to select COVID-19 patients at higher risk of pulmonary embolism, and practice computed tomography pulmonary angiography for the diagnosis of pulmonary thromboembolism especially in case of significant increase of D-dimer values. Anticoagulation could be a necessary therapy to control and reduce pro-thrombotic events, as well as to prevent pulmonary embolism [228].

8. Anticoagulation as a Key Therapy for COVID-19

The clinical course of COVID-19 consists of two main phases: viral infection and immune/inflammatory response (Figure 3), which require distinct therapeutic approaches. Strikingly, several drugs suggested as a potential therapeutic strategy for COVID-19 [229–231] have been shown to ameliorate endothelial function, including interleukin 6 (IL-6) receptor antagonists (e.g., tocilizumab [232]), colchicine [233], azithromycin [234], and famotidine [235].

Even the antimalaric agents chloroquine and hydroxychloroquine, initially proposed as a therapy for COVID-19 based on anecdotal data [229,236], have been shown to improve endothelial function [237,238]. If our theory is correct [239], other drugs that might be effective in treating COVID-19 patients through their beneficial effects on endothelial cells include α1 adrenergic receptor blockers (e.g., doxazosin) [240], modulators of Sigma receptors [241–243], metformin [244], indomethacin [245], and endothelin receptor antagonists (e.g., bosentan) [246]. However, data from randomized trials confirming the actual efficacy of these drugs are not (yet) available.

As discussed before, COVID-19 infection could cause endothelial dysfunction and a hyper-coagulation state. This condition is aggravated by hypoxia, which augments thrombosis by both increasing blood viscosity and hypoxia-inducible transcription factor-dependent signaling pathway [247]. Consequently, these phenomena could result in pulmonary embolism with occlusion and micro-thrombosis in pulmonary small vessels, as observed in critical COVID-19 patients [248]. Apart from cases of pulmonary embolism, COVID-19 can cause a sepsis-associated DIC, which is defined as "sepsis-induced coagulopathy" (SIC) [169]. Thus, there is an increasing interest in anticoagulant therapy to treat COVID-19 [249].

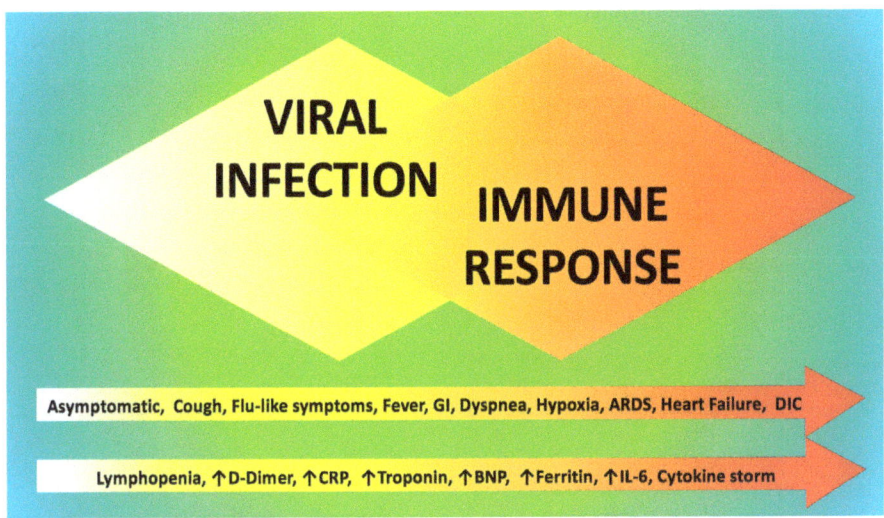

Figure 3. Clinical course of COVID-19 patients. Two main overlapping phases constitute the key pathogenic events in COVID-19: the acute phase represented by viral infection, followed by the immune/inflammatory response. Common clinical and laboratory findings are reported within the arrows at the bottom of the figure.

In a retrospective analysis conducted at Tongji Hospital of Huazhong University of Science and Technology in Wuhan, the authors examined 449 patients affected by severe COVID-19 [228]. The diagnosis of severe COVID-19 disease was made by evidence of respiratory rate ≥ 30 breaths/min, arterial oxygen saturation ≤ 93% at rest and PaO_2/FiO_2 ≤ 300 mmHg [228]. In these patients, they reviewed and compared the parameters of coagulation tests and clinical characteristics between survivors and non-survivors to evaluate the effects of heparin therapy [228]: 94 patients received low molecular weight heparin (LMWH, 40–60 mg enoxaparin/day) and 5 received unfractionated heparin (UFH, 10000–15000 U/day), without other anti-coagulants [228]. Heparin therapy significantly reduced mortality in patients with SIC score ≥4 (40.0% vs. 64.2%, $p < 0.05$), but not in those with SIC score < 4 (29.0% vs. 22.6%, $p > 0.05$) [228]. D-dimer, PT, and age were positively, while platelet count was negatively, correlated with 28-day mortality [228]. In addition, stratifying by D-dimer values the study population, the authors reported in heparin non-users a rise of mortality linked to the rising D-dimer, and 20% reduction of mortality for patients under heparin with D-dimer exceeding 3.0 µg/mL [228]. Therefore, heparin treatment appears to be associated with better prognosis in severe COVID-19 patients with coagulopathy. The beneficial effects of heparin-based therapies are also supported by the structural analogies between heparin and heparan-sulphate, which according to some investigators may confer heparin with antiviral properties [250–254]. In absence of contraindications, we suggest the use of enoxaparin 40 mg/day in all COVID-19 patients, to be raised up to 1 mg/kg every 12 h in case of D-dimer > 3.0 µg/mL; apixaban (5 mg every 12 h) could represent a useful alternative.

Of course, the full clinical evaluation of patients with COVID-19 infection cannot leave aside the analysis of laboratory and imaging data. We believe that PT/PTT, fibrinogen, and D-Dimer should be monitored daily and anticoagulation therapy should be recommended for COVID-19 patients when the D-Dimer value is four times higher than the normal upper limit, except for patients with anticoagulant contraindications. The confirmed diagnosis of severe COVID-19 disease in patients with hypercoagulation and organ failure could evidence an early stage of sepsis-induced DIC. On the other hand, anticoagulant may not benefit unselected patients. Consequently, further prospective studies are needed to confirm these findings in COVID-19 patients, also testing other anti-aggregants and anti-coagulants (at different doses).

Author Contributions: Conceptualization, G.S.; data curation, C.S., J.G., M.B.M., X.W., R.M. and G.S. and S.R.; writing—original draft preparation, C.S., J.G. and G.S.; writing—review and editing, J.G., M.B.M. and G.S.; visualization, M.B.M. and G.S.; supervision, G.S.; funding acquisition, G.S. and J.G. A preprint version of the manuscript was sent to preprints.org by on 9 April 2020: *Preprints* 2020, 2020040204 (doi:10.20944/preprints202004.0204.v1). All authors have read and agreed to the published version of the manuscript.

Funding: The Santulli's lab is supported in part by the NIH (R01-DK123259, R01-HL146691, R01-DK033823, and R00-DK107895 to G.S.) and by the American Heart Association (AHA-20POST35211151 to J.G.).

Conflicts of Interest: The authors declare no conflict of interest. The funders had no role in the design of the study; in the collection, analyses, or interpretation of data; in the writing of the manuscript, or in the decision to publish the paper.

References

1. Fauci, A.S.; Lane, H.C.; Redfield, R.R. Covid-19—Navigating the Uncharted. *N. Engl. J. Med.* **2020**, *382*, 1268–1269. [CrossRef] [PubMed]
2. Paules, C.I.; Marston, H.D.; Fauci, A.S. Coronavirus Infections-More Than Just the Common Cold. *JAMA* **2020**, *323*, 707. [CrossRef] [PubMed]
3. Hui, D.S.; Azhar, E.E.; Madani, T.A.; Ntoumi, F.; Kock, R.; Dar, O.; Ippolito, G.; McHugh, T.D.; Memish, Z.A.; Drosten, C.; et al. The continuing 2019-nCoV epidemic threat of novel coronaviruses to global health—The latest 2019 novel coronavirus outbreak in Wuhan, China. *Int. J. Infect. Dis.* **2020**, *91*, 264–266. [CrossRef] [PubMed]
4. Zhang, H.; Penninger, J.M.; Li, Y.; Zhong, N.; Slutsky, A.S. Angiotensin-converting enzyme 2 (ACE2) as a SARS-CoV-2 receptor: Molecular mechanisms and potential therapeutic target. *Intensive Care Med.* **2020**, *46*, 586–590. [CrossRef] [PubMed]
5. Zhou, P.; Yang, X.L.; Wang, X.G.; Hu, B.; Zhang, L.; Zhang, W.; Si, H.R.; Zhu, Y.; Li, B.; Huang, C.L.; et al. A pneumonia outbreak associated with a new coronavirus of probable bat origin. *Nature* **2020**, *579*, 270–273. [CrossRef]
6. Hamming, I.; Timens, W.; Bulthuis, M.L.; Lely, A.T.; Navis, G.; van Goor, H. Tissue distribution of ACE2 protein, the functional receptor for SARS coronavirus. A first step in understanding SARS pathogenesis. *J. Pathol.* **2004**, *203*, 631–637. [CrossRef]
7. Lovren, F.; Pan, Y.; Quan, A.; Teoh, H.; Wang, G.; Shukla, P.C.; Levitt, K.S.; Oudit, G.Y.; Al-Omran, M.; Stewart, D.J.; et al. Angiotensin converting enzyme-2 confers endothelial protection and attenuates atherosclerosis. *Am. J. Physiol. Circ. Physiol.* **2008**, *295*, H1377–H1384. [CrossRef]
8. Sluimer, J.C.; Gasc, J.M.; Hamming, I.; van Goor, H.; Michaud, A.; van den Akker, L.H.; Jutten, B.; Cleutjens, J.; Bijnens, A.P.; Corvol, P.; et al. Angiotensin-converting enzyme 2 (ACE2) expression and activity in human carotid atherosclerotic lesions. *J. Pathol.* **2008**, *215*, 273–279. [CrossRef]
9. Schiffrin, E.L.; Flack, J.; Ito, S.; Muntner, P.; Webb, C. Hypertension and COVID-19. *Am. J. Hypertens.* **2020**, *33*, 33–373. [CrossRef]
10. Richardson, S.; Hirsch, J.S.; Narasimhan, M.; Crawford, J.M.; McGinn, T.; Davidson, K.W. The Northwell COVID-19 Research Consortium. Presenting Characteristics, Comorbidities, and Outcomes among 5700 Patients Hospitalized With COVID-19 in the New York City Area. *JAMA* **2020**. [CrossRef]
11. Chen, T.; Wu, D.; Chen, H.; Yan, W.; Yang, D.; Chen, G.; Ma, K.; Xu, D.; Yu, H.; Wang, H.; et al. Clinical characteristics of 113 deceased patients with coronavirus disease 2019: Retrospective study. *BMJ* **2020**, *368*, m1091. [CrossRef] [PubMed]
12. Myers, L.C.; Parodi, S.M.; Escobar, G.J.; Liu, V.X. Characteristics of Hospitalized Adults With COVID-19 in an Integrated Health Care System in California. *JAMA* **2020**. [CrossRef] [PubMed]
13. Guan, W.J.; Liang, W.H.; Zhao, Y.; Liang, H.R.; Chen, Z.S.; Li, Y.M.; Liu, X.Q.; Chen, R.C.; Tang, C.L.; Wang, T.; et al. Comorbidity and its impact on 1590 patients with Covid-19 in China: A Nationwide Analysis. *Eur. Respir. J.* **2020**, 2000547. [CrossRef] [PubMed]

14. Zhou, F.; Yu, T.; Du, R.; Fan, G.; Liu, Y.; Liu, Z.; Xiang, J.; Wang, Y.; Song, B.; Gu, X.; et al. Clinical course and risk factors for mortality of adult inpatients with COVID-19 in Wuhan, China: A retrospective cohort study. *Lancet* **2020**, *395*, 1054–1062. [CrossRef]
15. Bikdeli, B.; Madhavan, M.V.; Jimenez, D.; Chuich, T.; Dreyfus, I.; Driggin, E.; Nigoghossian, C.; Ageno, W.; Madjid, M.; Guo, Y.; et al. Lip GYH. COVID-19 and Thrombotic or Thromboembolic Disease: Implications for Prevention, Antithrombotic Therapy, and Follow-up. *J. Am. Coll. Cardiol.* **2020**. [CrossRef]
16. Klok, F.A.; Kruip, M.; van der Meer, N.J.M.; Arbous, M.S.; Gommers, D.; Kant, K.M.; Kaptein, F.H.J.; van Paassen, J.; Stals, M.A.M.; Huisman, M.V.; et al. Incidence of thrombotic complications in critically ill ICU patients with COVID-19. *Thromb. Res.* **2020**. [CrossRef]
17. Durvasula, R.; Wellington, T.; McNamara, E.; Watnick, S. COVID-19 and Kidney Failure in the Acute Care Setting: Our Experience From Seattle. *Am. J. Kidney Dis.* **2020**. [CrossRef]
18. Ronco, C.; Reis, T. Kidney involvement in COVID-19 and rationale for extracorporeal therapies. *Nat. Rev. Nephrol.* **2020**, 1–3. [CrossRef]
19. Rotzinger, D.C.; Beigelman-Aubry, C.; von Garnier, C.; Qanadli, S.D. Pulmonary embolism in patients with COVID-19: Time to change the paradigm of computed tomography. *Thromb. Res.* **2020**, *190*, 58–59. [CrossRef]
20. Poissy, J.; Goutay, J.; Caplan, M.; Parmentier, E.; Duburcq, T.; Lassalle, F.; Jeanpierre, E.; Rauch, A.; Labreuche, J.; Susen, S. Pulmonary Embolism in COVID-19 Patients: Awareness of an Increased Prevalence. *Circulation* **2020**. [CrossRef]
21. Aggarwal, G.; Lippi, G.; Michael Henry, B. Cerebrovascular disease is associated with an increased disease severity in patients with Coronavirus Disease 2019 (COVID-19): A pooled analysis of published literature. *Int. J. Stroke* **2020**, 1747493020921664. [CrossRef] [PubMed]
22. Mao, L.; Jin, H.; Wang, M.; Hu, Y.; Chen, S.; He, Q.; Chang, J.; Hong, C.; Zhou, Y.; Wang, D.; et al. Neurologic Manifestations of Hospitalized Patients With Coronavirus Disease 2019 in Wuhan, China. *JAMA Neurol.* **2020**. [CrossRef] [PubMed]
23. Santulli, G.; Morelli, M.; Gambardella, J. Is Endothelial Dysfunction the Concealed Cornerstone of COVID-19? *BMJ* **2020**, in press.
24. Cooke, J.P. The endothelium: A new target for therapy. *Vasc. Med.* **2000**, *5*, 49–53. [CrossRef] [PubMed]
25. Aird, W.C. Endothelium as an organ system. *Crit. Care Med.* **2004**, *32*, S271–S279. [CrossRef] [PubMed]
26. Inagami, T.; Naruse, M.; Hoover, R. Endothelium as an endocrine organ. *Annu. Rev. Physiol.* **1995**, *57*, 171–189. [CrossRef] [PubMed]
27. Riphagen, S.; Gomez, R.; Gonzalez-Martinez, C.; Wilkinson, N.; Theocharis, P. Hyperinflammatory shock in children during COVID-19 pandemic. *Lancet* **2020**, in press. [CrossRef]
28. Letko, M.; Marzi, A.; Munster, V. Functional assessment of cell entry and receptor usage for SARS-CoV-2 and other lineage B betacoronaviruses. *Nat. Microbiol.* **2020**, *5*, 562–569. [CrossRef]
29. Wang, Q.; Zhang, Y.; Wu, L.; Niu, S.; Song, C.; Zhang, Z.; Lu, G.; Qiao, C.; Hu, Y.; Yuen, K.Y.; et al. Structural and Functional Basis of SARS-CoV-2 Entry by Using Human ACE2. *Cell* **2020**. [CrossRef]
30. Guzzi, P.H.; Mercatelli, D.; Ceraolo, C.; Giorgi, F.M. Master Regulator Analysis of the SARS-CoV-2/Human Interactome. *J. Clin. Med.* **2020**, *9*, 982. [CrossRef]
31. Xu, H.; Zhong, L.; Deng, J.; Peng, J.; Dan, H.; Zeng, X.; Li, T.; Chen, Q. High expression of ACE2 receptor of 2019-nCoV on the epithelial cells of oral mucosa. *Int. J. Oral Sci.* **2020**, *12*, 8. [CrossRef] [PubMed]
32. Jia, H.P.; Look, D.C.; Shi, L.; Hickey, M.; Pewe, L.; Netland, J.; Farzan, M.; Wohlford-Lenane, C.; Perlman, S.; McCray, P.B., Jr. ACE2 receptor expression and severe acute respiratory syndrome coronavirus infection depend on differentiation of human airway epithelia. *J. Virol.* **2005**, *79*, 14614–14621. [CrossRef] [PubMed]
33. Perico, L.; Benigni, A.; Remuzzi, G. Should COVID-19 Concern Nephrologists? Why and to What Extent? The Emerging Impasse of Angiotensin Blockade. *Nephron* **2020**, 1–9. [CrossRef] [PubMed]
34. Gheblawi, M.; Wang, K.; Viveiros, A.; Nguyen, Q.; Zhong, J.; Turner, A.T.; Raizada, M.K.; Grant, M.B.; Oudit, G.Y. Angiotensin Converting Enzyme 2: SARS-CoV-2 Receptor and Regulator of the Renin-Angiotensin System. *Circ. Res.* **2020**, *126*. [CrossRef] [PubMed]
35. Li, M.; Chen, L.; Zhang, J.; Xiong, C.; Li, X. The SARS-CoV-2 receptor ACE2 expression of maternal-fetal interface and fetal organs by single-cell transcriptome study. *PLoS ONE* **2020**, *15*, e0230295. [CrossRef]
36. Gallagher, T.M.; Buchmeier, M.J. Coronavirus spike proteins in viral entry and pathogenesis. *Virology* **2001**, *279*, 371–374. [CrossRef]

37. Matsuyama, S.; Nao, N.; Shirato, K.; Kawase, M.; Saito, S.; Takayama, I.; Nagata, N.; Sekizuka, T.; Katoh, H.; Kato, F.; et al. Enhanced isolation of SARS-CoV-2 by TMPRSS2-expressing cells. *Proc. Natl. Acad. Sci. USA* **2020**, *117*, 7001–7003. [CrossRef]
38. Sungnak, W.; Huang, N.; Becavin, C.; Berg, M.; Queen, R.; Litvinukova, M.; Talavera-Lopez, C.; Maatz, H.; Reichart, D.; Sampaziotis, F.; et al. SARS-CoV-2 entry factors are highly expressed in nasal epithelial cells together with innate immune genes. *Nat. Med.* **2020**. [CrossRef]
39. Tortorici, M.A.; Walls, A.C.; Lang, Y.; Wang, C.; Li, Z.; Koerhuis, D.; Boons, G.-J.; Bosch, B.-J.; Rey, F.A.; De Groot, R.J.; et al. Structural basis for human coronavirus attachment to sialic acid receptors. *Nat. Struct. Mol. Biol.* **2019**, *26*, 481–489. [CrossRef]
40. Hulswit, R.; Lang, Y.; Bakkers, M.J.G.; Li, W.; Li, Z.; Schouten, A.; Ophorst, B.; Van Kuppeveld, F.J.M.; Boons, G.-J.; Bosch, B.-J.; et al. Human coronaviruses OC43 and HKU1 bind to 9-O-acetylated sialic acids via a conserved receptor-binding site in spike protein domain A. *Proc. Natl. Acad. Sci. USA* **2019**, *116*, 2681–2690. [CrossRef]
41. Chen, Z.; Mi, L.; Xu, J.; Yu, J.; Wang, X.; Jiang, J.; Xing, J.; Shang, P.; Qian, A.; Li, Y.; et al. Function of HAb18G/CD147 in invasion of host cells by severe acute respiratory syndrome coronavirus. *J. Infect. Dis.* **2005**, *191*, 755–760. [CrossRef] [PubMed]
42. Ou, X.; Liu, Y.; Lei, X.; Li, P.; Mi, D.; Ren, L.; Guo, L.; Guo, R.; Chen, T.; Hu, J.; et al. Characterization of spike glycoprotein of SARS-CoV-2 on virus entry and its immune cross-reactivity with SARS-CoV. *Nat. Commun.* **2020**, *11*, 1620. [CrossRef] [PubMed]
43. Yang, J.; Feng, X.; Zhou, Q.; Cheng, W.; Shang, C.; Han, P.; Lin, C.-H.; Chen, H.-S.V.; Quertermous, T.; Chang, C.-P. Pathological Ace2-to-Ace enzyme switch in the stressed heart is transcriptionally controlled by the endothelial Brg1-FoxM1 complex. *Proc. Natl. Acad. Sci. USA* **2016**, *113*, E5628–E5635. [CrossRef] [PubMed]
44. Aimes, R.; Zijlstra, A.; Hooper, J.; Ogbourne, S.; Sit, M.-L.; Fuchs, S.; Gotley, D.; Quigley, J.P.; Antalis, T. Endothelial cell serine proteases expressed during vascular morphogenesis and angiogenesis. *Thromb. Haemost.* **2003**, *89*, 561–572. [CrossRef] [PubMed]
45. Huang, D.T.-N.; Lu, C.-Y.; Chi, Y.; Li, W.-L.; Chang, L.-Y.; Lai, M.-J.; Chen, J.-S.; Hsu, W.-M.; Huang, L.-M. Adaptation of influenza A (H7N9) virus in primary human airway epithelial cells. *Sci. Rep.* **2017**, *7*, 11300. [CrossRef]
46. Vanarsdall, A.L.; Pritchard, S.R.; Wisner, T.W.; Liu, J.; Jardetzky, T.S.; Johnson, D.C. CD147 Promotes Entry of Pentamer-Expressing Human Cytomegalovirus into Epithelial and Endothelial Cells. *mBio* **2018**, *9*, e00781-18. [CrossRef]
47. Im, E.; Venkatakrishnan, A.; Kazlauskas, A. Cathepsin B regulates the intrinsic angiogenic threshold of endothelial cells. *Mol. Biol. Cell.* **2005**, *16*, 3488–3500. [CrossRef]
48. Platt, M.O.; Shockey, W.A. Endothelial cells and cathepsins: Biochemical and biomechanical regulation. *Biochimie* **2016**, *122*, 314–323. [CrossRef]
49. Cai, J.; Zhong, H.; Wu, J.; Chen, R.-F.; Yang, H.; Al-Abed, Y.; Li, Y.; Li, X.; Jiang, W.; Montenegro, M.F.; et al. Cathepsin L promotes Vascular Intimal Hyperplasia after Arterial Injury. *Mol. Med.* **2017**, *23*, 92–100. [CrossRef]
50. Rivellese, F.; Prediletto, E. ACE2 at the centre of COVID-19 from paucisymptomatic infections to severe pneumonia. *Autoimmun. Rev.* **2020**, 102536. [CrossRef]
51. Touyz, R.M.; Li, H.; Delles, C. ACE2 the Janus-faced protein—From cardiovascular protection to severe acute respiratory syndrome-coronavirus and COVID-19. *Clin. Sci. (Lond.)* **2020**, *134*, 747–750. [CrossRef]
52. Leng, Z.; Zhu, R.; Hou, W.; Fengchun, Z.; Yangyang, Z.; Luchan, D.; Shan, G.; Meng, F.; Du, D.; Wang, S.; et al. Transplantation of ACE2(-) Mesenchymal Stem Cells Improves the Outcome of Patients with COVID-19 Pneumonia. *Aging Dis.* **2020**, *11*, 216–228. [CrossRef] [PubMed]
53. Brake, S.; Barnsley, K.; Lu, W.; McAlinden, K.; Eapen, M.S.; Sohal, S.S. Smoking Upregulates Angiotensin-Converting Enzyme-2 Receptor: A Potential Adhesion Site for Novel Coronavirus SARS-CoV-2 (Covid-19). *J. Clin. Med.* **2020**, *9*, 841. [CrossRef] [PubMed]
54. Jakovac, H. COVID-19-is the ACE2 just a foe? *Am. J. Physiol. Cell. Mol. Physiol.* **2020**. [CrossRef] [PubMed]
55. Zou, Z.; Yan, Y.; Shu, Y.; Gao, R.; Sun, Y.; Li, X.; Ju, X.; Liang, Z.; Liu, Q.; Zhao, Y.; et al. Angiotensin-converting enzyme 2 protects from lethal avian influenza A H5N1 infections. *Nat. Commun.* **2014**, *5*, 3594. [CrossRef] [PubMed]

56. Guo, J.; Huang, Z.; Lin, L.; Lv, J. Coronavirus Disease 2019 (COVID-19) and Cardiovascular Disease: A Viewpoint on the Potential Influence of Angiotensin-Converting Enzyme Inhibitors/Angiotensin Receptor Blockers on Onset and Severity of Severe Acute Respiratory Syndrome Coronavirus 2 Infection. *J. Am. Heart Assoc.* **2020**, *9*, e016219. [PubMed]
57. Mourad, J.-J.; Levy, B.I. Interaction between RAAS inhibitors and ACE2 in the context of COVID-19. *Nat. Rev. Cardiol.* **2020**, *17*, 313. [CrossRef]
58. South, A.M.; Diz, D.; Chappell, M.C. COVID-19, ACE2 and the Cardiovascular Consequences. *Am. J. Physiol. Heart Circ. Physiol.* **2020**. [CrossRef]
59. Chen, L.; Li, X.; Chen, M.; Feng, Y.; Xiong, C. The ACE2 expression in human heart indicates new potential mechanism of heart injury among patients infected with SARS-CoV-2. *Cardiovasc. Res.* **2020**, *116*, 1097–1100. [CrossRef]
60. Sommerstein, R.; Kochen, M.M.; Messerli, F.H.; Grani, C. Coronavirus Disease 2019 (COVID-19): Do Angiotensin-Converting Enzyme Inhibitors/Angiotensin Receptor Blockers Have a Biphasic Effect? *J. Am. Heart Assoc.* **2020**, *9*, e016509. [CrossRef]
61. Danser, A.J.; Epstein, M.; Batlle, D. Renin-Angiotensin System Blockers and the COVID-19 Pandemic: At Present There Is No Evidence to Abandon Renin-Angiotensin System Blockers. *Hypertension* **2020**, 12015082. [CrossRef] [PubMed]
62. Wang, M.; Hao, H.; Leeper, N.J.; Zhu, L. Thrombotic Regulation from the Endothelial Cell Perspectives. *Arter. Thromb. Vasc. Biol.* **2018**, *38*, e90–e95. [CrossRef] [PubMed]
63. Bernfield, M.; Götte, M.; Park, P.W.; Reizes, O.; Fitzgerald, M.L.; Lincecum, J.; Zako, M. Functions of cell surface heparan sulfate proteoglycans. *Annu. Rev. Biochem.* **1999**, *68*, 729–777. [CrossRef] [PubMed]
64. Mast, A.E. Tissue Factor Pathway Inhibitor: Multiple Anticoagulant Activities for a Single Protein. *Arter. Thromb. Vasc. Biol.* **2016**, *36*, 9–14. [CrossRef]
65. Martin, F.A.; Murphy, R.P.; Cummins, P.M. Thrombomodulin and the vascular endothelium: Insights into functional, regulatory, and therapeutic aspects. *Am. J. Physiol. Circ. Physiol.* **2013**, *304*, H1585–H1597. [CrossRef]
66. Oliver, J.; Webb, D.J.; Newby, D.E. Stimulated tissue plasminogen activator release as a marker of endothelial function in humans. *Arter. Thromb. Vasc. Biol.* **2005**, *25*, 2470–2479. [CrossRef]
67. Huber, D.; Cramer, E.M.; Kaufmann, J.E.; Meda, P.; Massé, J.-M.; Kruithof, E.K.O.; Vischer, U.M. Tissue-type plasminogen activator (t-PA) is stored in Weibel-Palade bodies in human endothelial cells both in vitro and in vivo. *Blood* **2002**, *99*, 3637–3645. [CrossRef]
68. Godo, S.; Shimokawa, H. Endothelial Functions. *Arter. Thromb. Vasc Biol.* **2017**, *37*, e108–e114. [CrossRef]
69. Vanhoutte, P.M.; Shimokawa, H.; Tang, E.H.; Feletou, M. Endothelial dysfunction and vascular disease. *Acta Physiol.* **2009**, *196*, 193–222. [CrossRef]
70. Boyce, S.; Lwaleed, B.; Kazmi, R. Homeostasis of Hemostasis: The Role of Endothelium. *Semin. Thromb. Hemost.* **2015**, *41*, 549–555. [CrossRef]
71. Loscalzo, J. Oxidative stress in endothelial cell dysfunction and thrombosis. *Pathophysiol. Haemost. Thromb.* **2002**, *32*, 359–360. [CrossRef] [PubMed]
72. Santulli, G. Endothelial cells: The heart attack of the Clones. *Sci. Transl. Med.* **2018**, *10*, eaar7529. [CrossRef] [PubMed]
73. Avogaro, A.; Albiero, M.; Menegazzo, L.; De Kreutzenberg, S.; Fadini, G.P. Endothelial dysfunction in diabetes: The role of reparatory mechanisms. *Diabetes Care* **2011**, *34* (Suppl. 2), S285–S290. [CrossRef] [PubMed]
74. Goligorsky, M.S. Vascular endothelium in diabetes. *Am. J. Physiol. Physiol.* **2017**, *312*, F266–F275. [CrossRef] [PubMed]
75. Kaur, R.; Kaur, M.; Singh, J. Endothelial dysfunction and platelet hyperactivity in type 2 diabetes mellitus: Molecular insights and therapeutic strategies. *Cardiovasc. Diabetol.* **2018**, *17*, 121. [CrossRef]
76. Maamoun, H.; Abdelsalam, S.S.; Zeidan, A.; Korashy, H.M.; Agouni, A. Endoplasmic Reticulum Stress: A Critical Molecular Driver of Endothelial Dysfunction and Cardiovascular Disturbances Associated with Diabetes. *Int. J. Mol. Sci.* **2019**, *20*, 1658. [CrossRef]
77. Eringa, E.C.; Serné, E.H.; Meijer, R.I.; Schalkwijk, C.G.; Houben, A.J.H.M.; Stehouwer, C.D.A.; Smulders, Y.M.; Van Hinsbergh, V.W.M. Endothelial dysfunction in (pre)diabetes: Characteristics, causative mechanisms and pathogenic role in type 2 diabetes. *Rev. Endocr. Metab. Disord.* **2013**, *14*, 39–48. [CrossRef]

78. Jansson, P.A. Endothelial dysfunction in insulin resistance and type 2 diabetes. *J. Intern. Med.* **2007**, *262*, 173–183. [CrossRef]
79. Gambardella, J.; Sardu, C.; Santulli, G. COVID-19 and endothelial dysfunction. *JAMA* **2020**, in press.
80. Esler, M.; Esler, D. Can angiotensin receptor-blocking drugs perhaps be harmful in the COVID-19 pandemic? *J. Hypertens.* **2020**, *38*, 781–782. [CrossRef]
81. Fang, L.; Karakiulakis, G.; Roth, M. Are patients with hypertension and diabetes mellitus at increased risk for COVID-19 infection? *Lancet Respir. Med.* **2020**, *8*, e21. [CrossRef]
82. Nascimento, I.J.B.D.; Cacic, N.; Abdulazeem, H.M.; Von Groote, T.; Jayarajah, U.; Weerasekara, I.; Esfahani, M.A.; Civile, V.T.; Marusic, A.; Jeroncic, A.; et al. Novel Coronavirus Infection (COVID-19) in Humans: A Scoping Review and Meta-Analysis. *Clin. Med.* **2020**, *9*, 941. [CrossRef] [PubMed]
83. Wu, J.T.; Leung, K.; Bushman, M.; Kishore, N.; Niehus, R.; De Salazar, P.M.; Cowling, B.J.; Lipsitch, M.; Leung, G.M. Estimating clinical severity of COVID-19 from the transmission dynamics in Wuhan, China. *Nat. Med.* **2020**, *26*, 506–510. [CrossRef] [PubMed]
84. Guan, W.-J.; Ni, Z.-Y.; Hu, Y.; Liang, W.-H.; Ou, C.-Q.; He, J.-X.; Liu, L.; Shan, H.; Lei, C.-L.; Hui, D.S.; et al. Clinical Characteristics of Coronavirus Disease 2019 in China. *N. Engl. J. Med.* **2020**, *382*, 1708–1720. [CrossRef] [PubMed]
85. Huang, C.; Wang, Y.; Li, X.; Ren, L.; Zhao, J.; Hu, Y.; Zhang, L.; Fan, G.; Xu, J.; Gu, X.; et al. Clinical features of patients infected with 2019 novel coronavirus in Wuhan, China. *Lancet* **2020**, *395*, 497–506. [CrossRef]
86. Wang, D.; Hu, B.; Hu, C.; Zhu, F.; Liu, X.; Zhang, J.; Wang, B.; Xiang, H.; Cheng, Z.; Xiong, Y.; et al. Clinical Characteristics of 138 Hospitalized Patients With 2019 Novel Coronavirus-Infected Pneumonia in Wuhan, China. *JAMA* **2020**, *323*, 1061. [CrossRef]
87. Zhang, J.-J.; Dong, X.; Cao, Y.-Y.; Yuan, Y.-D.; Yang, Y.-B.; Yan, Y.-Q.; Akdis, C.A.; Gao, Y.-D. Clinical characteristics of 140 patients infected with SARS-CoV-2 in Wuhan, China. *Allergy* **2020**. [CrossRef]
88. Williams, B.; Mancia, G.; Spiering, W.; Rosei, E.A.; Azizi, M.; Burnier, M.; Clement, D.L.; Coca, A.; De Simone, G.; Dominiczak, A.F.; et al. 2018 ESC/ESH Guidelines for the management of arterial hypertension. *Eur. Heart J.* **2018**, *39*, 3021–3104. [CrossRef]
89. Vaduganathan, M.; Vardeny, O.; Michel, T.; McMurray, J.J.V.; Pfeffer, M.A.; Solomon, S. Renin-Angiotensin-Aldosterone System Inhibitors in Patients with Covid-19. *N. Engl. J. Med.* **2020**, *382*, 1653–1659. [CrossRef]
90. Gurwitz, D. Angiotensin receptor blockers as tentative SARS-CoV-2 therapeutics. *Drug Dev. Res.* **2020**. [CrossRef]
91. Li, J.; Wang, X.; Chen, J.; Zhang, H.; Deng, A. Association of Renin-Angiotensin System Inhibitors With Severity or Risk of Death in Patients With Hypertension Hospitalized for Coronavirus Disease 2019 (COVID-19) Infection in Wuhan, China. *JAMA Cardiol.* **2020**. [CrossRef] [PubMed]
92. Ferrario, C.M.; Jessup, J.; Chappell, M.; Averill, D.B.; Brosnihan, K.B.; Tallant, E.A.; Diz, D.I.; Gallagher, P.E. Effect of angiotensin-converting enzyme inhibition and angiotensin II receptor blockers on cardiac angiotensin-converting enzyme 2. *Circulation* **2005**, *111*, 2605–2610. [CrossRef] [PubMed]
93. Jessup, J.A.; Gallagher, P.E.; Averill, D.B.; Brosnihan, K.B.; Tallant, E.A.; Chappell, M.C.; Ferrario, C.M. Effect of angiotensin II blockade on a new congenic model of hypertension derived from transgenic Ren-2 rats. *Am. J. Physiol. Circ. Physiol.* **2006**, *291*, H2166–H2172. [CrossRef] [PubMed]
94. Igase, M.; Strawn, W.B.; Gallagher, P.E.; Geary, R.L.; Ferrario, C.M. Angiotensin II AT1 receptors regulate ACE2 and angiotensin-(1-7) expression in the aorta of spontaneously hypertensive rats. *Am. J. Physiol. Circ. Physiol.* **2005**, *289*, H1013–H1019. [CrossRef]
95. South, A.M.; Tomlinson, L.; Edmonston, D.; Hiremath, S.; Sparks, M.A. Controversies of renin-angiotensin system inhibition during the COVID-19 pandemic. *Nat. Rev. Nephrol.* **2020**. [CrossRef]
96. Ferrario, C.M.; Ahmad, S.; Groban, L. Mechanisms by which angiotensin-receptor blockers increase ACE2 levels. *Nat. Rev. Cardiol.* **2020**. [CrossRef]
97. Ishiyama, Y.; Gallagher, P.E.; Averill, D.B.; Tallant, E.A.; Brosnihan, K.B.; Ferrario, C.M. Upregulation of angiotensin-converting enzyme 2 after myocardial infarction by blockade of angiotensin II receptors. *Hypertension* **2004**, *43*, 970–976. [CrossRef]
98. Jin, H.-Y.; Song, B.; Oudit, G.Y.; Davidge, S.T.; Yu, H.-M.; Jiang, Y.-Y.; Gao, P.-J.; Zhu, D.-L.; Ning, G.; Kassiri, Z.; et al. ACE2 deficiency enhances angiotensin II-mediated aortic profilin-1 expression, inflammation and peroxynitrite production. *PLoS ONE* **2012**, *7*, e38502. [CrossRef]

99. Soler, M.J.; Ye, M.; Wysocki, J.; William, J.; Lloveras, J.; Batlle, D. Localization of ACE2 in the renal vasculature: Amplification by angiotensin II type 1 receptor blockade using telmisartan. *Am. J. Physiol. Physiol.* **2009**, *296*, F398–F405. [CrossRef]
100. Patel, V.B.; Clarke, N.; Wang, Z.; Fan, D.; Parajuli, N.; Basu, R.; Putko, B.; Kassiri, Z.; Turner, A.J.; Oudit, G.Y. Angiotensin II induced proteolytic cleavage of myocardial ACE2 is mediated by TACE/ADAM-17: A positive feedback mechanism in the RAS. *J. Mol. Cell. Cardiol.* **2014**, *66*, 167–176. [CrossRef]
101. Yamamuro, M.; Yoshimura, M.; Nakayama, M.; Abe, K.; Sumida, H.; Sugiyama, S.; Saito, Y.; Nakao, K.; Yasue, H.; Ogawa, H. Aldosterone, but not angiotensin II, reduces angiotensin converting enzyme 2 gene expression levels in cultured neonatal rat cardiomyocytes. *Circ. J.* **2008**, *72*, 1346–1350. [CrossRef] [PubMed]
102. Keidar, S.; Gamliel-Lazarovich, A.; Kaplan, M.; Pavlotzky, E.; Hamoud, S.; Hayek, T.; Karry, R.; Abassi, Z. Mineralocorticoid Receptor Blocker Increases Angiotensin-Converting Enzyme 2 Activity in Congestive Heart Failure Patients. *Circ. Res.* **2005**, *97*, 946–953. [CrossRef] [PubMed]
103. Furuhashi, M.; Moniwa, N.; Mita, T.; Fuseya, T.; Ishimura, S.; Ohno, K.; Shibata, S.; Tanaka, M.; Watanabe, Y.; Akasaka, H.; et al. Urinary angiotensin-converting enzyme 2 in hypertensive patients may be increased by olmesartan, an angiotensin II receptor blocker. *Am. J. Hypertens.* **2015**, *28*, 15–21. [CrossRef] [PubMed]
104. Rice, G.I.; Thomas, D.A.; Grant, P.J.; Turner, A.J.; Hooper, N.M. Evaluation of angiotensin-converting enzyme (ACE), its homologue ACE2 and neprilysin in angiotensin peptide metabolism. *Biochem. J.* **2004**, *383*, 45–51. [CrossRef] [PubMed]
105. Nicholls, J.; Peiris, M. Good ACE, bad ACE do battle in lung injury, SARS. *Nat. Med.* **2005**, *11*, 821–822. [CrossRef] [PubMed]
106. Santos, R.A. Angiotensin-(1-7). *Hypertension* **2014**, *63*, 1138–1147. [CrossRef] [PubMed]
107. El-Hashim, A.Z.; Renno, W.M.; Raghupathy, R.; Abduo, H.T.; Akhtar, S.; Benter, I.F. Angiotensin-(1-7) inhibits allergic inflammation, via the MAS1 receptor, through suppression of ERK1/2- and NF-kappaB-dependent pathways. *Br. J. Pharmacol.* **2012**, *166*, 1964–1976. [CrossRef]
108. Kuba, K.; Imai, Y.; Rao, S.; Gao, H.; Guo, F.; Guan, B.; Huan, Y.; Yang, P.; Zhang, Y.; Deng, W.; et al. A crucial role of angiotensin converting enzyme 2 (ACE2) in SARS coronavirus-induced lung injury. *Nat. Med.* **2005**, *11*, 875–879. [CrossRef]
109. Povlsen, A.L.; Grimm, D.; Wehland, M.; Infanger, M.; Kruger, M. The Vasoactive Mas Receptor in Essential Hypertension. *J. Clin. Med.* **2020**, *9*, 267. [CrossRef]
110. Patel, A.B.; Verma, A. COVID-19 and Angiotensin-Converting Enzyme Inhibitors and Angiotensin Receptor Blockers: What Is the Evidence? *JAMA* **2020**. [CrossRef]
111. de Simone, G.; Mancusi, C. Speculation is not evidence: Antihypertensive therapy and COVID-19. *Eur. Heart J. Cardiovasc. Pharm.* **2020**. [CrossRef] [PubMed]
112. Iaccarino, G.; Borghi, C.; Cicero, A.F.G.; Ferri, C.; Minuz, P.; Muiesan, M.L.; Mulatero, P.; Mule, G.; Pucci, G.; Salvetti, M.; et al. Renin-Angiotensin System Inhibition in Cardiovascular Patients at the Time of COVID19: Much Ado for Nothing? A Statement of Activity from the Directors of the Board and the Scientific Directors of the Italian Society of Hypertension. *High Blood Press. Cardiovasc. Prev.* **2020**, *27*, 105–108. [CrossRef] [PubMed]
113. Sultana, J.; Trotta, F.; Addis, A.; Brown, J.S.; Gil, M.; Menniti-Ippolito, F.; Milozzi, F.; Suissa, S.; Trifiro, G. Healthcare Database Networks for Drug Regulatory Policies: International Workshop on the Canadian, US and Spanish Experience and Future Steps for Italy. *Drug Saf.* **2020**, *43*, 1–5. [CrossRef] [PubMed]
114. Talreja, H.; Tan, J.; Dawes, M.; Supershad, S.; Rabindranath, K.; Fisher, J.; Valappil, S.; van der Merwe, V.; Wong, L.; van der Merwe, W.; et al. A consensus statement on the use of angiotensin receptor blockers and angiotensin converting enzyme inhibitors in relation to COVID-19 (corona virus disease 2019). *N. Z. Med. J.* **2020**, *133*, 85–87.
115. Zhang, P.; Zhu, L.; Cai, J.; Lei, F.; Qin, J.J.; Xie, J.; Liu, Y.M.; Zhao, Y.C.; Huang, X.; Lin, L.; et al. Association of Inpatient Use of Angiotensin Converting Enzyme Inhibitors and Angiotensin II Receptor Blockers with Mortality Among Patients With Hypertension Hospitalized With COVID-19. *Circ. Res.* **2020**. [CrossRef]
116. Yang, G.; Tan, Z.; Zhou, L.; Yang, M.; Peng, L.; Liu, J.; Cai, J.; Yang, R.; Han, J.; Huang, Y.; et al. Effects Of ARBs And ACEIs On Virus Infection, Inflammatory Status And Clinical Outcomes In COVID-19 Patients With Hypertension: A Single Center Retrospective Study. *Hypertension* **2020**. [CrossRef]
117. Mehra, M.; Desai, S.; Kuy, S.; Henry, T.; Patel, A. Cardiovascular Disease, Drug Therapy, and Mortality in Covid-19. *NEJM* **2019**, in press. [CrossRef]

118. Reynolds, H.; Adhikari, S.; Pulgarin, C.; Troxel, A.; Iturrate, E.; Johnson, S.; Hausvater, A.; Newman, J.; Berger, J.; Bangalore, S.; et al. Renin–Angiotensin–Aldosterone System Inhibitors and Risk of Covid-19. *NEJM* **2019**, in press. [CrossRef]
119. Mancia, G.; Rea, F.; Ludergnani, M.; Apolone, G.; Corrao, G. Renin–Angiotensin–Aldosterone System Inhibitors and Risk of Covid-19. *NEJM* **2019**, in press.
120. Rajagopalan, S.; Harrison, D.G. Reversing endothelial dysfunction with ACE inhibitors. A new trend. *Circulation* **1996**, *94*, 240–243. [CrossRef]
121. Beckman, J.A.; Creager, M.A. The nonlipid effects of statins on endothelial function. *Trends Cardiovasc. Med.* **2006**, *16*, 156–162. [CrossRef]
122. Ruszkowski, P.; Masajtis-Zagajewska, A.; Nowicki, M. Effects of combined statin and ACE inhibitor therapy on endothelial function and blood pressure in essential hypertension—A randomised double-blind, placebo controlled crossover study. *J. Renin Angiotensin Aldosterone Syst.* **2019**, *20*, 1470320319868890. [CrossRef]
123. Blum, A.; Shamburek, R. The pleiotropic effects of statins on endothelial function, vascular inflammation, immunomodulation and thrombogenesis. *Atherosclerosis* **2009**, *203*, 325–330. [CrossRef]
124. Glowacka, I.; Bertram, S.; Herzog, P.; Pfefferle, S.; Steffen, I.; Muench, M.O.; Simmons, G.; Hofmann, H.; Kuri, T.; Weber, F.; et al. Differential downregulation of ACE2 by the spike proteins of severe acute respiratory syndrome coronavirus and human coronavirus NL63. *J. Virol.* **2010**, *84*, 1198–1205. [CrossRef]
125. Luque, M.; Martin, P.; Martell, N.; Fernandez, C.; Brosnihan, K.B.; Ferrario, C.M. Effects of captopril related to increased levels of prostacyclin and angiotensin-(1-7) in essential hypertension. *J. Hypertens.* **1996**, *14*, 799–805. [CrossRef]
126. Chen, L.; Hao, G. The role of angiotensin-converting enzyme 2 in coronaviruses/influenza viruses and cardiovascular disease. *Cardiovasc. Res.* **2020**. [CrossRef]
127. Murray, E.; Tomaszewski, M.; Guzik, T.J. Binding of SARS-CoV-2 and angiotensin-converting enzyme 2: Clinical implications. *Cardiovasc. Res.* **2020**. [CrossRef]
128. Sunden-Cullberg, J. Chronic Use of Angiotensin-Converting Enzyme Inhibitors and Angiotensin II Receptor Blockers Is High Among Intensive Care Unit Patients With Non-COVID-19 Sepsis but Carry a Moderately Increased Risk of Death. *Hypertension* **2020**. [CrossRef]
129. Fan, Z.; Wu, G.; Yue, M.; Ye, J.; Chen, Y.; Xu, B.; Shu, Z.; Zhu, J.; Lu, N.; Tan, X. Hypertension and hypertensive left ventricular hypertrophy are associated with ACE2 genetic polymorphism. *Life Sci.* **2019**, *225*, 39–45. [CrossRef]
130. Pinheiro, D.S.; Santos, R.S.; Jardim, P.; Silva, E.G.; Reis, A.A.S.; Pedrino, G.R.; Ulhoa, C.J. The combination of ACE I/D and ACE2 G8790A polymorphisms revels susceptibility to hypertension: A genetic association study in Brazilian patients. *PLoS ONE* **2019**, *14*, e0221248. [CrossRef]
131. Lackland, D.T. Racial differences in hypertension: Implications for high blood pressure management. *Am. J. Med. Sci.* **2014**, *348*, 135–138. [CrossRef] [PubMed]
132. Bonow, R.O.; Fonarow, G.C.; O'Gara, P.T.; Yancy, C.W. Association of Coronavirus Disease 2019 (COVID-19) With Myocardial Injury and Mortality. *JAMA Cardiol.* **2020**. [CrossRef] [PubMed]
133. Guo, T.; Fan, Y.; Chen, M.; Wu, X.; Zhang, L.; He, T.; Wang, H.; Wan, J.; Wang, X.; Lu, Z. Cardiovascular Implications of Fatal Outcomes of Patients With Coronavirus Disease 2019 (COVID-19). *JAMA Cardiol.* **2020**. [CrossRef]
134. De Filippo, O.; D'Ascenzo, F.; Angelini, F.; Bocchino, P.P.; Conrotto, F.; Saglietto, A.; Secco, G.G.; Campo, G.; Gallone, G.; Verardi, R.; et al. Reduced Rate of Hospital Admissions for ACS during Covid-19 Outbreak in Northern Italy. *New Engl. J. Med.* **2020**. [CrossRef]
135. Garcia, S.; Albaghdadi, M.S.; Meraj, P.M.; Schmidt, C.; Garberich, R.; Jaffer, F.A.; Dixon, S.; Rade, J.J.; Tannenbaum, M.; Chambers, J.; et al. Reduction in ST-Segment Elevation Cardiac Catheterization Laboratory Activations in the United States during COVID-19 Pandemic. *J. Am. Coll Cardiol.* **2020**. [CrossRef]
136. Yang, X.; Yu, Y.; Xu, J.; Shu, H.; Xia, J.; Liu, H.; Wu, Y.; Zhang, L.; Yu, Z.; Fang, M.; et al. Clinical course and outcomes of critically ill patients with SARS-CoV-2 pneumonia in Wuhan, China: A single-centered, retrospective, observational study. *Lancet Respir. Med.* **2020**, *8*, 475–481. [CrossRef]
137. Fanelli, V.; Fiorentino, M.; Cantaluppi, V.; Gesualdo, L.; Stallone, G.; Ronco, C.; Castellano, G. Acute kidney injury in SARS-CoV-2 infected patients. *Crit. Care* **2020**, *24*, 155. [CrossRef]
138. Cheng, Y.; Luo, R.; Wang, K.; Zhang, M.; Wang, Z.; Dong, L.; Li, J.; Yao, Y.; Ge, S.; Xu, G. Kidney disease is associated with in-hospital death of patients with COVID-19. *Kidney Int.* **2020**. [CrossRef]

139. Henry, B.M.; Lippi, G. Chronic kidney disease is associated with severe coronavirus disease 2019 (COVID-19) infection. *Int. Urol. Nephrol.* **2020**. [CrossRef]
140. Ye, M.; Wysocki, J.; William, J.; Soler, M.J.; Cokic, I.; Batlle, D. Glomerular localization and expression of Angiotensin-converting enzyme 2 and Angiotensin-converting enzyme: Implications for albuminuria in diabetes. *J. Am. Soc. Nephrol.* **2006**, *17*, 3067–3075. [CrossRef] [PubMed]
141. Han, L.; We, X.; Liu, C.; Volpe, G.; Wang, Z. Single-cell atlas of a non-human primate reveals new pathogenic mechanisms of COVID-19. *bioRXiv* **2020**. [CrossRef]
142. Varga, Z.; Flammer, A.J.; Steiger, P.; Haberecker, M.; Andermatt, R.; Zinkernagel, A.S.; Mehra, M.R.; Schuepbach, R.A.; Ruschitzka, F.; Moch, H. Endothelial cell infection and endotheliitis in COVID-19. *Lancet* **2020**, *395*, 1417–1418. [CrossRef]
143. Su, H.; Yang, M.; Wan, C.; Yi, L.X.; Tang, F.; Zhu, H.Y.; Yi, F.; Yang, H.C.; Fogo, A.B.; Nie, X.; et al. Renal histopathological analysis of 26 postmortem findings of patients with COVID-19 in China. *Kidney Int.* **2020**. [CrossRef] [PubMed]
144. Gentile, S.; Strollo, F.; Ceriello, A. COVID-19 Infection in italian people with diabetes: Lessons learned for our future (an experience to be used). *Diabetes Res. Clin. Pract.* **2020**, 108137. [CrossRef] [PubMed]
145. Ma, R.C.W.; Holt, R.I.G. COVID-19 and diabetes. *Diabet. Med.* **2020**, *37*, 723–725. [CrossRef] [PubMed]
146. Muniyappa, R.; Gubbi, S. COVID-19 Pandemic, Corona Viruses, and Diabetes Mellitus. *Am. J. Physiol. Endocrinol. Metab.* **2020**. [CrossRef]
147. Arentz, M.; Yim, E.; Klaff, L.; Lokhandwala, S.; Riedo, F.X.; Chong, M.; Lee, M. Characteristics and Outcomes of 21 Critically Ill Patients With COVID-19 in Washington State. *JAMA* **2020**, *323*, 1612. [CrossRef]
148. Bornstein, S.R.; Dalan, R.; Hopkins, D.; Mingrone, G.; Boehm, B.O. Endocrine and metabolic link to coronavirus infection. *Nat. Rev. Endocrinol.* **2020**. [CrossRef]
149. Remuzzi, A.; Remuzzi, G. COVID-19 and Italy: What next? *Lancet* **2020**, *395*, 1225–1228. [CrossRef]
150. Fadini, G.P.; Morieri, M.L.; Longato, E.; Avogaro, A. Prevalence and impact of diabetes among people infected with SARS-CoV-2. *J. Endocrinol. Investig.* **2020**. [CrossRef]
151. Li, B.; Yang, J.; Zhao, F.; Zhi, L.; Wang, X.; Liu, L.; Bi, Z.; Zhao, Y. Prevalence and impact of cardiovascular metabolic diseases on COVID-19 in China. *Clin. Res. Cardiol.* **2020**, *109*, 531–538. [CrossRef] [PubMed]
152. Yang, J.K.; Feng, Y.; Yuan, M.Y.; Yuan, S.Y.; Fu, H.J.; Wu, B.Y.; Sun, G.Z.; Yang, G.R.; Zhang, X.L.; Wang, L.; et al. Plasma glucose levels and diabetes are independent predictors for mortality and morbidity in patients with SARS. *Diabet. Med.* **2006**, *23*, 623–628. [CrossRef] [PubMed]
153. Simonnet, A.; Chetboun, M.; Poissy, J.; Raverdy, V.; Noulette, J.; Duhamel, A.; Labreuche, J.; Mathieu, D.; Pattou, F.; Jourdain, M. High prevalence of obesity in severe acute respiratory syndrome coronavirus-2 (SARS-CoV-2) requiring invasive mechanical ventilation. *Obesity (Silver Spring)* **2020**. [CrossRef] [PubMed]
154. Wang, A.; Zhao, W.; Xu, Z.; Gu, J. Timely blood glucose management for the outbreak of 2019 novel coronavirus disease (COVID-19) is urgently needed. *Diabetes Res. Clin. Pract.* **2020**, *162*, 108118. [CrossRef] [PubMed]
155. Yang, J.K.; Lin, S.S.; Ji, X.J.; Guo, L.M. Binding of SARS coronavirus to its receptor damages islets and causes acute diabetes. *Acta Diabetol.* **2010**, *47*, 193–199. [CrossRef] [PubMed]
156. Lu, C.L.; Wang, Y.; Yuan, L.; Li, Y.; Li, X.Y. The angiotensin-converting enzyme 2/angiotensin (1-7)/Mas axis protects the function of pancreatic beta cells by improving the function of islet microvascular endothelial cells. *Int. J. Mol. Med.* **2014**, *34*, 1293–1300. [CrossRef]
157. Xuan, X.; Gao, F.; Ma, X.; Huang, C.; Wang, Y.; Deng, H.; Wang, S.; Li, W.; Yuan, L. Activation of ACE2/angiotensin (1-7) attenuates pancreatic beta cell dedifferentiation in a high-fat-diet mouse model. *Metabolism* **2018**, *81*, 83–96. [CrossRef]
158. Shoemaker, R.; Yiannikouris, F.; Thatcher, S.; Cassis, L. ACE2 deficiency reduces beta-cell mass and impairs beta-cell proliferation in obese C57BL/6 mice. *Am. J. Physiol. Endocrinol. Metab.* **2015**, *309*, E621–E631. [CrossRef]
159. Bindom, S.M.; Lazartigues, E. The sweeter side of ACE2: Physiological evidence for a role in diabetes. *Mol. Cell Endocrinol.* **2009**, *302*, 193–202. [CrossRef]
160. Roca-Ho, H.; Riera, M.; Palau, V.; Pascual, J.; Soler, M.J. Characterization of ACE and ACE2 Expression within Different Organs of the NOD Mouse. *Int. J. Mol. Sci.* **2017**, *18*, 563. [CrossRef]

161. Blodgett, D.M.; Nowosielska, A.; Afik, S.; Pechhold, S.; Cura, A.J.; Kennedy, N.J.; Kim, S.; Kucukural, A.; Davis, R.J.; Kent, S.C.; et al. Novel Observations From Next-Generation RNA Sequencing of Highly Purified Human Adult and Fetal Islet Cell Subsets. *Diabetes* **2015**, *64*, 3172–3181. [CrossRef] [PubMed]
162. Wang, H.; Bender, A.; Wang, P.; Karakose, E.; Inabnet, W.B.; Libutti, S.K.; Arnold, A.; Lambertini, L.; Stang, M.; Chen, H.; et al. Insights into beta cell regeneration for diabetes via integration of molecular landscapes in human insulinomas. *Nat. Commun.* **2017**, *8*, 767. [CrossRef] [PubMed]
163. Li, J.; Wang, X.; Chen, J.; Zuo, X.; Zhang, H.; Deng, A. COVID-19 infection may cause ketosis and ketoacidosis. *Diabetes Obes. Metab.* **2020**. [CrossRef] [PubMed]
164. Stoian, A.P.; Banerjee, Y.; Rizvi, A.A.; Rizzo, M. Diabetes and the COVID-19 Pandemic: How Insights from Recent Experience Might Guide Future Management. *Metab. Syndr. Relat. Disord.* **2020**. [CrossRef] [PubMed]
165. Zhang, M.D.; Xiao, M.; Zhang, S.; Xia, P.; Caio, W.; Jiang, W. Coagulopathy and Antiphospholipid Antibodies in Patients with Covid-19. *NEJM* **2020**, *382*, e38. [CrossRef] [PubMed]
166. Zhou, B.; She, J.; Wang, Y.; Ma, X. Venous thrombosis and arteriosclerosis obliterans of lower extremities in a very severe patient with 2019 novel coronavirus disease: A case report. *J. Thromb. Thrombolysis* **2020**. [CrossRef]
167. Tang, N.; Li, D.; Wang, X.; Sun, Z. Abnormal coagulation parameters are associated with poor prognosis in patients with novel coronavirus pneumonia. *J. Thromb. Haemost.* **2020**, *18*, 844–847. [CrossRef]
168. Lin, L.; Lu, L.; Cao, W.; Li, T. Hypothesis for potential pathogenesis of SARS-CoV-2 infection-a review of immune changes in patients with viral pneumonia. *Emerg. Microbes Infect.* **2020**, *9*, 727–732. [CrossRef]
169. Iba, T.; Levy, J.H.; Warkentin, T.E.; Thachil, J.; van der Poll, T.; Levi, M. Scientific, Standardization Committee on DIC, the S, Standardization Committee on P, Critical Care of the International Society on T and Haemostasis. Diagnosis and management of sepsis-induced coagulopathy and disseminated intravascular coagulation. *J. Thromb. Haemost.* **2019**, *17*, 1989–1994. [CrossRef]
170. Escher, R.; Breakey, N.; Lammle, B. Severe COVID-19 infection associated with endothelial activation. *Thromb. Res.* **2020**, *190*, 62. [CrossRef]
171. McCormack, J.J.; Lopes da Silva, M.; Ferraro, F.; Patella, F.; Cutler, D.F. Weibel-Palade bodies at a glance. *J. Cell Sci.* **2017**, *130*, 3611–3617. [CrossRef] [PubMed]
172. Liu, Y.; Yang, Y.; Zhang, C.; Huang, F.; Wang, F.; Yuan, J.; Wang, Z.; Li, J.; Li, J.; Feng, C.; et al. Clinical and biochemical indexes from 2019-nCoV infected patients linked to viral loads and lung injury. *Sci. China Life Sci.* **2020**, *63*, 364–374. [CrossRef] [PubMed]
173. Williams, B.; Baker, A.Q.; Gallacher, B.; Lodwick, D. Angiotensin II increases vascular permeability factor gene expression by human vascular smooth muscle cells. *Hypertension* **1995**, *25*, 913–917. [CrossRef] [PubMed]
174. Victorino, G.P.; Newton, C.R.; Curran, B. Effect of angiotensin II on microvascular permeability. *J. Surg. Res.* **2002**, *104*, 77–81. [CrossRef] [PubMed]
175. Dielis, A.W.; Smid, M.; Spronk, H.M.; Hamulyak, K.; Kroon, A.A.; ten Cate, H.; de Leeuw, P.W. The prothrombotic paradox of hypertension: Role of the renin-angiotensin and kallikrein-kinin systems. *Hypertension* **2005**, *46*, 1236–1242. [CrossRef]
176. Watanabe, T.; Barker, T.A.; Berk, B.C. Angiotensin II and the endothelium: Diverse signals and effects. *Hypertension* **2005**, *45*, 163–169. [CrossRef]
177. Celi, A.; Cianchetti, S.; Dell'Omo, G.; Pedrinelli, R. Angiotensin II, tissue factor and the thrombotic paradox of hypertension. *Expert Rev. Cardiovasc. Ther.* **2010**, *8*, 1723–1729. [CrossRef]
178. Jagroop, I.A.; Mikhailidis, D.P. Angiotensin II can induce and potentiate shape change in human platelets: Effect of losartan. *J. Hum. Hypertens.* **2000**, *14*, 581–585. [CrossRef]
179. Ding, Y.A.; MacIntyre, D.E.; Kenyon, C.J.; Semple, P.F. Angiotensin II effects on platelet function. *J. Hypertens. Suppl.* **1985**, *3*, S251–S253. [CrossRef]
180. Larsson, P.T.; Schwieler, J.H.; Wallen, N.H. Platelet activation during angiotensin II infusion in healthy volunteers. *Blood Coagul. Fibrinolysis* **2000**, *11*, 61–69. [CrossRef]
181. Langeggen, H.; Berge, K.E.; Macor, P.; Fischetti, F.; Tedesco, F.; Hetland, G.; Berg, K.; Johnson, E. Detection of mRNA for the terminal complement components C5, C6, C8 and C9 in human umbilical vein endothelial cells in vitro. *Apmis* **2001**, *109*, 73–78. [CrossRef] [PubMed]
182. Langeggen, H.; Pausa, M.; Johnson, E.; Casarsa, C.; Tedesco, F. The endothelium is an extrahepatic site of synthesis of the seventh component of the complement system. *Clin. Exp. Immunol.* **2000**, *121*, 69–76. [CrossRef] [PubMed]

183. Dauchel, H.; Julen, N.; Lemercier, C.; Daveau, M.; Ozanne, D.; Fontaine, M.; Ripoche, J. Expression of complement alternative pathway proteins by endothelial cells. Differential regulation by interleukin 1 and glucocorticoids. *Eur. J. Immunol.* **1990**, *20*, 1669–1675. [CrossRef] [PubMed]
184. Warren, H.B.; Pantazis, P.; Davies, P.F. The third component of complement is transcribed and secreted by cultured human endothelial cells. *Am. J. Pathol.* **1987**, *129*, 9–13. [PubMed]
185. Johnson, E.; Hetland, G. Human umbilical vein endothelial cells synthesize functional C3, C5, C6, C8 and C9 in vitro. *Scand J. Immunol.* **1991**, *33*, 667–671. [CrossRef] [PubMed]
186. Shagdarsuren, E.; Wellner, M.; Braesen, J.H.; Park, J.K.; Fiebeler, A.; Henke, N.; Dechend, R.; Gratze, P.; Luft, F.C.; Muller, D.N. Complement activation in angiotensin II-induced organ damage. *Circ. Res.* **2005**, *97*, 716–724. [CrossRef]
187. Ruan, C.C.; Gao, P.J. Role of Complement-Related Inflammation and Vascular Dysfunction in Hypertension. *Hypertension* **2019**, *73*, 965–971. [CrossRef]
188. Fischetti, F.; Tedesco, F. Cross-talk between the complement system and endothelial cells in physiologic conditions and in vascular diseases. *Autoimmunity* **2006**, *39*, 417–428. [CrossRef]
189. Risitano, A.M.; Mastellos, D.C.; Huber-Lang, M.; Yancopoulou, D.; Garlanda, C.; Ciceri, F.; Lambris, J.D. Complement as a target in COVID-19? *Nat. Rev. Immunol.* **2020**. [CrossRef]
190. Schulz, C.; Engelmann, B.; Massberg, S. Crossroads of coagulation and innate immunity: The case of deep vein thrombosis. *J. Thromb. Haemost.* **2013**, *11* (Suppl. 1), 233–241. [CrossRef]
191. abret, N.; Britton, G.J.; Gruber, C.; Hegde, S.; Kim, J.; Kuksin, M.; Levantovsky, R.; Malle, L.; Moreira, A.; Park, M.D.; et al. The Sinai Immunology Review Project. Immunology of COVID-19: Current state of the science. *Immunity* **2020**. [CrossRef]
192. Steinberg, B.E.; Goldenberg, N.M.; Lee, W.L. Do viral infections mimic bacterial sepsis? The role of microvascular permeability: A review of mechanisms and methods. *Antiviral. Res.* **2012**, *93*, 2–15. [CrossRef] [PubMed]
193. Zeng, H.; Pappas, C.; Belser, J.A.; Houser, K.V.; Zhong, W.; Wadford, D.A.; Stevens, T.; Balczon, R.; Katz, J.M.; Tumpey, T.M. Human pulmonary microvascular endothelial cells support productive replication of highly pathogenic avian influenza viruses: Possible involvement in the pathogenesis of human H5N1 virus infection. *J. Virol.* **2012**, *86*, 667–678. [CrossRef] [PubMed]
194. Maniatis, N.A.; Orfanos, S.E. The endothelium in acute lung injury/acute respiratory distress syndrome. *Curr. Opin. Crit. Care* **2008**, *14*, 22–30. [CrossRef] [PubMed]
195. Polverino, F.; Celli, B.R.; Owen, C.A. COPD as an endothelial disorder: Endothelial injury linking lesions in the lungs and other organs? (2017 Grover Conference Series). *Pulm. Circ.* **2018**, *8*, 2045894018758528. [CrossRef] [PubMed]
196. Millar, F.R.; Summers, C.; Griffiths, M.J.; Toshner, M.R.; Proudfoot, A.G. The pulmonary endothelium in acute respiratory distress syndrome: Insights and therapeutic opportunities. *Thorax* **2016**, *71*, 462–473. [CrossRef]
197. Armstrong, S.M.; Wang, C.; Tigdi, J.; Si, X.; Dumpit, C.; Charles, S.; Gamage, A.; Moraes, T.J.; Lee, W.L. Influenza infects lung microvascular endothelium leading to microvascular leak: Role of apoptosis and claudin-5. *PLoS ONE* **2012**, *7*, e47323. [CrossRef]
198. Chan, M.C.; Chan, R.W.; Yu, W.C.; Ho, C.C.; Chui, W.H.; Lo, C.K.; Yuen, K.M.; Guan, Y.I.; Nicholls, J.M.; Peiris, J.S. Influenza H5N1 virus infection of polarized human alveolar epithelial cells and lung microvascular endothelial cells. *Respir. Res.* **2009**, *10*, 102. [CrossRef]
199. Lee, N.; Hui, D.; Wu, A.; Chan, P.; Cameron, P.; Joynt, G.M.; Ahuja, A.; Yung, M.Y.; Leung, C.B.; To, K.F.; et al. A major outbreak of severe acute respiratory syndrome in Hong Kong. *N. Engl. J. Med.* **2003**, *348*, 1986–1994. [CrossRef]
200. Wong, R.S.; Wu, A.; To, K.F.; Lee, N.; Lam, C.W.; Wong, C.K.; Chan, P.K.; Ng, M.H.; Yu, L.M.; Hui, D.S.; et al. Haematological manifestations in patients with severe acute respiratory syndrome: Retrospective analysis. *BMJ* **2003**, *326*, 1358–1362. [CrossRef]
201. Xiang-Hua, Y.; Le-Min, W.; Ai-Bin, L.; Zhu, G.; Riquan, L.; Xu-You, Z.; Wei-Wei, R.; Ye-Nan, W. Severe acute respiratory syndrome and venous thromboembolism in multiple organs. *Am. J. Respir. Crit. Care Med.* **2010**, *182*, 436–437. [CrossRef] [PubMed]
202. de Wit, E.; van Doremalen, N.; Falzarano, D.; Munster, V.J. SARS and MERS: Recent insights into emerging coronaviruses. *Nat. Rev. Microbiol.* **2016**, *14*, 523–534. [CrossRef] [PubMed]

203. Bunce, P.E.; High, S.M.; Nadjafi, M.; Stanley, K.; Liles, W.C.; Christian, M.D. Pandemic H1N1 influenza infection and vascular thrombosis. *Clin. Infect. Dis.* **2011**, *52*, e14–e17. [CrossRef]
204. Huzmeli, C.; Saglam, M.; Arikan, A.; Doner, B.; Akinci, G.; Candan, F. Infrarenal Aorta Thrombosis Associated with H1N1 Influenza A Virus Infection. *Case Rep. Infect. Dis.* **2016**, *2016*, 9567495. [CrossRef] [PubMed]
205. Ishiguro, T.; Matsuo, K.; Fujii, S.; Takayanagi, N. Acute thrombotic vascular events complicating influenza-associated pneumonia. *Respir. Med. Case Rep.* **2019**, *28*, 100884. [CrossRef] [PubMed]
206. Iwasaki, A.; Medzhitov, R. A new shield for a cytokine storm. *Cell* **2011**, *146*, 861–862. [CrossRef]
207. Tscherne, D.M.; Garcia-Sastre, A. Virulence determinants of pandemic influenza viruses. *J. Clin. Investig.* **2011**, *121*, 6–13. [CrossRef]
208. Canna, S.W.; Behrens, E.M. Making sense of the cytokine storm: A conceptual framework for understanding, diagnosing, and treating hemophagocytic syndromes. *Pediatr. Clin. N. Am.* **2012**, *59*, 329–344. [CrossRef]
209. Chaudhry, H.; Zhou, J.; Zhong, Y.; Ali, M.M.; McGuire, F.; Nagarkatti, P.S.; Nagarkatti, M. Role of cytokines as a double-edged sword in sepsis. *In Vivo* **2013**, *27*, 669–684.
210. Bracaglia, C.; Prencipe, G.; De Benedetti, F. Macrophage Activation Syndrome: Different mechanisms leading to a one clinical syndrome. *Pediatr. Rheumatol. Online J.* **2017**, *15*, 5. [CrossRef]
211. Hayden, A.; Park, S.; Giustini, D.; Lee, A.Y.; Chen, L.Y. Hemophagocytic syndromes (HPSs) including hemophagocytic lymphohistiocytosis (HLH) in adults: A systematic scoping review. *Blood Rev.* **2016**, *30*, 411–420. [CrossRef] [PubMed]
212. Mehta, P.; McAuley, D.F.; Brown, M.; Sanchez, E.; Tattersall, R.S.; Manson, J.J.; Hlh Across Speciality Collaboration UK. COVID-19: Consider cytokine storm syndromes and immunosuppression. *Lancet* **2020**, *395*, 1033–1034. [CrossRef]
213. Gattinoni, L.; Coppola, S.; Cressoni, M.; Busana, M.; Rossi, S.; Chiumello, D. Covid-19 Does Not Lead to a "Typical" Acute Respiratory Distress Syndrome. *Am. J. Respir. Crit. Care Med.* **2020**. [CrossRef] [PubMed]
214. Pedersen, S.F.; Ho, Y.C. SARS-CoV-2: A storm is raging. *J. Clin. Investig.* **2020**, *130*, 2202–2205. [CrossRef] [PubMed]
215. Staedtke, V.; Bai, R.Y.; Kim, K.; Darvas, M.; Davila, M.L.; Riggins, G.J.; Rothman, P.B.; Papadopoulos, N.; Kinzler, K.W.; Vogelstein, B.; et al. Disruption of a self-amplifying catecholamine loop reduces cytokine release syndrome. *Nature* **2018**, *564*, 273–277. [CrossRef]
216. Sinha, P.; Delucchi, K.L.; McAuley, D.F.; O'Kane, C.M.; Matthay, M.A.; Calfee, C.S. Development and validation of parsimonious algorithms to classify acute respiratory distress syndrome phenotypes: A secondary analysis of randomised controlled trials. *Lancet Respir. Med.* **2020**, *8*, 247–257. [CrossRef]
217. Qin, C.; Zhou, L.; Hu, Z.; Zhang, S.; Yang, S.; Tao, Y.; Xie, C.; Ma, K.; Shang, K.; Wang, W.; et al. Dysregulation of immune response in patients with COVID-19 in Wuhan, China. *Clin. Infect. Dis.* **2020**. [CrossRef]
218. Teijaro, J.R.; Walsh, K.B.; Cahalan, S.; Fremgen, D.M.; Roberts, E.; Scott, F.; Martinborough, E.; Peach, R.; Oldstone, M.B.; Rosen, H. Endothelial cells are central orchestrators of cytokine amplification during influenza virus infection. *Cell* **2011**, *146*, 980–991. [CrossRef]
219. Sorriento, D.; Santulli, G.; Del Giudice, C.; Anastasio, A.; Trimarco, B.; Iaccarino, G. Endothelial cells are able to synthesize and release catecholamines both in vitro and in vivo. *Hypertension* **2012**, *60*, 129–136. [CrossRef]
220. Xie, Y.; Wang, X.; Yang, P.; Shutong, Z. COVID-19 complicated by acute pulmonary embolism. *Radiology* **2020**, *2*, e200067. [CrossRef]
221. Danzi, G.B.; Loffi, M.; Galeazzi, G.; Gherbesi, E. Acute pulmonary embolism and COVID-19 pneumonia: A random association? *Eur. Heart J.* **2020**. [CrossRef]
222. Leonard-Lorant, I.; Delabranche, X.; Severac, F.; Helms, J.; Pauzet, C.; Collange, O.; Schneider, F.; Labani, A.; Bilbault, P.; Moliere, S.; et al. Acute Pulmonary Embolism in COVID-19 Patients on CT Angiography and Relationship to D-Dimer Levels. *Radiology* **2020**, 201561. [CrossRef]
223. Jolobe, O.M.P. Similarities Between Community-Acquired Pneumonia and Pulmonary Embolism. *Am. J. Med.* **2019**, *132*, e863. [CrossRef]
224. Santulli, G. MicroRNAs and Endothelial (Dys) Function. *J. Cell Physiol.* **2016**, *231*, 1638–1644. [CrossRef] [PubMed]
225. Yuan, Q.; Yang, J.; Santulli, G.; Reiken, S.R.; Wronska, A.; Kim, M.M.; Osborne, B.W.; Lacampagne, A.; Yin, Y.; Marks, A.R. Maintenance of normal blood pressure is dependent on IP3R1-mediated regulation of eNOS. *Proc. Natl. Acad. Sci. USA* **2016**, *113*, 8532–8537. [CrossRef] [PubMed]

226. Gando, S.; Levi, M.; Toh, C.H. Disseminated intravascular coagulation. *Nat. Rev. Dis. Primers.* **2016**, *2*, 16037. [CrossRef] [PubMed]
227. Walborn, A.; Rondina, M.; Mosier, M.; Fareed, J.; Hoppensteadt, D. Endothelial Dysfunction Is Associated with Mortality and Severity of Coagulopathy in Patients with Sepsis and Disseminated Intravascular Coagulation. *Clin. Appl. Thromb. Hemost.* **2019**, *25*, 1076029619852163. [CrossRef] [PubMed]
228. Tang, N.; Bai, H.; Chen, X.; Gong, J.; Li, D.; Sun, Z. Anticoagulant treatment is associated with decreased mortality in severe coronavirus disease 2019 patients with coagulopathy. *J. Thromb. Haemost.* **2020**. [CrossRef] [PubMed]
229. Rubin, E.J.; Baden, L.R.; Morrissey, S. Audio Interview: New Research on Possible Treatments for Covid-19. *New Engl. J. Med.* **2020**, *382*, e30. [CrossRef]
230. Ahn, D.G.; Shin, H.J.; Kim, M.H.; Lee, S.; Kim, H.S.; Myoung, J.; Kim, B.T.; Kim, S.J. Current Status of Epidemiology, Diagnosis, Therapeutics, and Vaccines for Novel Coronavirus Disease 2019 (COVID-19). *J. Microbiol. Biotechnol.* **2020**, *30*, 313–324. [CrossRef]
231. Xu, X.; Han, M.; Li, T.; Sun, W.; Wang, D.; Fu, B.; Zhou, Y.; Zheng, X.; Yang, Y.; Li, X.; et al. Effective treatment of severe COVID-19 patients with tocilizumab. *Proc. Natl. Acad. Sci. USA* **2020**, 202005615. [CrossRef] [PubMed]
232. Ruiz-Limon, P.; Ortega, R.; Arias de la Rosa, I.; Abalos-Aguilera, M.D.C.; Perez-Sanchez, C.; Jimenez-Gomez, Y.; Peralbo-Santaella, E.; Font, P.; Ruiz-Vilches, D.; Ferrin, G.; et al. Tocilizumab improves the proatherothrombotic profile of rheumatoid arthritis patients modulating endothelial dysfunction, NETosis, and inflammation. *Transl. Res.* **2017**, *183*, 87–103. [CrossRef] [PubMed]
233. Kajikawa, M.; Higashi, Y.; Tomiyama, H.; Maruhashi, T.; Kurisu, S.; Kihara, Y.; Mutoh, A.; Ueda, S.I. Effect of short-term colchicine treatment on endothelial function in patients with coronary artery disease. *Int. J. Cardiol.* **2019**, *281*, 35–39. [CrossRef] [PubMed]
234. Parchure, N.; Zouridakis, E.G.; Kaski, J.C. Effect of azithromycin treatment on endothelial function in patients with coronary artery disease and evidence of Chlamydia pneumoniae infection. *Circulation* **2002**, *105*, 1298–1303. [CrossRef] [PubMed]
235. Luo, T.; Chen, B.; Zhao, Z.; He, N.; Zeng, Z.; Wu, B.; Fukushima, Y.; Dai, M.; Huang, Q.; Xu, D.; et al. Histamine H2 receptor activation exacerbates myocardial ischemia/reperfusion injury by disturbing mitochondrial and endothelial function. *Basic Res. Cardiol.* **2013**, *108*, 342. [CrossRef] [PubMed]
236. Yazdany, J.; Kim, A.H.J. Use of Hydroxychloroquine and Chloroquine During the COVID-19 Pandemic: What Every Clinician Should Know. *Ann. Intern. Med.* **2020**. [CrossRef]
237. Le, N.T.; Takei, Y.; Izawa-Ishizawa, Y.; Heo, K.S.; Lee, H.; Smrcka, A.V.; Miller, B.L.; Ko, K.A.; Ture, S.; Morrell, C.; et al. Identification of activators of ERK5 transcriptional activity by high-throughput screening and the role of endothelial ERK5 in vasoprotective effects induced by statins and antimalarial agents. *J. Immunol.* **2014**, *193*, 3803–3815. [CrossRef]
238. Rahman, R.; Murthi, P.; Singh, H.; Gurusinghe, S.; Mockler, J.C.; Lim, R.; Wallace, E.M. The effects of hydroxychloroquine on endothelial dysfunction. *Pregnancy Hypertens.* **2016**, *6*, 259–262. [CrossRef]
239. Gambardella, J.; Morelli, M.; Sardu, C.; Santulli, G. Targeting Endothelial Dysfunction in COVID-19. *Nature* **2020**, in press.
240. Ciccarelli, M.; Santulli, G.; Campanile, A.; Galasso, G.; Cervero, P.; Altobelli, G.G.; Cimini, V.; Pastore, L.; Piscione, F.; Trimarco, B.; et al. Endothelial alpha1-adrenoceptors regulate neo-angiogenesis. *Br. J. Pharmacol.* **2008**, *153*, 936–946. [CrossRef]
241. Wilbert-Lampen, U.; Seliger, C.; Zilker, T.; Arendt, R.M. Cocaine increases the endothelial release of immunoreactive endothelin and its concentrations in human plasma and urine: Reversal by coincubation with sigma-receptor antagonists. *Circulation* **1998**, *98*, 385–390. [CrossRef] [PubMed]
242. Amer, M.S.; McKeown, L.; Tumova, S.; Liu, R.; Seymour, V.A.; Wilson, L.A.; Naylor, J.; Greenhalgh, K.; Hou, B.; Majeed, Y.; et al. Inhibition of endothelial cell Ca(2)(+) entry and transient receptor potential channels by Sigma-1 receptor ligands. *Br. J. Pharmacol.* **2013**, *168*, 1445–1455. [CrossRef] [PubMed]
243. Massamiri, T.; Duckles, S.P. Sigma receptor ligands inhibit rat tail artery contractile responses by multiple mechanisms. *J. Pharmacol. Exp. Ther.* **1991**, *259*, 22–29. [PubMed]
244. Hamidi Shishavan, M.; Henning, R.H.; van Buiten, A.; Goris, M.; Deelman, L.E.; Buikema, H. Metformin Improves Endothelial Function and Reduces Blood Pressure in Diabetic Spontaneously Hypertensive Rats Independent from Glycemia Control: Comparison to Vildagliptin. *Sci. Rep.* **2017**, *7*, 10975. [CrossRef]

245. Bolz, S.S.; Pohl, U. Indomethacin enhances endothelial NO release–evidence for a role of PGI2 in the autocrine control of calcium-dependent autacoid production. *Cardiovasc. Res.* **1997**, *36*, 437–444. [CrossRef]
246. Sfikakis, P.P.; Papamichael, C.; Stamatelopoulos, K.S.; Tousoulis, D.; Fragiadaki, K.G.; Katsichti, P.; Stefanadis, C.; Mavrikakis, M. Improvement of vascular endothelial function using the oral endothelin receptor antagonist bosentan in patients with systemic sclerosis. *Arthritis Rheum.* **2007**, *56*, 1985–1993. [CrossRef]
247. Gupta, N.; Zhao, Y.Y.; Evans, C.E. The stimulation of thrombosis by hypoxia. *Thromb. Res.* **2019**, *181*, 77–83. [CrossRef]
248. Xu, Z.; Shi, L.; Wang, Y.; Zhang, J.; Huang, L.; Zhang, C.; Liu, S.; Zhao, P.; Liu, H.; Zhu, L.; et al. Pathological findings of COVID-19 associated with acute respiratory distress syndrome. *Lancet Respir. Med.* **2020**, *8*, 420–422. [CrossRef]
249. Paranjpe, I.; Fuster, V.; Lala, A.; Russak, A.; Glicksberg, B.S.; Levin, M.A.; Charney, A.W.; Narula, J.; Fayad, Z.A.; Bagiella, E.; et al. Association of Treatment Dose Anticoagulation with In-Hospital Survival Among Hospitalized Patients with COVID-19. *J. Am. Coll. Cardiol.* **2020**. [CrossRef]
250. Basu, A.; Kanda, T.; Beyene, A.; Saito, K.; Meyer, K.; Ray, R. Sulfated homologues of heparin inhibit hepatitis C virus entry into mammalian cells. *J. Virol.* **2007**, *81*, 3933–3941. [CrossRef]
251. Lee, E.; Pavy, M.; Young, N.; Freeman, C.; Lobigs, M. Antiviral effect of the heparan sulfate mimetic, PI-88, against dengue and encephalitic flaviviruses. *Antiviral. Res.* **2006**, *69*, 31–38. [CrossRef] [PubMed]
252. Walker, S.J.; Pizzato, M.; Takeuchi, Y.; Devereux, S. Heparin binds to murine leukemia virus and inhibits Env-independent attachment and infection. *J. Virol.* **2002**, *76*, 6909–6918. [CrossRef] [PubMed]
253. Connell, B.J.; Lortat-Jacob, H. Human immunodeficiency virus and heparan sulfate: From attachment to entry inhibition. *Front. Immunol.* **2013**, *4*, 385. [CrossRef] [PubMed]
254. Nahmias, A.J.; Kibrick, S. Inhibitory effect of heparin on herpes simplex virus. *J. Bacteriol.* **1964**, *87*, 1060–1066. [CrossRef]

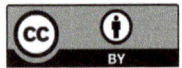

© 2020 by the authors. Licensee MDPI, Basel, Switzerland. This article is an open access article distributed under the terms and conditions of the Creative Commons Attribution (CC BY) license (http://creativecommons.org/licenses/by/4.0/).

MDPI
St. Alban-Anlage 66
4052 Basel
Switzerland
Tel. +41 61 683 77 34
Fax +41 61 302 89 18
www.mdpi.com

Journal of Clinical Medicine Editorial Office
E-mail: jcm@mdpi.com
www.mdpi.com/journal/jcm

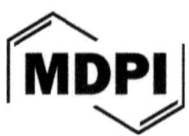